T0201251

Diseases and Conditions in Dentistry

Diseases and Conditions in Dentistry

An Evidence-Based Reference

Keyvan Moharamzadeh
School of Clinical Dentistry, University of Sheffield
Sheffield, UK

WILEY Blackwell

This edition first published 2018

Registered Offices
John Wiley & Sons, Inc., 111 River Street, Hoboken, NJ 07030, USA
John Wiley & Sons Ltd, The Atrium, Southern Gate, Chichester, West Sussex, PO19 8SQ, UK

Editorial Office
9600 Garsington Road, Oxford, OX4 2DQ, UK

For details of our global editorial offices, customer services, and more information about Wiley products visit us at www.wiley.com.

Wiley also publishes its books in a variety of electronic formats and by print-on-demand. Some content that appears in standard print versions of this book may not be available in other formats.

Library of Congress Cataloging-in-Publication Data

Names: Moharamzadeh, Keyvan, author.
Title: Diseases and conditions in dentistry : an evidence-based reference / Keyvan Moharamzadeh.
Description: Hoboken, NJ : Wiley, 2018. | Includes bibliographical references and index. |
Identifiers: LCCN 2018010426 (print) | LCCN 2018010630 (ebook) | ISBN 9781119312079 (pdf) | ISBN 9781119312116 (epub) | ISBN 9781119312031 (hardback)
Subjects: | MESH: Stomatognathic Diseases–diagnosis | Stomatognathic Diseases–therapy | Evidence-Based Dentistry
Classification: LCC RK301 (ebook) | LCC RK301 (print) | NLM WU 140 | DDC 617.5/22–dc23
LC record available at https://lccn.loc.gov/2018010426

Cover Design: Wiley
Cover Images: (Top, bottom middle, and bottom right) © Keyvan Moharamzadeh; (Bottom left) © Abdurahman El-Awa

Set in 10/12pt WarnockPro by SPi Global, Chennai, India

Printed in the UK by Bell & Bain Ltd, Glasgow.

10 9 8 7 6 5 4 3 2 1

Contents

Preface

This book has been written to address the current need for a comprehensive disease- and condition-based study guide in endodontics, periodontics, prosthodontics and restorative dentistry. It is the result of 7 years of hard work, including 5 years of specialty training in restorative dentistry, which enabled me to consolidate my knowledge and clinical skills, prepare and write the core content and appropriate clinical cases, followed by 2 additional years of further writing and updating the references to contain the most recent and relevant evidence from the literature. This book is an extract of thousands of pages of relevant dental books and articles presented in an easy-to-read style.

Each chapter starts with basic information regarding the definitions, prevalence, aetiology and pathogenesis of a particular disease or condition in dentistry which is suitable for undergraduate students and general dental practitioners (GDPs) who encounter these dental conditions commonly in their clinics. The chapters provide useful information on diagnosis and management strategies and then further evolve to include challenges, relevant evidence from the literature and advanced knowledge at the specialist level, making the book also suitable for postgraduate students, specialty trainees and specialists in restorative dentistry, periodontics, prosthodontics and endodontics.

The case studies at the end of each chapter demonstrate examples of diagnostic and management approaches combined with reflective discussions on the prognostic factors, challenges and rationale for the treatment provided to further enhance the reader's understanding of the condition, treatment planning and procedural steps for executing the planned treatment.

This 50-chapter book contains over 100 hours of continuing professional development reading for GDPs and specialists. It is also an excellent revision guide for undergraduate students in dentistry preparing for their finals, postgraduate students and monospecialty trainees in endodontics, periodontics and prosthodontics preparing for the Masters, MClinDent, DClinDent and MRD exams and specialty trainees in restorative dentistry sitting the Intercollegiate Specialty Fellowship Examinations.

Any suggestions for the current edition's further improvement will be greatly appreciated and incorporated in the next edition.

Acknowledgements

This book is dedicated to my mother, father and brother for their endless love and support throughout my life.

I would like to thank Dr Dewi Borkent for tremendous support and continued encouragement during this book project.

I would like to acknowledge Professor Ian Brook, Mr Abdurahman El-Awa, Dr Poyan Barabari, Dr Abdulrahman Elmougy, Dr Zaid Ali, Dr Badr Alghaithi and Dr Yusuf A. Alzayani for their contribution to some of the chapters of this book.

The completion of this book would not have been possible without the support of my colleagues during my specialty training programme in restorative dentistry. I would like to thank Professors Andrew Rawlinson, Nicolas Martin and Gareth Griffiths, Mr Phillip Wragg, Mr Ian Harris, Mr Raj Joshi, Miss Sandra Orr, Dr Ade Mosaku and Mr Raj Patel for being great teachers and for their valuable help and advice.

I am grateful to my colleagues in other restorative dentistry units in the UK, including Mr. Peter Briggs, Professor Craig Barclay, Mr Chris Butterworth, Mr Martin Chan, Miss Shiyana Eliyas, Mr Joe Vere, Dr Shashwat Bhakta, Mr Kushal Gadhia and Mr Karun Dewan for their kind help during my fellowship examination.

My sincere thanks go to the Wiley publishing team, including Jessica Evans, Jayadivya Saiprasad, Archana Rangaswamy, Erica Judisch, and everyone involved with the production and publication of this title.

I would like to thank friends, relatives and colleagues who helped and supported me during this project whose names may not all be enumerated. I acknowledge and sincerely appreciate their participation and assistance with this undertaking.

I am grateful to all my patients for giving me permission to use their clinical photographs and radiographs in this book.

Finally, I am grateful to God for giving me the gifts of talent, determination and the strength to be able to create this comprehensive textbook.

Image Contributors

Badr Alghaithi (Figures 11.2 and 11.3)
University of Sheffield, UK

Yusuf Alzayani (Figures 22.2 to 22.6)
University of Sheffield, Sheffield, UK

Poyan Barabari (Figure 23.2)
University of Sheffield, Sheffield, UK

Ian Brook (Figures 28.1 to 28.5)
University of Sheffield, Sheffield, UK

Abdul-Rahman Elmougy (Figures 5.1, 5.2, and 23.3 to 23.8)
University of Sheffield, Sheffield, UK

Zaid Ali (Figures 13.1 to 13.4)
University of Sheffield, Sheffield, UK

Abdurahman El-Awa (Figure 46.1)
Charles Clifford Dental Hospital, Sheffield, UK

Abbreviations

AA	*Actinobacillus actinomycetemcomitans*
AAP	acute apical periodontitis
ABG	alveolar bone graft
AFR	annual failure rate
AI	amelogenesis imperfecta
AIDS	acquired immunodeficiency syndrome
ALT	anterolateral thigh
APF	acidulated phosphate fluoride
BEWE	Basic Erosive Wear Examination
BMP	bone morphogenic protein
BOP	bleeding on probing
BPE	basic periodontal examination
BRONJ	bisphosphonate-related osteonecrosis of the jaw
BW	bitewing, biological width
CAA	cast adhesive onlay
CAD/CAM	computer-aided design/computer-assisted manufacturing
CAF	coronally advanced flap
CAL	clinical attachment level
CAP	chronic apical periodontitis
CBCT	cone beam computed tomography
CBT	cognitive behavioural therapy
CEJ	cementoenamel junction
CGRP	calcitonin gene-related peptide
CHS	Chediak–Higashi syndrome
CHX	chlorhexidine
CLP	cleft lip and palate
CNS	clinical nurse specialist
CO	centric occlusion
Co-Cr	cobalt-chromium
CPI	Community Periodontal Index
CR	centric relation
CS	combination syndrome
CT	computed tomography, connective tissue
DCIA	deep circumflex iliac artery
DD	dentine dysplasia
DGI	dentinogenesis imperfecta
DHS	dentine hypersensitivity
DI	dentinogenesis imperfecta
DO	distraction osteogenesis
DWI	diffusion-weighted imaging
EAL	electronic apex locator
EAO	European Association for Osseointegration
ED	ectodermal dysplasia
EDTA	ethylene-diamine tetra-acetic acid
EDS	Ehlers–Danlos syndrome
EFP	European Federation of Periodontology
ELISA	enzyme-linked immunosorbent assay
EMD	Emdogain
ENT	ear, nose and throat
EPT	electric pulp tester
ESE	European Society of Endodontology
FGG	full gold crown, free gingival graft
FMD	full-mouth disinfection
FWS	free-way space
GA	general anaesthesia
GAP	generalised aggressive periodontitis
GBR	guided bone regeneration
GCF	gingival crevicular fluid
GDP	general dental practitioner
GI	gastrointestinal
GIC	glass ionomer cement
GP	gutta-percha
GTR	guided tissue regeneration
HAART	highly active antiretroviral therapy
HBO	hyperbaric oxygen
HBOT	hyperbaric oxygen therapy
HED	hypohidrotic ectodermal dysplasia
HGF	hereditary gingival fibromatosis
HIV	human immunodeficiency virus
HPV	human papilloma virus
HRT	hormone replacement therapy
IADT	International Association of Dental Traumatology
ICP	intercuspal position
IGF	insulin-like growth factor
IL	interleukin
IMF	intermaxillary fixation
IMRT	intensity-modulated radiation therapy

INF interferon
INR international normalised ratio
IRM intermediate restorative material
ISQ implant stability quotient
IV intravenous
JE junctional epithelium
LA local anaesthesia
LAD leucocyte adhesion deficiency
LAP localised aggressive periodontitis
LCH Langerhans cell histiocytosis
LD lamina dura
LDF laser Doppler flowmetry
LPS lipopolysaccharide
MB mesiobuccal
MCN managed clinical network
MDT multidisciplinary team
MGJ mucogingival junction
MHC major histocompatibility complex
MIH molar-incisor hypomineralisation
MIST minimally invasive surgical technique
MMA methyl methacrylate
MMP matrix metalloproteinase
MRI magnetic resonance imaging
MRONJ medication-related osteonecrosis of the jaw
MTA mineral trioxide aggregate
NKA neurokinin A
NNT number needed to treat
NO nitric oxide
NSAID non-steroidal anti-inflammatory drug
OAF oral-antral fistula
OCD obsessive compulsive disorder
OHE oral hygiene education
OHI oral hygiene instructions
OHIP oral health impact profile
OHRQoL oral health-related quality of life
OMFS oral and maxillofacial surgeon
OPG osteoprotegerin
OPT oral panoramic radiograph
ORN osteoradionecrosis
OVD occlusal vertical dimension
PAI periapical index
PCR polymerase chain reaction
PD pocket depth
PDGF platelet-derived growth factor
PDL periodontal ligament
PEEK polyether-ether-ketone
PET positron emission tomography
PFM porcelain fused to metal
PG *Porphyromonas gingivalis*, prostaglandin
PLS Papillon–Lefèvre syndrome
PMH past medical history
PPD probing pocket depth
PRA periodontal risk assessment
RANKL receptor activator of NF-kappa B ligand
RBB resin-bonded bridge
RCP retruded contact position
RCT root canal treatment
RET regenerative endodontic treatment
RM-GIC resin-modified glass-ionomer cement
RPD removable partial denture
RSD root surface debridement
RSR root separation and resection
RTOG Radiation Therapy Oncology Group
SCC squamous cell carcinoma
SDA shortened dental arch
SLE systemic lupus erythematosus
SLT speech and language therapist
SP substance P
SPECT single photon emission computed tomography
SPT supportive periodontal therapy
SSC stainless steel crown
STSG soft tissue substitute graft
TAD temporary anchorage device
TDAA thoracodorsal angular artery
TGF transforming growth factor
TMD temporomandibular disorder
TMJ temporomandibular joint
TNF tumour necrosis factor
TSL tooth surface loss
VD vertical dimension
VP velopharyngeal
WHO World Health Organization
WL working length
ZOE zinc oxide eugenol

About the Companion Website

Don't forget to visit the companion website for this book:

www.wiley.com/go/moharamzadeh/diseases

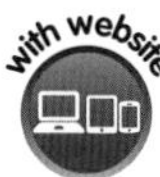

There you will find valuable material designed to enhance your learning, including:

- Clinical cases

Scan this QR code to visit the companion website:

1

Aggressive Periodontitis

1.1 Definition

Aggressive periodontitis can be defined based on the following primary and secondary features (Lang *et al.*, 1999).

1.1.1 Primary Features

- Non-contributory medical history; diagnosis requires the exclusion of systemic diseases.
- Rapid attachment loss and bone destruction.
- Familial aggregation of cases.

1.1.2 Secondary Features

- Amount of plaque is inconsistent with the severity of the disease.
- Elevated levels of *Actinobacillus actinomycetemcomitans* (AA) and *Porphyromonas gingivalis* (PG) in some population.
- Phagocyte abnormalities.
- Hyper-responsive macrophage phenotype, elevated prostaglandin (PG)-E_2, interleukin (IL)-1 beta in response to bacterial endotoxins.
- Progression of attachment and bone loss may be self-arresting.

1.2 Classification

Based on the 1999 International Workshop for Classification of Periodontal Diseases and Conditions, aggressive periodontitis can be classified into two main categories (Armitage, 1999): localised aggressive periodontitis (LAP) and generalised aggressive periodontitis (GAP).

Localised aggressive periodontitis is characterised by the following features.

- Circumpubertal onset.
- Localised first molar/incisor presentation with interproximal attachment loss on at least two permanent teeth, one of which is a first molar and involving no more than two teeth other than the first molars and incisors.
- Robust serum antibody response to infecting agents.

Generalised aggressive periodontitis is characterised by the following features.

- Usually affecting a person under 35 years of age but patients may be older.
- Generalised interproximal attachment loss affecting at least three permanent teeth other than the first molars and incisors.
- Pronounced episodic nature of the destruction.
- Poor serum antibody response to infecting agents.

There can be high heterogeneity in the clinical presentation of aggressive periodontitis. Some LAP cases may initially affect the primary dentition.

1.3 Prevalence

There is a wide variation in the prevalence of aggressive periodontitis between populations and differences in race/ethnicities can be a key factor (Susin *et al.*, 2014). Most studies show comparable disease prevalence in male and female subjects.

Aggressive periodontitis is most prevalent in Africa and in populations of African descent (around 1%), compared to Caucasians where the prevalence of LAP is 0.1%.

1.4 Aetiology and Pathogenesis

Aggressive periodontitis is a multifactorial disease. It shares most of the risk factors associated with chronic periodontitis, as discussed in Chapter 6. However, the

Diseases and Conditions in Dentistry: An Evidence-Based Reference, First Edition. Keyvan Moharamzadeh.

Companion website: www.wiley.com/go/moharamzadeh/diseases

following parameters play key roles in the onset and progression of the aggressive disease.

1.4.1 Bacteria

Actinobacillus actinomycetemcomitans (mainly serotype b) has been isolated from periodontal lesions in 90% of LAP patients. It can invade the soft tissue and produces virulence factors including leucotoxins, endotoxin (LPS), bacteriocin, immunosuppressive factors and collagenase, and causes chemotactic inhibition (Kononen and Muller, 2014).

Elevated serum antibodies against AA can be detected in LAP patients and there is a correlation between treatment outcomes and levels of AA after therapy.

On the other hand, GAP is associated with PG, *Bacteroides forsythus* and AA.

1.4.2 Genetic Susceptibility

Available data suggest that aggressive periodontitis is caused by mutations in multiple genes, combined with environmental effects (Vieira and Albandar, 2014). A hereditary pattern for susceptibility to aggressive periodontitis has been reported and the most likely mode of inheritance is autosomal dominant. The percentage of the affected siblings can be 40–50%.

Disease-modifying genes that have been studied in relation to periodontitis include:

- IL-1, IL-10 and tumour necrosis factor (TNF)-alpha gene polymorphism
- Fc gamma receptor gene polymorphism
- gene polymorphism in the innate immunity receptors
- vitamin D receptor gene polymorphism.

1.4.3 Smoking

Smoking is a major risk factor for periodontal disease and it further adds to the susceptibility for severe aggressive disease. Patients with aggressive periodontitis who are smokers show poorer response to treatment compared to non-smokers (Hughes *et al.*, 2006) (see also Chapter 6).

1.5 Screening

The most sensitive screening method for aggressive periodontitis in adults is the measurement of pocket depth by probing (attachment loss measurement).

In children with primary and mixed dentition, probing may not be a reliable method due to partial eruption of teeth and the presence of pseudo-pockets. Therefore, measurement of distance between the alveolar bone crest and the cementoenamel junction (CEJ) using bitewing (BW) radiographs can be an appropriate screening method in children. The median distance between the alveolar bone crest and the CEJ in 7–9-year-old children is 0.8–1.4 mm in primary molars and the normal range is less than 2 mm.

1.6 Diagnosis

Aggressive periodontitis can be differentiated from chronic periodontitis based on the primary and secondary features as described above, including the criteria for the classification of localised and generalised disease (Albandar, 2014).

The diagnosis of aggressive periodontitis can be confirmed by different approaches as listed below.

- *History, clinical, and radiographic examination* (see Chapter 6).
- *Microbiological testing*: bacterial testing alone cannot distinguish between chronic and aggressive periodontitis but it can provide useful information that can improve the outcome of periodontal therapy. It can help with the choice of antibiotics so it is best to postpone microbiological testing until after the initial treatment phase. It can also help to identify the presence of transmissible AA or PG in family members so that disease can be potentially prevented by early intervention.
- *Serological testing*: serum antibody levels against AA may be useful for differential diagnosis of GAP and LAP and in the early detection of LAP cases with high risk for progression.
- *Genetic diagnosis*: pedigree plotting can be essential for the diagnosis of aggressive periodontitis due to its familial aggregation.

1.7 Prognosis

General patient-level, site-level and tooth-level prognostic factors for periodontal disease are discussed in Chapter 6.

The prognosis for aggressive periodontitis specifically depends on early diagnosis, the extent and severity of the disease, directing treatment towards elimination of infecting pathogens and long-term maintenance.

1.8 Treatment

Non-surgical and even surgical periodontal treatments alone are not sufficient for the elimination of AA in LAP and in some chronic periodontitis patients. Therefore, oral hygiene instructions (OHI) and root surface debridement (RSD) supplemented with systemic antibiotics are recommended for the treatment of aggressive periodontitis patients.

1.8.1 Systemic Antibiotics

Systematic reviews show significantly larger adjunctive benefits of systemic antibiotics and greater clinical improvements and reduction in periodontal indices following systemic antibiotic administration upon completion of subgingival instrumentation in aggressive periodontitis cases compared to patients with chronic periodontitis (Haffajee *et al.*, 2003; Keestra *et al.*, 2015a; Rabelo *et al.*, 2015; Rajendra and Spivakovsky, 2016).

According to the American Academy of Periodontology and the British Society for Periodontology guidelines, patients who are likely to benefit from adjunctive systemic antibiotics are those diagnosed with aggressive periodontitis, those suffering from acute periodontal infections such as necrotising periodontal disease and periodontal abscesses with systemic involvement, certain medically compromised patients, and those for whom conventional mechanical treatment has proven ineffective (BSP, 2016).

Systemic antibiotics are not routinely prescribed for the treatment of chronic periodontitis due to the risk of resistance which is enhanced by the biofilm's protective nature and the risk of unwanted systemic side effects such as hypersensitivity, nausea, vomiting, gastrointestinal (GI) intolerance, and pseudomembranous colitis.

Different types and combinations of systemic antibiotics have been used for the treatment of periodontal disease (Herrera *et al.*, 2002, 2008; Keestra *et al.*, 2015b; Moreno Villagrana and Gomez Clavel, 2012; Renatus *et al.*, 2016; Santos *et al.*, 2016). Some examples of the most commonly prescribed regimens include:

- amoxicillin 500 mg, three times per day + metronidazole 500 mg, three times per day for 7 days
- metronidazole 500 mg, three times per day + ciprofloxacin 500 mg twice a day for 7 days
- clindamycin 300 mg, four times per day for 7 days
- doxycycline 200 mg, once a day for 7–14 days
- azithromycin 500 mg, once a day for 3 days.

It has been shown that metronidazole on its own does not eradicate AA but combination therapy with metronidazole and amoxicillin can be effective against AA.

There is a growing body of evidence that azithromycin used as an adjunct to RSD significantly improves the efficacy of non-surgical periodontal therapy in reducing probing pocket depth and other periodontal indices, particularly at the initially deep probing depth sites (Buset *et al.*, 2015; Renatus *et al.*, 2016; Zhang *et al.*, 2016). Azithromycin is an effective, safe and well-tolerated drug and has the advantage of a relatively short duration of therapy and therefore improved patient compliance and reduced potential side effects.

1.8.2 Local Antimicrobials

Local delivery of antibiotics can be beneficial in the control of localised ongoing periodontal disease in otherwise stable patients. It can also be useful in the management of non-responding sites following initial treatment.

The advantages of local antimicrobials include their ease of use, independence of patient co-operation, high dose at treated sites and reduced systemic adverse effects. The disadvantages include narrow distribution to other sites that may reinfect, potential washout, dilution within minutes and rapid clearance. Furthermore, local therapy may be less successful in patients with widespread lesions than those with localised lesions. It has been shown that local healing with locally delivered antibiotics is affected if the other diseased sites are left untreated (Mombelli *et al.*, 1997).

Local antimicrobial products most commonly used in the treatment of periodontal disease with the relevant studies on their efficacy are listed below.

- Minocycline ointment (Dentomycin) and microspheres (Arestin) (Williams *et al.*, 2001)
- Doxycycline hyclate in a biodegradable polymer (Atridox two-syringe system) (Wennstrom *et al.*, 2001)
- Metronidazole gel (Elyzol Dental Gel 25%) (Ainamo *et al.*, 1992)
- Tetracycline in a non-resorbable plastic co-polymer (Actisite periodontal fibre 25%) (Michalowicz *et al.*, 1995)
- Chlorhexidine in a gelatin chip (PerioChip) (Jeffcoat *et al.*, 1998)

A meta-analysis of 19 clinical trials indicated significant adjunctive pocket depth reduction for locally delivered minocycline gel, microencapsulated minocycline, chlorhexidine chip and doxycycline gel during non-surgical periodontal treatment compared to RSD alone (Hanes and Purvis, 2003).

In another systematic review, subgingival application of tetracycline fibres, sustained-release doxycycline and minocycline demonstrated a significant benefit in probing pocket depth reduction. The local application of chlorhexidine and metronidazole showed a minimal effect when compared with placebo (Matesanz-Perez *et al.*, 2013).

Locally delivered antibiotics, although extensively demonstrated to have clinical efficacy and microbiological benefits, are still debated regarding their cost-effectiveness and adequate indications (Herrera *et al.*, 2012; Kalsi *et al.*, 2011).

Finally, it is important to emphasise that mechanical debridement before the application of antimicrobial agents and mechanical plaque control after therapy are essential for treatment success. To limit the development of microbial antibiotic resistance in general, and to avoid the risk of unwanted systemic effects of antibiotics for the treated individual, a precautionary, restrictive attitude towards using antibiotics is recommended (Lang and Lindhe, 2015).

Case Study

A 34-year-old female patient was referred by the general dental practitioner for the management of periodontal disease and residual deep pockets despite repeated cycles of non-surgical periodontal treatment in the practice. The patient presented with painful gums, drifted upper front teeth, recurrent infections and loss of several teeth. She was a non-smoker, medically fit and well and reported a positive familial history of periodontal disease.

The patient's preoperative clinical photograph and radiographs are shown in Figures 1.1 and 1.2 respectively. Table 1.1 shows full periodontal charting at the baseline prior to any specialist treatment.

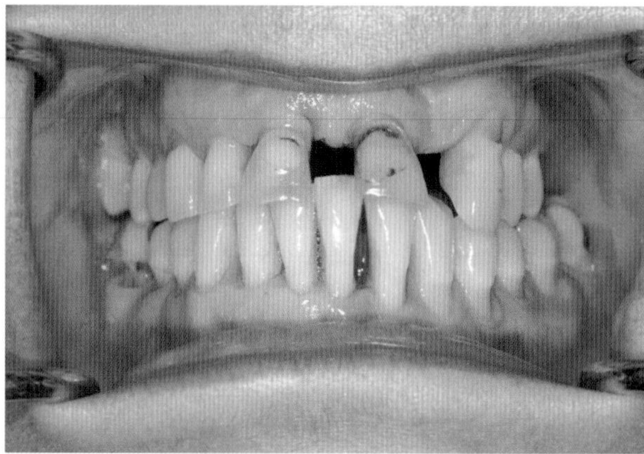

Figure 1.1 Preoperative clinical photograph.

Diagnoses

- Generalised aggressive periodontitis
- Secondary occlusal trauma to the incisor teeth
- Caries
- Chronic apical periodontitis UL1, UL3, LR5, LL1
- Missing teeth
- Cervical abrasion lesions

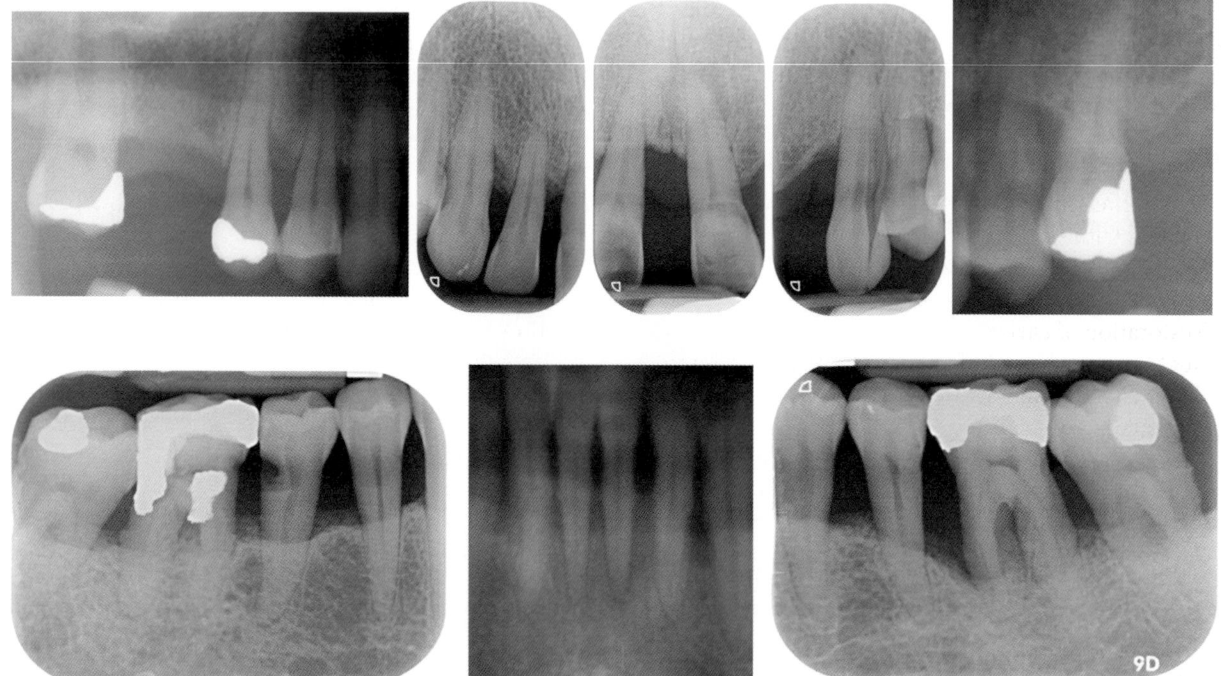

Figure 1.2 Preoperative full-mouth periapical radiographs showing the extent and severity of periodontal bone loss and presence of multiple periapical radiolucencies.

Table 1.1 Preoperative full periodontal charting.

Mobility	X		X					II	II	X	I	II	I	X	X	X
Recession	X		X		1	2		2	2	X	3	1		X	X	X
PPD (Buccal)	X	733	X	216	524	327	323	424	422	X	515	726	634	X	X	X
Upper teeth	8	7	6	5	4	3	2	1	1	2	3	4	5	6	7	8
PPD (Palatal)	X	533	X	236	535	336	433	345	522	X	656	656	543	X	X	X
Recession	X		X		1	1		2	2	X	1	1		X	X	X
Furcation	X		X							X				X	X	X

Mobility	X		I				I	I	III	I		I	II	I	I	X
Recession	X	1	1	1	2	1	2	4	5	3	2	2	1	2	1	X
PPD (Lingual)	X	455	335	534	524	355	333	233	326	423	554	636	535	943	576	X
Lower teeth	8	7	6	5	4	3	2	1	1	2	3	4	5	6	7	8
PPD (Buccal)	X	425	624	524	524	526	623	523	336	326	525	523	528	857	656	X
Recession	X	2	3	3	3	2	3	4	4	3	3	3	3	3	3	X
Furcation	X	I	II											III	I	X

Prognosis

The prognosis for LR6 and LL1 was hopeless. LR6 was non-vital as tested by the electric pulp tester and had large restoration with subgingival secondary caries and was non-restorable. This tooth also had advanced periodontal bone loss with furcation involvement.

LL1 had advanced periodontal bone loss and periapical radiolucency and was grade III mobile. The prognosis for the remaining teeth was questionable and would also depend on the patient's compliance

Treatment Strategy

- Initial non-surgical periodontal treatment supplemented with systemic antibiotics
- Extraction of non-restorable teeth with hopeless prognosis
- Restoration of caries
- Root canal treatment of teeth with apical periodontitis
- Surgical periodontal treatment in the lower left sextant
- Direct and indirect restoration of compromised teeth and replacement of missing teeth with fixed bridges
- Periodontal maintenance

Clinical Procedures Undertaken

1) Full periodontal assessment and recording indices.
2) Oral hygiene instructions including modified Bass and interdental brushing.
3) Full-mouth RSD under local anaesthesia (LA) in combination with systemic azithromycin 500 mg once a day for 3 days.
4) Extraction of LR6 and LL1.
5) Splinting of the extracted LL1 crown to LR1 using composite fibre splint.
6) Restoration of caries LR5, UR1, UL1 and cervical abrasion lesion UL3.
7) Root canal treatment (RCT) of UL1, UR1, UL3, LR5.
8) Periodontal reassessment. Significant improvement and reduction in the probing pocket depth was recorded. Deep residual pockets remained in the LL6 region.
9) Surgical periodontal treatment in the lower left sextant and tunnel preparation in the LL6 furcation area to facilitate cleaning of the furcation with an interdental brush.
10) Impressions and diagnostic wax-up of the upper anterior teeth to ideal crown position, shape and occlusion (Figure 1.3).
11) Preparation and fitting of porcelain fused to metal (PFM) crowns on UR1 and UR2 and a three-unit PFM bridge for UL1–UL3 to replace the missing UL2.
12) Three-monthly periodontal reassessment and supportive periodontal treatment.

Postoperative periodontal charting is shown in Table 1.2 and the postoperative clinical photograph and radiographs

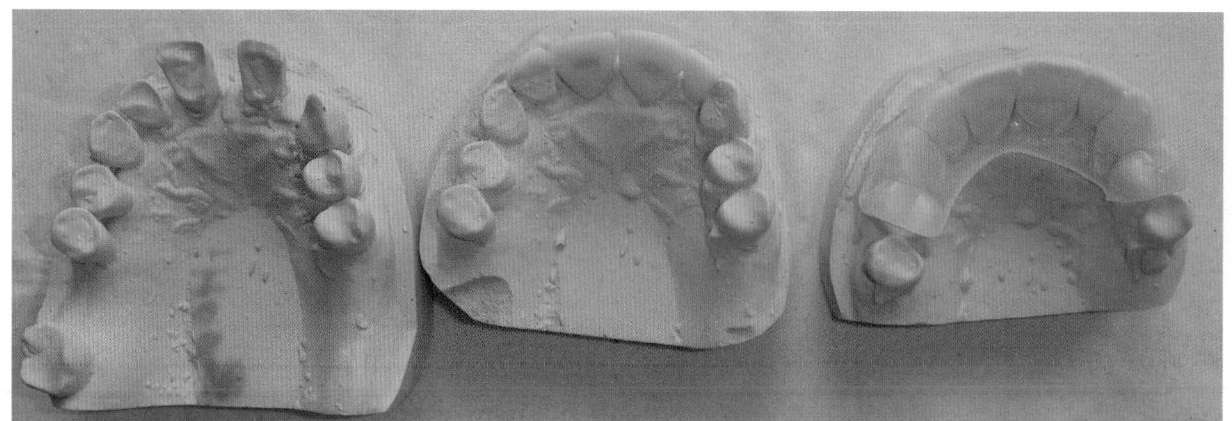

Figure 1.3 Diagnostic wax-up of the upper anterior teeth and fabrication of a clear stent to facilitate construction of provisional restorations.

of the root-treated teeth are demonstrated in Figures 1.4 and 1.5 respectively.

Discussion and Learning Points

The diagnosis of aggressive periodontitis was made for this case because of rapid disease progression in a relatively young patient, non-contributory medical history and positive familial history of periodontitis. Also, there was little plaque and calculus which was not commensurate with the severity of the disease.

The patient responded well to the RSD under LA supplemented with systemic azithromycin. She had shown a poorer response to repeated RSD alone in the dental practice previously. This shows the additional beneficial role of adjunctive systemic antibiotics in the treatment of aggressive periodontitis.

Extraction of LL1 with hopeless prognosis and splinting the extracted tooth to the adjacent tooth with composite fibre splint was a successful attempt to eliminate the infection, alleviate the patient's discomfort and restore function using the patient's own extracted tooth. Optimised bonding technique with appropriate moisture control and careful occlusal adjustment of the pontic tooth were the key factors in achieving a satisfactory outcome.

LR6 was also extracted as this tooth was not restorable. However, the patient did not want to replace this tooth and was satisfied with maintaining a shortened dental arch.

Table 1.2 Postoperative full periodontal charting.

Mobility	X		X		I		I	I	I	X		I	I	X	X	X
Recession	X	4	X	4	3	4				X	1	4	2	X	X	X
PPD (Buccal)	X	323	X	223	323	223	323	223	323	X	223	223	333	X	X	X
Upper teeth	8	7	6	5	4	3	2	1	1	2	3	4	5	6	7	8
PPD (Palatal)	X	323	X	223	333	223	333	222	222	X	333	323	332	X	X	X
Recession	X	4	X	3	2	3	1	1	1	X	1	3	1	X	X	X
Furcation	X		X							X				X	X	X

Mobility	X		X	I			I	I	X	I		I	II	II	II	X
Recession	X	4	X	5	3	2	3	4	X	4	4	3	3	5	4	X
PPD (Lingual)	X	333	X	323	322	222	222	222	X	221	212	323	333	333	233	X
Lower teeth	8	7	6	5	4	3	2	1	1	2	3	4	5	6	7	8
PPD (Buccal)	X	333	X	323	323	323	212	222	X	322	222	323	333	323	333	X
Recession	X	5	X	6	4	3	4	5	X	5	5	5	5	6	5	X
Furcation	X	I	X						X					III	I	X

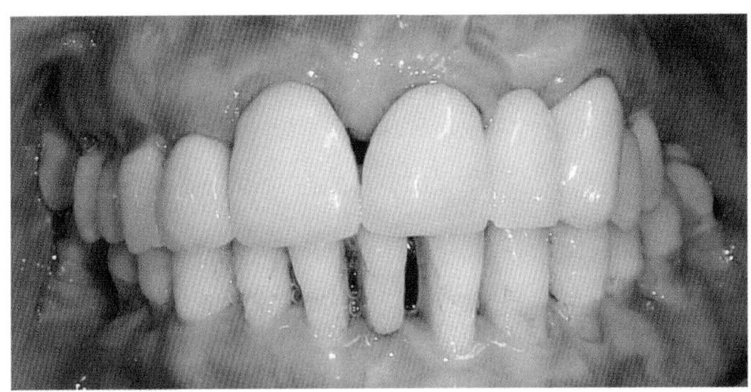

Figure 1.4 Postoperative clinical photograph.

Surgical periodontal treatment in the lower left sextant resulted in the elimination of the isolated residual deep periodontal pockets associated with LL6 which had grade III furcation involvement, and a tunnel preparation technique facilitated access for cleaning of the furcation area using an interdental brush. Management of teeth with furcation involvement is discussed in detail in Chapter 6.

The options regarding the drifted upper anterior teeth with spacing and poor aesthetics included: (a) keeping the teeth as they were with maintenance only; (b) extraction of the teeth and replacement by removable partial dentures or implant-retained prosthesis; and (c) RCT of non-vital teeth and UR1 and modification of the teeth using crowns and replacement of the spaces using fixed bridges. As the patient responded well to periodontal treatment and was well motivated to maintain her teeth, it was decided to restore the anterior teeth with crowns and bridges following root canal treatment. The use of a diagnostic wax-up (see Figure 1.3) to correct the position and alignment of the drifted teeth and recreate the ideal tooth shape, size and ratios was a very helpful approach.

The patient was very satisfied with the outcome of the treatment in terms of aesthetics, function and the resolution of symptoms associated with periodontal disease. Supportive periodontal therapy was extremely important in long-term maintenance of the patient's periodontal health.

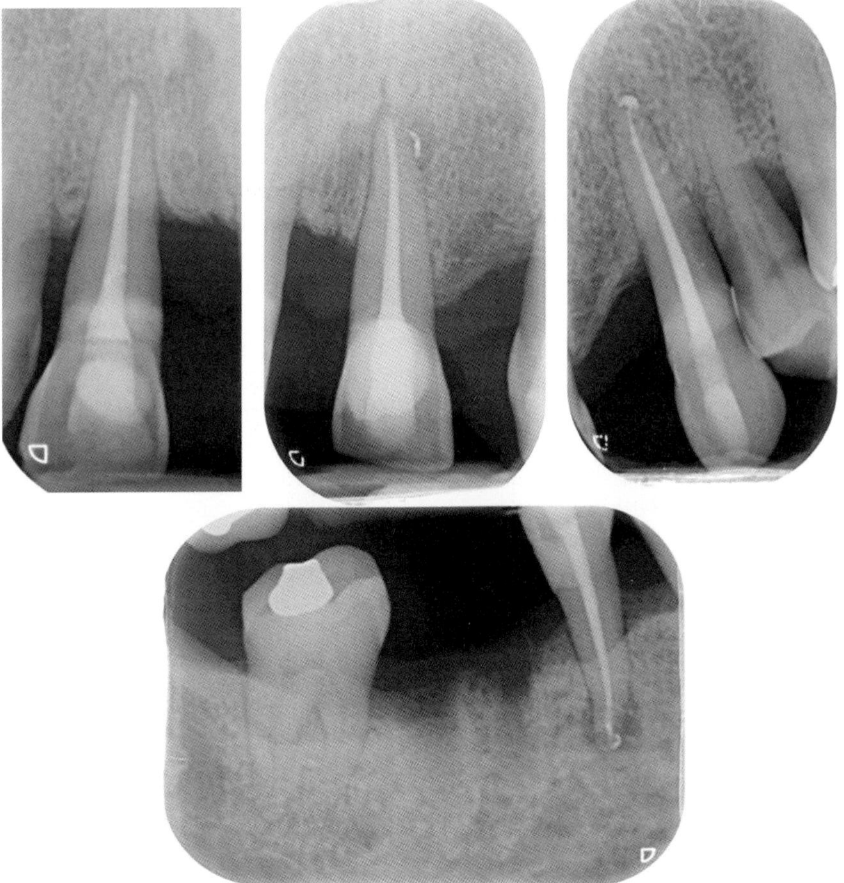

Figure 1.5 Postoperative periapical radiographs of the teeth following root canal treatment showing evidence of periapical healing.

References

Ainamo, J., Lie, T., Ellingsen, B.H. *et al.* (1992) Clinical responses to subgingival application of a metronidazole 25% gel compared to the effect of subgingival scaling in adult periodontitis. *J Clin Periodontol*, **19**, 723–729.

Albandar, J.M. (2014) Aggressive periodontitis: case definition and diagnostic criteria. *Periodontology 2000*, **65**, 13–26.

Armitage, G.C. (1999) Development of a classification system for periodontal diseases and conditions. *Ann Periodontol*, **4**, 1–6.

BSP (2016) *The Good Practitioner's Guide To Periodontology*, British Society of Periodontology, Selby.

Buset, S.L., Zitzmann, N.U., Weiger, R. and Walter, C. (2015) Non-surgical periodontal therapy supplemented with systemically administered azithromycin: a systematic review of RCTs. *Clin Oral Invest*, **19**, 1763–1775.

Haffajee, A.D., Socransky, S.S. and Gunsolley, J.C. (2003) Systemic anti-infective periodontal therapy. a systematic review. *Ann Periodontol*, **8**, 115–181.

Hanes, P.J. and Purvis, J.P. (2003) Local anti-infective therapy: pharmacological agents. A systematic review. *Ann Periodontol*, **8**, 79–98.

Herrera, D., Sanz, M., Jepsen, S., Needleman, I. and Roldan, S. (2002) A systematic review on the effect of systemic antimicrobials as an adjunct to scaling and root planing in periodontitis patients. *J Clin Periodontol*, **29**(suppl 3), 136–159; discussion 160–162.

Herrera, D., Alonso, B., Leon, R., Roldan, S. and Sanz, M. (2008) Antimicrobial therapy in periodontitis: the use of systemic antimicrobials against the subgingival biofilm. *J Clin Periodontol*, **35**, 45–66.

Herrera, D., Matesanz, P., Bascones-Martinez, A. and Sanz, M. (2012. Local and systemic antimicrobial therapy in periodontics. *J Evid Based Dent Pract*, **12**, 50–60.

Hughes, F.J., Syed, M., Koshy, B. *et al.* (2006) Prognostic factors in the treatment of generalized aggressive periodontitis: II. Effects of smoking on initial outcome. *J Clin Periodontol*, **33**, 671–676.

Jeffcoat, M.K., Bray, K.S., Ciancio, S.G. *et al.* (1998) Adjunctive use of a subgingival controlled-release chlorhexidine chip reduces probing depth and improves attachment level compared with scaling and root planing alone. *J Periodontol*, **69**, 989–997.

Kalsi, R., Vandana, K.L. and Prakash, S. (2011) Effect of local drug delivery in chronic periodontitis patients: a meta-analysis. *J Indian Soc Periodontol*, **15**, 304–309.

Keestra, J.A., Grosjean, I., Coucke, W., Quirynen, M. and Teughels, W. (2015a) Non–surgical periodontal therapy with systemic antibiotics in patients with untreated aggressive periodontitis: a systematic review and meta-analysis. *J Periodontal Res*, **50**, 689–706.

Keestra, J.A., Grosjean, I., Coucke, W., Quirynen, M. and Teughels, W. (2015b) Non–surgical periodontal therapy with systemic antibiotics in patients with untreated chronic periodontitis: a systematic review and meta-analysis. *J Periodontal Res*, **50**, 294–314.

Kononen, E. and Muller, H.P. (2014) Microbiology of aggressive periodontitis. *Periodontology* 2000, **65**, 46–78.

Lang, N.P. and Lindhe, J. (2015) *Clinical Periodontology and Implant Dentistry*, Wiley-Blackwell, Oxford.

Lang, N., Bartold, P.M., Cullinan, M. *et al.* (1999) Consensus report: aggressive periodontitis. *Ann Periodontol*, **4**, 53.

Matesanz-Perez, P., Garcia-Gargallo, M., Figuero, E., Bascones-Martinez, A., Sanz, M. and Herrera, D. (2013) A systematic review on the effects of local antimicrobials as adjuncts to subgingival debridement, compared with subgingival debridement alone, in the treatment of chronic periodontitis. *J Clin Periodontol*, **40**, 227–241.

Michalowicz, B.S., Pihlstrom, B.L., Drisko, C.L. *et al.* (1995) Evaluation of periodontal treatments using controlled–release tetracycline fibers: maintenance response. *J Periodontol*, **66**, 708–715.

Mombelli, A., Lehmann, B., Tonetti, M. and Lang, N.P. (1997) Clinical response to local delivery of tetracycline in relation to overall and local periodontal conditions. *J Clin Periodontol*, **24**, 470–477.

Moreno Villagrana, A.P. and Gomez Clavel, J.F. (2012) Antimicrobial or subantimicrobial antibiotic therapy as an adjunct to the nonsurgical periodontal treatment: a meta-analysis. *ISRN Dent*, **2012**, 581207.

Rabelo, C.C., Feres, M., Goncalves, C. *et al.* (2015) Systemic antibiotics in the treatment of aggressive periodontitis. A systematic review and a Bayesian network meta-analysis. *J Clin Periodontol*, **42**, 647–657.

Rajendra, A. and Spivakovsky, S. (2016) Antibiotics in aggressive periodontitis. Is there a clinical benefit? *Evid Based Dent*, **17**, 100.

Renatus, A., Herrmann, J., Schonfelder, A., Schwarzenberger, F. and Jentsch, H. (2016) Clinical efficacy of azithromycin as an adjunctive therapy to non-surgical periodontal treatment of periodontitis: a systematic review and meta-analysis. *J Clin Diagn Res*, **10**, Ze01–7.

Santos, R.S., Macedo, R.F., Souza, E.A., Soares, R.S., Feitosa, D.S. and Sarmento, C.F. (2016) The use of systemic antibiotics in the treatment of refractory periodontitis: a systematic review. *J Am Dent Assoc*, **147**, 577–585.

Susin, C., Haas, A.N. and Albandar, J.M. (2014) Epidemiology and demographics of aggressive periodontitis. *Periodontology* 2000, **65**, 27–45.

Vieira, A.R. and Albandar, J.M. (2014) Role of genetic factors in the pathogenesis of aggressive periodontitis. *Periodontology* 2000, **65**, 92–106.

Wennstrom, J.L., Newman, H.N., Macneill, S.R. *et al.* (2001) Utilisation of locally delivered doxycycline in non-surgical treatment of chronic periodontitis. A comparative multi-centre trial of 2 treatment approaches. *J Clin Periodontol*, **28**, 753–761.

Williams, R.C., Paquette, D.W., Offenbacher, S. *et al.* (2001) Treatment of periodontitis by local administration of minocycline microspheres: a controlled trial. *J Periodontol*, **72**, 1535–1544.

Zhang, Z., Zheng, Y. and Bian, X. (2016) Clinical effect of azithromycin as an adjunct to non-surgical treatment of chronic periodontitis: a meta-analysis of randomized controlled clinical trials. *J Periodontal Res*, **51**, 275–283.

2

Amelogenesis Imperfecta

2.1 Definition

Amelogenesis imperfecta (AI) can be defined as an inherited disease that affects the enamel of both the deciduous and permanent dentition and is associated with mutations in different genes with a wide range of clinical presentations (Gadhia *et al.*, 2012).

2.2 Aetiology

Different types of AI have been associated with mutations in different genes that control the process of amelogenesis. These genes include *AMEL* (amelogenin), *ENAM* (enamelin), *MMP20* (matrix metalloproteinase-20), *KLK4* (kallikrein-4) and *FAM83H* (Hart and Hart, 2009).

Depending on the timing of disruptions that can occur during amelogenesis, a diversity of enamel abnormalities can be observed in AI. Defects during formation of the dentinoenamel junction can result in an enamel layer that is weakly attached to the underlying dentine and can be easily sheared off. Secretory stage flaws result in insufficient crystal formation and therefore thin or hypoplastic enamel layer. Defects during the maturation stage produce a pathologically soft enamel layer with normal thickness (Hu *et al.*, 2007).

2.3 Epidemiology

The prevalence of AI varies from 1 in 700 to 1 in 14 000, depending on the populations studied (Crawford *et al.*, 2007).

2.4 Classification

Amelogenesis imperfecta was first explained in 1890 but later in 1938, Finn *et al.* classified it as a separate developmental disorder to dentinogenesis imperfecta (Witkop, 1988). AI classification can be based on different factors (Aldred *et al.*, 2003).

- *Mode of inheritance*: autosomal dominant, autosomal recessive, X-linked and isolated cases.
- *Molecular basis*: chromosomal localisation, locus, mutation.
- *Biochemical outcome*: putative result of mutation when known.
- *Phenotype* (the most common mode of classification): type I, hypoplastic; type II, hypocalcified; type III, hypomaturation; type IV, mixed – hypomaturation-hypoplastic with taurodontism (enlarged pulp chamber).

2.5 Diagnostic Clinical Features

Different phenotypes of AI can have distinct clinical presentations (Gadhia *et al.*, 2012):

2.5.1 Hypoplastic Type

The enamel has reduced thickness and often pitting and grooves are present on the surface. The enamel is hard and translucent and contrasts with normal dentine on radiographic examination.

2.5.2 Hypocalcified Type

The enamel is poorly calcified and weak. It has normal thickness and appears opaque or chalky. The teeth become stained and can wear down rapidly. Radiographically, the enamel layer is less radio-opaque than the underlying dentine layer.

2.5.3 Hypomaturation Type

Enamel has normal thickness but is mottled in appearance (resembling fluorosis). It is slightly softer than normal and is vulnerable to wear. The enamel shows similar radio-opacity compared to dentine.

Diseases and Conditions in Dentistry: An Evidence-Based Reference, First Edition. Keyvan Moharamzadeh.

Companion website: www.wiley.com/go/moharamzadeh/diseases

Other clinical features of AI include delayed eruption of teeth, crowding, microdontia and abnormal crown morphology, root resorption, pulp abnormalities, gingival and periodontal diseases. Additionally, there can be skeletal abnormalities such as anterior open bite and crossbites (Poulsen *et al.*, 2008).

2.6 Relevant History

The important aspects of the history with regard to AI patients are as follows.

- Family history.
- *Pedigree plotting*: a diagram that shows the occurrence and appearance or phenotypes of a particular gene from one generation to the next.
- Medical history which might have caused sufficient metabolic disturbance to affect enamel formation.
- Questions regarding the chronological distribution of appearance of the defect.

It is important to identify and exclude other causes of defects in enamel, both extrinsic and intrinsic, including tetracycline staining, dental fluorosis, enamel hypoplasia, trauma and molar-incisor hypomineralisation (MIH).

2.7 Relevant Investigations

The following special investigations can be useful for diagnosis and management of AI patients.

- Clinical photographs, articulated study models and diagnostic wax-up of worn teeth can be very helpful for restorative treatment planning.
- Radiographic assessment to detect caries and also to provide information regarding the thickness and quality of enamel, delayed eruption of teeth, taurodontism and idiopathic tooth tissue resorption. Periapical radiographs may also be indicated prior to crown lengthening surgery to assess root length and amount of available bone support.
- Periodontal and endodontic assessment of the teeth, including vitality testing of the compromised teeth, is important to diagnose and treat any associated periodontal disease or endodontic lesion.
- Genetic testing is not routinely carried out but can be useful as a research tool.

2.8 Prognosis

Challenging features of AI that can affect the prognosis are listed below (Patel *et al.*, 2013).

- Childhood issues and psychological problems
- Compromised periodontal health due to the rough tooth surfaces retaining plaque
- Hypersensitive teeth which can make cleaning difficult. Use of warm water during brushing and scaling of the teeth can be helpful
- High risk of developing dental caries
- Discoloured and pitted tooth surfaces
- Diminutive teeth with short clinical crown height
- Malformed teeth
- Congenitally missing teeth
- Pulp calcifications
- Taurodontism, large pulps and risk of pulpal exposure
- Root malformations
- Reduced inter-root space due to rapid loss of enamel post eruption and teeth drifting close together, which can make it difficult to prepare the teeth for crowns
- Anterior and posterior open bite
- Multiple posterior spacing
- Loss of occlusal vertical dimension due to rapid tooth surface loss
- Decreased bond strength of composite resin to enamel due to high protein content of enamel

2.9 Treatment Considerations

The aim of treatment will be early diagnosis of disease, management of pain, prevention and stabilisation, maintaining face height, restoration of teeth with defects, and regular maintenance.

2.9.1 Management of Children

It is important to see the patient as early as possible to establish good rapport. Using techniques of behavioural management and also sedation can be valuable for the clinician and patient. General anaesthesia (GA) may be necessary in children with very severe anxiety (McDonald *et al.*, 2012).

Prevention is essential in childhood. This includes oral hygiene education, diet advice and appropriate fluoride treatment in older children to reduce sensitivity and prevent caries.

Maintaining periodontal health may require several visits for scaling under LA due to sensitivity of the teeth.

The use of a non-latex rubber dam can help to reduce sensitivity during restorative treatment.

Where there is no evidence of wear on the teeth, minimal intervention and monitoring is the preferred treatment plan.

Interventions would become necessary if there is occlusal wear and the patient is complaining about sensitivity and poor aesthetics. Treatment may include:

- glass ionomer restorations or direct composite veneers on the anterior teeth
- stainless steel crowns (SSCs) or glass ionomer restorations on the occlusal surfaces of primary molars. Orthodontic separators between molar teeth will assist the placement of SSCs.

2.9.2 Mixed Dentition

During mixed dentition, teeth can take a long time to erupt and damage can occur while waiting. In this situation, placement of glass ionomer material on the occlusal surface of partially erupted teeth can be considered until the teeth fully erupt. Excising the residual soft tissue operculum to expose the whole crown can further facilitate restorative procedure.

Cast adhesive onlays (CAAs), SSCs or gold crowns on the first permanent molars can be considered when the teeth have fully erupted. The SSC can be cheaper and simpler to use but more tooth tissue is lost during preparation and fitting compared to CAAs. They both have similar longevity and quality when used in AI patients (Zagdwon *et al.*, 2003). However, the choice of restoration is dependent on the needs of each individual patient.

For the permanent incisor teeth, direct or indirect composite veneers will improve the aesthetics, reduce sensitivity and prevent incisal wear. This treatment should be provided as soon as possible but the child and parents should be warned that with continuing eruption and gingival maturation, the margins of any restoration may become visible and additional treatment will be required at intervals to maintain good aesthetics.

2.9.3 Permanent Dentition

In young patients, the adhesive approach is still preferred over preparing teeth for indirect restorations due to the risk of damage to the pulp with large size and to preserve tooth structure.

Definitive restorative management of the dentition would be best postponed until full dental and gingival maturity occurs.

Joint specialty clinics can be useful at this stage to ensure a multidisciplinary approach involving general dental practitioners, paediatric dentists, orthodontists, restorative specialists, hygienists and therapists (Arkutu *et al.*, 2012; Malik *et al.*, 2012).

2.9.4 Adulthood

The aim of treatment at this stage is to reduce pain and sensitivity, improve any malocclusion present such as anterior open bite and to restore function and aesthetics. This may include the following aspects.

- Prevention: OHI, diet advice and fluoride application.
- Periodontal treatment and maintenance (see Chapter 6).
- Treatment of any present caries or endodontic lesions.
- Multidisciplinary treatment planning, including assessment in joint restorative and orthodontics clinics as prior orthodontic treatment can significantly facilitate further prosthetic treatment in some AI patients (especially hypoplastic type).
- Management of tooth wear (see Chapter 50) which may require prior crown-lengthening surgery.
- Restoration of compromised anterior teeth.
  - Definitive direct composite restorations can be considered for the anterior teeth where the enamel is not too compromised or the discolouration is not too severe.
  - Dentine bonded crowns with minimal preparation of the upper anterior teeth can be an alternative option and would provide excellent aesthetic results.
- Restoration of mandibular incisor teeth.
  - Direct composite build-ups.
  - Indirect labial porcelain veneers.
  - Dentine bonded crowns if retention is a concern.
- Restoration of posterior teeth.
  - Posterior teeth may be allowed to erupt into the occlusion (Dahl approach) if the enamel is not too compromised.
  - Premolar teeth can be restored with direct or indirect restorations.
  - Molar teeth can be restored with gold onlays or crowns if protection of the tooth structure is required.
- Replacement of missing teeth. Treatment options would include removable partial denture, fixed bridges or dental implants (see Chapters 35, 37 and 38).
- Long-term maintenance should include oral hygiene and plaque control, periodontal health, occlusal stability and maintenance of any restorations and fixed or removable prostheses.
- Provision of an appropriate occlusal splint can be helpful for long-term protection of the restorations, especially in patients with parafunctional habits.

2.10 Survival of Restorations

In general, the survival of different types of restorations in patients with AI is considerably lower compared to the longevity of restorations on normal teeth. The type and severity of AI influence the survival of the restoration (Sabandal and Schafer, 2016).

The survival of coronal restorations in patients with AI has been shown to be as low as 50% (Pousette Lundgren and Dahllof, 2014), with 2.5 times higher replacement rate for defective restorations compared to unaffected patients. The hypoplastic type of AI shows a higher survival rate for restorations than other types.

Direct composite restorations have higher failure rates in patients with hypocalcified AI compared to other types. The longevity of composite restorations is also affected by the severity of AI (Koruyucu *et al.*, 2014).

Case Study

A 45-year-old male patient was referred by the GDP for treatment of worn dentition. The patient was concerned about the poor appearance of the teeth and sensitivity to cold and reported that the teeth had been small and yellow since childhood and were gradually worn over many years.

The patient also reported:

- positive familial history of developmental teeth disorders
- positive diet history as the patient used to drink a lot of carbonated beverages
- negative history of parafunctional habits such as bruxism and clenching
- negative history of any GI disorder, acid reflux disease or excessive vomiting.

The patient was medically fit and well. He was a former smoker and had low alcohol consumption.

Preoperative clinical photographs are shown in Figures 2.1–2.4 and the radiographs are shown in Figures 2.5 and 2.6.

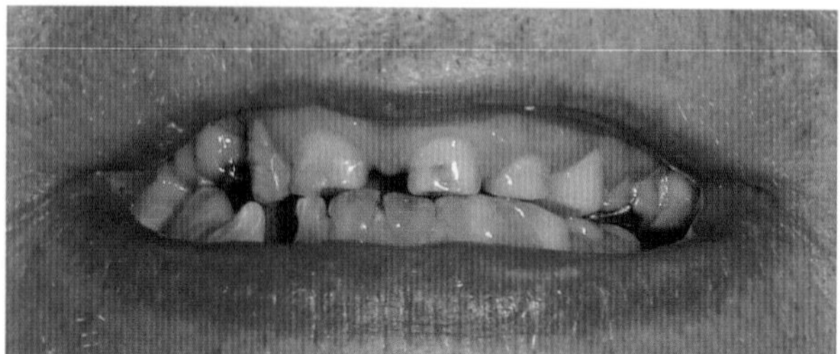

Figure 2.1 Preoperative photograph of the patient's smile.

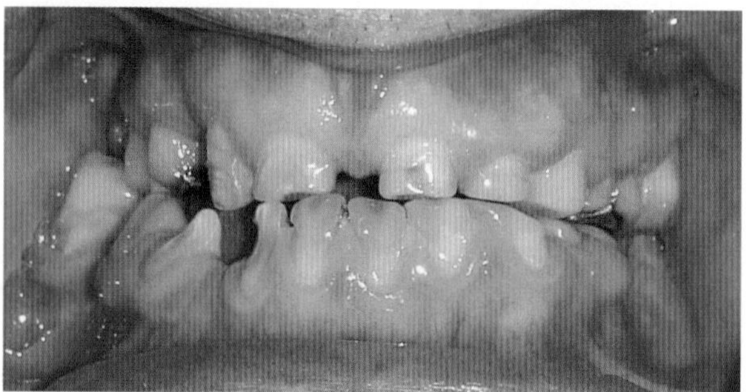

Figure 2.2 Preoperative photograph of occlusion.

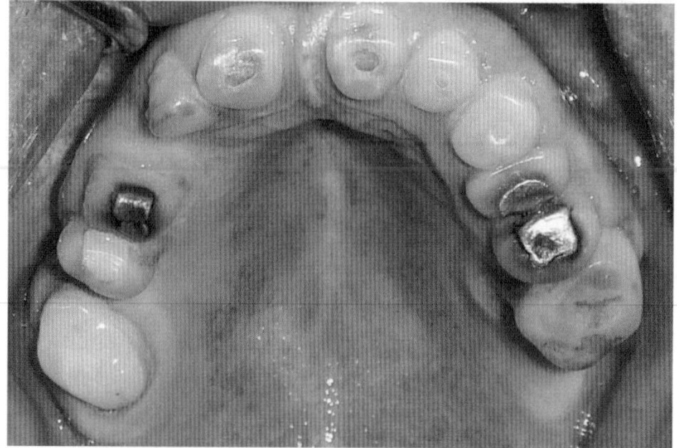

Figure 2.3 Preoperative photograph of the upper teeth.

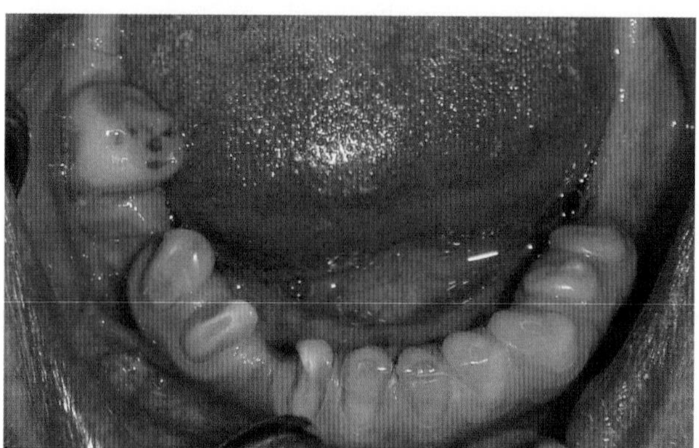

Figure 2.4 Preoperative photograph of the lower teeth.

Periodontal examination showed a healthy periodontium with shallow periodontal pockets and minimal bleeding on probing.

Sensibility testing using an electric pulp tester (EPT) showed that all the teeth were vital.

Diagnoses

Based on patient history, clinical and radiographic findings, the following diagnoses could be reached.

- Amelogenesis imperfecta
- Tooth wear due to a combination of erosion and attrition
- Impacted upper and lower right canine teeth with enlarged follicle of LR3 (dentigerous cyst)

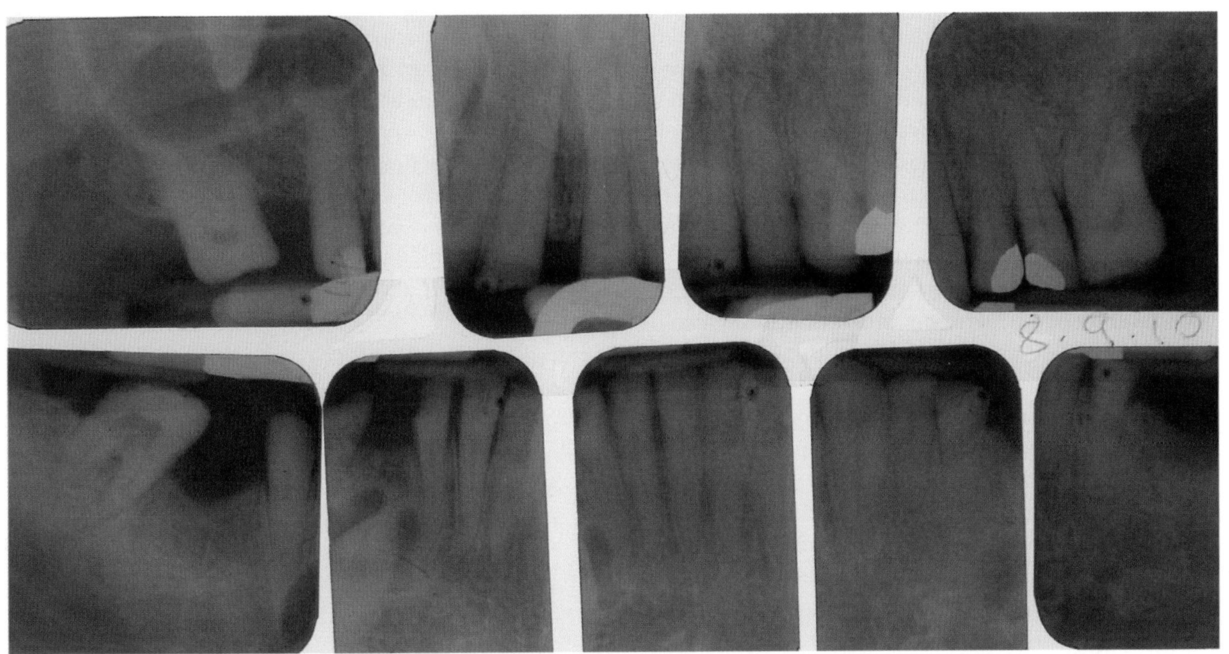

Figure 2.5 Preoperative periapical radiographs showing absence of enamel but normal appearance of dentine.

- Lost or missing teeth UR6, UR8, LR6, LR8, UL7–8, LL6–8

Treatment Options for the Upper Arch

- No treatment, but this option would not address the patient's concerns.
- Referral to oral surgery department for the assessment and treatment of impacted canine teeth which would be necessary prior to restorative treatment.
- Direct composite restoration of worn teeth. This is a conservative and reversible treatment option and would be preferred in children and young adults but the outcome would be unpredictable in the longterm due to the lack of enamel and weak bonding of resin to the AI affected teeth.
- Crown lengthening, crowns and a bridge to replace the UR3. This is a less conservative treatment option but is more predictable in the long term compared to direct restorations and would be preferred in this case considering the amount of excessive gingiva showing on the smile photograph (see Figure 2.1), adequate root length and bone support of the upper anterior teeth (see Figure 2.5).
- Reduction of the teeth and overdenture treatment. This is a very destructive and irreversible treatment option and may require root canal treatment (RCT) of the teeth. This is not recommended as the first treatment option in the upper arch as there are more conservative options available.
- Implant treatment for replacement of the UR3. This is not an ideal option due to the presence of the impacted UR3, which would need to be surgically removed prior to implant placement and would result in the loss of bone which would require further bone graft.

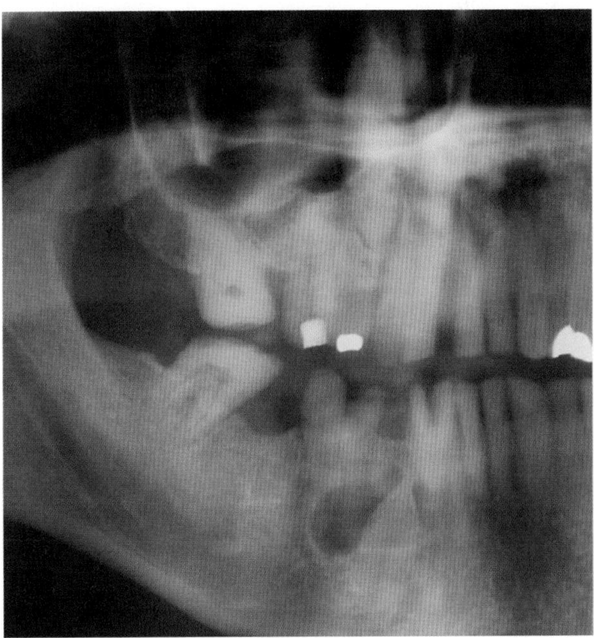

Figure 2.6 Preoperative half panoramic radiograph of the right side showing impacted unerupted upper and lower canine teeth.

Treatment Options for the Lower Arch

- No treatment.
- Referral to oral surgery department for the assessment and treatment of impacted canine teeth.
- Direct composite restorations which share the same above-mentioned limitations as the upper arch.
- Crown lengthening and crowns. This option is not recommended in the lower arch due to the presence of short roots of some of the lower teeth (see Figure 2.5). Preparation of narrow lower incisor teeth can also be very destructive and carries a high risk of damage to the pulp.
- Elective RCT and post crowns, which is an invasive option with unpredictable long-term prognosis and risk of vertical root fracture and tooth loss.
- Overdenture would be the preferred option in the lower arch due to severe wear and loss of coronal tooth structure which are not amenable to crown lengthening.

Aims of Treatment

- Management or removal of impacted teeth to avoid future complications and to facilitate restorative treatment.
- Restoration of function.
- Improvement of aesthetics.
- Reduction of sensitivity.
- Protection of teeth from further wear.

Treatment Procedures Undertaken

1) Preventive care, OHI and diet advice.
2) Referral to oral surgery department for the management of impacted canine teeth. The LR3 was surgically removed but it was decided to leave the UR3 as it was asymptomatic with no evidence of pathology.
3) Preparation of articulated study models, initial diagnostic wax-up and intraoral trial and fabrication of stent for crown lengthening (Figure 2.7).

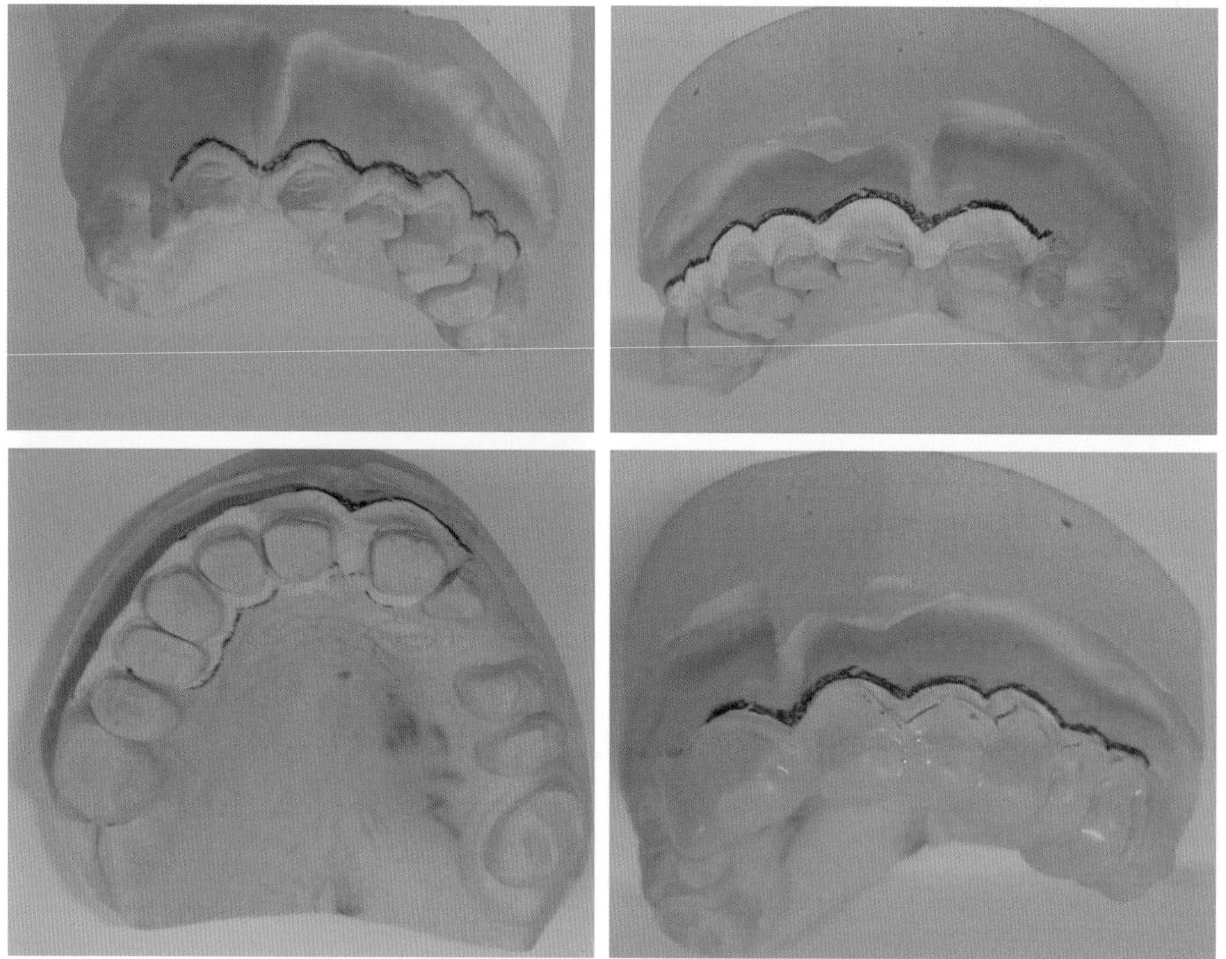

Figure 2.7 Study model for surgery by removing the stone from the marked gingivae around the teeth to be crown lengthened and fabrication of a surgical stent for crown lengthening.

4) Crown lengthening of upper anterior teeth UR1 to UL5 (Figure 2.8).
5) Impressions 6 weeks following crown lengthening, preparation of diagnostic wax-up of the upper teeth at an increased vertical dimension, intraoral trial of the upper wax-up and the wax try-in of the lower overdenture (Figure 2.9).
6) Preparation of upper anterior teeth for dentine bonded crowns and all ceramic bridge UR2 to UR4 (Figure 2.10) and fitting provisional crowns and bridge.
7) Fabrication and fitting of a temporary acrylic lower overdenture.

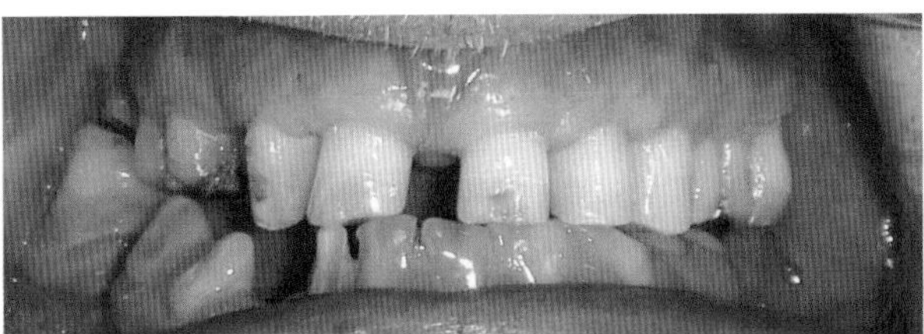

Figure 2.8 Clinical photograph of the teeth following crown lengthening.

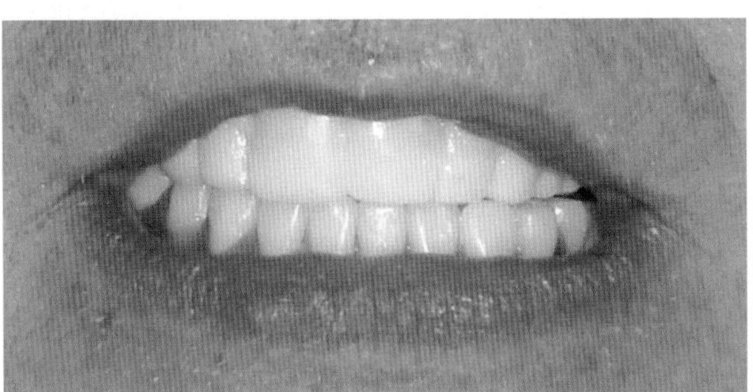

Figure 2.9 Simultaneous intraoral trial of the diagnostic wax-up of the upper teeth and overdenture wax try-in on the lower teeth.

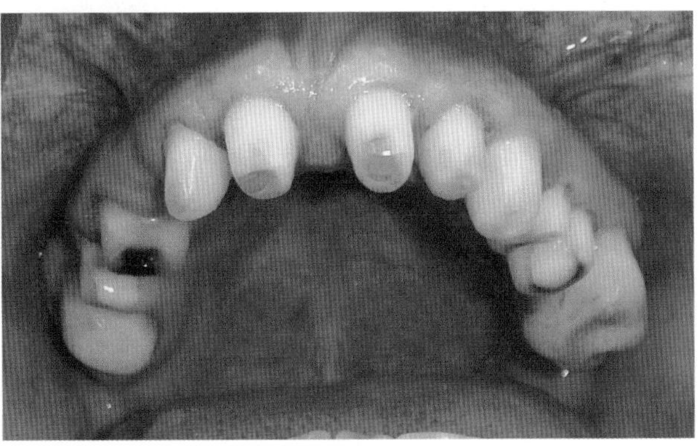

Figure 2.10 Prepared upper teeth for dentine bonded crowns and all ceramic bridge.

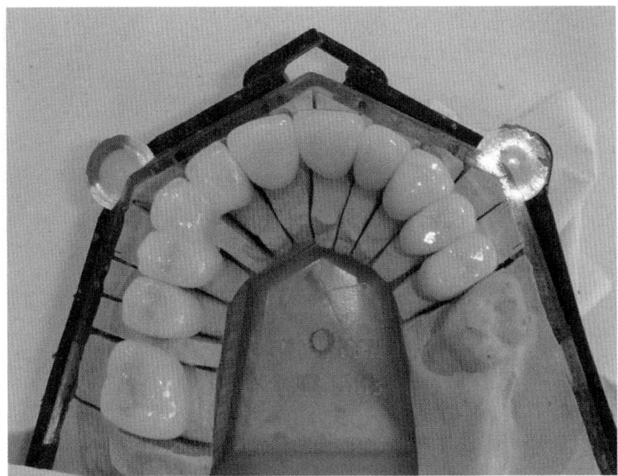

Figure 2.11 Dentine bonded crowns and all ceramic bridge.

8) Fabrication and fitting of definitive upper crowns and bridge (Figure 2.11).
9) Fabrication and fitting of a definitive lower Co-Cr overdenture.
10) Review and maintenance.

Postoperative clinical photographs are shown in Figures 2.12 and 2.13.

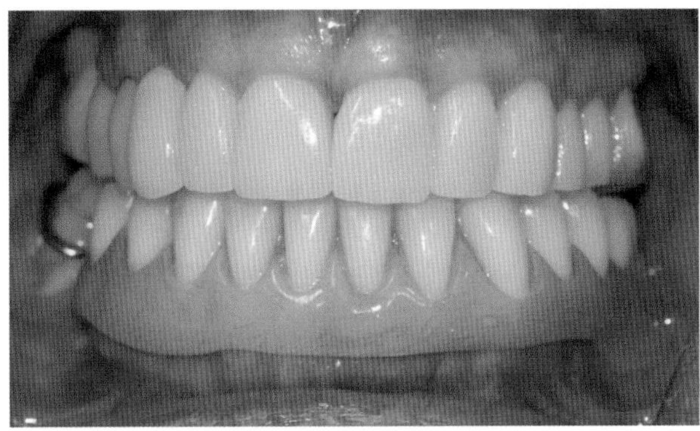

Figure 2.12 Postoperative clinical photograph of the upper crowns, bridge and lower overdenture.

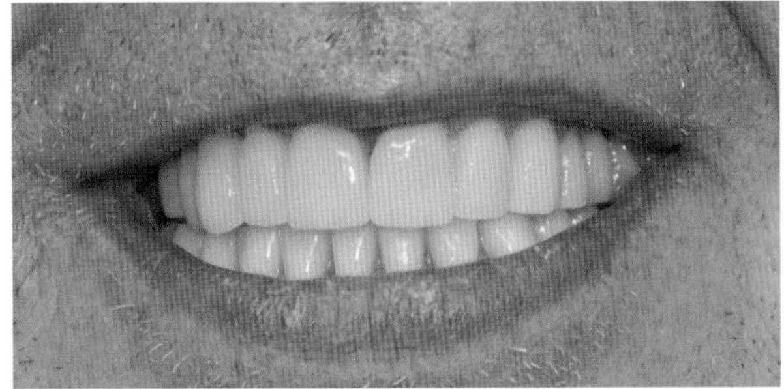

Figure 2.13 Postoperative photograph of the patient's smile.

Maintenance Requirements

The multiple upper crowns and bridge require careful maintenance in terms of oral hygiene, regular GDP visits, periodontal maintenance, repairs and replacements (if necessary due to fracture or secondary caries) in the long term.

Lower overdenture teeth are also subject to wear as they are opposing upper ceramic teeth.

The patient was made aware of these maintenance issues, including costs and the GDP's role.

References

Aldred, M.J., Savarirayan, R. and Crawford, P.J. (2003) Amelogenesis imperfecta: a classification and catalogue for the 21st century. *Oral Dis*, **9**, 19–23.

Arkutu, N., Gadhia, K., McDonald, S., Malik, K. and Currie, L. (2012) Amelogenesis imperfecta: the orthodontic perspective. *Br Dent J*, **212**, 485–489.

Crawford, P.J., Aldred, M. and Bloch-Zupan, A. (2007) Amelogenesis imperfecta. *Orphanet J Rare Dis*, **2**, 17.

Gadhia, K., McDonald, S., Arkutu, N. and Malik, K. (2012) Amelogenesis imperfecta: an introduction. *Br Dent J*, **212**, 377–379.

Hart, T.C. and Hart, P.S. (2009) Genetic studies of craniofacial anomalies: clinical implications and applications. *Orthod Craniofac Res*, **12**, 212–220.

Hu, J.C., Chun, Y.H., Al Hazzazzi, T. and Simmer, J.P. (2007) Enamel formation and amelogenesis imperfecta. *Cells Tissues Organs*, **186**, 78–85.

Koruyucu, M., Bayram, M., Tuna, E.B., Gencay, K. and Seymen, F. (2014) Clinical findings and long-term managements of patients with amelogenesis imperfecta. *Eur J Dent*, **8**, 546–552.

Malik, K., Gadhia, K., Arkutu, N., McDonald, S. and Blair, F. (2012) The interdisciplinary management of patients with amelogenesis imperfecta – restorative dentistry. *Br Dent J*, **212**, 537–542.

McDonald, S., Arkutu, N., Malik, K., Gadhia, K. and McKaig, S. (2012) Managing the paediatric patient with amelogenesis imperfecta. *Br Dent J*, **212**, 425–428.

Patel, M., McDonnell, S.T., Iram, S. and Chan, M.F. (2013) Amelogenesis imperfecta – lifelong management. Restorative management of the adult patient. *Br Dent J*, **215**, 449–457.

Poulsen, S., Gjorup, H., Haubek, D. *et al.* (2008) Amelogenesis imperfecta – a systematic literature review of associated dental and oro-facial abnormalities and their impact on patients. *Acta Odontol Scand*, **66**, 193–199.

Pousette Lundgren, G. and Dahllof, G. (2014) Outcome of restorative treatment in young patients with amelogenesis imperfecta. A cross-sectional, retrospective study. *J Dent*, **42**, 1382–1389.

Sabandal, M.M. and Schafer, E. (2016) Amelogenesis imperfecta: review of diagnostic findings and treatment concepts. *Odontology*, **104**, 245–256.

Witkop, C.J. Jr. (1988) Amelogenesis imperfecta, dentinogenesis imperfecta and dentin dysplasia revisited: problems in classification. *J Oral Pathol*, **17**, 547–553.

Zagdwon, A.M., Fayle, S.A. and Pollard, M.A. (2003) A prospective clinical trial comparing preformed metal crowns and cast restorations for defective first permanent molars. *Eur J Paediatr Dent*, **4**, 138–142.

3

Apical Periodontitis

3.1 Definitions and Classification

Apical periodontitis is an inflammatory disorder of periradicular tissues caused by irritants of endodontic origin, mostly of persistent microbes living in the root canal system of the affected tooth (Orstavik and Pitt Ford, 2007).

Based on the World Health Organization (WHO) *International Classification of Diseases and Related Health Problems* (ICD-10), diseases of periapical tissues can be classified into the following categories (WHO, 2016).

- Acute apical periodontitis (AAP)
- Chronic apical periodontitis (CAP)
- Periapical abscess with sinus to antrum, nasal cavity, oral cavity and skin
- Periapical abscess without sinus
- Radicular cyst

Different types of endodontic infections, based on the location and time of entry of bacteria, are listed below.

- Primary intraradicular infection is the virgin infection before any endodontic treatment.
- Secondary intraradicular infection is the reinfection during and after treatment. It can be due to contamination, leakage, remaining caries and poor isolation.
- Persistent intraradicular infection is caused by the resisting micro-organisms after treatment.
- Extraradicular infection is the invasion of bacteria to periradicular tissues. It can be dependent on intraradicular infection, such as acute apical abscess, or it can be independent from the root canal infection, such as apical actinomycosis.

Phoenix abscess or secondary acute apical periodontitis is the exacerbation of an existing chronic apical periodontitis.

Condensing apical periodontitis is reactive bone tissue formation at the apex of a tooth with chronic pulpal inflammation which may progress to CAP if not treated.

3.2 Relevant Anatomy

Root canal systems can have different morphologies. Various types of root canal configurations (type I–VIII) and canal isthmi (type I–V) were demonstrated by Vertucci (1984).

Myelinated A-fibres and non-myelinated C-fibres carry the pain sensation in pulp. Most nerves are located in the coronal pulp and less than 10% are in the root pulp (Byers, 1984).

Neuropeptides including calcitonin gene-related peptide (CGRP), substance P (SP) and neurokinin A (NKA) modulate pulp vascular tension and are associated with neurogenic inflammation of the pulp (Berggreen *et al.*, 2007).

Pulp stones or denticles can be present and are classified based on their structure as true or false stones, or based on their location as free, attached or embedded stones (Goga *et al.*, 2008).

Dentinal tubules can have different widths based on the Mjor and Nordahl classification, including major branches (0.5–1.0 micron), fine branches (300–700 nm), and microbranches (25–200 nm) (Mjor and Nordahl, 1996).

Accessory roots and canals can be present with variable distributions in the anterior and posterior teeth (Ahmed and Hashem, 2016).

3.3 Immunopathology

Defence systems in the pulp include dentine deposition by odontoblasts, the cellular defence system and the immune surveillance system including major histocompatibility complex (MHC) class II antigen-expressing cells such as dendritic cells and macrophages (Jontell *et al.*, 1998).

Defence systems in periapical tissues include dense fibrous tissues with sparsely distributed macrophage-lineage cells and rare lymphocytes; these are less mature than the pulp defence system (Morse, 1977).

Diseases and Conditions in Dentistry: An Evidence-Based Reference, First Edition. Keyvan Moharamzadeh.

Companion website: www.wiley.com/go/moharamzadeh/diseases

Major proinflammatory mediators associated with pulpal and periapical inflammation include IL-1 and TNF-alpha, true cytokines produced by macrophages. Other molecules such as nitric oxide (NO), prostaglandins (PGs), IL-2 and interferon (INF) gamma further promote pulpal and periapical inflammation (Stashenko *et al.*, 1998).

Receptor activator of NF-kappa B ligand (RANKL) and osteoprotegerin (OPG) play an important role in periapical bone and dental hard tissue destruction in pulp and periapical disease (Belibasakis *et al.*, 2013).

3.4 Aetiology

Aetiological factors that have been associated with periapical disease include:

- bacterial invasion
- caries
- progression of periodontal disease
- pulpal necrosis
- anachoresis of bacteria from blood or lymph
- exposure to endodontic materials, which can be debatable.

The anatomical complexity of the root canal and the ability of micro-organisms to form biofilms make it unlikely that a sterile canal system can be achieved by current technology used in endodontic treatment.

Persistent apical periodontitis following root canal treatment can be due to the following biological factors (Nair, 2006).

- Intraradicular infection persisting in the complex apical root canal system.
- Extraradicular infection, generally in the form of periapical actinomycosis.
- Extruded root filling or other exogenous materials that can cause foreign body reaction. Cellulose granuloma can develop as a foreign body reaction to extruded paper points.
- Accumulation of endogenous cholesterol crystals that irritate periapical tissues.
- True cystic lesions.
- Scar tissue healing of the periapical area.

3.5 Microbiology

In a classic study by Kakehashi *et al.* (1965), the effects of surgical exposure of dental pulps in germ-free rats and conventional laboratory rats were compared. In germ-free rats, pulp and dentine repair with no periapical infection was histologically evident. On the other hand, conventional laboratory rats developed pulpal and periapical disease which indicated the bacterial aetiology of apical periodontitis.

Bacteriological study of necrotic dental pulps by Sundqvist (1976) showed that necrotic pulps with apical periodontitis contained large amounts of bacteria, but necrotic pulps without apical periodontitis were aseptic.

The microflora of infected root canals are similar to those of deep periodontal pockets. These include *Prevotella, Fusobacterium, Lactobacillus, Streptococcus, Clostridium* and *Peptostreptococus* species as well as *Candida* and *Saccharomyces* yeasts, cocci, rods, filaments and spirochaetes. Dentinal tubules can also be penetrated by bacteria (Aw, 2016; Siqueira and Rocas, 2009).

It is now believed that endodontic disease is associated with bacterial biofilms, which are resistant to conventional antibacterial treatments. Most research has investigated *Enterococcus faecalis*, which is thought to be implicated in persistent or recurrent apical periodontitis (Jhajharia *et al.*, 2015).

Progression of the infection and development of symptoms can be due to the following factors: presence of virulent clonal types, microbial synergism or additism, number of microbial cells, environmental cues, host resistance and concomitant viral infections such as herpes (Baumgartner, 2004; Nair, 1997).

Bacterial virulence factors involved in the development and progression of apical periodontitis include lipopolysaccharide (LPS), peptidoglycan, teichoic and lipoteichoic acids, outer membrane proteins and vesicles, lipoproteins, fimbriae, exopolysaccharides, bacterial DNA, enzymes (proteinases), exotoxins, metabolic end-products and flagellae (Orstavik and Pitt Ford, 2007).

According to the focal infection theory, an infectious disorder can be caused by micro-organisms that have disseminated from a distant body site (e.g. through blood). There is no evidence that bacteraemia can arise spontaneously from infected root canals associated with chronic apical periodontitis lesion. However, it can occur in cases of acute apical abscesses and during treatment of infected root canals or periradicular surgery (Debelian *et al.*, 1995; Savarrio *et al.*, 2005). The reported chances of bacteraemia following dental procedures include 3% for RCT if the instrumentation extends beyond the apex and lasts for more than 10 minutes, 33% for periapical surgery (apicectomy), 83% for periodontal flap surgery and 100% for tooth extraction.

There is no concrete evidence that bacteria from root canals can cause systemic disease following bacteraemia. However, immunosuppressed patients and patients with indwelling catheters may be at risk and prophylactic antibiotics may be beneficial in these cases. A systematic review shows that there may be a moderate risk and correlation between some systemic diseases and apical periodontitis (Khalighinejad *et al.*, 2016).

Systemic antibiotics may be indicated in the following endodontic conditions (Segura-Egea *et al.*, 2018).

- Acute apical abscess with systemic involvement such as fever and lymphadenopathy.
- Spreading infections including cellulitis and diffuse swelling with trismus.
- Acute apical abscess in medically compromised patients.
- Replantation of avulsed teeth.
- Some cases of persistent exudation which are not resolved after revision of intracanal procedures.

Amoxicillin is the antibiotic of choice in most cases. Clavulanic acid or metronidazole can be added in more serious cases. Clindamycin is indicated if the patient has confirmed allergy to penicillin (Segura-Egea *et al.*, 2017).

3.6 Radiology

The most extensive investigation correlating the histology and radiology of apical periodontitis was Brynolf's study (Brynolf, 1967) which reached the following conclusions.

- The radiographic appearance of CAP is always smaller than the histological extent of the lesion.
- The absence of radiographic signs of CAP does not rule out its presence, whereas the presence of its key radiographic signs is virtually pathognomonic.
- The radiograph cannot be used reliably to distinguish between a periapical granuloma and a cyst.

Radiographic differential diagnosis for intrabony radiolucencies is detailed below.

- CAP associated with a necrotic non-vital tooth.
- Periodontic-endodontic lesion which is normally associated with a deep periodontal pocket.
- Osteomyelitis is characterised by bone destruction and sequestrum formation.
- Incisive canal cyst with normal vitality of the adjacent teeth.
- Periodontal cyst where there is continuous lamina dura (LD) and vital teeth.
- Dentigerous cyst forms around the crowns of unerupted teeth.
- Traumatic (simple) bone cyst is not a true cyst and there is no sign of root resorption or loss of vitality.
- Central giant cell granuloma (CGCG) is a large multilocular lesion.
- Osseous (cemental) dysplasia or periapical cementoma where the teeth are normally vital and occurs most commonly in the anterior mandible.
- Odontogenic keratocyst (OKC) most often affects the posterior mandible and has a high recurrence rate.
- Ameloblastoma is a multilocular lesion which often affects the posterior mandible and can cause root resorption and cortex expansion and perforation.
- Tumours such as lymphoma and multiple myeloma.
- Hyperparathyroidism that can be associated with lytic bone lesions.
- Eosinophilic granuloma is a form of Langerhans cell histiocytosis that can affect the bone.
- Medication-related osteonecrosis of jaw (see Chapter 4).

The periapical index (PAI) scoring system is a visual reference scale developed for assessing the health status of the root and is mainly used as a research tool.

- Score 1: little change in bone mineral content and any structural alteration
- Score 2: little change in bone mineral content but there is disorganisation of bone texture periapically
- Score 3: loss of mineral and shotgun appearance
- Score 4: all signs of classic CAP
- Score 5: elements indicating expansion of the lesion such as radiolucent streaks and structural disorganisation peripheral to body of the lesion

In addition to the standard radiographic examination, advanced imaging methods have been used for the diagnosis and management of endodontic diseases (Orstavik and Pitt Ford, 2007).

- Cone beam computed tomography (CBCT) can be very helpful in demonstrating details which may not be evident on the periapical radiograph (ESE *et al.*, 2014; Patel *et al.*, 2015).
- Magnetic resonance imaging (MRI) can be useful to identify oedema, dentigerous cyst, osteomyelitis, tumours, myxoma and large cysts.
- Medical (multidetector) CT can be useful for jaw lesions but carries a higher dose of radiation exposure compared to CBCT.
- Micro-CT is often used in laboratory *in vitro* studies.
- Tuned-aperture CT (TACT) is based on layering of images and is suitable for assessment of root resorption and root fractures.
- Ultrasound has also been used for the diagnosis of CAP.
- Nuclear scintigraphy can be used for localisation of active root canal infection that could not be localised clinically.

3.7 Diagnosis

An accurate and detailed pain history followed by clinical examination is essential to distinguish necrotic pulp and apical periodontitis from reversible and irreversible pulpitis.

Important special investigations to confirm the diagnosis of CAP include the following (Rowe and Pitt Ford, 1990).

- Sensibility testing by EPT.
  - EPT activates mainly A-delta nerve bundles in the pulp.
  - It has two modes: bipolar (which is more accurate) and monopolar (which is the most common).
  - 97% of cases with no response to EPT have complete or partially necrotic pulps.
  - EPT can be unreliable shortly after trauma or in immature teeth.
- Sensibility testing using thermal tests.
  - Cold test using ice (0 °C) and ethyl chloride (-4 °C) may not be cold enough to elicit an accurate pulp response. Refrigerant spray dichlorodifluoromethane (DDM) (-50 °C) and carbon dioxide ice (-78 °C) pencils are more reliable and safe.
  - Heat test using hot GP or rubber dam and hot water bath is less commonly used but can provide clinically relevant information as a positive test indicates severe inflammation of the pulp. However, application of excessive heat carries the risk of damage to the pulp.
- Mechanical tests include the percussion test which indicates periodontal and periapical involvement.
- Palpation can be useful to detect soft tissue swelling and tenderness, fluctuation, hardness or crepitus.
- Radiographic examination should ideally be carried out using film holders to allow parallelism and standardisation. The use of rubber bite blocks can facilitate comparative radiographs, allowing similar positioning of the film and the tube at different times.
- Laser Doppler flowmetry (LDF) is a commercially available pulpal blood flow assessment method. Its main limitation is false-positive or false-negative responses.

Rubber dam isolation is essential to avoid gingivae interference. It is objective, non-invasive and accurate in determining revascularisation of the pulp in young traumatised teeth.

Differential diagnoses for odontogenic pain are listed below (Orstavik and Pitt Ford, 2007).

- Temporomandibular joint (TMJ) dysfunction is often associated with chronic self-reported pain over 6 months in the face, TMJ and/or neck. Pain is deep and vague and does not have a very clear location. The muscles of mastication and the joint may also be tender to palpation. The teeth are normally vital.
- Sinusitis is characterised by diffuse pressure pain in the maxillae and if the trigeminal nerve is pressured then multiple teeth can be affected. Patients may report a history of nasal congestion or cold and pain which is worsened with sudden movements of head. Multiple teeth on the affected side may have a lower cold sensitivity threshold.
- Angina patients may report pain in the mandible with exercise or stress which is not localised to one tooth. Teeth are normally vital. Past medical history often reveals cardiac disease risk factors.
- Trigeminal neuralgia (TN) (tic douloureux) can be characterised by electric stabbing pain that comes in bursts and often has a trigger point and very short duration. It does not affect sleep and the teeth are usually vital.
- Atypical odontalgia or neuropathic pain is a dull, radiating, diffuse pain that may get worse with RCT or extraction. Obsessive compulsive disorder (OCD) is common in these patients. The teeth are normally vital.
- Herpes zoster is associated with pain that starts before herpetic vesicle development. Vitality testing can be inconclusive. It is important to assess relevant risk factors such as age, immune system and stress.
- Cluster headache is often associated with pain in suborbital or retro-orbital areas. Multiple teeth can hurt but the teeth are normally vital. Oxygen administration for up to 15 minutes usually eliminates the pain.
- Salivary gland disorders can be accompanied by pain when eating and start prior to eating. Reduced salivary flow can be confirmed using salivary flow rate tests. Teeth are normally vital.
- Eagle's syndrome can be associated with pain when swallowing, turning the head and opening the mouth wide. Palpation of the tonsillar fossa can cause a similar pain. Teeth are normally vital and the CT often shows stylohyoid ligament calcification.
- Psychological pain and Munchausen syndrome in patients with psychological disorders who are looking for unnecessary medical treatments. Patients are well read and the vitality tests are unreliable as the patients may deceive the clinician.
- Idiopathic (atypical) facial pain is a constant chronic orofacial discomfort or pain, defined by the International Headache Society as 'facial pain not fulfilling other criteria'. Pain is often of a deep, dull, boring or burning nature causing chronic discomfort, and persists for most or all of the day but does not wake the patient from sleep. Its diagnosis is reached only by the exclusion of organic disease. There are no physical signs and investigations (X-rays, cranial nerve exams, blood tests) are often all negative.

3.8 Epidemiology

The prevalence of apical periodontitis has been reported to be within the range of 1.8–7.2% of remaining teeth and 37–71% of individuals and it increases with age. This means approximately one tooth per individual is affected (Hamedy *et al.*, 2016; Pak *et al.*, 2012).

Maxillary lateral incisors, first premolars and mandibular first molars are the most commonly affected teeth. The risk of acute CAP exacerbation is less than 5% annually and approximately 50% within 10 years, and 75% of teeth affected with CAP demonstrate signs of disease within the first year (Orstavik and Pitt Ford, 2007).

3.9 Endodontic Treatment Considerations

3.9.1 Local Anaesthesia

Pain management before, during and after root canal treatment is an extremely important aspect of endodontic treatment. Inadequate anaesthesia can significantly hamper treatment and have distressing effects on both the patient and the clinician.

Different methods are available to establish and maintain effective pain relief, including various local anaesthesia techniques (such as local infiltration, nerve block, intraligamentary, intraosseous and intrapulpal anaesthesia), solutions (such as lidocaine and articaine) and orally administered pharmacological agents (including non-steroidal anti-inflammatory drugs (NSAIDs) and paracetamol or acetaminophen) (Kung *et al.*, 2015; Meechan, 2002; Shirvani *et al.*, 2017). The choice of the material and technique depends on individual patient need, diagnosis and treatment plan.

3.9.2 Isolation and Disinfection

It is universally agreed that appropriate rubber dam isolation is an essential requirement for endodontic treatment to be safe and successful (Ahmed *et al.*, 2014). Initial disinfection of the tooth surface with an appropriate antiseptic solution such as 30% hydrogen peroxide and 5% tincture of iodine can be helpful in achieving and maintaining an aseptic operating field (Malmberg *et al.*, 2016).

3.9.3 Access Cavity Preparation

Preparation of an adequate, clean and caries-free access cavity is an essential prerequisite for successful endodontic treatment. An access cavity with optimal design which allows straight-line access to the apical third of the root canal would facilitate exploration of the root canal system, subsequent preparation, debridement and obturation of the root canals.

The common features of the root canal anatomy of different teeth and principles of access cavity preparation have been described in previous publications (Adams and Tomson, 2014; Darcey *et al.*, 2015a).

3.9.4 Magnification

Magnification devices such as operating microscopes, magnifying loupes and endoscopes have been used increasingly to improve visualisation of the operating field. The use of magnification can be significantly helpful in many aspects of primary and secondary root canal treatment procedures, including:

- identification of the canal orifices
- exploration of the root canal system
- negotiation of the canal blockages
- removal of different types of root-filling materials and broken instruments
- visualisation and repair of perforations
- obturation of canals with specific anatomy.

There is still insufficient high-quality evidence to prove if or how magnification devices improve the outcomes of endodontic treatment (Congiusta and Veitz-Keenan, 2016; del Fabbro *et al.*, 2015).

3.9.5 Working Length Determination

Although the exact landmark for termination of root canal preparation remains controversial, there is general agreement that the apical constriction is the most appropriate. Recommended working length for root canals with necrotic pulp is 1 mm from the radiographic apex and for root canals with vital pulp is 1–2 mm from the radiographic apex (Orstavik and Pitt Ford, 2007).

The European Society of Endodontology (ESE) recommends two methods of measurement of the root canal length: electronic and radiographic (ESE, 2006). Some literature suggests there is no significant difference between the accuracy of the electronic apex locator (EAL) and radiographic working length measurement (Kim and Lee, 2004) but systematic reviews suggest that apex locators are more accurate than the radiographic method (Mello, 2014). It is recommended that a combination of the electronic and radiographic methods would be the most accurate approach for determination of the working length.

The use of an EAL may prevent unintentional overinstrumentation. Despite having an accuracy of 80–90% in most root canals, their performance can be affected by the device and type of irrigation. The status of the pulp has no effect on accuracy (Tsesis *et al.*, 2015).

3.9.6 Root Canal Preparation Techniques

Several techniques have been developed for the preparation and instrumentation of root canal systems (Darcey *et al.*, 2015b). These include the stepback technique (Mullaney, 1979), step-down technique (Goerig *et al.*, 1982), double-flared technique (Fava, 1983) and crown down technique (Morgan and Montgomery, 1984). It is claimed that the development of nickel-titanium rotary instruments has increased the efficiency and speed of root canal preparation (Carrotte, 2004a).

The author's preferred method of root canal preparation is a combination of the Pro Taper technique (Ruddle, 2001) with the use of ultrasonic instruments. This technique is very quick and efficient and produces greater coronal taper and adequate apical size preparation and increases the effectiveness of irrigation. Furthermore, the use of rotary files, crown down technique and ultrasonic instruments extrudes less debris to the apex compared to hand instrumentation and the step-back technique.

3.9.7 Irrigation and Debridement

Preparation of the root canal should be undertaken carefully with copious amounts of irrigation to eliminate endodontic micro-organisms, remove debris, lubricate the canal and dissolve organic deposits without the risk of extrusion of the irrigant into periapical tissues (Eliyas *et al.*, 2010; Darcey *et al.*, 2016a).

The recommended technique includes slow passive irrigation using a freely placed 27 or 31 gauge side-venting needle in the apical third of the root canal within 1–3 mm of the working length. Sodium hypochlorite is considered to be the most effective and most commonly used antibacterial irrigant with increased tissue dissolving ability at high concentrations (Haapasalo *et al.*, 2014). Thepreferred concentration of hypochlorite solution for the initial RCT is 1% and for endodontic retreatment is 5% to eradicate resistant bacteria. 2% Chlorhexidine is less toxic than 5% hypochlorite and is effective against resistance micro-organisms such as *E. faecalis* but it does not dissolve necrotic tissues. There is inadequate evidence to determine which of the above two irrigants is superior to the other (Goncalves *et al.*, 2016).

Removal of the smear layer with a decalcifying agent such as 15% ethylene-diamine tetracetic acid (EDTA) solution prior to obturation allows penetration of the sealer into tubules and accessory canals (Mohammadi *et al.*, 2013). MTAD is another irrigant which is a mixture of doxycycline, citric acid and Tween 80. It gently removes the smear layer and disinfects the root canal but can cause discolouration (Mohammadi, 2012).

Evidence shows that ultrasonic agitation significantly enhances the irrigant's effectiveness (Mozo *et al.*, 2012).

It is important not to mix different irrigants during debridement of the root canal to avoid the risk of chemical reaction between the irrigants and precipitation of by-products in the root canal.

3.9.8 Interappointment Medication

Calcium hydroxide $Ca(OH)_2$ is believed to be the best intracanal medicament for the management of apical periodontitis (Law and Messer, 2004). It can eliminate bacteria within 7 days, and its antibacterial effect and LPS inactivation help apical healing. However, it is not effective against *E. faecalis*. Other intracanal medicaments used in endodontic procedures are listed below.

- Ledermix is a mixture of 1% triamcinolone and 3% demclocycline. It can be used in trauma cases to control root resorption but it is not superior to $Ca(OH)_2$.
- Chlorhexidine gel can be effective against *E. faecalis*.
- Triple antibiotic paste including ciprofloxacin, metronidazole and minocycline is proven to effectively disinfect the root canal. It has been used in regenerative endodontic treatment for revascularisation of immature necrotic teeth. Tetracycline staining of crown is one of the disadvantages of this paste.
- Phenol derivatives such as CMCP have been used in the past. They have short duration and are inefficient and toxic.
- Iodine and chlorine have also been used in the past. They are less effective than $Ca(OH)_2$.

3.9.9 Obturation Techniques

Gutta-percha (GP) is the material of choice for root canal obturation. GP cone is composed of 20% GP, 60–70% zinc oxide (for opacity and antimicrobial effect), 10% resins, waxes and metal sulfates.

Different sealers have been developed to fill the spaces around the GP.

- Zinc oxide eugenol (ZOE)-based sealers including Rickets, Proco-sol, Grosman, Wach and Tubli seal are the most commonly used sealers.
- GIC-based sealers such as Ketac-endo are able to adhere to dentine.
- Polymer sealers including Endofill and AH products contain epoxy resins and have good handling and flow properties.
- $Ca(OH)_2$-based sealers such as Sealapex, Apexit and CRCS are developed to release alkaline ions but there is weak evidence to support their advantages as the material does not ionise and may dissolve and leave voids in the root canal (Orstavik and Pitt Ford, 2007).

- Chlorpercha is a mixture of GP and chloroform, which is toxic and shrinks, and its use is not recommended.
- N2 sealer contained formaldehyde and is not used now due to its toxicity, ability to cause necrosis and delayed healing.

Different obturation techniques have been developed for filling root canal systems (Carrotte, 2004b; Darcey *et al.*, 2016b).

- Cold lateral condensation of GP cones
- Lateral compaction of warm GP cones
- Obturation with single GP point and sealer
- Thermal compaction of GP
- Heated carrier-based GP obturation such as Thermafil
- Vertical compaction of warm GP using continuous wave of heat (such as System-B)
- Injection of thermoplasticised GP (such as Obtura II)
- Coronal backfill (initial obturation of the apical 5–7 mm of the root canal with a fitted GP cone using System-B and then backfill with thermoplasticised GP using the Obtura gun)

A review of the literature shows that clinical studies have still not identified the superiority of one obturation technique over the others (Tortini *et al.*, 2011).

3.9.10 Coronal Restoration

Coronal restoration should be placed as soon as possible after root filling to maintain the coronal seal. Evidence shows that both coronal seal and apical root canal seal in combination are essential factors to achieve a successful and predictable endodontic treatment outcome (Williams and Williams, 2010).

Restoration of endodontically treated teeth is discussed in detail in Chapter 18.

3.9.11 Review

Clinical and radiographic follow-up should take place 12 months after RCT to determine the outcome of treatment. The period of observation can be extended up to 4 years in CAP cases due to slow healing in some cases.

Success criteria and terms that are commonly used in endodontic literature include the following (Chugal *et al.*, 2017).

- *Strict (robust) criteria*: where success means the absence of radiolucency and absence of signs and symptoms.
- *Lenient (flexible) criteria*: where success means the absence of clinical signs and symptoms.

Using the above criteria can sometimes lead to outcome categories such as uncertain, questionable, doubtful and improved, which can be confusing and misleading. Therefore, it is recommended that some of the disease-based terms be replaced with more patient-centred values and expressions, such as chance of healing.

- *Healed (success)*: no clinical signs or symptoms and absence of radiolucency.
- *Healing (success)*: no clinical signs or symptoms and radiolucency decreasing in size.
- *Survival (continuing disease state)*: no clinical signs or symptoms but persisting radiolucency that has increased or not decreased in size.
- *Failure*: symptomatic and persisting radiolucency.

3.9.12 Exacerbation

Exacerbation can occur in 3–5% of primary endodontic treatment and 15% of retreatment cases (Orstavik and Pitt Ford, 2007). The causes include:

- mechanical irritation due to overinstrumentation
- underinstrumentation
- immunological factors
- psychological factors such as low pain threshold.

Different treatment modalities for endodontic exacerbation include the following.

- Pain can be relieved with NSAID medication and relieving occlusion.
- Apical abscess can be treated by reopening the coronal access and draining through the root canal. A fluctuant swelling that does not drain through the root canal can be managed by incision and drainage.
- Diffuse swellings with systemic involvement and fever can be treated with systemic antibiotics such as penicillin. Where there is no improvement in 48 hours, metronidazole can be added. In case of penicillin allergy , clindamycin can be prescribed.
- Extraradicular refractory infection can be treated by either endodontic retreatment combined with systemic antibiotics following culture and sensitivity of the exudate from the canal or endodontic retreatment followed by surgery which is a more reliable option.

3.10 Endodontic Retreatment

Endodontic retreatment is indicated on previously root-treated teeth with persistent periapical disease if the tooth is still restorable and is amenable to non-surgical treatment. The objective is to re-enter the pulp chamber, remove any present root-filling materials and address and repair any pathological or iatrogenic deficiencies or defects (Ruddle, 2004).

There are different methods for removing GP from the root canal (Good and McCammon, 2012).

- Thermal methods using heat pluggers, Nd:YAG lasers and frictional heat generated by rotary instruments.
- Mechanical methods using hand files, rotary files designed for retreatment and ultrasonic tips.
- Use of solvents and chemicals, including chloroform (the most commonly used), methylchloroform, halothane, turpentine oil, orange oil, xylol, eucalyptol, d-limonene and ethyl acetate.

It is important to be aware of the potential toxicity of these solvents and care must be taken to ensure safe use to avoid extrusion of the agents into periapical tissues.

Methods for removing fractured endodontic instruments and posts are discussed in detail in Chapters 20 and 21.

3.11 Prognosis and Outcome of Non-Surgical Endodontic Treatment

Based on epidemiological studies, the success rate for root canal treatment is reported to be 35–78%. However, based on clinical trials, the reported success rate is increased to 77–95%. The reason for the difference in reported success rates may be the superior skills of operators who provide the treatment in clinical trials (Chugal *et al.*, 2017; Ng *et al.*, 2007; Pak *et al.*, 2012).

Prognosis of healed outcome for non-surgical endodontic treatment of teeth without apical periodontitis (vital pulp, irreversible pulpitis or poor RCT with no periapical radiolucency) is 93–98% from various studies, and all studies show poorer outcome (10–25% lower success) if apical radiolucency is present before treatment. Prognosis of healed outcome of non-surgical endodontic treatment of teeth with apical periodontitis is 73–86% (73–90% for initial RCT, 56–86% for re-RCT) (de Chevigny *et al.*, 2008a, b; Farzaneh *et al.*, 2004; Friedman *et al.*, 2003; Marquis *et al.*, 2006; Ng *et al.*, 2008a, b, 2010).

Potential factors that may affect the prognosis of non-surgical endodontic treatment include the following (Ng *et al.*, 2011a, b; Orstavik and Pitt Ford, 2007).

3.11.1 Preoperative Factors

- Patient's systemic health: healing is poorer in patients with uncontrolled diabetes.
- Clinical signs and symptoms such as pain and discharging sinus tract.
- Presence of apical periodontitis negatively affects the outcome.
- Size of the radiolucent lesion: the prognosis is improved if the lesion is smaller than 5 mm.
- Status of periodontal tissues: there is a higher chance of tooth loss if there is periodontal disease.
- Quality of previous root treatment: the prognosis is better if the previous RCT is poor and it can be improved significantly by new treatment but prognosis is poorer if there is a pre-existing perforation.

3.11.2 Intraoperative Factors

- Apical extent of the root filling is not an outcome predictor in vital teeth but in teeth with apical periodontitis, the outcome is improved if the root filling is within 0–2 mm short of the root end.
- Achieving apical patency can improve the prognosis.
- Efficiency of irrigation and disinfection can also affect the prognosis.
- Treatment complications such as perforations, instrument breakage and large extrusion of the root filling into the periapical area negatively affect prognosis.

3.11.3 Post-Treatment Factors

Maintaining coronal seal is an important factor for successful endodontic treatment.

3.12 Surgical Endodontic Treatment

3.12.1 Indications

Surgical endodontic treatment of apical periodontitis can be indicated in the following circumstances.

- Perforations in the apical part of the root when it is not possible to manage conservatively.
- Broken instrument at the apical part of the canal when it is not possible to remove it or bypass with an orthograde approach.
- A large post in the canal of a tooth that supports a large fixed prosthesis and there is a high risk of root fracture during post removal.
- Root canal obliteration by calcification or inaccessible canals.
- Biopsy of a suspected malignancy in the periapical region.
- Persisting radiolucency following good-quality non-surgical root canal treatment.
- To investigate possible root fracture.

3.12.2 Contraindications

Surgical endodontic treatment is contraindicated in the following conditions.

- Teeth with inadequate periodontal bone support, short roots and advanced periodontal bone loss.
- Non-restorable teeth.
- Poor surgical access.
- Medical conditions such as bleeding disorders, haemophilia or endocarditis, which would require special precautions.

3.12.3 Flap Design

Different designs for surgical incisions have been proposed for use in surgical endodontic procedures (Board, 2008).

- Sulcular incision provides good access and good healing but may result in gingival recession and damage to the interdental papillae.
- Papillae-base incision prevents the loss of interdental papillae height and shows significant less recession compared to sulcular incision.
- Submarginal incision (Luebke–Ochsenbein) in attached gingivae requires wide attached gingivae to allow a 3 mm band of attached gingivae above the incision to prevent ischaemia. It provides limited surgical access and results in some scarring.
- Semilunar incision provides very limited access, disrupts blood supply and causes flap shrinkage. It can increase swelling and pain and shows slow healing and scarring due to exposure of the granulation tissue.
- Vertical incision provides limited access to large lesions and carries the risk of infection as the incision lies over the blood clot.

3.12.4 Specific Anatomy

Specific anatomy that needs to be considered in surgical endodontic treatment includes maxillary sinus, palatine neurovascular bundle, inferior alveolar nerve and mental nerve, which must be identified and preserved.

3.12.5 Bone Removal

Bone can be removed using a round surgical bur and sterile isotonic coolant.

The use of piezoelectric surgery devices enables selective cutting of bone, reducing the risk of damage to adjacent tissues without generating heat and providing a clear operative field (Abella *et al.*, 2014).

In mandibular molars, the bony lid approach can be used. This involves removal of the buccal bone window and replacement after root end surgery.

3.12.6 Root End Preparation

Root end preparation considerations include the following.

- The use of microscope magnification can assist visualisation of the cross-sectional canal morphology of the resected root end to enhance the quality of retrograde preparation and filling. However, there is still a lack of high-quality evidence on the effect of magnification on the outcome of surgical endodontic treatment (del Fabbro *et al.*, 2015).
- It is important to avoid bevelling the root end as this would expose more dentinal tubules and has an adverse effect on healing.
- Root end resection level should be 3 mm from the apex.
- Root end preparation with ultrasonic tips is safer and more effective cleaning is achieved with angled ultrasonic tips than with traditional burs.
- The preparation should extend to well-condensed GP or the apical end of the post. If this distance is too long, the root canal should be treated by the orthograde approach first.

3.12.7 Root End Filling

Different materials that have been used for retrograde filling are listed below (Tang *et al.*, 2010; Torabinejad and Pitt Ford, 1996).

- Amalgam has the following disadvantages: leakage, lack of biocompatibility, corrosion, staining and poor performance.
- GP is difficult to use.
- Zinc oxide eugenol has better outcome than amalgam. Super-EBA and intermediate restorative material (IRM) are more biocompatible than the other forms and are less soluble, show less leakage and have good antibacterial action.
- GIC has questionable sealing ability.
- Composite resin has shown good clinical results but success is dependent on excellent moisture control.
- Cavit is a combination of zinc oxide and calcium sulfate that can self-harden with moisture. It has similar biocompatibility to zinc oxide eugenol.
- Diaket is calcium chelate reinforced with polyvinyl resin. It has high sealing ability and shows good healing.
- Mineral trioxide aggregate (MTA) shows less leakage and less inflammation than the other materials. Studies show good clinical outcomes with evidence of cementum formation over MTA (Tang *et al.*, 2010; Torabinejad and Pitt Ford, 1996).

3.12.8 Prognosis and Outcomes

The outcome of surgical endodontic treatment has been described in the following terms.

- Complete healing with resolution of periapical radiolucency.
- Incomplete healing with scar tissue showing bone trabeculae radiating from a centre that may remain radiolucent indefinitely.
- Uncertain healing with no symptoms.
- Failure with persistent or increasing radiolucency and clinical signs and symptoms.

Based on the literature prior to 2005, reported success rates for surgical endodontic treatment ranged from 60% to 78% (Orstavik and Pitt Ford, 2007). However, with the introduction of microsurgical techniques (Eliyas *et al.*, 2014), the outcome of surgical endodontic treatment has improved and the reported figures indicate 72–96% success rates (Evans *et al.*, 2012; Friedman, 2011; Setzer *et al.*, 2010; Tsesis *et al.*, 2013).

Systematic reviews comparing non-surgical with surgical endodontic treatment indicate a significantly higher success rate for microsurgery treatment at short-term follow-up (1–2 years) but no significant difference between surgical and non-surgical treatment at long-term follow-up (more than 4 years) (Kang *et al.*, 2015; Torabinejad *et al.*, 2009).

Reported prognostic factors that can affect the outcome of surgical endodontic treatment include the list below, although there is still a need for high-quality evidence to produce reliable guidelines (del Fabbro *et al.*, 2016; Serrano-Gimenez *et al.*, 2015).

3.12.8.1 Preoperative Factors

- Tooth location (better outcome for the maxillary anterior and premolar teeth).
- Clinical signs and symptoms (better outcome for asymptomatic teeth).
- Lesion size (better outcome for periapical lesions smaller than 5–10 mm).
- Supporting bone loss (poorer outcome for periodontally involved teeth).
- Repeat surgery (poorer outcome for second surgery than initial surgery unless a better technique is used).

3.12.8.2 Intraoperative Factors

- Level of apical resection (better outcome for more radical and right-angled resection).
- Root end management (better outcome with ultrasonic preparation).
- Root-end filling material (favourable outcome with MTA, similar to IRM, and EBA).
- Operator skill.

Case Study

A 50-year-old male patient was referred from the undergraduate student clinic for endodontic retreatment of UR1 and UR3. The patient reported history of pain and frequent swellings associated with previously root-treated upper right central incisor and canine teeth.

The patient was medically fit and well.

Periodontal examination showed mild periodontal bone loss in the anterior region but no deep pockets were present. The UR1 was grade I mobile.

Soft tissue examination showed presence of palpable swelling on the labial mucosa between the roots of UR1 and UR3.

Clinical examination showed UR2 was missing and both UR1 and UR3 were tender to percussion and the buccal sulcus was tender.

Radiographic examination showed a large periapical radiolucency associated with the apices of UR1 and UR3 which both had poor-quality root canal fillings (Figure 3.1).

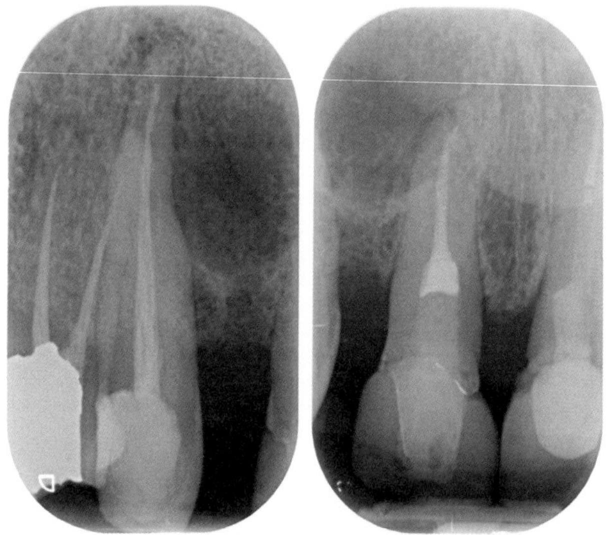

Figure 3.1 Preoperative radiographs of UR1 and UR3.

Diagnosis

Based on the clinical and radiographic findings, a diagnosis of chronic apical periodontitis of UR1 and UR3 was made.

Prognosis

Important preoperative prognostic factors in this case included the large area of periapical radiolucency and reduced periodontal bone support for UR1.

Treatment Strategy

Initially, non-surgical endodontic retreatment was carried out on both UR1 and UR3. Previous root-filling material was removed from the coronal part of the root canal using rotary instruments. Hand files and solvent were used to remove the GP from the apical parts of the canal. Following preparation and shaping of the root canal using ProTaper technique and effective irrigation and debridement, UR3 with a long root canal was obturated with Thermafil and UR1 was obturated with GP using System-B and Obtura. A direct adhesive fibre post was cemented into the previously enlarged coronal part of the root canal to support the core and improve retention of the crown.

UR3 responded well to non-surgical retreatment whereas UR1 remained symptomatic following the treatment. The patient did not want to lose his tooth and therefore the option of surgical endodontic treatment to remove the large periapical lesion was discussed with the patient (including risks and benefits).

Periapical surgery was carried out using microsurgical techniques, including the use of an operating microscope, ultrasonic tip for retrograde root end preparation, and MTA as root end-filling material.

The immediate postoperative radiograph of UR1 and postoperative radiograph of UR3 are shown in Figure 3.2.

At 1-year review, the patient had remained asymptomatic and clinical examination showed no signs of swelling or infection. One-year follow-up radiographic examination (Figure 3.3) showed evidence of periapical healing with bony infill of the defect and resolution of periapical radiolucency associated with UR1 and UR3.

Clinical and radiographic findings indicate successful outcome of the surgical endodontic treatment of UR1 and non-surgical root canal treatment of UR3.

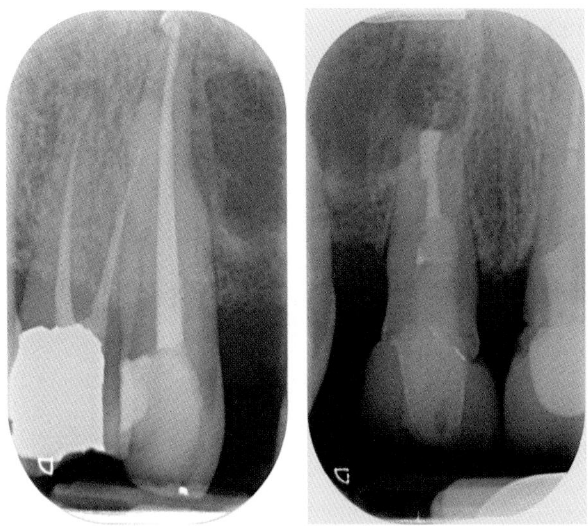

Figure 3.2 Periapical radiographs of UR1 immediately following periapical surgery and UR3 following non-surgical endodontic treatment.

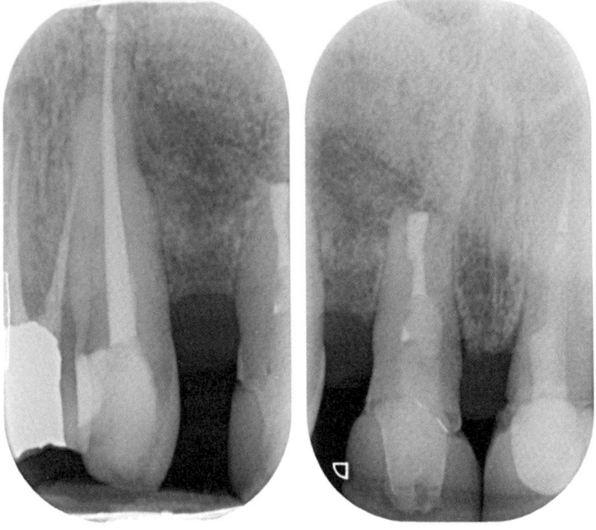

Figure 3.3 Postoperative periapical radiographs of UR1 and UR3 at 1 year follow-up.

References

Abella, F., de Ribot, J., Doria, G., Duran-Sindreu, F. and Roig, M. (2014) Applications of piezoelectric surgery in endodontic surgery: a literature review. *J Endod*, **40**, 325–332.

Adams, N. and Tomson, P.L. (2014) Access cavity preparation. *Br Dent J*, **216**, 333–339.

Ahmed, H.M. and Hashem, A.A. (2016) Accessory roots and root canals in human anterior teeth: a review and clinical considerations. *Int Endod J*, **49**, 724–736.

Ahmed, H.M., Cohen, S., Levy, G., Steier, L. and Bukiet, F. (2014) Rubber dam application in endodontic practice: an update on critical educational and ethical dilemmas. *Aust Dent J*, **59**, 457–463.

Aw, V. (2016) Discuss the role of microorganisms in the aetiology and pathogenesis of periapical disease. *Aust Endod J*, **42**, 53–59.

Baumgartner, J.C. (2004) Microbiologic aspects of endodontic infections. *J Calif Dent Assoc*, **32**, 459–468.

Belibasakis, G.N., Rechenberg, D.K. and Zehnder, M. (2013) The receptor activator of NF-kappaB ligand-osteoprotegerin system in pulpal and periapical disease. *Int Endod J*, **46**, 99–111.

Berggreen, E., Bletsa, A. and Heyraas, K.J. (2007) Circulation in normal and inflamed dental pulp. *Endodontic Topics*, **17**, 2–11.

Board, J.O.E.E. (2008) Endodontic surgery: an online study guide. *J Endod*, **34**, e53–63.

Brynolf, I. (1967) A histological and roentgenological study of the periapical region of human upper incisors. *Odonto Revy*, Supplement **11**, 1–176.

Byers, M.R. (1984) Dental sensory receptors. *Int Rev Neurobiol*, **25**, 39–94.

Carrotte, P. (2004a) Endodontics: Part 7. Preparing the root canal. *Br Dent J*, **197**, 603–613.

Carrotte, P. (2004b) Endodontics: Part 8. Filling the root canal system. *Br Dent J*, **197**, 667–672.

Chugal, N., Mallya, S.M., Kahler, B. and Lin, L.M. (2017) Endodontic treatment outcomes. *Dent Clin North Am*, **61**, 59–80.

Congiusta, M. and Veitz-Keenan, A. (2016) No evidence that magnification devices improve the success of endodontic therapy. *Evid Based Dent*, **17**, 84–85.

Darcey, J., Taylor, C., Roudsari, R.V., Jawad, S. and Hunter, M. (2015a) Modern Endodontic Planning Part 2: Access and Strategy. *Dent Update*, **42**, 709–710, 712–714, 717–718 passim.

Darcey, J., Taylor, C., Roudsari, R.V., Jawad, S. and Hunter, M. (2015b) Modern Endodontic Principles Part 3: Preparation. *Dent Update*, **42**, 810–812, 815–818, 821–822.

Darcey, J., Taylor, C., Roudsari, R.V., Jawad, S. and Hunter, M. (2016a) Modern Endodontic Principles Part 4: Irrigation. *Dent Update*, **43**, 20–22, 25–26, 28–30 passim.

Darcey, J., Taylor, C., Roudsari, R.V., Jawad, S. and Hunter, M. (2016b) Modern Endodontic Principles. Part 5: Obturation. *Dent Update*, **43**, 114–116, 119–120, 123–126 passim.

Debelian, G.J., Olsen, I. and Tronstad, L. (1995) Bacteremia in conjunction with endodontic therapy. *Endod Dent Traumatol*, **11**, 142–149.

de Chevigny, C., Dao, T.T., Basrani, B.R. *et al.* (2008a) Treatment outcome in endodontics: the Toronto study – phase 4: initial treatment. *J Endod*, **34**, 258–263.

de Chevigny, C., Dao, T.T., Basrani, B.R. *et al.* (2008b) Treatment outcome in endodontics: the Toronto study – phases 3 and 4: orthograde retreatment. *J Endod*, **34**, 131–137.

del Fabbro, M., Taschieri, S., Lodi, G., Banfi, G. and Weinstein, R.L. (2015) Magnification devices for endodontic therapy. *Cochrane Database Syst Rev*, **3**, CD005969.

del Fabbro, M., Corbella, S., Sequeira-Byron, P. *et al.* (2016) Endodontic procedures for retreatment of periapical lesions. *Cochrane Database Syst Rev*, **10**, CD005511.

Eliyas, S., Briggs, P.F. and Porter, R.W. (2010) Antimicrobial irrigants in endodontic therapy: 1. Root canal disinfection. *Dent Update*, **37**, 390–392, 395–397.

Eliyas, S., Vere, J., Ali, Z. and Harris, I. (2014) Micro-surgical endodontics. *Br Dent J*, **216**, 169–177.

ESE (2006) Quality guidelines for endodontic treatment: consensus report of the European Society of Endodontology. *Int Endod J*, **39**, 921–930.

ESE, Patel, S., Durack, C., Abella, F. *et al.* (2014) European Society of Endodontology position statement: the use of CBCT in endodontics. *Int Endod J*, **47**, 502–504.

Evans, G.E., Bishop, K. and Renton, T. (2012) Update of guidelines for surgical endodontics – the position after ten years. *Br Dent J*, **212**, 497–498.

Farzaneh, M., Abitbol, S., Lawrence, H.P., Friedman, S. and Toronto, S. (2004) Treatment outcome in endodontics – the Toronto Study. Phase II: initial treatment. *J Endod*, **30**, 302–309.

Fava, L.R. (1983) The double-flared technique: an alternative for biomechanical preparation. *J Endod*, **9**, 76–80.

Friedman, S. (2011) Outcome of endodontic surgery: a meta-analysis of the literature – part 1: comparison of traditional root-end surgery and endodontic microsurgery. *J Endod*, **37**, 577–578; author reply 578–580.

Friedman, S., Abitbol, S. and Lawrence, H.P. (2003) Treatment outcome in endodontics: the Toronto Study. Phase 1: initial treatment. *J Endod*, **29**, 787–793.

Goerig, A.C., Michelich, R.J. and Schultz, H.H. (1982) Instrumentation of root canals in molar using the step-down technique. *J Endod*, **8**, 550–554.

Goga, R., Chandler, N.P. and Oginni, A.O. (2008) Pulp stones: a review. *Int Endod J*, **41**, 457–468.

Goncalves, L.S., Rodrigues, R.C., Andrade Jr, C.V., Soares, R.G. and Vettore, M.V. (2016) The effect of sodium hypochlorite and chlorhexidine as irrigant solutions for root canal disinfection: a systematic review of clinical trials. *J Endod*, **42**, 527–532.

Good, M.L. and McCammon, A. (2012) An removal of gutta-percha and root canal sealer: a literature review and an audit comparing current practice in dental schools. *Dent Update*, **39**, 703–708.

Haapasalo, M., Shen, Y., Wang, Z. and Gao, Y. (2014) Irrigation in endodontics. *Br Dent J*, **216**, 299–303.

Hamedy, R., Shakiba, B., Pak, J.G., Barbizam, J.V., Ogawa, R.S. and White, S.N. (2016) Prevalence of root canal treatment and periapical radiolucency in elders: a systematic review. *Gerodontology*, **33**, 116–127.

Jhajharia, K., Parolia, A., Shetty, K.V. and Mehta, L.K. (2015) Biofilm in endodontics: a review. *J Int Soc Prev Community Dent*, **5**, 1–12.

Jontell, M., Okiji, T., Dahlgren, U. and Bergenholtz, G. (1998) Immune defense mechanisms of the dental pulp. *Crit Rev Oral Biol Med*, **9**, 179–200.

Kakehashi, S., Stanley, H.R. and Fitzgerald, R.J. (1965) The effects of surgical exposures of dental pulps in germ-free and conventional laboratory rats. *Oral Surg Oral Med Oral Pathol*, **20**, 340–349.

Kang, M., In Jung, H., Song, M., Kim, S.Y., Kim, H.C. and Kim, E. (2015) Outcome of nonsurgical retreatment and endodontic microsurgery: a meta-analysis. *Clin Oral Invest*, **19**, 569–582.

Khalighinejad, N., Aminoshariae, M.R., Aminoshariae, A., Kulild, J.C., Mickel, A. and Fouad, A.F. (2016) Association between systemic diseases and apical periodontitis. *J Endod*, **42**, 1427–1434.

Kim, E. and Lee, S.J. (2004. Electronic apex locator. *Dent Clin North Am*, **48**, 35–54.

Kung, J., McDonagh, M. and Sedgley, C.M. (2015. Does articaine provide an advantage over lidocaine in patients with symptomatic irreversible pulpitis? A systematic review and meta-analysis. *J Endod*, **41**, 1784–1794.

Law, A. and Messer, H. (2004) An evidence-based analysis of the antibacterial effectiveness of intracanal medicaments. *J Endod*, **30**, 689–694.

Malmberg, L., Bjorkner, A.E. and Bergenholtz, G. (2016) Establishment and maintenance of asepsis in endodontics – a review of the literature. *Acta Odontol Scand*, **74**, 431–435.

Marquis, V.L., Dao, T., Farzaneh, M., Abitbol, S. and Friedman, S. (2006) Treatment outcome in endodontics: the Toronto Study. Phase III: initial treatment. *J Endod*, **32**, 299–306.

Meechan, J.G. (2002) Supplementary routes to local anaesthesia. *Int Endod J*, **35**, 885–896.

Mello, I. (2014) Use of electronic apex locators may improve determination of working length. *Evid Based Dent*, **15**, 120.

Mjor, I.A. and Nordahl, I. (1996) The density and branching of dentinal tubules in human teeth. *Arch Oral Biol*, **41**, 401–412.

Mohammadi, Z. (2012) MTAD: a review of a promising endodontic irrigant. *N Y State Dent J*, **78**, 47–53.

Mohammadi, Z., Shalavi, S. and Jafarzadeh, H. (2013) Ethylenediaminetetraacetic acid in endodontics. *Eur J Dent*, **7**, S135–142.

Morgan, L.F. and Montgomery, S. (1984) An evaluation of the crown-down pressureless technique. *J Endod*, **10**, 491–498.

Morse, D.R. (1977) Immunologic aspects of pulpal–periapical diseases. A review. *Oral Surg Oral Med Oral Pathol*, **43**, 436–451.

Mozo, S., Llena, C. and Forner, L. (2012) Review of ultrasonic irrigation in endodontics: increasing action of irrigating solutions. *Med Oral Patol Oral Cir Bucal*, **17**, e512–516.

Mullaney, T.P. (1979) Instrumentation of finely curved canals. *Dent Clin North Am*, **23**, 575–592.

Nair, P.N. (1997) Apical periodontitis: a dynamic encounter between root canal infection and host response. *Periodontology* 2000, **13**, 121–148.

Nair, P.N. (2006) On the causes of persistent apical periodontitis: a review. *Int Endod J*, **39**, 249–281.

Ng, Y.L., Mann, V., Rahbaran, S., Lewsey, J. and Gulabivala, K. (2007) Outcome of primary root canal treatment: systematic review of the literature – part 1. Effects of study characteristics on probability of success. *Int Endod J*, **40**, 921–939.

Ng, Y.L., Mann, V. and Gulabivala, K. (2008a) Outcome of secondary root canal treatment: a systematic review of the literature. *Int Endod J*, **41**, 1026–1046.

Ng, Y.L., Mann, V., Rahbaran, S., Lewsey, J. and Gulabivala, K. (2008b) Outcome of primary root canal treatment: systematic review of the literature – Part 2. Influence of clinical factors. *Int Endod J*, **41**, 6–31.

Ng, Y.L., Mann, V. and Gulabivala, K. (2010) Tooth survival following non-surgical root canal treatment: a systematic review of the literature. *Int Endod J*, **43**, 171–189.

Ng, Y.L., Mann, V. and Gulabivala, K. (2011a) A prospective study of the factors affecting outcomes of non-surgical root canal treatment: part 2: tooth survival. *Int Endod J*, **44**, 610–625.

Ng, Y.L., Mann, V. and Gulabivala, K. (2011b) A prospective study of the factors affecting outcomes of nonsurgical root canal treatment: part 1: periapical health. *Int Endod J*, **44**, 583–609.

Orstavik, D. and Pitt Ford, T.R. (2007) *Essential Endodontology: Prevention and Treatment of Apical Periodontitis*, 2nd edn, Wiley-Blackwell, Oxford.

Pak, J.G., Fayazi, S. and White, S.N. (2012) Prevalence of periapical radiolucency and root canal treatment: a systematic review of cross-sectional studies. *J Endod*, **38**, 1170–1176.

Patel, S., Durack, C., Abella, F., Shemesh, H., Roig, M. and Lemberg, K. (2015) Cone beam computed tomography in endodontics – a review. *Int Endod J*, **48**, 3–15.

Rowe, A.H. and Pitt Ford, T.R. (1990) The assessment of pulpal vitality. *Int Endod J*, **23**, 77–83.

Ruddle, C.J. (2001) The ProTaper technique: endodontics made easier. *Dent Today*, **20**, 58–64, 66–68.

Ruddle, C.J. (2004) Nonsurgical endodontic retreatment. *J Calif Dent Assoc*, **32**, 474–484.

Savarrio, L., Mackenzie, D., Riggio, M., Saunders, W.P. and Bagg, J. (2005) Detection of bacteraemias during non-surgical root canal treatment. *J Dent*, **33**, 293–303.

Segura-Egea, J.J., Gould, K., Sen, B.H. *et al.* (2017a) Antibiotics in endodontics: a review. *Int Endod J*, **50**, 1169–1184.

Segura-Egea, J.J., Gould, K., Sen, B.H. *et al.* (2018) European Society of Endodontology position statement: the use of antibiotics in endodontics. *Int Endod J*, **51**, 20–25.

Serrano-Gimenez, M., Sanchez-Torres, A. and Gay-Escoda, C. (2015) Prognostic factors on periapical surgery: a systematic review. *Med Oral Patol Oral Cir Bucal*, **20**, e715–722.

Setzer, F.C., Shah, S.B., Kohli, M.R., Karabucak, B. and Kim, S. (2010) Outcome of endodontic surgery: a meta-analysis of the literature – part 1: Comparison of traditional root-end surgery and endodontic microsurgery. *J Endod*, **36**, 1757–1765.

Shirvani, A., Shamszadeh, S., Eghbal, M.J., Marvasti, L.A. and Asgary, S. (2017) Effect of preoperative oral analgesics on pulpal anesthesia in patients with irreversible pulpitis – a systematic review and meta-analysis. *Clin Oral Invest*, **21**, 43–52.

Siqueira, J.F. Jr and Rocas, I.N. (2009) Diversity of endodontic microbiota revisited. *J Dent Res*, **88**, 969–981.

Stashenko, P., Teles, R. and d'Souza, R. (1998) Periapical inflammatory responses and their modulation. *Crit Rev Oral Biol Med*, **9**, 498–521.

Sundqvist, G. (1976) Bacteriological studies of necrotic dental pulps. *Umae Univ Odontological Dissertations*, **7**, 1–93.

Tang, Y., Li, X. and Yin, S. (2010) Outcomes of MTA as root-end filling in endodontic surgery: a systematic review. *Quintessence Int*, **41**, 557–566.

Torabinejad, M. and Pitt Ford, T.R. (1996) Root end filling materials: a review. *Endod Dent Traumatol*, **12**, 161–178.

Torabinejad, M., Corr, R., Handysides, R. and Shabahang, S. (2009) Outcomes of nonsurgical retreatment and endodontic surgery: a systematic review. *J Endod*, **35**, 930–937.

Tortini, D., Grassi, M., Re Cecconi, D., Colombo, M. and Gagliani, M. (2011) Warm gutta-percha obturation technique: a critical review. *Minerva Stomatol*, **60**, 35–50.

Tsesis, I., Rosen, E., Taschieri, S., Telishevsky Strauss, Y., Ceresoli, V. and del Fabbro, M. (2013) Outcomes of surgical endodontic treatment performed by a modern technique: an updated meta-analysis of the literature. *J Endod*, **39**, 332–339.

Tsesis, I., Blazer, T., Ben-Izhack, G. *et al.* (2015) The precision of electronic apex locators in working length determination: a systematic review and meta-analysis of the literature. *J Endod*, **41**, 1818–1823.

Vertucci, F.J. (1984) Root canal anatomy of the human permanent teeth. *Oral Surg Oral Med Oral Pathol*, **58**, 589–599.

WHO (2016) *International Classification of Diseases* (ICD), 10th Revision, World Health Organization, Geneva.

Williams, J.V. and Williams, L.R. (2010) Is coronal restoration more important than root filling for ultimate endodontic success? *Dent Update*, **37**, 187–193.

4

Bisphosphonates and Medication-Related Osteonecrosis of the Jaw

4.1 Definition and Staging

Medication-related osteonecrosis of the jaw (MRONJ), previously known as bisphosphonate-related osteonecrosis of the jaw (BRONJ), can be defined as exposed bone or bone that can be probed through an intraoral or extraoral fistula(e) in the maxillofacial region that has persisted for more than 8 weeks in a patient with current or previous treatment with antiresorptive or antiangiogenic agents and no history of radiation therapy to the jaws or obvious metastatic disease to the jaws (Ruggiero *et al.*, 2014).

MRONJ has three stages (Ruggiero, 2015).

- Stage 1: Asymptomatic exposed, necrotic bone with no evidence of infection.
- Stage 2: Exposed, necrotic bone with evidence of infection and pain.
- Stage 3: Exposed, necrotic bone in patients with pain, infection and one of the following features: extension beyond the alveolar bone, pathological fracture, extraoral fistula, oral-antral/oral-nasal communication, or osteolysis extending to the inferior border of the mandible or maxillary sinus floor.

Radiographic changes may not be evident until there is significant bone involvement. Widening of the periodontal ligament space may also be an early radiographic sign of the condition.

4.2 Pathogenesis

The pathophysiology of MRONJ has not been fully explained. It is believed that bisphosphonates and some other antiresorptive (denosumab) and antiangiogenic medications can impair osteoclast function and inhibit endothelial cell function, and therefore interfere with normal bone turnover and resorption. Inflammation and infection are also important factors that can contribute to the development and progression of MRONJ (Katsarelis *et al.*, 2015; Lombard *et al.*, 2016).

Antiresorptive medications include alendronate (Fosamax®), risedronate (Actonel®), ibandronate (Boniva®), pamidronate (Aredia®), zolendronate (Zometa® and Reclast®), and denosumab (Xgeva® and Prolia®).

Antiangiogenic medications include sunitinib (Sutent®), sorafenib (Nexavar®), bevacizumab (Avastin®) and sirolimus (Rapamune®).

Patient characteristics and associated risk factors include (Brock *et al.*, 2011; Peer and Khamaisi, 2015; Turner *et al.*, 2016):

- a patient with cancer and metastatic bone disease (multiple myeloma, lung, breast, prostate, cancer), osteopenia or osteoporosis
- a patient on antiresorptive and antiangiogenic medication for any reason
- the use of intravenous formulations for a minimum of several months to 1 year or the use of oral formulations for a minimum of 3–4 years
- a patient who is taking long-term corticosteroids and is on oral bisphosphonate therapy for osteopenia or osteoporosis
- diabetic patients are at higher risk for developing MRONJ
- history of dentoalveolar trauma.

The risk of MRONJ is significantly higher in cancer patients receiving antiresorptive medication compared to treatment regimens for osteoporosis (Gaudin *et al.*, 2015; Ruggiero *et al.*, 2014).

4.3 Prevalence

Oral delivery of antiresoptive medication is associated with a low incidence of MRONJ (reported as between 1 in 10 000 and 1 in 100 000 patients). However, less commonly prescribed intravenous delivery is associated with

Diseases and Conditions in Dentistry: An Evidence-Based Reference, First Edition. Keyvan Moharamzadeh.

Companion website: www.wiley.com/go/moharamzadeh/diseases

a much higher incidence of MRONJ (1 in 10 to 1 in 100 patients) (Dodson, 2015).

The mandible is at least twice as likely to be affected as the maxilla. MRONJ is also more common in areas with thin mucosa covering a bony prominence (Brock *et al.*, 2011).

4.4 Prevention

The following preventtive measures are recommended prior to commencement of the medication (Brock *et al.*, 2011; Ruggiero *et al.*, 2014).

- Initiation of antiresorptive therapy should be delayed, if possible, until dental health is optimised.
- Non-restorable teeth and teeth with a poor prognosis should be extracted and any other necessary elective dentoalveolar surgery should be completed at this stage.
- Antiresorptive therapy should be delayed at least 4–6 weeks to ensure adequate osseous healing.
- Preventive dental care, including caries prevention and periodontal maintenance, must be continued indefinitely.
- Patients with complete or partial dentures should be assessed for areas of mucosal trauma.
- Patients should be educated to maintain good oral hygiene and regular dental visits and to report any pain, swelling or exposed bone.

After the initiation of antiresorptive treatment, the following preventive measures are recommended (Ruggiero *et al.*, 2014).

- Maintaining good oral hygiene and dental care.
- Extraction and surgical trauma can be avoided by endodontic treatment of the retained roots.
- Placement of dental implants should be avoided in oncology patients receiving intravenous antiresorptive therapy or antiangiogenic medications.
- Discontinuation of the oral bisphosphonate (drug holiday) by the prescribing provider for at least 2 months prior to oral surgery can be considered in patients taking bisphosphonate for more than 4 years, if systemic conditions permit.

4.5 Assessment and Investigations

It is essential to obtain an accurate history and carry out thorough clinical and radiographic assessment of the oral and dental tissues.

Bacterial culture and sensitivity can be helpful in infected cases for appropriate antibiotic selection.

Tissue biopsy is indicated only if metastatic disease is suspected.

4.6 Treatment Considerations

The objectives of treatment are to alleviate pain, control the infection, reduce the progression of osteonecrosis and prevent development of new sites of bone necrosis. Therefore, elective dentoalveolar surgery should be avoided in patients with established MRONJ. Areas of necrotic bone that potentially irritate the soft tissues can be gently removed. However, surgical intervention should be delayed if possible (Williams and O'Ryan, 2015).

The American Association of Oral and Maxillofacial Surgeons recommended the following stage-specific treatment guidelines for MRONJ (Ruggiero *et al.*, 2014).

- Stage 1: Patient education, daily antimicrobial mouthwash, regular clinical follow-ups, assessment of the need for continuation of bisphosphonate medication.
- Stage 2: Antiseptic mouthwash, systemic antibiotics, pain control, localised debridement.
- Stage 3: Antimicrobial mouthwash, systemic antibiotics, pain control, surgical debridement including resection and long-term rehabilitation.

Case Study

An 82-year-old female patient presented with an ulcerating defect on the right side of the palate and the alveolar ridge, causing communication between the oral and nasal cavity and difficulty with eating and drinking.

The patient had been taking long-term oral bisphosphonate medication (risedronate) for the management of osteoporosis. Her preoperative intraoral photograph is shown in Figure 4.1.

Clinical examination showed a small mouth opening and presence of an oral-antral communicating defect with necrosis of alveolar bone and soft tissue inflammation on the maxillary right premolar region. Only carious maxillary central incisor teeth were present in the upper arch. The patient had a lower shortened dental arch.

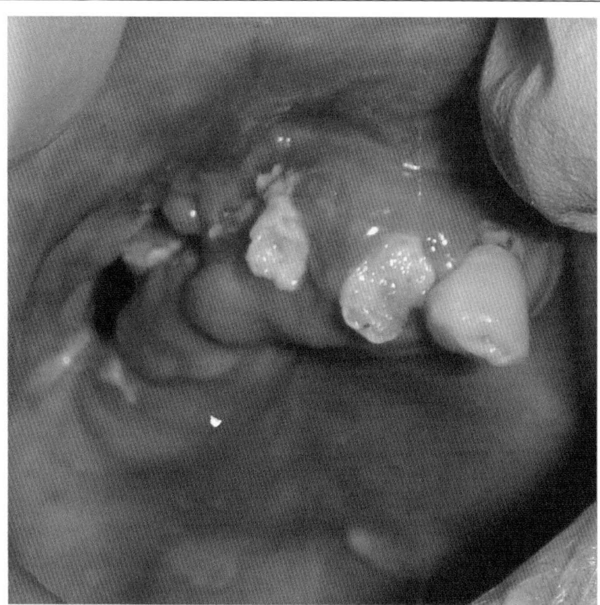

Figure 4.1 Preoperative photograph of the defect showing necrotic bone and oral-antral communication.

Diagnoses

Medication-related osteonecrosis of jaw (stage 3), caries and missing teeth.

Treatment Strategy

1) Prevention and oral hygiene education.
2) Analgesia and systemic antibiotics to control pain and infection.
3) Removal and stabilisation of dental caries.
4) Local debridement and trimming of necrotic bone to minimise soft tissue irritation.
5) Impression of the palate and fabrication of a well-fitting clear acrylic baseplate obturator (Figure 4.2) in the first instance to seal the defect and help with eating and drinking.
6) Chairside addition of the anterior teeth on wax to the baseplate.
7) Processing and fitting of the final obturator with teeth.
8) Review and maintenance.

The patient's postoperative photograph is shown in Figure 4.3.

Treatment Challenges

This was an extremely challenging case due to the following issues.

- The patient could not be placed in a supine position and had to be treated in an upright position in a wheelchair. Therefore, it was decided to add the teeth to the baseplate chairside, which was very challenging.
- The access was very difficult due to the small mouth.
- The buccal sulcus was very shallow in the upper arch and the retention of the obturator was compromised.
- The patient also had dry mouth and the prescription of an oral moisturising gel helped to reduce the discomfort and improve retention of the obturator.
- Compromised healing due to bisphosphonate medication and tenderness in the defect region further complicated the treatment process.

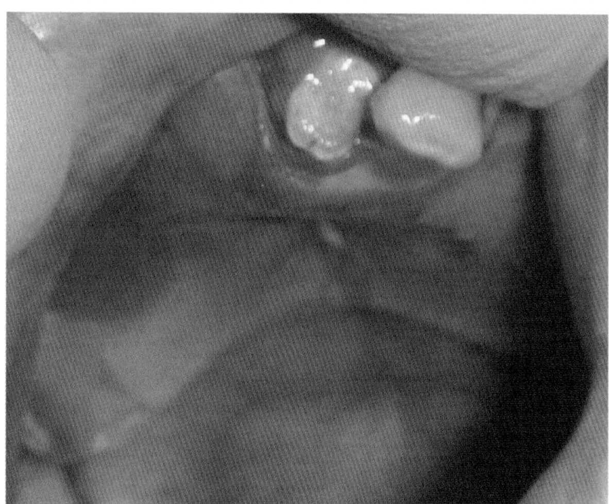

Figure 4.2 Clear acrylic baseplate obturator sealing the maxillary defect.

The patient was satisfied with the outcome of the treatment as it reduced her pain, controlled the infection, separated the oral and nasal communication and restored the patient's masticatory function and aesthetics.

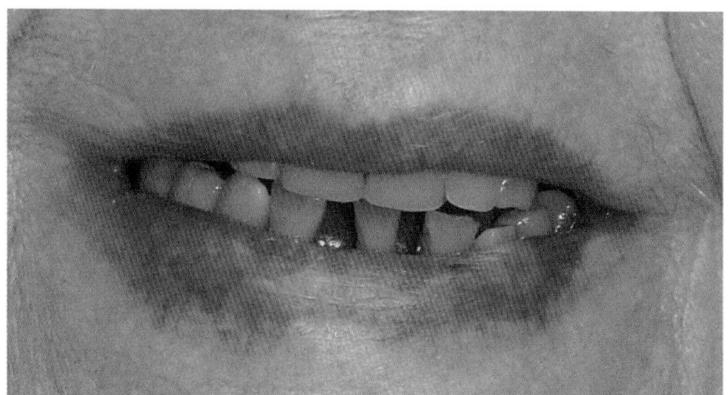

Figure 4.3 Postoperative photograph of the patient's smile.

References

Brock, G., Barker, K., Butterworth, C.J. and Rogers, S. (2011) Practical considerations for treatment of patients taking bisphosphonate medications: an update. *Dent Update*, **38**, 313–314, 317–318, 321–324 passim.

Dodson, T.B. (2015) The frequency of medication-related osteonecrosis of the jaw and its associated risk factors. *Oral Maxillofac Surg Clin North Am*, **27**, 509–516.

Gaudin, E., Seidel, L., Bacevic, M., Rompen, E. and Lambert, F. (2015) Occurrence and risk indicators of medication-related osteonecrosis of the jaw after dental extraction: a systematic review and meta-analysis. *J Clin Periodontol*, **42**, 922–932.

Katsarelis, H., Shah, N.P., Dhariwal, D.K. and Pazianas, M. (2015) Infection and medication-related osteonecrosis of the jaw. *J Dent Res*, **94**, 534–539.

Lombard, T., Neirinckx, V., Rogister, B., Gilon, Y. and Wislet, S. (2016) Medication-related osteonecrosis of the jaw: new insights into molecular mechanisms and cellular therapeutic approaches. *Stem Cells Int*, **2016**, 8768162.

Peer, A. and Khamaisi, M. (2015) Diabetes as a risk factor for medication-related osteonecrosis of the jaw. *J Dent Res*, **94**, 252–260.

Ruggiero, S. L. (2015) Diagnosis and staging of medication-related osteonecrosis of the jaw. *Oral Maxillofac Surg Clin North Am*, **27**, 479–487.

Ruggiero, S.L., Dodson, T.B., Fantasia, J. *et al.* (2014) American Association of Oral And Maxillofacial Surgeons position paper on medication-related osteonecrosis of the jaw – 2014 update. *J Oral Maxillofac Surg*, **72**, 1938–1956.

Turner, B., Drudge-Coates, L., Ali, S. *et al.* (2016) Osteonecrosis of the jaw in patients receiving bone-targeted therapies: an overview – part I. *Urol Nurs*, **36**, 111–116, 154.

Williams, W.B. and O'Ryan, F. (2015) Management of medication-related osteonecrosis of the jaw. *Oral Maxillofac Surg Clin North Am*, **27**, 517–525.

5

Caries

Abdul-Rahman Elmougy - Case study

5.1 Definition and Aetiology

Dental caries is a bacterial infection that causes demineralization of the tooth tissue and can result in destruction of enamel, dentin and cementum.

According to the chemo-parasitic or acidogenic theory proposed by Miller in 1980, dental caries is caused by acid production due to fermentation of dietary sugars by non-specific bacteria found in plaque (Herschfeld, 1978).

The well-known Stephan curve shows that plaque pH drops from 6.8 to 5 within 2–3 minutes of sugar intake and it takes approximately 40 minutes to return to the original pH. Although the Stephan curve has been a crucial element of cariology research, the effects of alkali production within plaque have recently been investigated (Bowen, 2013).

5.2 Pathogenesis

Dental caries develops and progresses in several dynamic stages (Featherstone, 2008; Zero, 1999).

- *Initial lesion*: white spot or brown spot development on the surface of enamel due to microscopic removal of mineral material.
- *Early lesion*: subsurface spread of demineralisation without cavity formation. Early lesion is reversible and can be remineralised.
- *Enamel caries*: irreversible breakdown of the enamel surface due to continuous demineralisation and cavity formation.
- *Dentine caries*: destruction and demineralisation of dentine due to bacterial invasion.

The bacteria most responsible for development and progression of dental caries are *Streptococcus mutans, Streptococcus sobrinus* and lactobacilli (Asikainen and Alaluusua, 1993; Takahashi and Nyvad, 2011).

5.3 Epidemiology

The prevalence and extent of caries have fallen significantly since the late 1970s. However, caries remains a problem in preschool children in many countries. According to the UK Child Dental Health Survey, in 2013, 28% of children aged 5 and 39% of children aged 8 had untreated dental caries and 31% of children had experienced caries by the time they were 5 years old (NHS, 2013).

5.4 Classification

Different types of dental caries have been described based on their clinical presentation, location, time of development, rate of progression and aetiological factors.

- Tidemark caries are previously non-cavitated caries parallel to the gingiva that have been remineralised following tooth eruption and gingival recession.
- Early childhood caries, or baby bottle caries or nursing bottle mouth, is a type of caries found on deciduous teeth in young children, due to consumption of sugar-containing liquids in feeding bottles.
- Rampant caries is extensive and rapidly progressing caries affecting multiple surfaces of many teeth.
- Radiation-induced caries is rampant caries as a result of previous radiation to the head and neck (Aguiar *et al.*, 2009). Several factors contribute to the development of radiation-induced caries in cancer patients, including compromised plaque control, reduced quantity and quality of saliva, changes in oral microbial flora, cariogenic diet and direct effects of radiotherapy on enamel and dentine.
- Recurrent caries or secondary caries is frequently found on the margins of restorations where caries was present previously.

Diseases and Conditions in Dentistry: An Evidence-Based Reference, First Edition. Keyvan Moharamzadeh.

Companion website: www.wiley.com/go/moharamzadeh/diseases

- Incipient caries is caries at a location without any previous caries.
- Arrested caries are remineralised lesions on teeth that were previously demineralised without causing a cavitation.

5.5 Relevant History

The following aspects of the patient's history can be relevant to dental caries.

- Diet history and frequency of sugar intake.
- History of dry mouth and medical conditions causing xerostomia such as Sjögren's syndrome, diabetes, relevant medications including antihistamines and antidepressants.
- History of radiotherapy to head and neck.
- Smoking can increase the risk of root-surface caries.

5.6 Clinical Examination of Caries

There are several methods for investigating caries (Gimenez *et al.*, 2013, 2015; Gomez, 2015; Schwendicke *et al.*, 2015).

- Visual examination has high specificity and low sensitivity but good overall performance.
- Visual tactile examination is the most commonly used method of caries detection.
- BW radiography has highly accuracy for detecting cavitated interproximal caries, and can also be suitable for detection of dentine caries.
- Electrical resistance has high sensitivity and specificity for fissure caries but can be sensitive to moisture.
- Fibre-optic transillumination can be helpful in detecting early enamel lesions.
- Laser fluorescence is less sensitive to moisture but may not distinguish caries from plaque or stain.

A recent systematic review and meta-analysis showed visual examination, radiographic assessment and laser fluorescence detection to be the most useful tools to detect secondary carious lesions (Brouwer *et al.*, 2016).

5.7 Differential Diagnosis

The differential diagnosis for dental caries includes dental fluorosis (see Chapter 19), developmental dental defects and cervical root resorption (see Chapter 17).

Developmental defects usually follow the incremental lines of enamel and, unlike caries, affect the cusp tips or incisal edges.

5.8 Prevention

The four main preventive measures to control caries are plaque control, diet, fluoride and fissure sealing.

5.8.1 Tooth Brushing and Mechanical Plaque Control

Different methods of mechanical plaque control, including tooth brushing and interdental cleaning, are thoroughly discussed in Chapter 6.

5.8.2 Diet

Sucrose is the most cariogenic sugar, followed by glucose, fructose and maltose.

Non-milk extrinsic sugars, added sugars and freesugars should be the focus of preventive diet advice. Milk sugars such as lactose and intrinsic sugars found in fruit and vegetables have much lower cariogenic potential compared to non-milk extrinsic sugars. Non-sugar sweeteners can also be safe (Moynihan, 2016).

Sugar-free chewing gums have the potential to decrease dental caries by enhancing plaque removal and stimulating saliva flow but may increase the risk of dental erosion (Nadimi *et al.*, 2011).

Dietary assessment should include general advice for every patient to reduce the amount and frequency of non-milk extrinsic sugars and specific advice for children with caries problem. It should be carried out over three sessions, including an initial appointment to give the patient a diet diary to be filled in, a follow-up session to collect the diet diary, and a further appointment to provide advice and target setting.

5.8.3 Fluoride

Fluoride has the ability to increase remineralisation of enamel and its resistance to demineralisation and reduce plaque acid production (Rosin-Grget *et al.*, 2013).

It is widely believed that water fluoridation at 1 ppm can significantly reduce caries rates. However, a recent Cochrane review showed that there is a lack of high-quality evidence and the available evidence is subject to a high risk of bias in previous studies (Iheozor-Ejiofor *et al.*, 2015).

There is also low-quality evidence suggesting that milk fluoridation may be beneficial in terms of caries prevention but less effective than water fluoridation (Yeung *et al.*, 2015). Salt fluoridation has been shown to be a cheaper alternative (Marthaler, 2013).

Fluoride diet supplements can also be provided in the form of tablets, drops, lozenges or chewing gums. There is good evidence to support the effectiveness of this approach in caries prevention (Tubert-Jeannin *et al.*,

2011). Fluoride supplements are indicated in areas with low water fluoride.

The most important vehicle for effective fluoride delivery is toothpaste. Recommended toothpaste fluoride content for children aged 1–5 years is 500 ppm, 6–9 years is 1000 ppm, and over 9 years old is 1500 ppm (Walsh *et al.*, 2010; Wright *et al.*, 2014).

Fluoride mouthwash can be effective in caries prevention and reduction if used daily at 0.05% or weekly at 0.2% concentrations (Marinho *et al.*, 2016). It can also be recommended for patients wearing orthodontic appliances. Fluoride mouthwashes are contraindicated in children less than 6 years of age. Mouthrinse use by older children and adolescents must be under supervision.

Topical fluoride gels such as 2% stannous fluoride or acidulated phosphate fluoride (APF) gels applied in trays for 4 minutes every 6 months can have caries-inhibiting effects in both primary and permanent dentition (Marinho *et al.*, 2015). Daily self-application of fluoride gel following application of high-calcium phosphate-containing products has also been recommended for head and neck oncology patients receiving radiotherapy who are at risk of developing radiation-induced caries (Jawad *et al.*, 2015b; Noone and Barclay, 2017).

Fluoride varnishes such as 5% sodium fluoride (Duraphat®, Colgate) varnish can be effective and quick for treatment and remineralisation of incipient caries in both primary and permanent dentition (Lenzi *et al.*, 2016).

It is extremely important to be aware of the safety risks associated with topical and systemic fluorides, including risks of ingestion, overdose, systemic toxicity and development of fluorosis. Appropriate precautions must be taken by parents and childcare providers to prevent and minimise the risk of fluoride ingestion in children (Moharamzadeh, 2016).

5.8.4 Fissure Sealing

Fissure sealing can be particularly indicated in the following groups of patients.

- Children with special needs would benefit from fissure sealing of all the occlusal surfaces of their permanent teeth.
- Children with extensive caries in their primary teeth would require fissure sealing of all their permanent molar teeth as soon as they erupt.

Resin-based fissure sealants are the best performing materials with median survival of at least 5 years. GIC sealants may be less retentive than resin sealants but early fluoride release can be good for newly erupted teeth in patients with high caries rates (Wright *et al.*, 2016).

5.9 Treatment Considerations

Parents should be encouraged to bring their child for dental check-up as soon as the child develops teeth, to enable prevention. Preschool children should be examined 2–3 times per year and more frequently for those with high caries risk. Thorough caries risk assessment must be carried out and appropriate caries management protocols should be implemented for each risk category at different ages (AAPD, 2014). The Department of Health (DoH) and Public Health England (PHE) have also recommended a useful evidence-based prevention toolkit for clinical teams entitled *Delivering Better Oral Health* (DoH and PHE, 2017).

5.9.1 Primary Teeth

Caries in primary teeth can be treated by hand excavation and restoration with a GIC-based restorative material. Step-wise excavation can be effective in the management of deeply carious primary teeth to reduce the risk of pulp exposure (Ricketts *et al.*, 2013).

It has been shown that well-sealed lesions of carious dentine do not progress and indirect pulp capping has a good success rate in posterior primary teeth (Bressani *et al.*, 2013).

Primary molars with caries affecting more than two surfaces without irreversible pulp involvement can be restored with Hall crowns if there is sufficient tooth structure remaining. The Hall technique is a novel method of managing carious primary molars by cementing preformed metal crowns over the tooth. The technique does not require local anaesthesia, caries removal or any tooth preparation and is preferred by the majority of children, carers and dentists (Innes *et al.*, 2007, 2009).

In cases of carious pulp exposure, it is important to maintain the vitality of the radicular pulp as immune cells from the pulp are involved in physiological root resorption. Treatment of pulpitis in extensively carious primary teeth includes excavation of caries and pulpotomy (Smail-Faugeron *et al.*, 2014). Extractions are indicated for unrestorable primary teeth.

5.9.2 Permanent Teeth

5.9.2.1 Minimally Invasive Techniques

Advances in adhesive technology have led to the development of minimally invasive approaches for caries treatment (Banerjee, 2013; Featherstone and Domejean, 2012; Marending *et al.*, 2016).

Resin infiltration into a carious tooth structure is an innovative, minimally invasive technique that can be useful for the treatment of non-cavitated early carious lesions. It involves etching of demineralised areas, rinsing, drying, dehydration with ethanol, application of infiltration resin and light polymerisation (Lasfargues *et al.*, 2013).

Atraumatic restorative treatment is another modality indicated for deeply carious teeth, particularly in children and patients with special needs as well as those living in areas with poor socioeconomic conditions and limited access to conventional dental rotary instruments. This technique involves the excavation of infected soft dentine and placement of an adhesive restoration with simultaneous sealing of the adjacent pits and fissures (Holmgren *et al.*, 2013).

Minimally invasive operative caries removal techniques are summarised below (Banerjee, 2013).

- Mechanical rotary using handpiece and burs
- Mechanical non-rotary such as hand excavators, air abrasion, air polishing, sonoabrasion and ultrasonic instruments
- Chemomechanical approach using agents such as Carisolv, Caridex and enzymes
- Laser ablation
- Photoactive and ozone disinfection

Minimally invasive techniques using adhesive restorative materials can also be beneficial for the management of patients with radiation-induced dental caries.

5.9.2.2 Treatment of Exposed Pulp in Permanent Teeth

Indirect pulp capping and step-wise excavation can be used in the management of deeply carious permanent teeth with normal pulps and without visible exposure (Bjorndal, 2008; Ricketts *et al.*, 2013).

Direct pulp capping is indicated for the management of permanent teeth with normal pulp and small carious or mechanical exposure. Calcium hydroxide and MTA are commonly used for direct pulp capping. Systematic reviews indicate a higher clinical success rate with MTA compared to calcium hydroxide (Schwendicke *et al.*, 2016; Zhu *et al.*, 2015).

Partial (Cvek) pulpotomy is indicated in teeth with traumatic vital pulp exposure and in young permanent teeth with carious pulp exposure in which the affected pulp is not too deep (1.5–2 mm) and pulpal bleeding is controlled within several minutes. The tooth must be vital, with a diagnosis of normal pulp or reversible pulpitis (Mejare and Cvek, 1993). The outcome of this treatment may be compromised in teeth with luxation injuries (Bimstein and Rotstein, 2016).

Pulpotomy can be carried out in exposed carious permanent teeth with incomplete roots where the affected pulp is deep. Management of teeth with open apices is discussed in detail in Chapter 34.

Root canal treatment is recommended for large carious exposures and large traumatic exposures in fully developed teeth (see Chapter 3).

Extractions are indicated for non-restorable teeth with extensive caries.

Case Study

A 65-year-old male patient presented with dry mouth, cavities on multiple teeth, broken-down teeth and poor aesthetics. The teeth were asymptomatic with no history of pain or swellings.

He reported a history of radiotherapy 10 years ago for the treatment of left tonsilar squamous cell carcinoma (SCC).

Clinical examination showed slight limitation in mouth opening. The soft tissues were normal and the periodontium was healthy.

Examination of the dentition showed a shortened dental arch and extensive caries affecting the anterior teeth and remaining posterior teeth. Except for the retained second premolar roots, the other teeth gave a positive response to electric pulp testing.

A preoperative clinical photograph of the anterior teeth is shown is Figure 5.1.

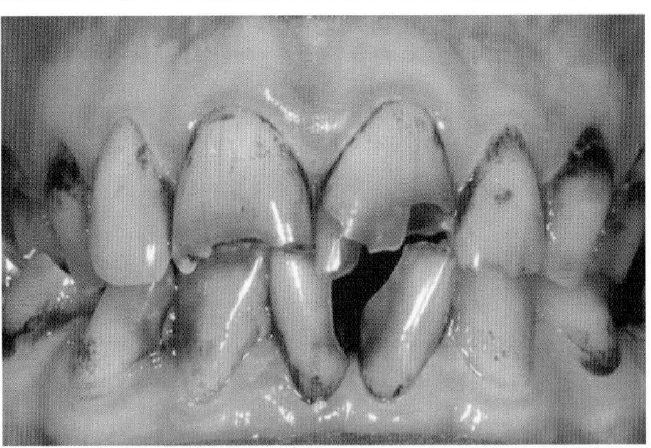

Figure 5.1 Preoperative clinical photograph showing extensive radiation-induced caries.

Diagnoses
Based on the patient's history and clinical findings, the following diagnoses were made.

- Radiation-induced dental caries
- Retained carious roots
- Xerostomia
- Trismus (mild) which can be another side effect of radiotherapy (Jawad *et al.*, 2015a)

Treatment Strategy
Preventive measures included oral hygiene education (modified Bass tooth brushing and interdental cleaning), dietary advice, prescription of high-fluoride toothpaste (Duraphat 5000 ppm) and daily applications of Tooth Mousse (GC) on the teeth for 5 minutes (to increase calcium and phosphate levels) followed by wearing custom-made applicator trays filled with a pea-sized amount of fluoride toothpaste (Duraphat 5000) for 30 min to enhance remineralisation.

The patient was also advised to take frequent sips of water and was recommended to use commercially available, sugar-free, neural pH, fluoride-containing saliva substitutes such as BioXtra (RIS Products), to relieve the symptoms of xerostomia.

Restorative treatment included removal of caries and direct restorations with composite resin.

The patient was informed about the hopeless prognosis of the non-restorable retained roots which may need to be extracted in the future if they become symptomatic. He was also warned about the risk of developing osteoradionecrosis (see Chapter 36) due to the history of radiotherapy.

The patient's postoperative clinical photograph is shown in Figure 5.2.

The patient was advised to see his general dental practitioner for regular dental care and maintenance.

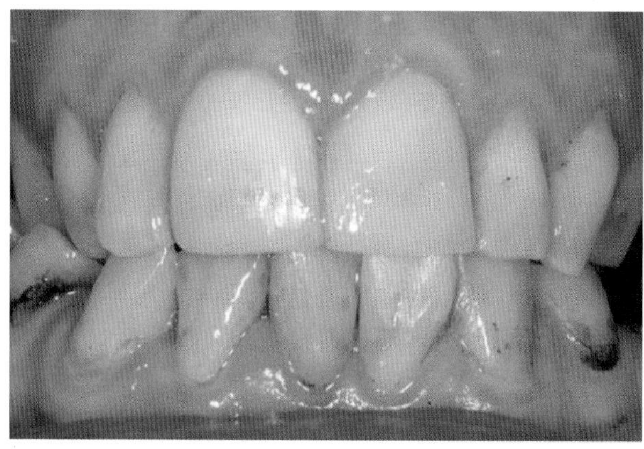

Figure 5.2 Postoperative photograph of the restored anterior teeth.

References

AAPD (2014) *Guideline on Caries-risk Assessment and Management for Infants, Children, and Adolescents.* Available at: www.aapd.org/media/policies_guidelines/g_cariesriskassessment.pdf (accessed 14 December 2017).

Aguiar, G.P., Jham, B.C., Magalhaes, C.S., Sensi, L.G. and Freire, A.R. (2009) A review of the biological and clinical aspects of radiation caries. *J Contemp Dent Pract*, **10**, 83–89.

Asikainen, S. and Alaluusua, S. (1993) Bacteriology of dental infections. *Eur Heart J*, **14**(Suppl K), 43–50.

Banerjee, A. (2013) Minimal intervention dentistry: part 7. Minimally invasive operative caries management: rationale and techniques. *Br Dent J*, **214**, 107–111.

Bimstein, E. and Rotstein, I. (2016) Cvek pulpotomy – revisited. *Dent Traumatol*, **32**, 438–442.

Bjorndal, L. (2008) Indirect pulp therapy and stepwise excavation. *J Endod*, **34**, S29–33.

Bowen, W.H. (2013) The Stephan Curve revisited. *Odontology*, **101**, 2–8.

Bressani, A.E., Mariath, A.A., Haas, A.N., Garcia-Godoy, F. and de Araujo, F.B. (2013) Incomplete caries removal and indirect pulp capping in primary molars: a randomized controlled trial. *Am J Dent*, **26**, 196–200.

Brouwer, F., Askar, H., Paris, S. and Schwendicke, F. (2016) Detecting secondary caries lesions: a systematic review and meta-analysis. *J Dent Res*, **95**, 143–151.

DOH and PHE (2017) *Delivering Better Oral Health: An Evidence-Based Toolkit for Prevention*, Department of Health and Public Health England, London.

Featherstone, J.D. (2008) Dental caries: a dynamic disease process. *Aust Dent J*, **53**, 286–291.

Featherstone, J.D. and Domejean, S. (2012) Minimal intervention dentistry: part 1. From 'compulsive' restorative dentistry to rational therapeutic strategies. *Br Dent J*, **213**, 441–445.

Gimenez, T., Braga, M.M., Raggio, D.P., Deery, C., Ricketts, D.N. and Mendes, F.M. (2013) Fluorescence-based methods for detecting caries lesions: systematic review, meta-analysis and sources of heterogeneity. *PLoS One*, **8**, e60421.

Gimenez, T., Piovesan, C., Braga, M.M. *et al.* (2015) Visual inspection for caries detection: a systematic review and meta-analysis. *J Dent Res*, **94**, 895–904.

Gomez, J. (2015) Detection and diagnosis of the early caries lesion. *BMC Oral Health*, **15**(Suppl 1), S3.

Herschfeld, J.J. (1978) W.D. Miller and the "chemico-parasitic" theory of dental caries. *Bull Hist Dent*, **26**, 11–20.

Holmgren, C.J., Roux, D. and Domejean, S. (2013) Minimal intervention dentistry: part 5. Atraumatic restorative treatment (ART) – a minimum intervention and minimally invasive approach for the management of dental caries. *Br Dent J*, **214**, 11–18.

Iheozor-Ejiofor, Z., Worthington, H.V., Walsh, T. *et al.* (2015) Water fluoridation for the prevention of dental caries. *Cochrane Database Syst Rev*, **6**, CD010856.

Innes, N.P., Evans, D.J. and Stirrups, D.R. (2007) The Hall Technique; a randomized controlled clinical trial of a novel method of managing carious primary molars in general dental practice: acceptability of the technique and outcomes at 23 months. *BMC Oral Health*, **7**, 18.

Innes, N., Evans, D. and Hall, N. (2009) The Hall Technique for managing carious primary molars. *Dent Update*, **36**, 472–474, 477–478.

Jawad, H., Hodson, N.A. and Nixon, P.J. (2015a) A review of dental treatment of head and neck cancer patients, before, during and after radiotherapy: part 1. *Br Dent J*, **218**, 65–68.

Jawad, H., Hodson, N.A. and Nixon, P.J. (2015b) A review of dental treatment of head and neck cancer patients, before, during and after radiotherapy: part 2. *Br Dent J*, **218**, 69–74.

Lasfargues, J.J., Bonte, E., Guerrieri, A. and Fezzani, L. (2013) Minimal intervention dentistry: part 6. Caries inhibition by resin infiltration. *Br Dent J*, **214**, 53–59.

Lenzi, T.L., Montagner, A.F., Soares, F.Z. and de Oliveira Rocha, R. (2016) Are topical fluorides effective for treating incipient carious lesions? A systematic review and meta-analysis. *J Am Dent Assoc*, **147**, 84–91 e1.

Marending, M., Attin, T. and Zehnder, M. (2016) Treatment options for permanent teeth with deep caries. *Swiss Dent J*, **126**, 1007–1027.

Marinho, V.C., Worthington, H.V., Walsh, T. and Chong, L.Y. (2015) Fluoride gels for preventing dental caries in children and adolescents. *Cochrane Database Syst Rev*, **6**, CD002280.

Marinho, V.C., Chong, L.Y., Worthington, H.V. and Walsh, T. (2016) Fluoride mouthrinses for preventing dental caries in children and adolescents. *Cochrane Database Syst Rev*, **7**, CD002284.

Marthaler, T.M. (2013) Salt fluoridation and oral health. *Acta Med Acad*, **42**, 140–155.

Mejare, I. and Cvek, M. (1993) Partial pulpotomy in young permanent teeth with deep carious lesions. *Endod Dent Traumatol*, **9**, 238–242.

Moharamzadeh, K. (2016) Biocompatibility of oral care products, in *Biocompatibility of Dental Biomaterials* (ed. R. Shelton), Woodhead Publishing, Cambridge, pp. 113–129.

Moynihan, P. (2016) Sugars and dental caries: evidence for setting a recommended threshold for intake. *Adv Nutr*, **7**, 149–56.

Nadimi, H., Wesamaa, H., Janket, S. J., Bollu, P. and Meurman, J.H. (2011) Are sugar-free confections really beneficial for dental health? *Br Dent J*, **211**, E15.

NHS (2013) *Child Dental Health Survey, England, Wales and Northern Ireland*. Available at: https://digital.nhs.uk/catalogue/PUB17137 (accessed 14 December 2017).

Noone, J. and Barclay, C. (2017) Head and neck cancer patients – information for the general dental practitioner. *Dent Update*, **44**, 209–215.

Ricketts, D., Lamont, T., Innes, N.P., Kidd, E. and Clarkson, J.E. (2013) Operative caries management in adults and children. *Cochrane Database Syst Rev*, **3**, CD003808.

Rosin-Grget, K., Peros, K., Sutej, I. and Basic, K. (2013) The cariostatic mechanisms of fluoride. *Acta Med Acad*, **42**, 179–188.

Schwendicke, F., Tzschoppe, M. and Paris, S. (2015) Radiographic caries detection: a systematic review and meta-analysis. *J Dent*, **43**, 924–933.

Schwendicke, F., Brouwer, F., Schwendicke, A. and Paris, S. (2016) Different materials for direct pulp capping: systematic review and meta-analysis and trial sequential analysis. *Clin Oral Invest*, **20**, 1121–1132.

Smail-Faugeron, V., Courson, F., Durieux, P. *et al.* (2014) Pulp treatment for extensive decay in primary teeth. *Cochrane Database Syst Rev*, **8**, CD003220.

Takahashi, N. and Nyvad, B. (2011) The role of bacteria in the caries process: ecological perspectives. *J Dent Res*, **90**, 294–303.

Tubert-Jeannin, S., Auclair, C., Amsallem, E. *et al.* (2011) Fluoride supplements (tablets, drops, lozenges or chewing gums) for preventing dental caries in children. *Cochrane Database Syst Rev*, **12**, CD007592.

Walsh, T., Worthington, H.V., Glenny, A.M. *et al.* (2010) Fluoride toothpastes of different concentrations for preventing dental caries in children and adolescents. *Cochrane Database Syst Rev*, **1**, CD007868.

Wright, J.T., Hanson, N., Ristic, H. *et al.* (2014) Fluoride toothpaste efficacy and safety in children younger than 6 years: a systematic review. *J Am Dent Assoc*, **145**, 182–189.

Wright, J.T., Tampi, M.P., Graham, L. *et al.* (2016) Sealants for preventing and arresting pit-and-fissure occlusal caries in primary and permanent molars: a systematic review of randomized controlled trials – a report of the

American Dental Association and the American Academy of Pediatric Dentistry. *J Am Dent Assoc*, **147**, 631–645 e18.

Yeung, C.A., Chong, L.Y. and Glenny, A.M. (2015) Fluoridated milk for preventing dental caries. *Cochrane Database Syst Rev*, **8**, CD003876.

Zero, D.T. (1999) Dental caries process. *Dent Clin North Am*, **43**, 635–664.

Zhu, C., Ju, B. and Ni, R. (2015) Clinical outcome of direct pulp capping with MTA or calcium hydroxide: a systematic review and meta-analysis. *Int J Clin Exp Med*, **8**, 17055–17060.

6

Chronic Periodontitis

6.1 Definition and Classification

According to the consensus report from the 5th European Workshop on Periodontology, a two-level definition for periodontitis can be described (Tonetti *et al.*, 2005).

- Proximal attachment loss of greater than 3 mm in two or more non-adjacent teeth. This definition is suitable for defining incipient localised cases.
- Proximal attachment loss equal to or greater than 5 mm in more than 30% of teeth present. This definition is suitable for defining generalised cases with substantial extent and severity.

The 1989 classification of periodontal diseases has many shortcomings including considerable overlap in disease categories, absence of a gingival disease component, inappropriate emphasis on age of onset of disease and rates of progression, and inadequate or unclear classification criteria. In 1999, at the International Workshop for Classification of Periodontal Disease and Conditions, the following categories were defined (Armitage, 1999).

- Gingival diseases
- Chronic periodontitis
- Aggressive periodontitis
- Periodontitis as a manifestation of systemic disease
- Necrotising periodontal diseases
- Abscesses of the periodontium
- Periodontitis associated with endodontic lesions
- Developmental or acquired deformities and conditions

In 2017, the World Workshop on the Classification of Periodontal and Peri-Implant Diseases and Conditions, organised by the European Federation of Periodontology (EFP) and the American Academy of Periodontology (AAP), revisited the classification of periodontal and peri-implant diseases. The reader is encouraged to refer to the proceedings of this workshop for details of the new classification when it becomes available.

6.2 Clinical Features and Characteristics

Chronic periodontitis often has the following common clinical features.

- Colour, texture and volume alterations of marginal gingivae
- Bleeding on probing (BOP)
- Periodontal pocket formation
- Periodontal attachment loss
- Bone loss
- Furcation exposure
- Drifting and exfoliation of teeth

Main characteristics of chronic periodontitis include the following.

- Prevalent in adults but can occur in children as well.
- Amount of destruction is commensurate with plaque level, local predisposing factors, smoking, stress and systemic factors.
- Gingivitis usually precedes the onset of periodontitis.
- Subgingival calculus is often present in diseased sites.
- Host factors determine the pathogenesis and progression.
- Rate of progression in most cases is slow to moderate.
- Extent and severity of periodontitis are the most useful predictors of future disease progression.

6.3 Periodontal Indices

Several index systems have been developed for the assessment of periodontal disease. Periodontal indices that evaluate and record the inflammatory status and the level of plaque and bleeding include the following.

- Gingival Index (Loe, 1967)
  - Score 0: Entire absence of inflammation
  - Score 1: Slight change in the colour and texture of gingivae

Diseases and Conditions in Dentistry: An Evidence-Based Reference, First Edition. Keyvan Moharamzadeh.

Companion website: www.wiley.com/go/moharamzadeh/diseases

  - Score 2: Visual inflammation at gingival margin and BOP
  - Score 3: Significant inflammation and spontaneous bleeding
- Plaque Index (Silness and Loe, 1964)
  - Score 0: Absence of plaque
  - Score 1: Plaque disclosed after running the probe
  - Score 2: Visible plaque
  - Score 3: Abundant plaque
- Combined Gingival and Plaque Index: Dichotomised scoring (Ainamo and Bay, 1975)
  - Score 0: Absence of BOP and no visible plaque
  - Score 1: BOP and visible plaque
- Gingival Sulcus Bleeding Index to assess subgingival inflammation (Muhlemann and Son, 1971)
  - Score 0: Absence of bleeding within 15 seconds of probing to the depth of the pocket
  - Score 1: Bleeding within 15 seconds of probing to the depth of the pocket

Absence of BOP gives a high negative predictive value (98.5%) and is an important indicator of periodontal stability.

Periodontal indices based on attachment level loss include the following.

- Periodontal Index (Russell, 1956)
  - Score 0: Healthy periodontium
  - Score 1: Gingivitis around only one part
  - Score 2: Gingivitis encircling the tooth
  - Score 6: Pocket formation
  - Score 8: Loss of function due to mobility
- Periodontal Disease Index (Ramfjord, 1959)
  - Scores 0–3: Healthy periodontium to gingivitis
  - Scores 4–6: Various levels of attachment loss
- Extent and Severity Index (Carlos *et al.*, 1986)
  - Extent (percentage): Proportion of affected tooth sites with periodontitis
  - Severity (mm): Amount of attachment loss in the affected site

Indices based on periodontal treatment needs include the following.

- World Health Organization (WHO) Community Periodontal Index for Treatment Needs (CPITN), later modified to Community Periodontal Index (CPI) (Ainamo *et al.*, 1982)
  - Score 0: No bleeding, no calculus, no pocketing (no specific need for treatment)
  - Score 1: BOP (OHI was recommended)
  - Score 2: Plaque retentive factors present (OHI and supragingival scaling recommended)
  - Score 3: Periodontal pockets 4–5 mm present (OHI and subgingival scaling recommended)
  - Score 4: Periodontal pockets equal to or greater than 6 mm present (complex periodontal treatment recommended)

This index tended to overestimate the disease in epidemiological studies and contained only partial data compared to full-mouth recordings.

A commonly used index for screening of periodontal disease is the Basic Periodontal Examination (BPE) developed by the British Society of Periodontology in 1986 and further modified recently (BSP, 2016). The BPE index is a rapid and simple screening tool that indicates the level of further assessment and treatment needed. The dentition is divided into six sextants and the highest score in each sextant is recorded according to the following criteria.

- Code 0: Pockets <3.5 mm and healthy periodontal tissues
- Code 1: Pockets <3.5 mm and BOP
- Code 2: Pockets <3.5 mm and supra- or subgingival calculus or plaque retention factor
- Code 3: Probing depth 3.5–5.5 mm
- Code 4: Probing depth >5.5 mm
- Code *: Furcation involvement

For sextants with code 3, detailed periodontal charting is indicated following the initial therapy. If code 4 is present in any sextant, detailed periodontal charting is required for the entire dentition at the baseline and following treatment.

Furcation involvement can be assessed using a curved Naber's furcation probe and is classified based on the horizontal probing depth (Hamp *et al.*, 1975).

- Grade I: Horizontal probing depth equal to or less than 3 mm from one or two furcation entrances
- Grade II: Horizontal probing depth greater than 3 mm in at least one furcation entrance or in combination with grade I furcation involvement
- Grade III: Horizontal probing depth greater than 3 mm in two or more furcation entrances (through and through)

Furcation defects can also be classified based on the amount of bone loss in the furcation areas.

- Degree I: Horizontal bone loss less than one-third of the width of tooth
- Degree II: Horizontal bone loss more than one-third of the width of tooth but less than the total width
- Degree III: Through-and-through furcation bone loss

Tooth mobility can be categorised according to Miller's classification (Laster *et al.*, 1975).

- Degree 0: Physiological mobility 0.1–0.2 mm
- Degree 1: 1 mm horizontal mobility

- Degree 2: Greater than 1 mm horizontal mobility
- Degree 3: Severe mobility greater than 2 mm in horizontal direction or vertical mobility

6.4 Epidemiology

In a landmark study by Loe *et al.* (1986), the progression of periodontal disease in 480 untreated patients aged 14–31 in Sri Lanka (recruited in 1970 and reassessed in 1985) was assessed. Three progression patterns were reported: rapid progression (0.1–1 mm attachment loss per year) in 8% of the patients, no progression beyond gingivitis in 11% and moderate progression (0.05–0.5 mm attachment loss per year) in 81%.

A wide range of epidemiological studies on periodontitis in adults show that disease parameters increase significantly with age (Papapanou, 1999). Gingivitis and mild chronic periodontitis affect a large proportion of people and the severe form of periodontitis affects approximately 11% of the world population (Richards, 2014).

6.5 Risk Factors

Risk factors for periodontal disease can be divided into local factors and systemic risk factors.

6.5.1 Local Risk Factors

Local risk factors include plaque and plaque retentive factors such as calculus, restorations with poor margins or contour, malpositioned teeth, tooth surface defects and concavities, and plaque retentive fixed or removable prostheses.

6.5.2 Systemic Risk Factors

Systemic risk factors for periodontal disease are discussed below.

6.5.2.1 Smoking Tobacco

A substantial number of studies have established the association of smoking with poor periodontal status, and smoking is considered as a significant risk for periodontal progression in longitudinal studies (Linden and Mullally, 1994). Smoking is the second most important risk factor after poor oral hygiene and the risk of periodontal disease is increased by 2.5–7-fold in smokers (Salvi *et al.*, 1997).

Smokers have deeper periodontal pockets, larger numbers of deep pockets, more attachment loss (including recession, bone loss and furcation involvement) and more tooth loss compared to non-smokers. However, smokers show less degree of gingivitis and less BOP (due to decrease in vascularity of the gingival tissue) compared to non-smokers. Smokers also often have poor oral hygiene (Lang and Lindhe, 2015).

Smoking has a profound effect on the immune and inflammatory system, including adverse effects on polymorphonuclear leucocyte (PMN) and neutrophil function. It impairs tissue healing by affecting the microvasculature, fibroblasts, connective tissue matrix, bone (enhances osteoporosis) and the root surface (Lang and Lindhe, 2015).

Smokers show poorer response to all treatment modalities, including non-surgical, surgical and regeneration compared to former smokers and non-smokers (Garcia, 2005; Kotsakis *et al.*, 2015; Patel *et al.*, 2012).

Quitting smoking can significantly reduce the progression of periodontal disease and has an additional beneficial influence on the reduction of pocket depths following non-surgical treatment (Preshaw *et al.*, 2005). Therefore, smoking cessation should be considered an important part of periodontal treatment (Chambrone *et al.*, 2013).

6.5.2.2 Diabetes

Literature shows that diabetes is a significant and major risk factor for periodontitis (Preshaw *et al.*, 2010). Both type 1 and type 2 diabetes increase periodontal disease's prevalence, extent and severity in children and adults. Susceptibility to periodontitis is increased by approximately threefold in people with diabetes. There is a clear relationship between degree of hyperglycaemia and severity of periodontitis, with a strong positive association between HbA1c levels and periodontitis (Chapple *et al.*, 2014; Preshaw and Bissett, 2013).

Several studies show a two-way relationship between diabetes and periodontitis as insulin resistance can develop in response to chronic bacterial infection (Casanova *et al.*, 2014; Chapple *et al.*, 2013).

Diabetes can affect the following parameters which can influence the progression of periodontal disease (Taylor *et al.*, 2013).

- Oral microbiota can change with increased number of spirochaetes and motile rods (Marigo *et al.*, 2011).
- Host response is affected due to reduced PMN leucocyte function and chemotaxis, increased level of cytokines (IL-1, TNF) and PGE_2 in crevicular fluid, and reduced growth and synthesis of connective tissue (Sonnenschein and Meyle, 2015).
- Healing and treatment response are affected as a result of impaired wound healing due to delayed vascularisation, decreased collagen synthesis, increased

degradation by collagenase and decrease in growth factor production (Abiko and Selimovic, 2010).

There is low-quality evidence suggesting that non-surgical periodontal treatment results in reduction of HbA1c level in the short term (Simpson *et al.*, 2015)

The outcome of periodontal treatment in poorly controlled diabetic patients is poorer than that of non-diabetic patients but treatment outcome in well-controlled diabetic patients is similar to non-diabetic patients (Lang and Lindhe, 2015).

6.5.2.3 Genetics

Evidence from classic twin studies (Michalowicz *et al.*, 1991b) suggests that genetic determinants are significant modifiers of the periodontitis phenotype. Chronic periodontitis has approximately 50% heritability (Michalowicz *et al.*, 1991a). Kornman *et al.* (1997) showed the association of severe periodontitis with a composite genotype based on specific polymorphisms in the IL-1 gene cluster.

6.5.2.4 Osteoporosis

Studies have suggested increased susceptibility to periodontitis in postmenopausal osteoporotic women due to reduced bone density and strength (Martinez-Maestre *et al.*, 2010). Smoking can further reduce the oestrogen level and further weaken the bone in patients with osteoporosis. Oestrogen hormone replacement therapy (HRT) reduces the chance of tooth loss in patients with osteoporosis (Krall, 2001).

6.5.2.5 Psychosocial Factors

Evidence supports an association between psychosocial stress and chronic periodontitis (Preeja *et al.*, 2013). Stress can affect interactions among the nervous, endocrine and immune systems and therefore periodontal health as well as the response to treatment. Stress, depression and behavioural changes may also affect oral hygiene and smoking habits.

6.5.2.6 Other Considerations

Literature suggests a strong association between periodontal infections and cardiovascular disease (Scannapieco *et al.*, 2003). Risk of cardiovascular disease is increased by 20% in patients with periodontal disease. The risk of cardiorenal mortality is three times higher in diabetic patients with severe periodontitis compared to diabetic patients without severe periodontitis. Various factors such as LPS, immune system disorders, cytokines, oral bacteria in atheromatic plaque lesions, blood markers and immunoglobulins have been investigated (Nguyen *et al.*, 2015).

Periodontitis has also been associated with pregnancy complications such as late miscarriage, stillbirth and early spontaneous preterm birth. Possible mechanisms include distant infection, bacteraemia and LPS effects (Zi *et al.*, 2014).

6.6 Microbiology

Microbial aetiology of periodontal disease has been established in studies of experimental gingivitis (Loe *et al.*, 1965; Theilade *et al.*, 1966) and experimental animal models of periodontitis (Lindhe *et al.*, 1973).

The non-specific plaque theory hypothesised plaque as a mass to be the cause of periodontal disease (Theilade, 1986). However, according to the specific plaque theory, periodontal disease is due to overgrowth of specific bacterial pathogens (Loesche, 1979).

Dental plaque is formed by primary colonisation by gram-positive facultative bacteria such as *Streptococcus sanguis*, followed by gram-negative anaerobes such as *Porphyromonas gingivalis*. Dental plaque is a true biofilm which consists of bacteria in a matrix composed mainly of extracellular bacterial polymers (exopolysaccharides 50–95%) and salivary and/or gingival exudate products. Biofilm protects the bacteria from antimicrobial agents due to slow growth, nutritional status, temperature, pH, barrier and buffering (Socransky and Haffajee, 2005). Communication between periodontal pathogens is further enhanced by quorum sensing, which is signalling between bacteria and regulation of expression of specific genes (Plancak *et al.*, 2015). This emphasises the importance of mechanical removal of plaque.

The composition of subgingival plaque is similar to supragingival plaque in healthy patients but it changes when a periodontal pocket develops and different bacteria colonise on the tooth side and the tissue side of the pocket (Palmer, 2010). The composition of subgingival biofilm is altered following periodontal therapy (Haffajee *et al.*, 2006).

Dental calculus can be formed in 2 weeks after plaque accumulation and is a secondary aetiological factor for periodontitis by acting as a plaque retentive factor (White, 1997).

Different experimental techniques have been used for bacterial detection in plaque samples, including microscopy, bacterial culturing, enzyme-linked immunosorbent assay (ELISA), and molecular biological methods such as polymerase chain reaction (PCR) and DNA–DNA hybridization (Russell, 1992).

Haffajee and Socransky adapted Koch's postulates for identification of periodontal pathogens and proposed the following criteria (Haffajee and Socransky, 1994; Socransky and Haffajee, 1994).

- Association by elevated odds ratios in disease
- Elimination by conversion of disease to health when bacteria are suppressed

- Development of host response
- Presence of virulence factors
- Evidence from animal studies corroborating the observations in humans
- Support from risk assessment studies

Based on the above criteria, the consensus report of the 1996 World Workshop on Periodontics identified three species – AA, PG and *Bacteroides forsythus* – as causative factors for periodontitis.

Aggregatibacter (formerly *Actinobacillus) actinomycetemcomitans* is a gram-negative, saccharolytic, capnophilic, round-ended rod. It can invade gingival epithelial cells and elevated levels of AA are found in localised aggressive periodontitis. It has six serotypes: a–g (Henderson *et al.*, 2010).

Porphyromonas gingivalis is a gram-negative anaerobic, asaccharolytic rod. Its levels are elevated in destructive and actively progressing periodontitis lesions. It uses a number of virulence factors such as LPS, fimbriae, capsule and gingipains to invade tissue and evade host defence mechanisms (How *et al.*, 2016; Mysak *et al.*, 2014).

Tannerella forsythia is a gram-negative anaerobic, spindle-shaped pleomorphic rod. It produces trypsin-like proteolytic activity and its levels are elevated in actively progressing lesions and in subjects with refractory periodontitis (Sharma, 2010).

Other bacterial species associated with periodontitis include spirochaetes, *Prevotella intermedia, Fusobacterium nucleatum, Campylobacter rectus, Eikenella corrodens, Peptostreptococcus micros, Selenomonas, Eubacterium* and *Milleri* streptococci (Papapanou, 2002).

Mechanisms of bacterial pathogenicity include adhesins, co-aggregation, multiplication, interbacterial relationships, overcoming host defences, tissue damage by producing hydrogen sulfide, endotoxins (LPS), enzymes (protease and collagenase) and tissue invasion.

Factors affecting the composition of subgingival plaque include (Lang and Lindhe, 2015):

- periodontal disease status
- local environment, including pocket depth
- host factors, including genetic background, smoking, diet, diabetes and obesity
- transmission of bacteria – both vertical (parents to children) and horizontal (within married couples) have been recognised.

Prerequisites for periodontal disease initiation and progression are listed below.

- Presence of virulent periodontal pathogens of adequate number, type, site and the possession of necessary genetic elements.
- Local environment factors such as poor plaque control to accommodate the bacterial pathogens.
- Host susceptibility such as diabetes and smoking.

6.7 Pathogenesis

Pathogenesis of chronic periodontitis includes four phases of progression of gingival and periodontal lesions (Page and Schroeder, 1976).

1) The initial lesion develops within 24 hours in the presence of plaque and is characterised by vasodilation, increased permeability and gingival crevicular fluid (GCF) flow and PMN migration in the gingival tissue.
2) The early lesion develops after several days of plaque accumulation and is characterised by an increased number of active capillaries, increased redness of gingivae, PMN infiltration, collagen breakdown and junctional epithelium (JE) proliferation.
3) In the established lesion, JE is replaced with pocket epithelium harbouring leucocytes and PMNs with plasma cell domination.
4) The advanced lesion is characterised by deep periodontal pockets, loss of connective tissue attachment and periodontal bone loss.

Inflammatory cytokines, including IL-1 and TNF-alpha, produced as a result of plaque-induced inflammation, can cause bone resorption. PGE_2 also activates osteoclasts to produce matrix metalloproteinases (MMPs) and cause tissue destruction (Gemmell *et al.*, 1997). Receptor activator of nuclear factor kappa-B ligand (RANKL) is also a cytokine from the TNF family that promotes activation of osteoclasts and bone resorption (Cochran, 2008).

6.8 Role of Occlusal Trauma

Occlusal trauma can be classified into two main categories.

- Primary occlusal trauma is an injury to a periodontium of normal height as a result of excessive occlusal force.
- Secondary occlusal trauma is an injury to a periodontium of reduced height as a result of excessive occlusal force.

There is controversy in the literature over whether abnormal occlusal forces can change the course of plaque-induced periodontal disease and cause angular bony defects in teeth with periodontitis (Glickman's concept) (Glickman, 1965) or if angular bony defects and pockets develop equally in teeth with or without occlusal trauma (Waerhaug's concept) (Waerhaug, 1979).

Occlusal forces can be classified into two main categories: orthodontic type force and jiggling-type trauma. Studies show that in the absence of inflammatory disease, jiggling forces do not affect supracrestal connective tissue attachments and do not cause pocket formation in healthy periodontium (Green and Levine, 1996). They may cause periodontal ligament (PDL) widening and increased mobility (physiological adaptation) which may be reversed following occlusal adjustment and elimination of the traumatic force (Foz *et al.*, 2012). However, long-term high-intensity jiggling-type trauma to teeth with active plaque-associated inflammatory periodontal disease may act as a destructive co-factor and enhance the rate of disease progression (Polson and Zander, 1983).

6.9 Treatment

6.9.1 Treatment Goals

The aims of periodontal treatment include:

- elimination of pain and symptoms associated with periodontal disease
- addressing major periodontal risk factors such as poor plaque control, smoking and uncontrolled diabetes
- reduction or resolution of gingivitis and bleeding on probing
- reduction in probing pocket depth; no residual pockets greater than 5 mm should be present
- elimination of furcation defects in multirooted teeth and establishing access for cleaning furcation areas
- restoration of aesthetics and function.

6.9.2 Treatment Phases

Periodontal treatment includes four main stages – systemic phase, initial hygiene phase, corrective phase and maintenance – which are discussed in detail below.

6.9.2.1 Systemic Phase

The aim of this treatment phase is to eliminate or decrease the influence of systemic risk factors and to protect the patient and dental care provider against infectious hazard (Scully, 2014). Measures include the following.

- Cross-infection control and appropriate immunisation.
- Appropriate precautions for patients with serious systemic conditions such as cardiovascular or cerebrovascular disease, diabetes and patients with history of allergic reactions.
- It is important to control anxiety and pain with effective local anaesthesia and appropriate postoperative analgesia. Premedication can be indicated in anxious patients.
- Patients with bleeding disorders (receiving anticoagulants, liver disease, haemophilia) will require medical consultation and INR check and may need factor replacement and tranexamic acid mouthwash use following treatment. Atraumatic practice is recommended in this group of patients with the use of appropriate wound dressings to reduce the risk of bleeding.
- Smoking cessation programme following careful assessment of the patient's smoking history. This may include pharmacotherapy and using smoking cessation approaches such as the 5As (ask, advise, assess, assist, arrange), AAR (ask-advise-refer) and AAC (ask-advise-connect) (Vidrine *et al.*, 2013).

6.9.2.2 Initial Hygiene Phase

This phase aims to eliminate the infection in the oral cavity by complete removal of all soft and hard deposits on the root surfaces, including plaque retentive factors. It also aims to motivate the patient using approaches such as motivational interviewing (MI) and giving oral hygiene education (OHE) to perform optimal plaque control according to the methods described below (Lang and Lindhe, 2015).

6.9.2.2.1 Mechanical Supragingival Plaque Control

Tooth Brushing Different brushing techniques are used by patients, including horizontal, vertical, circular, scrubbing, sulcular (Bass) (cleaning under the gingival margin at 45°), vibratory (Stillman), vibratory (Charters), roll, and modified Bass/Stillman techniques (with added roll stroke). No method has been proven to be superior to any other. However, the modified Bass technique is recommended for subgingival cleaning in patients with deep periodontal pockets.

An ideal toothbrush should have appropriate handle size, head size, end-rounded nylon or polymer filaments not larger than 0.23 mm (0.009 inches) in diameter, soft-medium filament as defined by ISO, and appropriate filament pattern.

The quality of cleaning is more important than its frequency. Minimum frequency of brushing to reverse gingivitis is once a day and twice a day is generally recommended. Duration of brushing is consistently correlated with the amount of plaque removal and the optimum duration according to studies is 2 minutes.

Modern electric toothbrushes with oscillating rotating brush technology have become more effective at removing supragingival plaque than manual toothbrushes and enhance patient compliance (Rosema *et al.*, 2016; Sicilia *et al.*, 2002; Yaacob *et al.*, 2014).

A single-tufted toothbrush is ideal for cleaning the distal surfaces of the molar teeth, crowded or spaced teeth, around fixed bridge abutments and orthodontic appliances, and furcation and recession defects.

Interdental Cleaning Interdental brushes are the most effective method of interdental plaque removal (Salzer *et al.*, 2015). The largest size of interdental brush that fits in the interdental space should be selected for effective cleaning in patients with periodontitis. Interdental brushing is also useful for cleaning concave root surfaces and grade III furcation defects.

Dental floss and tape can be used in areas with tight contacts between the teeth and where it is difficult or impossible to use interdental brushes.

Woodsticks are less effective than interdental brushes in cleaning the lingual side of interproximal surfaces and their long-term use can cause permanent loss of interdental papillae.

Adjunctive Aids Dental water jet is a safe and effective oral hygiene aid that has an additional benefit in reducing gingivitis. Pulsating devices are more effective than jets with continuous flow (Jahn, 2010).

Tongue cleaning is recommended daily. Tongue scrapers and cleaners are more efficient than toothbrushes for tongue cleaning and are effective in control of oral halitosis (Outhouse *et al.*, 2006).

Plaque-disclosing agents such as erythrosine, fuchsin or fluorescin-containing dyes are useful to demonstrate the plaque to the patient before and after tooth brushing and calculate the plaque score.

6.9.2.2.2 Chemical Supragingival Plaque Control

Toothpastes are the most practical and cost-effective method of chemical plaque control for most people.

Antiseptic mouthwashes are also used for chemical plaque control. Chlorhexidine (CHX) is the most studied and effective antiseptic for plaque inhibition and prevention of gingivitis (James *et al.*, 2017). Phenols and essential oil mouthwashes also have similar antibacterial effects (Araujo *et al.*, 2015).

Biological aspects of different oral care products, including efficacy, biocompatibility and side effects of different types of toothpastes and mouthwashes, have been thoroughly discussed elsewhere (Moharamzadeh, 2016).

6.9.2.3 Non-Surgical Therapy

The aim of non-surgical treatment is to eliminate both microbial biofilm and calculus from the root surface and adjacent soft tissues.

Since bacterial toxins do not penetrate subsurface cementum, there is no need for aggressive root surface substance removal. Also, curettage of the granulation tissue has no added benefit over root surface debridement alone (Lindhe and Nyman, 1985).

Hand instrumentation offers good tactile sensation and minimises the risk of aerosol production. However, it is more time-consuming and technique sensitive and can lead to excessive tooth surface tissue removal. The sickle and hoe are used for supragingival scaling and the curette is suitable for subgingival scaling. Modified pen grasp with finger rest is recommended for hand instruments.

Ultrasonic scalers use an electric current of 18 000–45 000 Hz and have two types: magnetostrictive (magnetic field causes expansion and contraction of the insert) and piezoelectric (works by dimensional changes in the handpiece). There is no significant difference in clinical performance between the two types according to clinical studies (Sculean *et al.*, 2004).

Hand instrumentation and ultrasonic scaling produce similar periodontal healing in terms of improvement in pocket depth (PD), BOP and clinical attachment level (CAL) (Ioannou *et al.*, 2009). Sonic and ultrasonic scalers are faster and less technique sensitive, produce less tooth surface damage and provide better access in deep pockets and furcation areas with flushing effect compared to hand instruments. However, clinical improvement is less pronounced in furcation sites than in other locations following non-surgical therapy regardless of the type of instrument used (Loos *et al.*, 1989).

Root surface debridement (RSD) results in decreased total number of subgingival bacteria and a shift in the relative proportion of different microbial species and reduction of periodontal pathogens (Haffajee *et al.*, 1997).

Full-mouth disinfection (FMD) includes full-mouth RSD within 24 hours combined with subgingival irrigation with 1% CHX, tongue brushing with CHX 1% gel, and continued use of 0.2% CHX mouthwash for 2 weeks following treatment (Quirynen *et al.*, 1995). Studies have shown modest additional short-term improvement in periodontal condition using the FMD protocol compared to conventional treatment (Eberhard *et al.*, 2015; Fang *et al.*, 2016).

Adjunctive laser therapy is capable of removing plaque and calculus with low mechanical stress and no smear layer formation. However, lasers may cause eye damage, tissue damage and excessive destruction, and have high costs. Some studies have shown comparable clinical results to RSD alone with no adjunctive benefits (Slot *et al.*, 2014; Zhao *et al.*, 2014) but more recent systematic reviews have reported additional short-term benefits of adjunctive diode laser treatment (Qadri *et al.*, 2015) and photodynamic therapy (Xue *et al.*, 2017) compared to RSD alone.

Side effects of non-surgical therapy include the following.

- Pain which is often mild to moderate, peaks 2–8 hours after treatment and can be more severe in anxious patients. The use of NSAIDs can be helpful in reduction of postoperative pain.
- Root dentine sensitivity is usually moderate in most cases and reduces over 4 weeks following treatment.
- Recession can occur following reduction in pocket depth and patients should be informed of this prior to initial treatment.

Healing following non-surgical therapy occurs within the first 3 months. Re-evaluation at 3 months should include plaque scores, BOP, suppuration on probing, probing pocket depth (PPD), recession, CAL and mobility assessment.

Outcome predictors for non-surgical therapy include (Claffey and Egelberg, 1995; Claffey *et al.*, 1990) the following.

- The extent and severity of the disease at baseline.
- The number of sites with residual pockets equal to or greater than 6 mm at re-evaluation bears a direct relationship to future periodontal breakdown.
- BOP is a moderate predictor of future attachment loss and the absence of BOP is a good indicator of periodontal health and stability.

6.9.2.3.1 *Management of Tooth Mobility*

Tooth mobility can be physiological or pathological. Physiological mobility is characterised by increased occlusal load and PDL widening in the absence of any active inflammatory disease.

Pathological and progressive mobility is often associated with actively progressing inflammatory periodontal disease and can be characterised by the following features.

- Increasing tooth mobility, tooth migration or drifting.
- Fremitus defined by the movement of a tooth or teeth subjected to *functional* occlusal forces.
- Persistent discomfort on eating.

Teeth with physiological mobility and normal periodontal bone height as well as the mobile tooth with increased PDL width and reduced bone height after successful treatment of periodontal disease can be managed by occlusal adjustment if necessary (Foz *et al.*, 2012).

A mobile tooth with normal PDL width but reduced bone height in the absence of inflammatory periodontal disease can be managed without any treatment if it is asymptomatic or can be splinted to adjacent teeth if the mobility is causing discomfort for the patient (Forabosco *et al.*, 2006).

Teeth with progressive pathological mobility, active bone loss and inflammatory disease often have a poorer prognosis and management options include:

- maintaining the tooth and treatment of the inflammatory periodontal disease and considering splinting the tooth to reduce mobility
- extraction and replacement of the tooth.

6.9.2.4 Corrective Phase (Additional Therapy)

This phase includes periodontal surgery, endodontic therapy, restorative and prosthetic treatment.

6.9.2.4.1 *Periodontal Surgery*

Periodontal surgery is indicated in the following circumstances.

- Impaired access for RSD mainly when there are residual pockets deeper than 5 mm after repeated non-surgical RSD.
- Impaired access for self-performed plaque control including gingival enlargement and overhanging restoration margins.

Periodontal surgery can be contraindicated in the following conditions.

- Poor patient co-operation with plaque control as surgery in plaque-contaminated patients may cause additional destruction of the periodontium (Lindhe and Nyman, 1975).
- Medically compromised patients, including those with severe cardiovascular disease, blood disorders, patients with organ transplantation, severely immunosuppressed patients, and neurological disorders including multiple sclerosis and Parkinson's disease.
- Smokers show poor response to all treatment modalities.

Different surgical techniques have been developed for open flap debridement which can be categorised into two main groups.

- Flaps that position the gingival margin apically, including original Widman flap, Neumann flap, apically repositioned flaps and the distal wedge technique (Lang and Lindhe, 2015). These flaps can be suitable for posterior teeth with no aesthetic concerns and when the aim of surgery is resective pocket elimination.
- Flaps that are maintained coronally, including Kirkland flap, modified Widman flap (Ramfjord and Nissle, 1974) and papillae preservation flaps (Cortellini *et al.*, 1995). These flaps are suitable for the anterior aesthetic region and where the aim of surgery is periodontal regeneration.

Different suturing techniques for closure of periodontal flaps include the following.

- Interrupted interdental sutures provide close adaptation of the soft tissue to the bone.
- Horizontal mattress sutures can be useful when there are large distances between the tissues.
- Vertical mattress sutures can be indicated where the wound edges tend to evert.
- Suspensory sutures are used when surgery involves only the buccal or lingual aspect of the teeth and also when the buccal and lingual flaps are repositioned at different levels.
- Continuous sutures are used when flaps involving several teeth are to be repositioned apically.

Suture materials can be classified into natural or synthetic, absorbable or non-absorbable, multifilament (braided) or monofilament sutures.

Recommended postoperative care following open flap debridement includes:

- appropriate analgesia
- suture removal 7–10 days
- CHX 0.2% mouthrinse twice a day for the first 2–3 weeks. Patient not to perform mechanical cleaning and not to chew in the treated area during this period
- use of soft toothbrush and toothpicks for interdental areas after the above period
- two-weekly dental visits to monitor plaque control.

6.9.2.4.2 *Outcome of Periodontal Surgery*

Classic longitudinal studies by the Michigan group (Ramfjord *et al.*, 1987) and Gothenburg group (Lindhe *et al.*, 1984) evaluated the outcome of surgical and non-surgical periodontal treatment and the following observations were made.

- All surgical procedures resulted in a decrease in PD with greater reduction at initially deeper sites.
- Surgical therapy created greater short-term reduction of PD than non-surgically performed RSD but long-term (5–8 years) results showed variability in outcomes.
- In sites with shallow initial probing depth, both short- and long-term data show that surgery creates a greater loss of clinical attachment than non-surgical treatment, whereas in sites with initially deep (>7 mm) pockets, a greater gain of clinical attachment is generally obtained with surgery. Irrespective of treatment modality used, initially deeper pocket sites will experience more pronounced signs of recession.
- In molar sites, the outcome of surgical approach was better than non-surgical treatment.
- Surgery without osseous recontouring results in equal or greater clinical attachment gain than surgery with osseous recontouring.
- Deliberate excision of the pocket epithelium and soft tissue lesion by curettage did not improve the healing result.
- Patients with good postoperative plaque control maintained clinical attachment levels and PD reductions after surgery more consistently than patients with poor oral hygiene. There was no difference in longitudinal maintenance of clinical attachment levels between non-surgical and surgical treatments.

6.9.2.4.3 *Treatment of Teeth with Furcation Involvement*

This section focuses on the management of teeth with furcation involvement due to periodontal disease only. Management of periodontic-endodontic lesions is discussed in Chapter 42.

The aim of treatment is to eliminate microbial plaque from the root complex and establish an anatomy of the affected root surfaces that enables access for cleaning by the patient.

Recommended treatment options include the following.

- Degree I furcation involvement: RSD and furcation plasty
- Degree II furcation involvement: Furcation plasty, tunnel preparation, root resection and regeneration in mandibular molars
- Degree III furcation involvement: Tunnel preparation, root resection and extraction

Factors to consider when choosing the treatment option include:

- tooth-related factors, such as degree of furcation involvement, amount of remaining bone support, probing depth, tooth mobility, endodontic condition, available sound tooth structure, tooth position and occlusion
- patient-related factors, such as strategic value of the tooth, patient's function and aesthetics demand, patient's age and health, oral hygiene.

Furcation plasty involves odontoplasty and osteoplasty at the level of the furcation entrance and is often used in buccal or lingual furcations. It carries the risk of root sensitivity in vital teeth.

Tunnel preparation is indicated for deep degree II and III defects in mandibular molars with short root trunk, wide separation angle and long divergence between the roots. It involves widening the furcation area by removing some inter-radicular bone and apical repositioning of the flap. The associated risks include sensitivity and root caries. Therefore, topical application of CHX and fluoride varnish in the maintenance phase is recommended.

Root separation and resection (RSR) is suitable for teeth with long, wide and divergent roots and short root trunk with adequate bone support for the remaining roots. In maxillary molars, the disto-buccal root is the shortest and is often removed. The mesio-buccal root is preferred to the palatal root as it has a large surface area and is aligned with premolar teeth and located centrally. However, RCT is more difficult in the mesio-buccal than the palatal root. In mandibular molars, the mesial root is bigger but it is more difficult to manage due to the presence of concavity and two canals with thin walls. The distal root has one canal and a large root with more dentine and is a better candidate for a post crown. Also, retention of the distal root results in a longer dental arch than retention of the mesial root.

Clinical stages for RSR include the following.

- Endodontic treatment prior to RSR.
- Fabrication of provisional restorations.
- Root separation and resection and preparation of the remaining root cones to allow maximum separation with adequate parallelism of the walls.
- Periodontal surgery, osseous recontouring and elimination of hard and soft tissue deposits and existing undercuts.
- Relining of the provisional restorations with cold-cured acrylic resin and cementation of the temporary crowns. Margins of the crown must be at least 3 mm above the alveolar bone crest.
- Suture removal in 1 week and oral hygiene instructions.
- Final prosthetic restoration.

The outcome of RSR was evaluated in a 10-year clinical trial showing 93% survival rate of root resected furcation-involved teeth and 99% survival of non-furcation-involved teeth (Carnevale *et al.*, 1998).

Long-term (8–12 year) prognosis of teeth with furcation involvement treated by resective versus non-resective approaches was assessed by Svardstrom and Wennstrom (2000). Data collected from a total of 1313 first and second molars in 222 patients revealed that 96% of the molars were still in function without RSR treatment. The survival rate for molar teeth with RSR treatment was 89%. It was concluded that a conservative approach to the treatment of molars with even deep furcation involvement may offer a high long-term survival rate with appropriate maintenance.

Regeneration of furcation defects is indicated in class II furcation defects (Reddy *et al.*, 2015). The outcome of regeneration improves in the following conditions.

- The interproximal bone is located at a level close to the CEJ of the proximal surfaces (keyhole type of degree II involvement).
- Thorough RSD is carried out in the furcation area.
- A meticulous plaque control programme is put in place.
- Thick gingival biotype with at least 1 mm gingival thickness is present.

Different regeneration approaches are described in detail in the following section.

6.9.2.4.4 Periodontal Regeneration

Regenerative procedures are indicated for aesthetics, recession and sensitivity treatment, and management of furcation involvement (Lang and Lindhe, 2015).

Periodontal intrabony defects can be classified as three-wall, two-wall, one-wall and interproximal crater. Defect morphology can be assessed prior to surgery by clinical and radiographic evaluation, use of transgingival probing and bone sounding, and is confirmed after flap elevation.

Prognostic factors for periodontal regeneration are listed below.

- Poor plaque control, BOP and high bacterial load are associated with poor outcome for regeneration.
- Smoking significantly impairs regenerative outcome (Patel *et al.*, 2012).
- Defect morphology including the number of walls, the angle, depth and width of the defect, may affect the outcome. Three-wall and narrow deep defects often regenerate better than wide one-wall defects. However, the relevance of defect morphology parameters may be diminished with the use of appropriate regenerative technique.
- Tooth factors: tooth mobility (greater than grade I) negatively affects the outcome of regeneration (Cortellini *et al.*, 2001).

Different approaches that have been use for periodontal regeneration are discussed below.

Bone Grafts Bone grafts include autologous grafts harvested from intraoral or extraoral sites, allogeneic grafts such as freeze-dried or decalcified bone, xenogeneic grafts, such as processed bovine bone, and alloplastic materials such as hydroxyapatite, beta-tricalcium phosphate, polymers and bioactive glass (Almela *et al.*, 2017; Paknejad *et al.*, 2017).

Evidence shows that the implantation of alloplastic bone graft materials alone in periodontal defects may offer limited or even no periodontal regeneration (Sculean *et al.*, 2015).

Guided Tissue Regeneration (GTR) The use of guided tissue regeneration membranes offers good results but variable data are available due to factors such as the amount of remaining PDL, morphology of the defect, technical difficulties, gingival recession and bacterial contamination of the membrane and wound infection.

Membrane exposure and bacterial contamination are major complications and can be reduced significantly using a modified papillae preservation flap (Cortellini *et al.*, 1995). The use of local or systemic antibiotics can reduce the risk of infection. Membrane collapse into the defect also results in decreased regeneration.

Guided tissue regeneration membranes can be divided into two main categories.

- Non-absorbable materials such as e-PTFE (Gore-Tex) reinforced with titanium are capable of maintaining their shape and avoiding collapse of the membrane, especially in one-wall defects.
- Bioabsorbable materials such as bovine or porcine collagen carry the risk of disease transmission and complications such as early degradation, epithelial downgrowth and early loss of material.

Evidence shows that GTR results in greater improvement in periodontal indices and offers higher regenerative potential than open flap surgery alone in the treatment of intrabony defects. However, there is a marked degree of variability between different studies (Aichelmann-Reidy and Reynolds, 2008; Needleman *et al.*, 2006).

Enamel Matrix Proteins Application of Emdogain (EMD), enamel matrix protein derived from pigs, following EDTA conditioning of the root surface has been shown to enhance new cementum formation with inserting collagen fibres and new bone formation within the periodontal defect. EMD offers great potential for regeneration in three-wall defects. Compared to open flap debridement alone, faster healing has been reported with EMD. EMD provides comparable regeneration outcomes to the use of GTR membranes but is associated with less postoperative pain and swelling and less gingival recession (Esposito *et al.*, 2009; Koop *et al.*, 2012; Mueller *et al.*, 2013).

Other biologically active regenerative materials, including growth factors such as platelet-derived growth factor (PDGF), insulin-like growth factor (IGF), transforming growth factor (TGF) and bone morphogenic proteins (BMPs), have been shown to encourage bone formation and have positive effects on periodontal regeneration (Calin and Patrascu, 2016; Trombelli and Farina, 2008).

According to a systematic review by the American Academy of Periodontology (AAP) Regeneration Workshop, biologics including a combination of EMD and recombinant human PDGF-BB with beta-tricalcium phosphate produce regeneration outcomes comparable to a combination of demineralised freeze-dried bone allograft and GTR. The results of these combination therapies are superior to those of open flap debridement alone in terms of improvement in clinical parameters in the treatment of intrabony defects (Kao *et al.*, 2015).

Combination approaches now appear to provide the best outcomes for periodontal regeneration (Sculean *et al.*, 2015).

6.9.2.5 Maintenance Phase

The aim of supportive periodontal therapy (SPT) is the prevention of reinfection and disease recurrence. Numerous studies have shown that the risk of recurrence is very high in the absence of SPT (Axelsson and Lindhe, 1981).

The time interval between visits during the maintenance phase depends on the periodontal risk assessment (PRA) established at recall after the corrective phase. The continuous multilevel risk assessment matrix developed by Lang and Tonetti (2003) is a useful tool to establish and monitor periodontal risk throughout SPT. According to this system, important risk parameters include:

- percentage of sites with BOP
- number of residual pockets greater than 4 mm
- the number of teeth lost, not including wisdom teeth
- bone loss in relation to age in the worst affected site
- systemic conditions such as diabetes
- environmental factors such as cigarette smoking.

Tooth-level risk factors include tooth position (crowding), furcation involvement, iatrogenic factors such as overhanging restorations, residual periodontal support and mobility.

Site-level risk factors include:

- BOP, as the absence of BOP is a reliable indicator of periodontal stability
- PD and attachment loss indicate the extent and severity of the disease
- suppuration is a positive predictive factor for disease progression and indicates an exacerbation period.

The recall system must include medical and smoking history update, oral hygiene assessment, full periodontal charting and recording indices, sensibility testing of suspected teeth, reinforcement of oral hygiene, instrumentation of the sites with residual deep pockets (≥4 mm) under LA if necessary, and fluoride application on the exposed root surfaces to prevent dental caries. Regular assessment of prosthetic restorations and radiographic evaluation may also be indicated.

Case Study

A 62-year-old male patient referred by his general dental practitioner presented with pain associated with the lower left molar and upper right premolar and molar teeth, bleeding gums, paraesthesia of the lower lip on the left side and mobility of teeth.

The patient was medically fit and well. He had been smoking 5–10 cigarettes per day for the past 15 years.

Clinical examination showed generalised gingival inflammation and enlargement, recession on canine teeth, BOP and suppuration. Generalised subgingival and supragingival plaque and calculus were found.

The patient's preoperative clinical photograph and radiographs are shown in Figures 6.1 and 6.2 respectively. Table 6.1 shows full periodontal charting at the baseline.

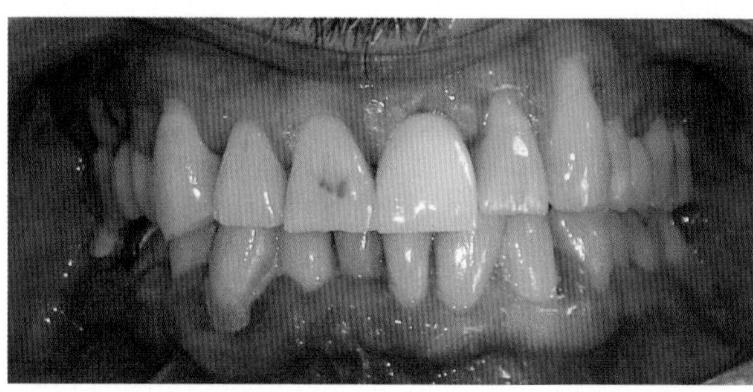

Figure 6.1 Preoperative clinical photograph showing gingival inflammation, swelling and recession.

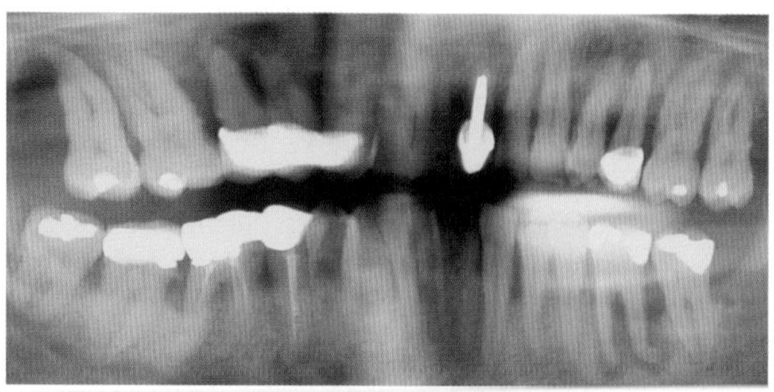

Figure 6.2 Preoperative panoramic radiograph showing periodontal bone loss with generalised extent, moderate to advanced severity and vertical pattern, interproximal calculus deposits and periapical radiolucencies associated with multiple teeth.

Diagnoses

- Generalised moderate to advanced chronic periodontitis and gingival recession
- Periodontic-endodontic lesions LL6, UR5, UR7
- Chronic apical periodontitis UR4

Prognosis

The prognosis for LL6 and UR7 was hopeless due to advanced periodontal bone loss, furcation involvement, presence of periodontic-endodontic lesion and grade III mobility of these teeth. The prognosis of UR5 was also hopeless due to advanced bone loss, periodontic-endodontic lesion and grade III mobility.

Table 6.1 Preoperative full periodontal charting showing generalised deep periodontal pockets, mobility and furcation involvement of several teeth.

Mobility	III	I	III	II	I			I			I	I		I
Recession	2	2			2					5			3	3
PPD (Buccal)	11-10-4	569	12-12-10	5-4-10	825	525	427	736	623	427	835	659	939	974
Upper teeth	7	6	5	4	3	2	1	1	2	3	4	5	6	7
PPD (Palatal)	9-11-8	356	757	727	746	534	447	626	625	578	826	829	747	537
Recession	3	5											5	5
Furcation	F3	F1											F1	F1

Mobility	I			I										III	
Recession		1				1								1	
PPD (Lingual)	756	545	637	638	634	736	753	434	722	323	328	733	227	578	443
Lower teeth	8	7	6	5	4	3	2	1	1	2	3	4	5	6	7
PPD (Buccal)	555	636	827	837	627	727	323	527	732	223	228	822	225	4-11-11	324
Recession		1				3			1	1		2		2	
Furcation	F1		F1											F3	

The prognosis for the maxillary molar teeth, with advanced vertical bone loss and furcation involvement, was better than the other molar teeth with less bone loss and no furcation involvement.

The prognosis for the teeth with moderate periodontal bone loss was questionable (guarded) and would depend on the patient's compliance with oral hygiene and smoking cessation.

Treatment Strategy

- Initial hygiene phase and smoking cessation advice
- Extraction of hopeless symptomatic teeth
- Non-surgical therapy
- Periodontal reassessment
- Corrective phase including root canal treatment of UR4 and surgical open flap debridement of upper left quadrant
- Reassessment and SPT

Clinical Procedures Undertaken

1) OHE including modified Bass technique and interdental brushing.
2) Smoking cessation advice.
3) Extraction of hopeless symptomatic infected LL6 (which was also causing lip paraesthesia due to proximity to the ID nerve) and painful UR5, and UR7 with periodontic-endodontic lesions.
4) Full-mouth RSD under local anaesthesia.
5) Review of oral hygiene in 1 month and full periodontal reassessment 3 months following RSD.
6) Repeated cycle of non-surgical RSD under LA in sites with residual pockets of ≥4 mm deep.
7) Periodontal reassessment following two cycles of non-surgical treatment showed significant improvement in periodontal condition and reduction in PD and BOP. The patient showed satisfactory compliance with oral hygiene and smoking cessation. However, residual deep periodontal pockets (greater than 5 mm) were present only in the upper left canine to molar sites.
8) RCT of UR4 was carried out to treat chronic apical periodontitis.
9) Surgical open flap debridement was performed in UL3–UL6 to treat residual deep pockets and vertical intrabony defects (Figure 6.3).

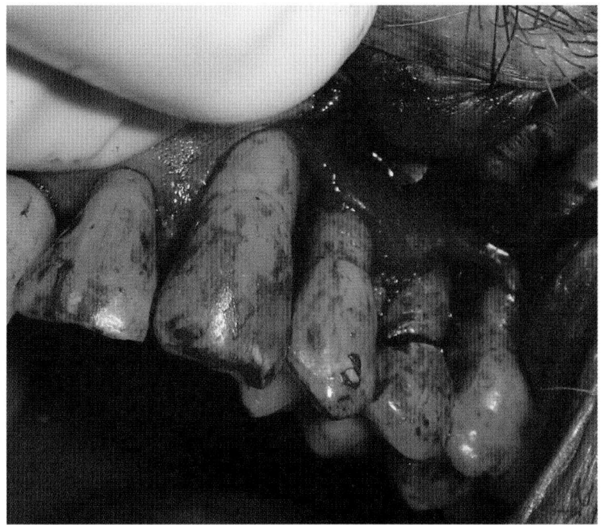

Figure 6.3 Photograph of the intrabony defects associated with the teeth in the upper left quadrant following flap elevation and removal of granulation tissue.

Periodontal reassessment showed further improvement and reduction in PD and periodontal indices. The patient was discharged back to the general dental practitioner for SPT and periodontal maintenance.

The postoperative periodontal charting is shown in Table 6.2 and the postoperative clinical photograph in Figure 6.4.

Table 6.2 Postoperative full periodontal charting showing significant improvement and reduction in PD.

Mobility	X	I	X	I	I			I			I	I		I
Recession	X	5	X	5	5			1	2	6	3	4	5	5
PPD (Buccal)	X	323	X	323	333	233	323	313	212	212	322	333	323	323
Upper teeth	7	6	5	4	3	2	1	1	2	3	4	5	6	7
PPD (Palatal)	X	323	X	322	212	323	333	323	323	322	323	222	323	223
Recession	X	6	X	3	3				1	4	2	3	6	6
Furcation	X	F1	X											

Mobility	I			I										X	
Recession		1				1								X	
PPD (Lingual)	433		323	313	322	223	313	323	322	323	323	322	223	X	334
Lower teeth	8	7	6	5	4	3	2	1	1	2	3	4	5	6	7
PPD (Buccal)	423	323	213	322	323	213	333	333	333	223	322	313	323	X	323
Recession		1				3			1	1		2		X	
Furcation	F1		F1											X	

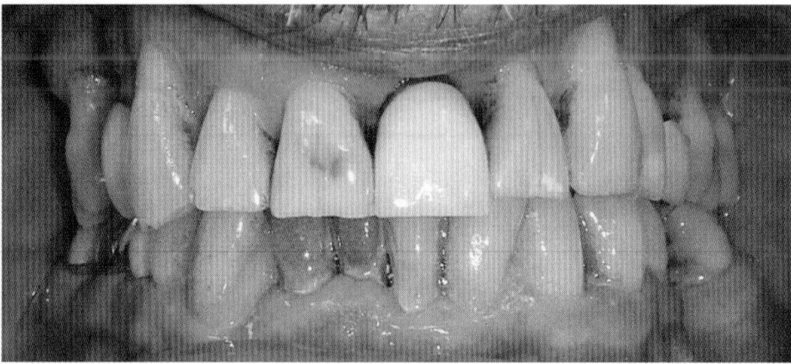

Figure 6.4 Postoperative clinical photograph.

References

(No authors) Proceedings of the 1996 World Workshop in Periodontics. Lansdowne, Virginia, July 13–17, 1996. *Ann Periodontol*, **1**, 1–947.

Abiko, Y. and Selimovic, D. (2010) The mechanism of protracted wound healing on oral mucosa in diabetes. Review. *Bosn J Basic Med Sci*, **10**, 186–191.

Aichelmann-Reidy, M.E. and Reynolds, M.A. (2008) Predictability of clinical outcomes following regenerative therapy in intrabony defects. *J Periodontol*, **79**, 387–393.

Ainamo, J. and Bay, I. (1975) Problems and proposals for recording gingivitis and plaque. *Int Dent J*, **25**, 229–235.

Ainamo, J., Barmes, D., Beagrie, G. *et al.* (1982) Development of the World Health Organization (WHO) community periodontal index of treatment needs (CPITN). *Int Dent J*, **32**, 281–291.

Almela, T., Brook, I. and Moharamzadeh, K. (2017) Bone tissue engineering in maxillofacial region, in *Biomaterials for Oral and Dental Tissue Engineering* (eds L. Tayebi and K. Moharamzadeh), Woodhead Publishing, Cambridge, pp. 387–404.

Araujo, M.W., Charles, C.A., Weinstein, R.B. *et al.* (2015) Meta-analysis of the effect of an essential oil-containing mouthrinse on gingivitis and plaque. *J Am Dent Assoc*, **146**, 610–622.

Armitage, G.C. (1999) Development of a classification system for periodontal diseases and conditions. *Ann Periodontol*, **4**, 1–6.

Axelsson, P. and Lindhe, J. (1981) The significance of maintenance care in the treatment of periodontal disease. *J Clin Periodontol*, **8**, 281–294.

BSP (2016) *The Good Practitioner's Guide to Periodontology*, British Society of Periodontology, Selby.

Calin, C. and Patrascu, I. (2016) Growth factors and beta-tricalcium phosphate in the treatment of periodontal intraosseous defects: a systematic review and meta-analysis of randomised controlled trials. *Arch Oral Biol*, **66**, 44–54.

Carlos, J.P., Wolfe, M.D. and Kingman, A. (1986) The extent and severity index: a simple method for use in epidemiologic studies of periodontal disease. *J Clin Periodontol*, **13**, 500–505.

Carnevale, G., Pontoriero, R. and di Febo, G. (1998) Long-term effects of root-resective therapy in furcation-involved molars. A 10-year longitudinal study. *J Clin Periodontol*, **25**, 209–214.

Casanova, L., Hughes, F.J. and Preshaw, P.M. (2014) Diabetes and periodontal disease: a two-way relationship. *Br Dent J*, **217**, 433–437.

Chambrone, L., Preshaw, P.M., Rosa, E.F. *et al.* (2013) Effects of smoking cessation on the outcomes of non-surgical periodontal therapy: a systematic review and individual patient data meta-analysis. *J Clin Periodontol*, **40**, 607–615.

Chapple, I.L., Genco, R. and Joint EFP/AAP Workshop on Periodontitis and Systemic Diseases (2013) Diabetes and periodontal diseases: consensus report of the Joint EFP/AAP Workshop on Periodontitis and Systemic Diseases. *J Periodontol*, **84**, S106–112.

Chapple, I.L., Borgnakke, W.S. and Genco, R.J. (2014) Hemoglobin A1c levels among patients with diabetes receiving nonsurgical periodontal treatment. *JAMA*, **311**, 1919–1920.

Claffey, N. and Egelberg, J. (1995) Clinical indicators of probing attachment loss following initial periodontal treatment in advanced periodontitis patients. *J Clin Periodontol*, **22**, 690–696.

Claffey, N., Nylund, K., Kiger, R., Garrett, S. and Egelberg, J. (1990) Diagnostic predictability of scores of plaque, bleeding, suppuration and probing depth for probing attachment loss. 3 1/2 years of observation following initial periodontal therapy. *J Clin Periodontol*, **17**, 108–114.

Cochran, D.L. (2008) Inflammation and bone loss in periodontal disease. *J Periodontol*, **79**, 1569–1576.

Cortellini, P., Prato, G.P. and Tonetti, M.S. (1995) The modified papilla preservation technique. A new surgical approach for interproximal regenerative procedures. *J Periodontol*, **66**, 261–266.

Cortellini, P., Tonetti, M.S., Lang, N.P. *et al.* (2001) The simplified papilla preservation flap in the regenerative treatment of deep intrabony defects: clinical outcomes and postoperative morbidity. *J Periodontol*, **72**, 1702–1712.

Eberhard, J., Jepsen, S., Jervoe-Storm, P.M., Needleman, I. and Worthington, H.V. (2015) Full-mouth treatment modalities (within 24 hours) for chronic periodontitis in adults. *Cochrane Database Syst Rev*, CD004622.

Esposito, M., Grusovin, M.G., Papanikolaou, N., Coulthard, P. and Worthington, H.V. (2009) Enamel matrix derivative (Emdogain(R)) for periodontal tissue regeneration in intrabony defects. *Cochrane Database Syst Rev*, **4**, CD003875.

Fang, H., Han, M., Li, Q.L., Cao, C.Y., Xia, R. and Zhang, Z.H. (2016) Comparison of full-mouth disinfection and quadrant-wise scaling in the treatment of adult chronic periodontitis: a systematic review and meta-analysis. *J Periodontal Res*, **51**, 417–430.

Forabosco, A., Grandi, T. and Cotti, B. (2006) The importance of splinting of teeth in the therapy of periodontitis. *Minerva Stomatol*, **55**, 87–97.

Foz, A.M., Artese, H.P., Horliana, A.C., Pannuti, C.M. and Romito, G.A. (2012) Occlusal adjustment associated with periodontal therapy – a systematic review. *J Dent*, **40**, 1025–1035.

Garcia, R.I. (2005) Smokers have less reductions in probing depth than non-smokers following nonsurgical periodontal therapy. *Evid Based Dent*, **6**, 37–38.

Gemmell, E., Marshall, R.I. and Seymour, G.J. (1997) Cytokines and prostaglandins in immune homeostasis and tissue destruction in periodontal disease. *Periodontology* 2000, **14**, 112–143.

Glickman, I. (1965) Clinical significance of trauma from occlusion. *J Am Dent Assoc*, **70**, 607–618.

Green, M.S. and Levine, D.F. (1996) Occlusion and the periodontium: a review and rationale for treatment. *J Calif Dent Assoc*, **24**, 19–27.

Haffajee, A.D. and Socransky, S.S. (1994) Microbial etiological agents of destructive periodontal diseases. *Periodontology* 2000, **5**, 78–111.

Haffajee, A.D., Cugini, M.A., Dibart, S. *et al.* (1997) The effect of SRP on the clinical and microbiological parameters of periodontal diseases. *J Clin Periodontol*, **24**, 324–334.

Haffajee, A.D., Teles, R.P. and Socransky, S.S. (2006) The effect of periodontal therapy on the composition of the subgingival microbiota. *Periodontology* 2000, **42**, 219–258.

Hamp, S.E., Nyman, S. and Lindhe, J. (1975) Periodontal treatment of multirooted teeth. Results after 5 years. *J Clin Periodontol*, **2**, 126–135.

Henderson, B., Ward, J.M. and Ready, D. (2010) Aggregatibacter (Actinobacillus) actinomycetemcomitans: a triple A* periodontopathogen? *Periodontology* 2000, **54**, 78–105.

How, K.Y., Song, K.P. and Chan, K.G. (2016) Porphyromonas gingivalis: an overview of periodontopathic pathogen below the gum line. *Front Microbiol*, **7**, 53.

Ioannou, I., Dimitriadis, N., Papadimitriou, K. *et al.* (2009) Hand instrumentation versus ultrasonic debridement in the treatment of chronic periodontitis: a randomized clinical and microbiological trial. *J Clin Periodontol*, **36**, 132–141.

Jahn, C.A. (2010) The dental water jet: a historical review of the literature. *J Dent Hyg*, **84**, 114–120.

James, P., Worthington, H.V., Parnell, C. *et al.* (2017) Chlorhexidine mouthrinse as an adjunctive treatment for gingival health. *Cochrane Database Syst Rev*, **3**, CD008676.

Kao, R.T., Nares, S. and Reynolds, M.A. (2015) Periodontal regeneration – intrabony defects: a systematic review from the AAP Regeneration Workshop. *J Periodontol*, **86**, S77–104.

Koop, R., Merheb, J. and Quirynen, M. (2012) Periodontal regeneration with enamel matrix derivative in reconstructive periodontal therapy: a systematic review. *J Periodontol*, **83**, 707–720.

Kornman, K.S., Crane, A., Wang, H.Y. *et al.* (1997) The interleukin-1 genotype as a severity factor in adult periodontal disease. *J Clin Periodontol*, **24**, 72–77.

Kotsakis, G.A., Javed, F., Hinrichs, J.E., Karoussis, I.K. and Romanos, G.E. (2015) Impact of cigarette smoking on clinical outcomes of periodontal flap surgical procedures: a systematic review and meta-analysis. *J Periodontol*, **86**, 254–263.

Krall, E.A. (2001) The periodontal-systemic connection: implications for treatment of patients with osteoporosis and periodontal disease. *Ann Periodontol*, **6**, 209–213.

Lang, N.P. and Lindhe, J. (2015) *Clinical Periodontology and Implant Dentistry*, Wiley-Blackwell, Oxford.

Lang, N.P. and Tonetti, M.S. (2003) Periodontal risk assessment (PRA) for patients in supportive periodontal therapy (SPT). *Oral Health Prev Dent*, **1**, 7–16.

Laster, L., Laudenbach, K.W. and Stoller, N.H. (1975) An evaluation of clinical tooth mobility measurements. *J Periodontol*, **46**, 603–607.

Linden, G.J. and Mullally, B.H. (1994) Cigarette smoking and periodontal destruction in young adults. *J Periodontol*, **65**, 718–723.

Lindhe, J. and Nyman, S. (1975) The effect of plaque control and surgical pocket elimination on the establishment and maintenance of periodontal health. A longitudinal study of periodontal therapy in cases of advanced disease. *J Clin Periodontol*, **2**, 67–79.

Lindhe, J. and Nyman, S. (1985) Scaling and granulation tissue removal in periodontal therapy. *J Clin Periodontol*, **12**, 374–388.

Lindhe, J., Hamp, S. and Loe, H. (1973) Experimental periodontitis in the beagle dog. *J Periodontal Res*, **8**, 1–10.

Lindhe, J., Westfelt, E., Nyman, S., Socransky, S.S. and Haffajee, A.D. (1984) Long-term effect of surgical/non-surgical treatment of periodontal disease. *J Clin Periodontol*, **11**, 448–458.

Loe, H. (1967) The Gingival Index, the Plaque Index and the Retention Index systems. *J Periodontol*, **38**(Suppl), 610–616.

Loe, H., Theilade, E. and Jensen, S.B. (1965) Experimental gingivitis in man. *J Periodontol*, **36**, 177–187.

Loe, H., Anerud, A., Boysen, H. and Morrison, E. (1986) Natural history of periodontal disease in man. Rapid, moderate and no loss of attachment in Sri Lankan laborers 14 to 46 years of age. *J Clin Periodontol*, **13**, 431–445.

Loesche, W.J. (1979) Clinical and microbiological aspects of chemotherapeutic agents used according to the specific plaque hypothesis. *J Dent Res*, **58**, 2404–2412.

Loos, B., Nylund, K., Claffey, N. and Egelberg, J. (1989) Clinical effects of root debridement in molar and non-molar teeth. A 2-year follow-up. *J Clin Periodontol*, **16**, 498–504.

Marigo, L., Cerreto, R., Giuliani, M. *et al.* (2011) Diabetes mellitus: biochemical, histological and microbiological aspects in periodontal disease. *Eur Rev Med Pharmacol Sci*, **15**, 751–758.

Martinez-Maestre, M.A., Gonzalez-Cejudo, C., Machuca, G., Torrejon, R. and Castelo-Branco, C. (2010) Periodontitis and osteoporosis: a systematic review. *Climacteric*, **13**, 523–529.

Michalowicz, B.S., Aeppli, D., Virag, J.G. *et al.* (1991a) Periodontal findings in adult twins. *J Periodontol*, **62**, 293–299.

Michalowicz, B.S., Aeppli, D.P., Kuba, R.K. *et al.* (1991b) A twin study of genetic variation in proportional radiographic alveolar bone height. *J Dent Res*, **70**, 1431–1435.

Moharamzadeh, K. (2016) Biocompatibility of oral care products, in *Biocompatibility of Dental Biomaterials* (ed. R. Shelton), Woodhead Publishing, Cambridge, pp. 113–129.

Mueller, V.T., Welch, K., Bratu, D.C. and Wang, H.L. (2013) Early and late studies of EMD use in periodontal intrabony defects. *J Periodontal Res*, **48**, 117–125.

Muhlemann, H.R. and Son, S. (1971) Gingival sulcus bleeding – a leading symptom in initial gingivitis. *Helv Odontol Acta*, **15**, 107–113.

Mysak, J., Podzimek, S., Sommerova, P. *et al.* (2014) Porphyromonas gingivalis: major periodontopathic pathogen overview. *J Immunol Res*, **2014**, 476068.

Needleman, I.G., Worthington, H.V., Giedrys-Leeper, E. and Tucker, R.J. (2006) Guided tissue regeneration for periodontal infra-bony defects. *Cochrane Database Syst Rev*, **2**, CD001724.

Nguyen, C.M., Kim, J.W., Quan, V.H., Nguyen, B.H. and Tran, S.D. (2015) Periodontal associations in cardiovascular diseases: the latest evidence and understanding. *J Oral Biol Craniofac Res*, **5**, 203–206.

Outhouse, T.L., Fedorowicz, Z., Keenan, J.V. and Al-Alawi, R. (2006) A Cochrane systematic review finds tongue scrapers have short-term efficacy in controlling halitosis. *Gen Dent*, **54**, 352–359; 360, 367–368; quiz 360.

Page, R.C. and Schroeder, H.E. (1976) Pathogenesis of inflammatory periodontal disease. A summary of current work. *Lab Invest*, **34**, 235–249.

Paknejad, Z., Jafart, M., Nazeman, P., Rezai Rad, M. and Khojasteh, A. (2017) Periodontal and peri-implant hard tissue regeneration, in *Biomaterials for Oral and Dental Tissue Engineering* (eds L. Tayebi and K. Moharamzadeh), Woodhead Publishing, Cambridge, pp. 405–428.

Palmer, R.J. Jr (2010) Supragingival and subgingival plaque: paradigm of biofilms. *Compend Contin Educ Dent*, **31**, 104–106, 108, 110 passim; quiz 124, 138.

Papapanou, P.N. (1999) Epidemiology of periodontal diseases: an update. *J Int Acad Periodontol*, **1**, 110–116.

Papapanou, P.N. (2002) Population studies of microbial ecology in periodontal health and disease. *Ann Periodontol*, **7**, 54–61.

Patel, R.A., Wilson, R.F. and Palmer, R.M. (2012) The effect of smoking on periodontal bone regeneration: a systematic review and meta-analysis. *J Periodontol*, **83**, 143–155.

Plancak, D., Music, L. and Puhar, I. (2015) Quorum sensing of periodontal pathogens. *Acta Stomatol Croat*, **49**, 234–241.

Polson, A.M. and Zander, H.A. (1983) Effect of periodontal trauma upon intrabony pockets. *J Periodontol*, **54**, 586–591.

Preeja, C., Ambili, R., Nisha, K.J., Seba, A. and Archana, V. (2013) Unveiling the role of stress in periodontal etiopathogenesis: an evidence-based review. *J Invest Clin Dent*, **4**, 78–83.

Preshaw, P.M. and Bissett, S.M. (2013) Periodontitis: oral complication of diabetes. *Endocrinol Metab Clin North Am*, **42**, 849–867.

Preshaw, P.M., Heasman, L., Stacey, F. *et al.* (2005) The effect of quitting smoking on chronic periodontitis. *J Clin Periodontol*, **32**, 869–879.

Preshaw, P.M., de Silva, N., McCracken, G.I. *et al.* (2010) Compromised periodontal status in an urban Sri Lankan population with type 2 diabetes. *J Clin Periodontol*, **37**, 165–171.

Qadri, T., Javed, F., Johannsen, G. and Gustafsson, A. (2015) Role of diode lasers (800–980 nm) as adjuncts to scaling and root planing in the treatment of chronic periodontitis: a systematic review. *Photomed Laser Surg*, **33**, 568–575.

Quirynen, M., Bollen, C.M., Vandekerckhove, B.N. *et al.* (1995) Full- vs. partial-mouth disinfection in the treatment of periodontal infections: short-term clinical and microbiological observations. *J Dent Res*, **74**, 1459–1467.

Ramfjord, S.P. (1959) Indices for prevalence and incidence of periodontal disease. *J Periodontol*, **30**, 51–59.

Ramfjord, S.P. and Nissle, R.R. (1974) The modified Widman flap. *J Periodontol*, **45**, 601–607.

Ramfjord, S.P., Caffesse, R.G., Morrison, E.C. *et al.* (1987) 4 modalities of periodontal treatment compared over 5 years. *J Clin Periodontol*, **14**, 445–452.

Reddy, M.S., Aichelmann-Reidy, M.E., Avila-Ortiz, G. *et al.* (2015) Periodontal regeneration – furcation defects: a consensus report from the AAP Regeneration Workshop. *J Periodontol*, **86**, S131–133.

Richards, D. (2014) Review finds that severe periodontitis affects 11% of the world population. *Evid Based Dent*, **15**, 70–71.

Rosema, N., Slot, D.E., van Palenstein Helderman, W.H. *et al.* (2016) The efficacy of powered toothbrushes following a brushing exercise: a systematic review. *Int J Dent Hyg*, **14**, 29–41.

Russell, A.L. (1956) A system of classification and scoring for prevalence surveys of periodontal disease. *J Dent Res*, **35**, 350–359.

Russell, R.R. (1992) Bacteriology of periodontal disease. *Curr Opin Dent*, **2**, 66–71.

Salvi, G.E., Lawrence, H.P., Offenbacher, S. and Beck, J.D. (1997) Influence of risk factors on the pathogenesis of periodontitis. *Periodontology* 2000, **14**, 173–201.

Salzer, S., Slot, D.E., van der Weijden, F.A. and Dorfer, C.E. (2015) Efficacy of interdental mechanical plaque control in managing gingivitis – a meta-review. *J Clin Periodontol*, **42**(Suppl 16), S92–105.

Scannapieco, F.A., Bush, R.B. and Paju, S. (2003) Associations between periodontal disease and risk for atherosclerosis, cardiovascular disease, and stroke. A systematic review. *Ann Periodontol*, **8**, 38–53.

Sculean, A., Schwarz, F., Berakdar, M. *et al.* (2004) Non-surgical periodontal treatment with a new ultrasonic device (Vector-ultrasonic system) or hand instruments. *J Clin Periodontol*, **31**, 428–433.

Sculean, A., Nikolidakis, D., Nikou, G. *et al.* (2015) Biomaterials for promoting periodontal regeneration in human intrabony defects: a systematic review. *Periodontology* 2000, **68**, 182–216.

Scully, C. (2014) *Scully's Medical Problems in Dentistry*, 7th edn, Churchill Livingstone, Edinburgh.

Sharma, A. (2010) Virulence mechanisms of Tannerella forsythia. *Periodontology* 2000, **54**, 106–116.

Sicilia, A., Arregui, I., Gallego, M., Cabezas, B. and Cuesta, S. (2002) A systematic review of powered vs manual toothbrushes in periodontal cause-related therapy. *J Clin Periodontol*, **29**(Suppl 3), 39–54; discussion 90–91.

Silness, J. and Loe, H. (1964) Periodontal disease in pregnancy. II. Correlation between oral hygiene and periodontal condition. *Acta Odontol Scand*, **22**, 121–135.

Simpson, T.C., Weldon, J.C., Worthington, H.V. *et al.* (2015) Treatment of periodontal disease for glycaemic control in people with diabetes mellitus. *Cochrane Database Syst Rev*, **11**, CD004714.

Slot, D.E., Jorritsma, K.H., Cobb, C.M. and van der Weijden, F.A. (2014) The effect of the thermal diode laser (wavelength 808–980 nm) in non-surgical periodontal therapy: a systematic review and meta-analysis. *J Clin Periodontol*, **41**, 681–692.

Socransky, S.S. and Haffajee, A.D. (1994) Evidence of bacterial etiology: a historical perspective. *Periodontology* 2000, **5**, 7–25.

Socransky, S.S. and Haffajee, A.D. (2005) Periodontal microbial ecology. *Periodontology* 2000, **38**, 135–187.

Sonnenschein, S.K. and Meyle, J. (2015) Local inflammatory reactions in patients with diabetes and periodontitis. *Periodontology* 2000, **69**, 221–254.

Svardstrom, G. and Wennstrom, J.L. (2000) Periodontal treatment decisions for molars: an analysis of influencing factors and long-term outcome. *J Periodontol*, **71**, 579–585.

Taylor, J.J., Preshaw, P.M. and Lalla, E. (2013) A review of the evidence for pathogenic mechanisms that may link periodontitis and diabetes. *J Periodontol*, **84**, S113–134.

Theilade, E. (1986) The non-specific theory in microbial etiology of inflammatory periodontal diseases. *J Clin Periodontol*, **13**, 905–911.

Theilade, E., Wright, W.H., Jensen, S.B. and Loe, H. (1966) Experimental gingivitis in man. II. A longitudinal clinical and bacteriological investigation. *J Periodont Res*, **1**, 1–13.

Tonetti, M.S., Claffey, N. and European Workshop in Periodontology Group (2005) Advances in the progression of periodontitis and proposal of definitions of a periodontitis case and disease progression for use in risk factor research. Group C consensus report of the 5th European Workshop in Periodontology. *J Clin Periodontol*, **32**(Suppl 6), 210–213.

Trombelli, L. and Farina, R. (2008) Clinical outcomes with bioactive agents alone or in combination with grafting or guided tissue regeneration. *J Clin Periodontol*, **35**, 117–135.

Vidrine, J.I., Shete, S., Cao, Y. *et al.* (2013) Ask–Advise–Connect: a new approach to smoking treatment delivery in health care settings. *JAMA Intern Med*, **173**, 458–464.

Waerhaug, J. (1979) The angular bone defect and its relationship to trauma from occlusion and downgrowth of subgingival plaque. *J Clin Periodontol*, **6**, 61–82.

White, D.J. (1997) Dental calculus: recent insights into occurrence, formation, prevention, removal and oral health effects of supragingival and subgingival deposits. *Eur J Oral Sci*, **105**, 508–522.

Xue, D., Tang, L., Bai, Y., Ding, Q., Wang, P. and Zhao, Y. (2017) Clinical efficacy of photodynamic therapy adjunctive to scaling and root planing in the treatment of chronic periodontitis: a systematic review and meta-analysis. *Photodiagnosis Photodyn Ther*, **18**, 119–127.

Yaacob, M., Worthington, H.V., Deacon, S.A. *et al.* (2014) Powered versus manual toothbrushing for oral health. *Cochrane Database Syst Rev*, **6**, CD002281.

Zhao, Y., Yin, Y., Tao, L., Nie, P., Tang, Y. and Zhu, M. (2014) Er:YAG laser versus scaling and root planing as alternative or adjuvant for chronic periodontitis treatment: a systematic review. *J Clin Periodontol*, **41**, 1069–1079.

Zi, M.Y., Longo, P.L., Bueno-Silva, B. and Mayer, M.P. (2014) Mechanisms involved in the association between periodontitis and complications in pregnancy. *Front Public Health*, **2**, 290.

7

Cleft Lip and Palate

7.1 Introduction

Cleft lip and palate is the most common craniofacial abnormality, affecting 1 in 650 live births. Twenty percent to 30% of the cases are cleft lip only, 30–45% are cleft palate only, and 35–50% are combined cleft lip and palate (CLP). It is more common in males than females (Panamonta *et al.*, 2015).

Cleft lip is caused by failure of unilateral or bilateral fusion of the medial nasal and maxillary processes during embryonic development. Cleft palate is due to the failure in merging of the palatal shelves (Sperber and Sperber, 2013).

The aetiology of CLP is multifactorial, including genetic and prenatal environmental factors such as smoking, alcohol and drugs during pregnancy, and vitamin deficiency (Dixon *et al.*, 2011).

Cleft lip and palate can be associated with other congenital anomalies or may occur as part of a syndrome. Over 400 syndromes may exhibit features of cleft lip and palate (Cohen, 1978).

Different classification systems have been used in the past (Allori *et al.*, 2017), including Veau's simple classification (Veau, 1931), Pfeifer's symbolic classification (Pfeifer *et al.*, 1974), Kernahan and Stark's striped Y classification (Kernahan and Stark, 1958), and Kriens' LAHSHAL classification (Kriens, 1989).

7.2 Complications

Patients with cleft lip and palate experience several functional and morphological problems, depending on the type and extent of the cleft.

- Feeding and swallowing in a baby with CLP can be challenging due to oronasal communication, reduced sucking efficiency and additional structural, airway and neuromotor problems (Miller, 2011).
- Mastication problems due to the presence of malocclusion which can affect the patient's quality of life (Dimberg *et al.*, 2015).
- Hearing problems due to middle ear infections and hearing loss (Timmermans *et al.*, 2006).
- Speech difficulties can be due to residual clefts/fistulae, velopharyngeal (VP) insufficiency, nasal obstruction and abnormal neuromotor and psychosocial development (Mildinhall, 2012).
- Craniofacial growth may be impaired and can result in midface retrusion (Will, 2000).
- The main cause of maxillary hypoplasia is scarring from primary palate surgery which restricts facial growth (Weinzweig *et al.*, 2006).
- Nasal deformity is also a common problem in CLP patients, affecting quality of life (Henry *et al.*, 2014).
- Aesthetic issues due to clefting and protruded premaxillae can further contribute to sociopsychological problems experienced by CLP patients (Kapp-Simon, 2004; Tobiasen and Hiebert, 1993).

7.3 Dental Abnormalities

Tooth formation can be disturbed in the area surrounding the cleft site and result in malformed crowns/roots, enamel hypoplasia, absent or ectopic teeth and supernumerary formation (Tannure *et al.*, 2012). Maxillary lateral incisors are the teeth most affected (Ranta, 1986).

Constricted maxillary dental arch, cross-bite and malocclusion are significantly increased in cleft patients (McCance *et al.*, 1990).

These patients also have a high incidence of dental caries and gingivitis (Dahllof *et al.*, 1989).

7.4 Management of Patients with CLP

The Clinical Standards Advisory Group (CSAG) 1998 report (di Biase and Markus, 1998) showed that the outcome of cleft care within UK was poorer than in other

Diseases and Conditions in Dentistry: An Evidence-Based Reference, First Edition. Keyvan Moharamzadeh.

Companion website: www.wiley.com/go/moharamzadeh/diseases

European countries. Therefore, to improve cleft care and outcomes, centralised regional cleft services were developed with multidisciplinary (MDT) teams including paediatricians, plastic surgeons, oral and maxillofacial surgeons, dentists, orthodontists, ear, nose and throat (ENT) physicians, psychiatrists and psychologists, restorative dentistry specialists, speech and language therapists, audiologists and co-ordinators (Colbert *et al.*, 2015).

7.4.1 Infancy and Primary Dentition Stage

Management of CLP during infancy includes the following aspects (Habel *et al.*, 1996; Madahar *et al.*, 2013; Sandler *et al.*, 2014).

- Prenatal diagnosis (Cockell and Lees, 2000) and referral to the regional CLP team.
- At birth, support is provided by specialist nurses to ensure normal bonding and feeding. Further infant feeding interventions may include fabrication of a feeding obturator and premaxilla repositioning appliances to retract and rotate the malposed premaxillae segment in bilateral cleft palate cases (Goyal *et al.*, 2014).
- Lip repair surgery is carried out at 3–6 months after birth to shift the premaxillae back and close the cleft lip.
- Palate repair surgery is performed at 12–18 months of age.
- Formal speech assessment is carried out at 18 months and is monitored throughout childhood.
- Closure of residual fistula and correction of velopharyngeal insufficiency at 4–5 years of age may be necessary to aid speech development.
- Preventive dental care, including oral hygiene education and dietary advice, is an important part of dental management at this stage.

7.4.2 Mixed Dentition

Bony defect of the maxillary alveolus can result in a variety of problems at mixed dentition stage, including displacement, rotation and tipping of the adjacent teeth and their failure to erupt (often maxillary canine). Bony defect can also result in collapse of the maxillary dental arch with loss of alveolar contour. Bony support around the base of nose can be compromised and in bilateral cleft cases, there can be instability and mobility of the premaxilla. Residual oronasal fistulae can also cause functional problems. Therefore, alveolar bone graft (ABG) surgery is carried out at the age of 8–10 years (prior to the eruption of maxillary canines) to address the above problems and restore the continuity and stability of the maxillary arch. Orthodontic differential expansion of the collapsed maxillary arch and some alignment of maxillary incisors can be considered prior to ABG surgery. Cancellous bone harvested from the iliac crest has been shown to provide the best outcome (Cho-Lee *et al.*, 2013).

7.4.3 Permanent Dentition

Treatment during permanent dentition may include orthodontic treatment, orthognathic surgery, distraction osteogenesis and finally restorative management.

7.4.3.1 Orthodontic Treatment

The extent and nature of orthodontic treatment depend on the severity of the malocclusion and the skeletal class III pattern. Orthodontic treatment alone, including dental camouflaging, alignment and retention, may be considered if the skeletal discrepancy is mild. Presurgical orthodontic treatment by simple maxillary dental alignment to improve the dental appearance in patients who require surgical correction of the skeletal problem is often indicated. Postsurgery orthodontic treatment may be required for final alignment of teeth and also can be indicated following any relapse (Cash, 2012).

7.4.3.2 Orthognathic Surgery

Le Fort I maxillary advancement osteotomy with or without mandibular set-back surgery is indicated for the correction of skeletal class III pattern due to maxillary hypoplasia in CLP patients following completion of growth.

Complications of orthognathic surgery in CLP patients include the following.

- Increased risk of postoperative infection and ischaemic complications.
- Maxillary advancement can compromise VP function, producing hyponasal speech.
- Retromaxillary scarring can occur following surgery.
- Relapse rate (both horizontal and vertical relapse) is much greater than in the non-cleft population and ranges from 30% to 65% (Saltaji *et al.*, 2012).

7.4.3.3 Distraction Osteogenesis (DO)

Distraction osteogenesis is used in patients with severe maxillary retrusion which is beyond correction with conventional orthognathic surgery.

Following presurgical orthodontic treatment, Le Fort I osteotomy cuts are placed and the maxillae is mobilised to enable placement of the distraction device, which can be either a rigid external (RED) or internal device. The latency period is normally 4–5 days to allow callus formation. Bone lengthening is achieved by gradual mechanical distraction at a rate of 1 mm/day with a consolidation period of 3 months (Wong *et al.*, 2008).

The advantages of DO are as follows (Kloukos *et al.*, 2016).

- Larger corrective movements than orthognathic surgery.
- Decreased postsurgical relapse.
- Fewer postoperative problems with speech and language.
- It can be used in growing patients but overcorrection is required.

The disadvantages of DO include the following.

- Precise movements and vector control are difficult to achieve, especially with internal DO.
- Multiple review appointments are required during the distraction phase.
- It can induce anxiety and stress.
- Scarring associated with the RED.
- Risk of infection.
- Encumbrance of the device can affect the quality of life.
- Second general anaesthesia is required to remove the device.

7.4.3.4 Restorative Treatment

Restorative dentistry specialists provide the final active treatment in CLP patients and provide restorative advice to the cleft team (Kantorowicz, 1990).

The aim of restorative treatment is to prevent relapse following orthognathic surgery and orthodontic treatment, restore masticatory function and improve speech and aesthetics.

Restorative challenges in CLP patients include the following.

- Discrepancy in the maxillo-mandibular relationship.
- Malposition and partial eruption of teeth.
- Malformation and tipping of teeth.
- Caries.
- Flat palate resulting from severe scarring.
- Presence of frenula, absence of keratinised mucosa, gingival recession, shallow vestibule and difficult hygiene.
- Poor condition of supporting periodontal tissues.

Prevention, including fluoride, dietary advice and oral hygiene education, is an integral part of any restorative treatment. Several factors contribute to the difficulty in maintaining oral hygiene of teeth close to the cleft area, including presence of gingival recessions, frenula, tooth malpositioning, dental anomalies and extended use of fixed orthodontic appliances.

Non-surgical and surgical periodontal treatments may be indicated. Surgical therapies include gingivoplasty, gingivectomy, gingival grafts, removal of frenula and restoration of biological dimensions.

Different types of prosthodontic treatment can be indicated for replacing the missing teeth and restoring the compromised dentition in CLP patients.

- Tooth reshaping and composite additions (see Chapter 29).
- Veneers (see Chapter 18).
- Crowns (see Chapter 18).
- Resin-bonded bridges (see Chapter 25).
- Conventional bridges (see Chapter 25).
- Removable partial dentures can be a temporary solution for replacing the missing teeth or can be a definitive treatment option when fixed restorative options are not possible (see Chapter 38).
- Osseointegrated implants can be successfully used in CLP patients but often require further bone grafting (de Barros Ferreira *et al.*, 2010; Wang *et al.*, 2014) (see Chapters 37 and 46).
- Overdentures and overlay dentures can be useful in extreme cases with severe maxillary hypoplasia and retrusion causing a large skeletal discrepancy that is not amenable to surgical and orthodontic treatment. Dentures can help to replace missing teeth, cover malpositioned teeth, recover the maxillary arch, close the anterior open bite and provide lip support (Turkyilmaz, 2008).
- Complete dentures are indicated in edentulous patients (see Chapter 9). Challenges of complete denture treatment in CLP patients include compromised denture stability and retention due to the alveolar ridge anatomy, physical factors (impaired adhesion, surface tension and cohesion) and presence of residual fistula or unrepaired cleft, which would allow the penetration of air and compromise the seal.
- Obturators are indicated for rehabilitation of untreated cleft patients and in patients with residual oronasal communication in large defects following surgery. Obturators can also eliminate hypernasality and improve speech. Obturators are discussed in detail in Chapter 33.
- Palatal lift prosthesis is indicated when there is velopharyngeal incompetency following soft palate repair. This is a removable appliance that extends to the soft palate and helps to lift the soft palate to achieve closure to improve speech (Dhakshaini *et al.*, 2015).
- Speech aids and speech bulbs can be useful when the soft palate has inadequate length and is unable to close, leading to velopharyngeal incompetency. The appliance covers the hard palate and the bulb extends posteriorly to the soft palate, providing velopharyngeal closure and therefore improving speech (Dhakshaini *et al.*, 2015; Shelton *et al.*, 1968).

Case Study

A 50-year-old male patient referred by a general dental practitioner to the restorative dentistry department presented with history of cleft lip and palate, multiple cleft repair surgeries in the past, a residual existing oronasal communication and an unstable and non-retentive maxillary acrylic removable partial denture (RPD). The patient had been wearing the denture for 6 years.

The patient was medically fit and well and a non-smoker.

The patient's remaining teeth in the maxillary arch were UR3, UR4, UR5, UR6, UL4 and UL6 (Figure 7.1). UL4 had a metal ceramic crown with no obvious endodontic pathology and the teeth were vital. Oral hygiene was good and the periodontium was healthy with mild gingival recession.

Diagnoses

- Repaired unilateral cleft lip and palate and residual oronasal communication
- Missing teeth
- Mild generalised gingival recession
- Unstable and non-retentive mucosa-borne maxillary acrylic RPD

Prognosis

The prognosis for the remaining teeth was good as they had adequate periodontal support with no active caries or endodontic disease.

The prognosis for surgical closure of the oronasal communication was poor due to previously failed surgery and presence of scar tissue and the patient did not want any further surgical treatment.

The prognosis for dental implant treatment was also compromised due to inadequate amounts of bone in the cleft site. Bone grafting would be complicated by the presence of scar tissue and inadequate soft tissue to cover the graft material in the cleft region.

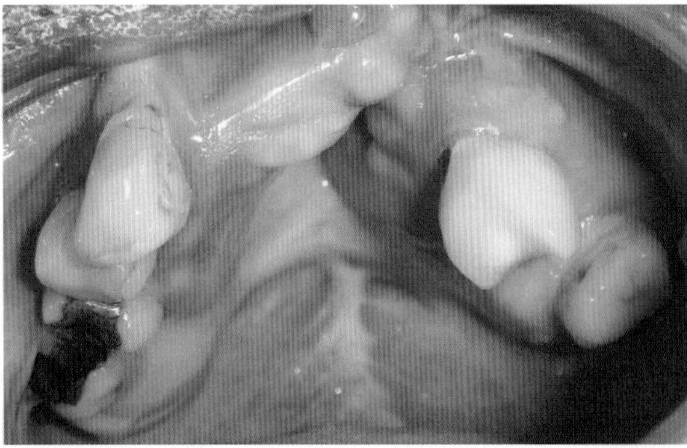

Figure 7.1 Preoperative clinical photograph of the maxillary arch showing the scarring from the previous cleft repair and residual oronasal communication.

The prognosis for treatment with a new cobalt-chromium (Co-Cr) RPD was good as the abutment teeth were suitable to support a partial denture with an incorporated obturator to seal the oronasal defect.

Treatment Provided

- Primary impressions with alginate impression material. A Vaseline-impregnated gauze was placed over the defect to avoid extrusion of alginate into the defect.
- Bite registration with an upper wax block.
- Preparation of articulated study models, surveying the casts and designing the RPD.
- Initial wax try-in of the maxillary anterior teeth to determine the anterior extension of the metal framework.
- Rest seat preparation on the abutment teeth and secondary impression with a special tray in two steps (Figure 7.2).
  1) Impression of the narrow palatal defect by injection of light-body silicone impression material.
  2) Overimpression with regular-body silicone impression material.
- Metal framework (Figure 7.3) try-in.
- Final try-in of teeth on wax on metal framework.
- RPD obturator insertion (Figure 7.4).
- Review and maintenance.

Further Learning Points

The two-stage approach using silicone impression material was an efficient impression technique that resulted in an accurate recording of the defect in the palate without the danger of extruding the material into the nasal cavity.

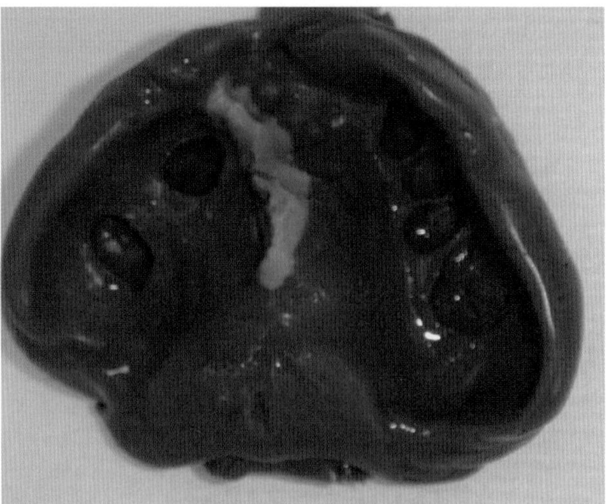

Figure 7.2 Impression of the maxillary arch showing the details of the cleft recorded by the light-body impression material in the centre while the rest of the palate and the teeth are recorded by the regular-body impression material.

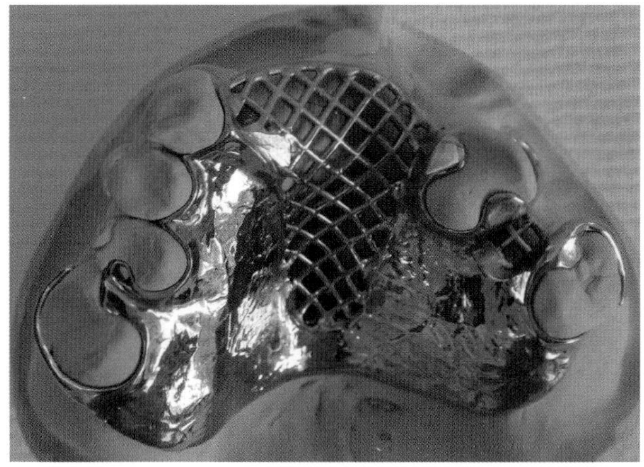

Figure 7.3 Co-Cr framework on the maxillary cast with a mesh metal structure over the central palate defect to enable mechanical retention for acrylic resin to obturate the defect. Maximum support, retention and reciprocation are achieved using the remaining upper teeth.

Covering the defect area with metal mesh and filling the defect with acrylic resin obturator was very effective in sealing the cleft communication.

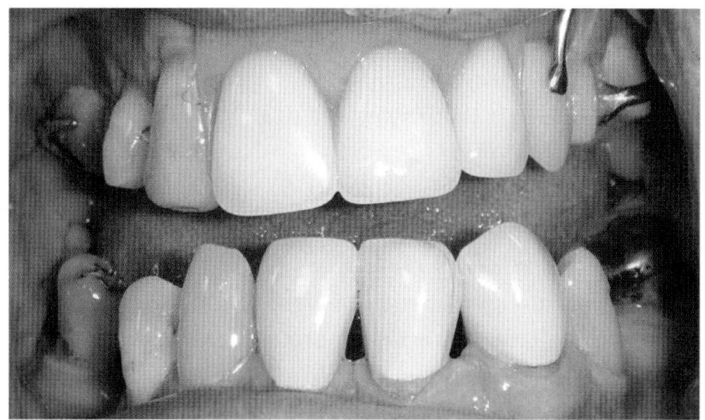

Figure 7.4 Postoperative clinical photograph following insertion of the upper Co-Cr RPD with incorporated central acrylic obturator.

The design of the partial denture was further complicated due to severe class III occlusal relationship and the position of the remaining upper teeth.

Denture teeth shade and mould selection were governed by patient preference for large maxillary anterior teeth with similar shade to the mandibular anterior crowns.

The patient was very satisfied with the new denture.

References

Allori, A.C., Mulliken, J.B., Meara, J.G., Shusterman, S. and Marcus, J.R. (2017) Classification of cleft lip/palate: then and now. *Cleft Palate Craniofac J*, **54**, 175–188.

Cash, A.C. (2012) Orthodontic treatment in the management of cleft lip and palate. *Front Oral Biol*, **16**, 111–123.

Cho-Lee, G.Y., Garcia-Diez, E.M., Nunes, R.A., Marti-Pages, C., Sieira-Gil, R. and Rivera-Baro, A. (2013) Review of secondary alveolar cleft repair. *Ann Maxillofac Surg*, **3**, 46–50.

Cockell, A. and Lees, M. (2000) Prenatal diagnosis and management of orofacial clefts. *Prenat Diagn*, **20**, 149–151.

Cohen, M.M. Jr (1978) Syndromes with cleft lip and cleft palate. *Cleft Palate J*, **15**, 306–328.

Colbert, S.D., Green, B., Brennan, P.A. and Mercer, N. (2015) Contemporary management of cleft lip and palate in the United Kingdom. Have we reached the turning point? *Br J Oral Maxillofac Surg*, **53**, 594–598.

Dahllof, G., Ussisoo-Joandi, R., Ideberg, M. and Modeer, T. (1989) Caries, gingivitis, and dental abnormalities in preschool children with cleft lip and/or palate. *Cleft Palate J*, **26**, 233–237; Discussion 237–238.

de Barros Ferreira, S. Jr, Esper, L.A., Sbrana, M.C., Ribeiro, I.W. and de Almeida, A.L. (2010) Survival of dental implants in the cleft area – a retrospective study. *Cleft Palate Craniofac J*, **47**, 586–590.

Dhakshaini, M.R., Pushpavathi, M., Garhnayak, M. and Dhal, A. (2015) Prosthodontic management in conjunction with speech therapy in cleft lip and palate: a review and case report. *J Int Oral Health*, **7**, 106–111.

Di Biase, D. and Markus, A. (1998) Cleft lip and palate care in the Uk: the CSAG Report. *Br Dent J*, **185**, 320–321.

Dimberg, L., Arnrup, K. and Bondemark, L. (2015) The impact of malocclusion on the quality of life among children and adolescents: a systematic review of quantitative studies. *Eur J Orthod*, **37**, 238–247.

Dixon, M.J., Marazita, M.L., Beaty, T.H. and Murray, J.C. (2011) Cleft lip and palate: understanding genetic and environmental influences. *Nat Rev Genet*, **12**, 167–178.

Goyal, M., Chopra, R., Bansal, K. and Marwaha, M. (2014) Role of obturators and other feeding interventions in patients with cleft lip and palate: a review. *Eur Arch Paediatr Dent*, **15**, 1–9.

Habel, A., Sell, D. and Mars, M. (1996. Management Of Cleft Lip and Palate. *Arch Dis Child*, **74**, 360–6.

Henry, C., Samson, T. and Mackay, D. (2014) Evidence-based medicine: the cleft lip nasal deformity. *Plast Reconstr Surg*, **133**, 1276–1288.

Kantorowicz, G.F. (1990) Role of the restorative dentist in the management of cleft palate patients: discussion paper. *J R Soc Med*, **83**, 29.

Kapp-Simon, K.A. (2004) Psychological issues in cleft lip and palate. *Clin Plast Surg*, **31**, 347–352.

Kernahan, D.A. and Stark, R.B. (1958) A new classification for cleft lip and cleft palate. *Plast Reconstr Surg Transplant Bull*, **22**, 435–441.

Kloukos, D., Fudalej, P., Sequeira-Byron, P. and Katsaros, C. (2016) Maxillary distraction osteogenesis versus orthognathic surgery for cleft lip and palate patients. *Cochrane Database Syst Rev*, **9**, CD010403.

Kriens, O. (1989) Lahshal: an easy clinical system of cleft lip, alveolus and palate documentation, in Proceedings of the Advanced Workshop: "What's A Cleft?", Thieme, Stuttgart.

Madahar, A., Murray, A., Orr, R. and Sandler, P.J. (2013) The long and winding road – the journey of a cleft lip and palate patient part 1. *Dent Update*, **40**, 791–794, 796–798.

McCance, A.M., Roberts-Harry, D., Sherriff, M., Mars, M. and Houston, W.J. (1990) A study model analysis of adult unoperated Sri Lankans with unilateral cleft lip and palate. *Cleft Palate J*, **27**, 146–154; discussion 174–175.

Mildinhall, S. (2012) Speech and language in the patient with cleft palate. *Front Oral Biol*, **16**, 137–146.

Miller, C.K. (2011) Feeding issues and interventions in infants and children with clefts and craniofacial syndromes. *Semin Speech Lang*, **32**, 115–126.

Panamonta, V., Pradubwong, S., Panamonta, M. and Chowchuen, B. (2015) Global birth prevalence of orofacial clefts: a systematic review. *J Med Assoc Thai*, **98**(Suppl 7), S11–21.

Pfeifer, G., Schlote, H.H. and von Kreybig, T. (1974) Clefts of the face in animal experiments. *J Maxillofac Surg*, **2**, 230–238.

Ranta, R. (1986) A review of tooth formation in children with cleft lip/palate. *Am J Orthod Dentofacial Orthop*, **90**, 11–18.

Saltaji, H., Major, M.P., Alfakir, H., Al-Saleh, M.A. and Flores-Mir, C. (2012) Maxillary advancement with conventional orthognathic surgery in patients with cleft lip and palate: is it a stable technique? *J Oral Maxillofac Surg*, **70**, 2859–2866.

Sandler, P.J., Murray, A., Orr, R. and Madahar, A.K. (2014) The long and winding road part 2. The CLP patient's journey, 0–21 years. *Dent Update*, **41**, 20–22, 24–26.

Shelton, R.L., Lindquist, A.F., Chisum, L., Arndt, W.B., Youngstrom, K.A. and Stick, S.L. (1968) Effect of prosthetic speech bulb reduction on articulation. *Cleft Palate J*, **5**, 195–204.

Sperber, G.H. and Sperber, S.M. (2013) Embryogenetics of cleft lip and palate, in *Cleft Lip and Palate: Diagnosis and Management* (ed. S. Berkowitz), Springer, Heidelberg, pp. 3–33.

Tannure, P.N., Oliveira, C.A., Maia, L.C., Vieira, A.R., Granjeiro, J.M. and Costa M.C. (2012) Prevalence of dental anomalies in nonsyndromic individuals with cleft lip and palate: a systematic review and meta-analysis. *Cleft Palate Craniofac J*, **49**, 194–200.

Timmermans, K., Vander Poorten, V., Desloovere, C. and Debruyne, F. (2006) The middle ear of cleft palate patients in their early teens: a literature study and preliminary file study. *B–Ent*, **2**(Suppl 4), 95–101.

Tobiasen, J.M. and Hiebert, J.M. (1993) Clefting and psychosocial adjustment. *Influence of facial aesthetics. Clin Plast Surg*, **20**, 623–631.

Turkyilmaz, I. (2008) Prosthodontic management of patient with cleft lip/palate using maxillary overdenture and swing-lock attachment mechanism. Clinical report. *N Y State Dent J*, **74**, 62–64.

Veau, V. (1931) *Division Palatine*, Masson, Paris.

Wang, F., Wu, Y., Zou, D., Wang, G. and Kaigler, D. (2014) Clinical outcomes of dental implant therapy in alveolar cleft patients: a systematic review. *Int J Oral Maxillofac Implants*, **29**, 1098–1105.

Weinzweig, J., Panter, K.E., Seki, J., Pantaloni, M., Spangenberger, A. and Harper, J.S. (2006) The fetal cleft palate: IV. Midfacial growth and bony palatal development following in utero and neonatal repair of the congenital caprine model. *Plast Reconstr Surg*, **118**, 81–93.

Will, L.A. (2000) Growth and development in patients with untreated clefts. *Cleft Palate Craniofac J*, **37**, 523–526.

Wong, G.B., Ciminello, F.S. and Padwa, B.L. (2008) Distraction osteogenesis of the cleft maxilla. *Facial Plast Surg*, **24**, 467–471.

8

Combination Syndrome

8.1 Defining Features

Combination syndrome (CS) can occur when a maxillary complete denture opposes a mandibular distal extension removable partial denture or a dentate mandibular arch. Characteristic features of CS include (Kelly, 1972):

- bone loss in the anterior maxilla which is often replaced by a flabby ridge
- downgrowth of the maxillary tuberosity
- palatal papillary hyperplasia
- overeruption of the mandibular anterior teeth
- bone loss in the mandibular distal extension areas under the removable partial denture bases.

Other changes may include poor adaptation of the prostheses, epulis formation, discrepancies of the occlusal plane, decrease in the vertical dimension (VD) and forward posturing of the mandible and periodontal problems associated with the remaining mandibular anterior teeth.

Different classifications have been proposed for categorising combination syndrome based on the complete or partial edentulous status of the maxilla and/or mandible. The common feature of most CS cases is an edentulous premaxilla with advanced ridge resorption in the anterior maxilla and overeruption of the mandibular anterior teeth (Rajendran, 2012; Tolstunov, 2007).

8.2 Pathogenesis

Ridge resorption in the mandibular distal extension areas can occur much faster (by four times) than the maxillae due to a smaller bearing area (Tallgren, 1972). This process, combined with the wear of posterior artificial teeth over time, would lead to the loss of posterior support in the mandible, encouraging the forward posturing of the mandible and significantly shifting the occlusal loads to the anterior region.

In response to the increased occlusal loads, the resorption of the anterior maxillary alveolar ridge can occur, and a flabby ridge can replace the hard bony ridge. A maxillary denture would then displace in the superior and anterior direction, reducing the occlusal VD, and the upper occlusal plane would drop posteriorly, resulting in downgrowth of fibrous tissue in the tuberosity region. Tuberosity pneumatisation can also occur due to an unknown mechanism. Inflammatory papillary hyperplasia of the palate can occur as a result of poor denture adaptation and poor oral hygiene.

Epulis can also form in the anterior maxilla due to the irritation caused by the upper denture's labial flange. Retention of the maxillary denture can then progressively deteriorate.

Due to the shift of the occlusal loads and changes in the occlusal plane, the remaining mandibular anterior teeth may drift or overerupt and become mobile, especially if the teeth have poor periodontal condition. The trauma caused by the lower partial denture can also cause gingival recession on the lingual aspect of the mandibular anterior teeth (Palmqvist *et al.*, 2003; Tolstunov, 2011).

8.3 Clinical Assessment

Clinical assessment of a patient with a complete denture includes:

- thorough history of the existing dentures and assessment of the denture's stability, retention, extension, occlusion, wear, aesthetics, phonetics and freeway space (FWS)
- extraoral examination, including temporomandibular joints (TMJ), muscles of mastication and lip support
- intraoral assessment including soft tissues, alveolar ridge height, width, flabby tissues, sulcus depth, neutral zone space available, tongue size and movements

Diseases and Conditions in Dentistry: An Evidence-Based Reference, First Edition. Keyvan Moharamzadeh.

Companion website: www.wiley.com/go/moharamzadeh/diseases

- assessment of any remaining teeth in terms of periodontal, caries and periapical disease
- panoramic radiograph and three-dimensional imaging if necessary to assess the bone available for potential implant treatment and periapical radiographs of remaining teeth if there is any suspected periapical or periodontal pathology.

8.4 Prevention

Patient education is an important aspect of prevention and includes maintaining good plaque control and periodontal health of the remaining anterior teeth, denture care instructions to leave the prostheses out of the mouth at night and regular recall and maintenance.

Ridge resorption can be minimised in denture wearers by considering the following provisions:

- retaining roots as overdenture abutments
- broad stress distribution
- bilaterally balanced occlusion
- minimising anterior contacts
- effective border seal.

Altered cast impression technique by taking an impression of the free-end saddle areas under controlled pressure can minimise displacement of the denture under occlusal loads. In this technique, close-fitting baseplates are constructed on the metal framework to take impression of the distal extension areas while the metal framework is seated and the pressure is applied only on the rest seat areas. The saddle areas of the master cast are then sectioned and removed in the laboratory and the new saddle areas are poured with the framework in place (Sajjan, 2010).

It has been shown that appropriate conventional impression taking using completely extended impression, use of magnification, adjustment of the framework to ensure complete seating, and coverage of the retromolar pads and buccal shelves can produce comparable impression outcomes to the altered cast impression technique (Frank *et al.*, 2004).

8.5 Treatment Considerations

The following considerations can be useful in management of patients with CS (Cabianca, 2003; Langer *et al.*, 1995; Lynch and Allen, 2004; Schmitt, 1985).

- Adopting a shortened dental arch approach with or without fixed bridges in the lower arch.
- Restoration of the posterior mandible with implant-retained fixed prosthesis.
- Correction of occlusal plane discrepancies and vertical dimension problems prior to definitive treatment.
- Fabrication of a heat-cured transparent baseplate prior to occlusal registration to assess the stability, retention and fit of the denture base at an early stage.
- Accurate bite registration, use of face-bow transfer to enable suitable orientation of the occlusal plane and mounting the casts on a semi-adjustable articulator to ensure balanced articulation.
- Selection of teeth with shallow-angled cusps and hardened surfaces for the posterior teeth and avoiding steep anterior incisal guidance.
- Careful assessment of occlusion and the need for check record and occlusal adjustment if necessary.

8.6 Management of Flabby Ridge

Surgical removal of the flabby tissue prior to denture fabrication may result in reduced sulcus depth and is not often recommended as a present flabby ridge would be better than an absent ridge.

Several impression techniques have been introduced for mucostatic recording of denture bearing areas that contain displaceable flabby tissues (Allen, 2005).

- The minimally displacive technique involves the use of a single impression tray that has a window or multiple perforations over the flabby area. Impression of the compressible tissues is recorded using a heavy-body silicone or zinc-oxide eugenol (ZOE) impression material. The flabby tissue is recorded with minimal displacement using a low-viscosity silicone impression or plaster impression material in the windowed or perforated areas of the impression tray (Lynch and Allen, 2006).
- The two-tray technique uses two separate impression trays to record the flabby and non-flabby areas separately which are then related intraorally (Bindhoo *et al.*, 2012).
- The selective pressure technique involves selective manipulation of the thermoplastic greenstick compound impression material and application of pressure over compressible areas and no pressure on the flabby tissues (Duncan *et al.*, 2004).
- The copy denture technique copies the patient's existing prosthesis, maintaining the polished surface and perforation of the base over the area of the flabby tissues when recording the master impression. It is advisable to fabricate a clear acrylic baseplate following the master impression to check the mucosal contacts prior to adding wax blocks for bite registration.

8.7 Management of Denture-Induced Stomatitis

Denture-induced stomatitis is a common condition that can occur due to inflammation of oral mucosa under the denture. Its aetiology is multifactorial and in approximately 90% of cases, fungal infections such as *Candida* species are involved. Prolonged trauma from the denture with poor hygiene and dry mouth can exacerbate the condition.

Denture-induced stomatitis can be divided into three categories according to Newton's classification.

- Type 1 is characterised by localised inflammation or small area with erythema.
- Type 2 is diffused erythema of the mucosa covered by the denture.
- Type 3 is inflammatory papillary or nodular hyperplasia of the palate.

Treatment for denture-induced stomatitis includes the following.

- Oral hygiene and denture care instructions to remove the dentures at night, clean, disinfect and store them in an antiseptic solution overnight (Lombardi and Budtz-Jorgensen, 1993).
- Treatment of any underlying disease such as diabetes and HIV infection.
- Application of topical antifungal medications in the form of oral gels, suspensions and lozenges. Antifungal medications can be effectively mixed with commercially available tissue conditioners to be used under the dentures (Iqbal and Zafar, 2016).
- The use of an antiseptic mouthrinse such as chlorhexidine is also recommended.

Case Study

A 57-year-old female patient presented with an edentulous maxillary arch and unstable and non-retentive 10-year-old upper complete denture against a dentate mandibular dental arch.

Clinical examination confirmed the diagnosis of combination syndrome and a flabby ridge in the anterior maxillae (Figure 8.1).

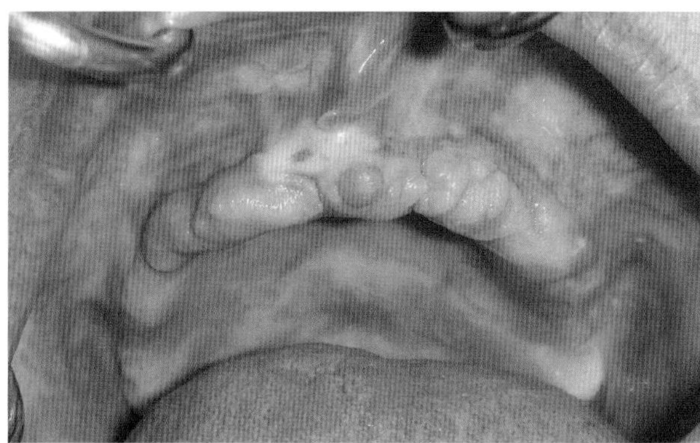

Figure 8.1 Edentulous maxillary arch with a flabby ridge in the anterior region.

Treatment procedures included the following.

- Primary impression with alginate material.
- Fabrication of a special tray with a window over the flabby ridge area (Figure 8.2). The special tray was spaced in the anterior region with displaceable tissues but close-fitting in the posterior compressible areas of the palate and the alveolar ridge.

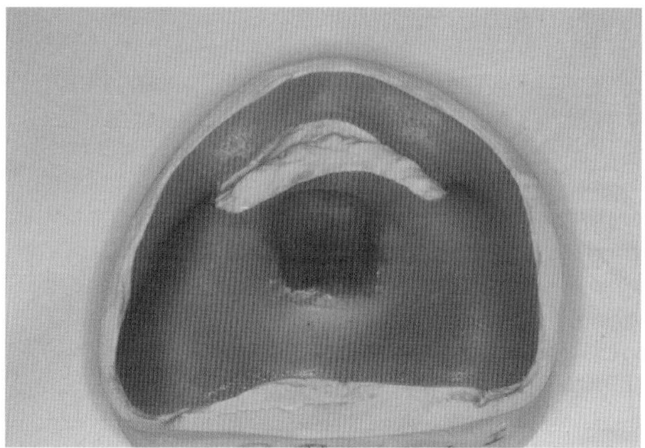

Figure 8.2 Special tray with a window over the flabby ridge.

- Adjustment and border moulding of the special tray and secondary impression using a combination of ZOE impression material in the compressible areas and light-body silicone impression material over the flabby ridge area in the anterior region (Figure 8.3).
- A clear acrylic baseplate was fabricated and tried in to assess the tissue contacts and the stability, retention and fit of the denture base at an early stage.
- Bite registration using wax blocks added onto the baseplate.
- Wax try-in and carving the post dam.
- Denture insertion and occlusal adjustment using a pre-centric check record.
- Review and maintenance.

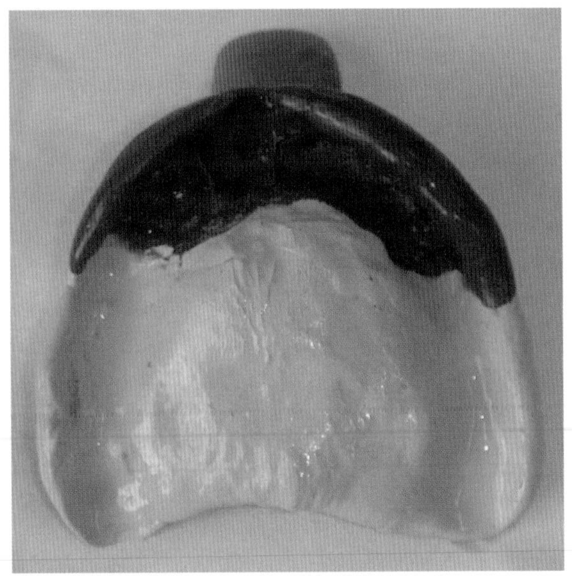

Figure 8.3 Master impression using a combination of ZOE and light-body silicone impression materials.

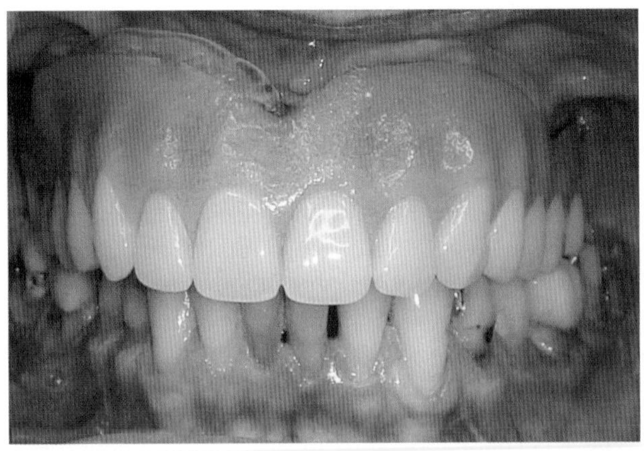

Figure 8.4 Postoperative clinical photograph of the denture in occlusion.

A postoperative clinical photograph of the denture in occlusion is shown in Figure 8.4 and the patient's smile is shown is Figure 8.5.

The flabby ridge impression technique used in this case resulted in an accurate impression of the ridge without displacement of the flabby areas. The assessment of the interface between the ZOE and the light-body silicon impression materials showed nice blending of the two materials without any steps or inaccuracies.

Due to the lingual inclination of the mandibular premolar teeth and a narrow mandibular arch, the maxillary premolar teeth were widened palatally to provide occlusion with the mandibular teeth while maintaining the wide maxillary arch-form.

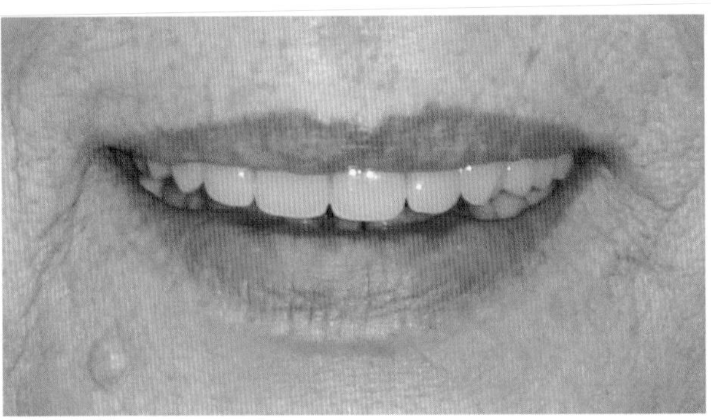

Figure 8.5 Postoperative photograph of the patient's smile.

With careful adjustment of the wax rim, a satisfactory lip support was achieved with a favourable smile line.

The patient was very satisfied with the aesthetics, retention and function of the new maxillary denture.

References

Allen, F. (2005) Management of the flabby ridge in complete denture construction. *Dent Update*, **32**, 524–526, 528.

Bindhoo, Y.A., Thirumurthy, V.R. and Kurien, A. (2012) Complete mucostatic impression: a new attempt. *J Prosthodont*, **21**, 209–214.

Cabianca, M. (2003) Combination syndrome: treatment with dental implants. *Implant Dent*, **12**, 300–305.

Duncan, J.P., Raghavendra, S. and Taylor, T.D. (2004) A selective-pressure impression technique for the edentulous maxilla. *J Prosthet Dent*, **92**, 299–301.

Frank, R.P., Brudvik, J.S. and Noonan, C.J. (2004) Clinical outcome of the altered cast impression procedure compared with use of a one–piece cast. *J Prosthet Dent*, **91**, 468–476.

Iqbal, Z. and Zafar, M.S. (2016) Role of antifungal medicaments added to tissue conditioners: a systematic review. *J Prosthodont Res*, **60**, 231–239.

Kelly, E. (1972) Changes caused by a mandibular removable partial denture opposing a maxillary complete denture. *J Prosthet Dent*, **90**, 213–219.

Langer, Y., Laufer, B.Z. and Cardash, H.S. (1995) Modalities of treatment for the combination syndrome. *J Prosthodont*, **4**, 76–81.

Lombardi, T. and Budtz-Jorgensen, E. (1993) Treatment of denture-induced stomatitis: a review. *Eur J Prosthodont Restor Dent*, **2**, 17–22.

Lynch, C.D. and Allen, P.F. (2004) The 'combination syndrome' revisited. *Dent Update*, **31**, 410–412, 415–416, 419–420.

Lynch, C.D. and Allen, P.F. (2006) Management of the flabby ridge: using contemporary materials to solve an old problem. *Br Dent J*, **200**, 258–261.

Palmqvist, S., Carlsson, G.E. and Owall, B. (2003) The combination syndrome: a literature review. *J Prosthet Dent*, **90**, 270–275.

Rajendran, S. (2012) Combination syndrome. *Int J Prosthodont Restor Dent*, **2**, 156–160.

Sajjan, C. (2010) An altered cast procedure to improve tissue support for removable partial denture. *Contemp Clin Dent*, **1**, 103–106.

Schmitt, S.M. (1985) Combination syndrome: a treatment approach. *J Prosthet Dent*, **54**, 664–671.

Tallgren, A. (1972) The continuing reduction of the residual alveolar ridges in complete denture wearers: a mixed-longitudinal study covering 25 years. *J Prosthet Dent*, **89**, 427–435.

Tolstunov, L. (2007) Combination syndrome: classification and case report. *J Oral Implantol*, **33**, 139–151.

Tolstunov, L. (2011) Combination syndrome symptomatology and treatment. *Compend Contin Educ Dent*, **32**, 62–66.

9

Complete Edentulism

9.1 Introduction

Complete edentulism is a highly prevalent condition globally and affects 0.1–14.5% of people below the age of 50 years and 2.1–32.3% of older people worldwide (Tyrovolas *et al.*, 2016). Edentulism is associated with depression and poor self-rated health in young age groups.

Complete dentures have been the prosthetic treatment of choice for edentulism for a long time and are indicated for the rehabilitation of edentulous patients to improve comfort, aesthetics, occlusal and facial support, masticatory function and speech.

A majority of edentulous patients report satisfaction with complete dentures although a small group of patients find it difficult to adapt to conventional complete dentures (Carlsson and Omar, 2010). Advances in implant dentistry and the introduction of implant-supported overdentures have significantly improved patient satisfaction and quality of life, especially in those with resorbed mandible where retention and stability of the conventional complete denture are compromised (Thomason *et al.*, 2012).

This chapter focuses on the treatment of edentulous patients with conventional complete dentures. Implant- and magnet-supported overdentures are discussed in detail in Chapter 45.

9.2 Treatment Stages

Management of edentulous patients with conventional complete dentures involves the stages listed below.

- Visit 1: Assessment, diagnosis and treatment planning.
- Visit 2: Primary impressions (clinical) and fabrication of special trays (laboratory).
- Visit 3: Adjustment of the special trays, border moulding, working impressions (clinical) and fabrication of record base and wax blocks (laboratory).
- Visit 4: Registration of jaw relation, selection of shade and mould for teeth (clinical) and setting up the teeth on wax (laboratory).
- Visit 5: Trial insertion, marking the post dam (clinical), carving the post dam and processing the denture (laboratory).
- Visit 6: Denture insertion (clinical) and check record if necessary (laboratory).
- Visit 7: Review and maintenance in subsequent visits (clinical).

Readers are strongly recommended to refer to the British Society for the Study of Prosthetic Dentistry (BSSPD) guidelines (Ogden, 1996) on standards for complete dentures in relation to clinical practice and procedures of complete prosthodontics, including the technical aspects of complete denture construction.

Additional aspects of complete denture treatment are discussed in the following sections.

9.3 Denture Support

Primary denture support areas are the hard palate for the maxillary denture and buccal shelves and the pear-shaped pads for the mandibular denture (Jacobson and Krol, 1983).

Secondary denture support areas are the ridge crests (maxillary and mandibular denture) and genial tubercles (mandibular denture).

Relief area includes the palatal midline suture (maxillary denture). Other areas including peripheral tissues (maxillary denture) and ridge inclines (mandibular denture) do not contribute to support and may require relief.

9.4 Challenging Conditions

Several conditions pose challenges for the treatment of edentulous patients with complete dentures, and

Diseases and Conditions in Dentistry: An Evidence-Based Reference, First Edition. Keyvan Moharamzadeh.

Companion website: www.wiley.com/go/moharamzadeh/diseases

alternative restorative approaches may be indicated in some of these situations.

- Paget's disease is characterised by ongoing enlargement and alteration of the anatomy of bones and can involve the maxillary arch, complicating denture treatment.
- Mucous membrane diseases, including vesiculobullous diseases, pemphigus, pemphigoid and atrophic lichen planus, where slight frictional trauma from dentures can lead to the development of oral lesions such as vesicles, bullae and painful ulcerations.
- Patients with uncontrolled Parkinson's disease may experience difficulties with dentures due to severe tremor and facial rigidity.
- Patients with uncontrolled epilepsy can be at risk of denture fracture and inhalation of the fragments during epileptic attacks.
- Complete denture wear must be avoided immediately after radiotherapy that involves the oral cavity due to the risk of development of radiation-induced mucositis.
- Restricted mouth opening (trismus) can be due to several conditions, including trauma, temporomandibular joint dysfunction (TMD), oral cancer surgery, radiotherapy, cleft lip and palate, scarring from burn, scleroderma, Plummer–Vinson syndrome and oral submucous fibrosis. These conditions can severely restrict access and may require significantly reduced or sectional impression trays and jaw registration bases. Alternative approaches would be making two-part dentures with two interlocking halves. Mouth-opening exercises using a bundle of tongue depressors can be helpful in some cases to improve the vertical opening. Patients with microstomia and small mouth opening may also require different techniques and modifications of complete dentures (Cura *et al.*, 2003; Hajimahmoudi and Mostafavi, 2014; Hegde *et al.*, 2012; Sharma *et al.*, 2013).
- Enlarged ridges can cause aesthetic problems and provide inadequate interocclusal space. Removable treatment options may include surgical reduction or prescription of thin cast metal bases for the dentures.
- Allergy to denture base acrylic material can be confirmed by patch testing. Hypoallergenic denture base materials such as methyl methacrylate (MMA)-free resins, vulcanite-based or polycarbonate dentures can be alternative options.

9.5 Complete Denture Occlusion

9.5.1 Measuring Occlusal Vertical Dimension (OVD)

Achieving an ideal FWS of 2–4 mm depends on accurate measurement of the rest face height and the OVD. Below are some of the methods of measuring the rest face height.

- Niswonger's method: placing markers on the nose and chin and using dividers to measure the rest face height after the patient relaxes the jaw following swallowing or saying 'M' repeatedly.
- Willis gauge: which has a high interoperator variability due to soft tissue compression.
- Silverman's closest speaking distance: by trimming the wax rims until the patient can say 'S' without the wax rims touching each other (2 mm space). This technique requires experience, confidence and reduction of the width of the anterior wax rims.
- Boos bimeter method: using intraoral strain gauges to detect the maximum biting force point (power point) which indicates the OVD.
- Using a screw-jack until the patient reports that the OVD is comfortable and is not too high or too overclosed.

9.5.2 Registration of Centric Relation (CR)

Registering the jaw relationship in CR is another important step to achieve satisfactory occlusal outcome. Methods for CR positioning of the mandible are listed below.

- Raising the tongue as far back as possible to touch the soft palate and biting.
- Jaw manipulation by chin guiding or bimanual technique to retrude the mandible.
- Intraoral gothic arch tracing can be an accurate and consistent method of mandibular positioning when the patient cannot be persuaded to close the mouth at CR (Rubel and Hill, 2011). An adjustable pointer is attached to the maxillary block and a scribing plate is attached to the mandibular block. A V-shaped tracing is produced by anteroposterior and then lateral movements of mandible. The apex of the V is the CR (Figure 9.1).

9.5.3 Complete Denture Occlusal Schemes

Ideal occlusion for a patient with complete dentures differs from ideal occlusion for a dentate patient. Unlike normal dentition, in complete denture, it is desirable to maintain the occlusal contacts during lateral excursions (balanced dynamic occlusion or balanced articulation) to enhance the stability of the dentures.

Different occlusal schemes for complete dentures are discussed below.

9.5.3.1 Bilateral Balanced Occlusion

Balanced occlusion in both lateral and protrusive excursions is desirable for complete dentures when there are well-developed residual ridges, with skeletal class I relation. The components of bilateral balanced occlusion include the following.

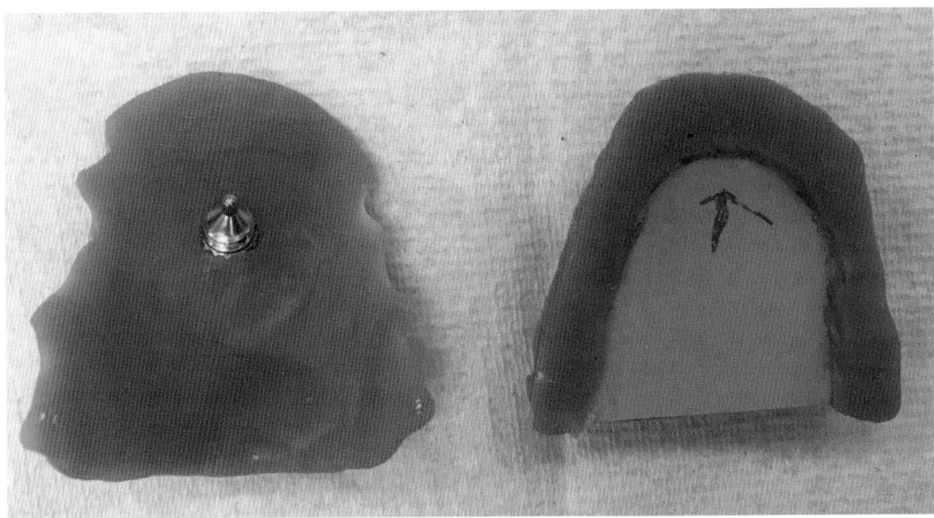

Figure 9.1 Gothic arch tracing using a pointer attached to the maxillary block and a scribing plate attached to the mandibular block.

- Anatomic denture teeth (with cusp angles of 20°) are set in an anteroposterior compensating curve (downwards curve) so that the teeth are tilted to form working cusp angles integrated with incisal guidance angle (10°) and condylar guidance angles (40°).
- Denture teeth are set in a lateral compensating curve where the maxillary teeth are tilted buccally to form working cusp angles integrated with the lateral translation movements of the mandible condyle.
- Bennet side shifts would affect the influence of condylar and incisal guidance and the geometry of the compensating curves (see Chapter 31).

When there is a highly resorbed or flat ridge or mandibular implant-supported complete denture against a maxillary complete denture, other occlusal schemes described below are recommended to improve the stability of the denture.

9.5.3.2 Monoplane Scheme of Occlusion

The monoplane scheme of occlusion with cuspless (flat-cusped, non-anatomic) teeth is set so that the anterior teeth provide the aesthetics, the premolars and first molars are used for chewing, and the second molars do not occlude although sometimes they are specifically used to establish bilateral contacts in lateral movements. This occlusal scheme provides better stability but has inefficient chewing and poor aesthetics.

9.5.3.3 Linear Occlusion Scheme

Linear contacts created by this occlusal scheme are the pinpoint contacts of the tips of the cusps of the bladed teeth in one arch against cuspless teeth that create a plane in the opposite arch. The specific design for positioning the modified teeth on the maxillary denture and non-anatomic teeth on the mandibular denture is called lingualised occlusion, which is characterised by contacts of only the palatal cusps of the maxillary teeth with the occlusal surfaces of the mandibular teeth. The lingualised occlusal scheme provides better aesthetics than the monoplane occlusion scheme, and better stability than the bilateral occlusion scheme of anatomic teeth in the case of resorbed residual ridges (Abduo, 2013).

9.5.4 Occlusal Adjustment

Where there is a large occlusal discrepancy, a precentric check record is essential to achieve a balanced occlusion by articulation and adjustment of dentures in the laboratory.

Slight discrepancies can be adjusted chairside by marking the premature contacts using articulating paper or occlusal indicator wax.

Premature contacts in CR can be corrected by deepening the opposing fossa to preserve the cusp. Premature contacts in lateral excursions can be eliminated by cusp reduction according to the BULL rule: Buccal cusp of the Upper teeth and Lingual cusp of the Lower teeth. Premature contacts in protrusive movements can be corrected by adjusting the distal slope of the maxillary buccal cusps and the mesial slopes of the mandibular lingual cusps (Davies *et al.*, 2001).

9.6 Setting Up the Teeth in Complete Denture

The upper incisor teeth are positioned to provide lip support with an average nasolabial angle of 90° with the incisal edges at 3–5 mm below the smile line.

The upper lip line, the smile line, alatragal and interpapillary lines are the most commonly used landmarks for the positioning, inclination and parallelism of the upper anterior and posterior occlusal planes. Other maxillary anatomical landmarks include the parotid papillae and the hamular notch-incisive papillae line (Shetty *et al.*, 2013).

Ismail and Bowman (1968) showed that the level of the pre-extraction mandibular natural dentition is at two-thirds of the retromolar pad and therefore it is recommended to position the lower occlusal plane extending from the corner of the lip.

A straight line connecting the inner canthus of the eye to the alar cartilages on each sides indicates the position of the tips of the maxillary canine teeth and the canine eminence which provides support for the angle of the mouth.

Biometric guidelines can be helpful in identifying the correct position of the teeth and a biometric special tray can be made accordingly. The labial surface of the incisor teeth is placed 6 mm labial to the palatal gingival vestige (a raised fibrous ridge on the palate). This measurement for the canine teeth is 8 mm and for the buccal surfaces of the premolars and molars is 10 mm and 12 mm respectively.

The incisive papilla is another important landmark, with the tips of the central incisor teeth being placed 8–10 mm in front of the central point of the papilla. This distance can be accurately measured on the denture using a Schottlander Alma gauge (Isa and Abdulhadi, 2012).

A lip index using silicone impression material can also be made to record the anterior neutral zone to aid positioning of maxillary anterior teeth.

9.7 Tooth Size and Shape

Factors affecting the tooth size and shape selection for complete denture are listed below.

- Interalar width, which is the distance between the midpoints of canines.
- Golden ratio of the width of the central incisor to the lateral incisor, which is 5:3.
- Patient's face shape which can be tapered, round or square.
- Shape of the maxillary ridge; for example, narrow teeth are suitable for a narrow ridge.
- Gender: women generally prefer curved and rounded features on their teeth.
- Age: attrition features and gingival recession can be incorporated into the denture teeth in older patients.

9.8 Soft Liners and Tissue Conditioners

Denture base relining with hard acrylic resin-based material can be indicated in cases of immediate dentures after the healing period and where the alveolar ridge resorption has resulted in poor denture adaptation. It is important to be aware of the risk that the relining procedure may increase the VD and the level of the incisal plane in the maxillary denture, which can cause occlusal and aesthetic problems. Using a closed-mouth silicone impression technique with escape holes in the denture can reduce this risk.

Soft liners can be useful to engage the ridge undercuts and cushion the underlying sharp and uneven edentulous ridges that are not amenable to relief.

Soft liners are categorised into two groups: highly plasticised acrylic liners (such as Eversoft, Coe-soft, Coe-comfort and Visco-Geland) and silicone-based soft liners (such as GC Reline Soft, Luci-soft, Molloplast B and Tokuyama). In terms of longevity, soft liners can be used in the short term as tissue conditioners or long term as semi-permanent reline materials (Rickman *et al.*, 2012).

Soft liners are associated with several problems, including biodegradation, hardening or softening, staining, roughening and delamination which can limit their long-term use (McCord *et al.*, 2011).

Tissue conditioners can be used to improve the fit of the denture temporarily and for cushioning of an existing denture to relieve soft tissue inflammation and trauma prior to the fabrication of new dentures. They can also be used for functional impression taking (see Chapter 45).

9.9 Copy Denture

The copy denture technique is intended to replace the patient's old dentures which have developed faults over time while maintaining or slightly modifying the position of the teeth, shape of the polished surface, base extension and OVD that the patient has been accustomed to, therefore improving patient acceptance of the new dentures (Davis, 1994).

The steps for the copy denture technique are described below (Soo and Cheng, 2014; Treasure, 1992).

1) Impression of the old dentures with alginate impression material using the flask technique and occlusal registration if necessary.
2) Denture replicates (models of acrylic bases with added acrylic teeth) are tried in and a closed-mouth silicone impression is taken. If there is a need to increase the VD, copy templates are made of acrylic bases with wax teeth first and are tried in the mouth. Then wax is added to the surface of the templates at

this stage to correct the VD. The acrylic teeth are then added and tried in the mouth in a subsequent visit.

3) Denture insertion.

9.10 Complete Denture Troubleshooting

Commonly encountered problems associated with complete denture wear include the following (LaBarre *et al.*, 2007; Pentel and Teichman, 1948).

- Poor retention can be due to dry mouth, anatomical issues (such as resorbed ridge, shallow sulcus), clinical faults (such as underextension, inadequate border seal) or technical fault. The underlying cause should be carefully identified and addressed. Saliva substitutes in patients with dry mouth and denture adhesives in patients with resorbed ridges may improve the retention of complete dentures. However, there is a need for standardised guidelines with regard to their application, removal and recall (Duqum *et al.*, 2012). Biological aspects of denture care products have been discussed in a separate publication (Moharamzadeh, 2016). Implant-supported solutions offer significant improvement in the retention of complete dentures as discussed in Chapter 45.
- Unstable denture can be due to problems with fitting surface (poor adaptation), occlusal surface (unbalanced occlusion), polishing surface (bulky or overextended), neutral zone (teeth placed out of neutral zone), anatomy (shallow sulcus), physiology (strong gag reflex) or pathology such as neuromuscular disease.
- Pain in the denture-bearing surface can be due to overextension, occlusal discrepancy, unstable denture, inadequate FWS (which may require remaking the dentures), allergy to denture-base materials, dry mouth, superficial mental foramen (which may require relief), sharp bony edges (which may require surgical correction or soft liners if the patient is not suitable for surgery).
- Pain from the tongue can be due to irregular lingual surface of the denture (which may require smoothing), inadequate tongue space (which can be improved by trimming the lingual aspect of the teeth or fabrication of new dentures), or burning mouth syndrome.
- Cheek biting can be due to excessive FWS or inadequate overjet. It can be corrected by trimming the buccal surfaces of the buccal cusps of the mandibular posterior teeth. Lip biting can be corrected by trimming the labial surfaces of the mandibular anterior teeth. If there is an edge-to-edge occlusion and minor adjustment does not solve the problem, the anterior mandibular teeth should be removed and new mandibular anterior teeth in retroclined position should be placed on the denture.
- Nausea can be caused by several factors in complete denture patients.
  - If nausea is recent and the patient has been wearing the dentures for a long time, it could be due to systemic or gastrointestinal disease.
  - Nausea can also be due to a bulky denture that may require thinning of the posterior palate to provide extra tongue space.
  - It can be due to a non-retentive maxillary denture falling on the tongue. Denture adhesives or dental implants can be helpful in these cases.
  - If the patient has never worn a denture previously, a gradual habituation approach can be helpful, using a horseshoe-shaped baseplate first, and then adding the anterior teeth, followed by the addition of the posterior teeth without lingual cusps.
  - If the patient cannot tolerate the impression taking, controlled breathing exercises or psychotherapy involving hypnosis or behavioural therapy can be useful alternative approaches.
- Poor speech can be due to the following factors.
  - Inadequate FWS that can affect the pronunciation of 's', 'sh' and 'th' and can cause denture clicking when the patient speaks.
  - Thick palate can affect the pronunciation of 'ch' and 't'.
  - Anterior misplaced teeth can affect 'f' and 'v' pronunciation.
  - Inadequate tongue space can also cause general difficulty with speech.
  - Excessive tongue space can cause hissing when saying 'L'.

Case Study

A 71-year-old male edentulous patient was referred from the oral and maxillofacial surgery department following the removal of T3 N0 M0 squamous cell carcinoma (SCC) of tongue involving partial glossectomy and reconstruction of the soft tissues with a right radial forearm free flap and postoperative adjuvant radiotherapy (50 Gy conventional external beam radiotherapy).

The patient was unable to wear his old dentures due to changes in the denture-bearing tissues following surgery and radiotherapy.

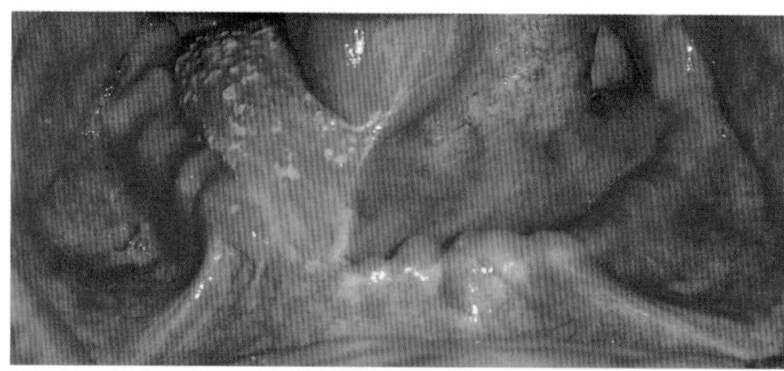

Figure 9.2 Preoperative clinical photograph of the edentulous mandible showing reduced sulcus depth and the radial forearm free flap on the right side of the floor of the mouth.

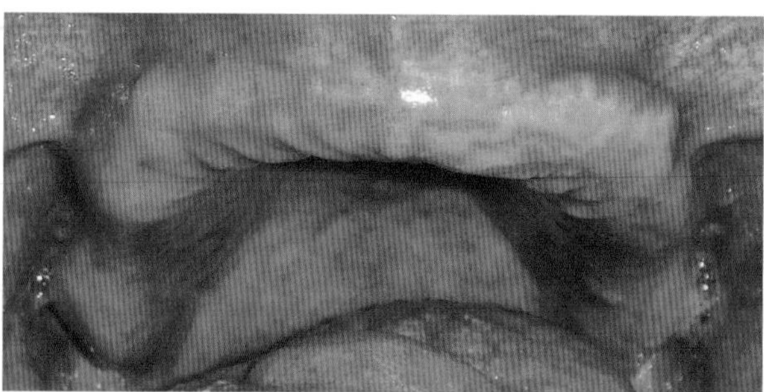

Figure 9.3 Preoperative photograph of the edentulous maxilla showing satisfactory ridge width and height.

The patient's preoperative clinical photographs are shown in Figures 9.2 and 9.3.

The patient had good mouth opening, reduced but satisfactory residual tongue function and no problems with swallowing. The decision was made to restore the patient's missing teeth with a set of new conventional complete dentures first.

The prognosis for the maxillary arch was good due to the presence of an alveolar ridge with adequate bone width and height. However, the prognosis for the complete denture in the mandible was compromised due to the resorbed ridge, reduced sulcus depth, presence of the flap and reduced tongue function. Therefore, it was decided to initially rehabilitate the mandible with an acrylic baseplate only to assess the patient's adaptability to the prosthesis in the mandibular arch.

Procedures Undertaken

1) Primary impressions with alginate impression material using stock trays.
2) Adjustment and border moulding of the close-fitting special trays with green stick material and secondary impressions using ZOE impression material.
3) Wax rim adjustment for the maxillary denture to achieve ideal lip support, anterior and posterior occlusal planes and the midline.
4) Wax try-in of the maxillary teeth only.
5) Insertion of the maxillary complete denture and a mandibular acrylic baseplate only.
6) At the review appointment, the patient showed good adaptation to the new maxillary denture and satisfactory compliance with wearing the mandibular baseplate.
7) Addition of wax rim to the baseplate, and bite registration to achieve an ideal occlusion, OVD and FWS.
8) Wax try-in of the mandibular teeth.
9) Denture insertion.
10) Review.

The patient's postoperative photographs are shown in Figures 9.4 and 9.5.

This was a challenging case due to the altered anatomy following partial glossectomy and the presence of a radial forearm flap.

Adjusting and border moulding the special trays was an important step in recording the accurate sulcus depth and width to improve retention and stability of the dentures.

Fabrication of the mandibular baseplate was very helpful to allow the patient to adapt to the baseplate as a transitional stage before fabricating the mandibular complete denture.

The patient was very satisfied with the maxillary denture, but the retention of the mandibular denture was compromised due to the anatomical limitations described above. The use of denture adhesives improved retention

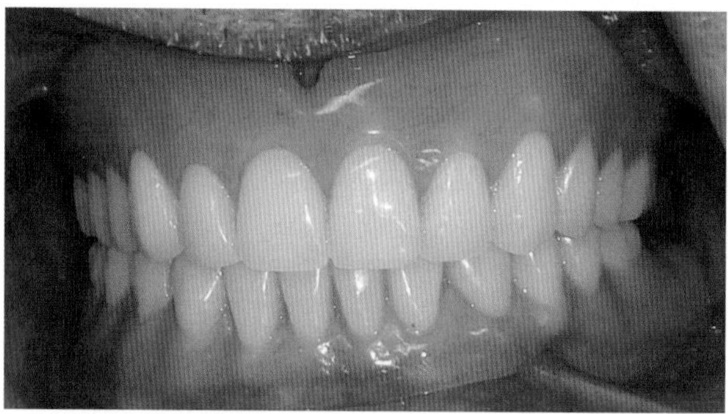

Figure 9.4 Postoperative photograph of the complete dentures.

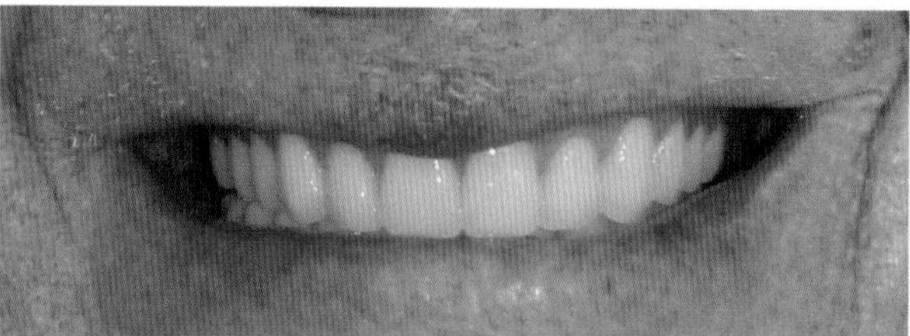

Figure 9.5 Postoperative photograph of the smile.

of the denture. The option of mandibular implants to support an overdenture was discussed with the patient, including the risks and benefits. The limitations of implant treatment in this case included reduced bone volume in the mandible, poor-quality soft tissues and the increased risk of implant failure and development of osteoradionecrosis due to the history of high-dose external beam radiotherapy in the mandible.

Restorative rehabilitation of oncology patients is discussed in Chapters 32 and 33.

References

Abduo, J. (2013) Occlusal schemes for complete dentures: a systematic review. *Int J Prosthodont*, **26**, 26–33.

Carlsson, G.E. and Omar, R. (2010) The future of complete dentures in oral rehabilitation. A critical review. *J Oral Rehabil*, **37**, 143–156.

Cura, C., Cotert, H.S. and User, A. (2003) Fabrication of a sectional impression tray and sectional complete denture for a patient with microstomia and trismus: a clinical report. *J Prosthet Dent*, **89**, 540–543.

Davis, D.M. (1994) Copy denture technique: a critique. *Dent Update*, **21**, 15–20.

Davies, S.J., Gray, R.M. and Mccord, J.F. (2001) Good occlusal practice in removable prosthodontics. *Br Dent J*, **191**, 491–494, 497–502.

Duqum, I., Powers, K.A., Cooper, L. and Felton, D. (2012) Denture adhesive use in complete dentures: clinical recommendations and review of the literature. *Gen Dent*, **60**, 467–477; quiz 478–479.

Hajimahmoudi, M. and Mostafavi, A.S. (2014) A simple and effective method for prosthetic rehabilitation in scleroderma patients: a clinical report. *Int J Prosthodont*, **27**, 169–173.

Hegde, C., Prasad, K., Prasad, A. and Hegde, R. (2012) Impression tray designs and techniques for complete dentures in cases of microstomia – a review. *J Prosthodont Res*, **56**, 142–146.

Isa, Z.M. and Abdulhadi, L.M. (2012) Relationship of maxillary incisors in complete dentures to the incisive papilla. *J Oral Sci*, **54**, 159–163.

Ismail, Y.H. and Bowman, J.F. (1968) Position of the occlusal plane in natural and artificial teeth. *J Prosthet Dent*, **20**, 407–411.

Jacobson, T.E. and Krol, A.J. (1983) A contemporary review of the factors involved in complete dentures. Part III: support. *J Prosthet Dent*, **49**, 306–313.

Labarre, E., Giusti, L. and Pitigoi-Aron, G. (2007) Addressing problems in complete dentures. *Compend Contin Educ Dent*, **28**, 538–540, 542.

McCord, J.F., Donaldson, A.C. and Lamont, T.J. (2011) A contemporary update on 'soft' linings. *Dent Update*, **38**, 102–104.

Moharamzadeh, K. (2016) Biocompatibility of oral care products, in *Biocompatibility Of Dental Biomaterials* (ed. R. Shelton), Woodhead Publishing, Cambridge, pp. 113–129.

Ogden, A. (1996) *British Society for the Study of Prosthetic Dentistry: Guidelines in Prosthetic and Implant Dentistry*, Quintessence Publishing, New Malden.

Pentel, L. and Teichman, S.G. (1948) Troubleshooting in complete denture prosthesis. *N Y State Dent J*, **14**, 551–565.

Rickman, L.J., Padipatvuthikul, P. and Satterthwaite, J.D. (2012) Contemporary denture base resins: part 2. *Dent Update*, **39**, 176–178, 180–182, 184 passim.

Rubel, B. and Hill, E.E. (2011) Intraoral gothic arch tracing. *N Y State Dent J*, **77**, 40–43.

Sharma, A., Arora, P. and Wazir, S.S. (2013) Hinged and sectional complete dentures for restricted mouth opening: a case report and review. *Contemp Clin Dent*, **4**, 74–77.

Shetty, S., Zargar, N.M., Shenoy, K. and Rekha, V. (2013) Occlusal plane location in edentulous patients: a review. *J Indian Prosthodont Soc*, **13**, 142–148.

Soo, S. and Cheng, A.C. (2014) Complete denture copy technique – a practical application. *Singapore Dent J*, **35**, 65–70.

Thomason, J.M., Kelly, S.A., Bendkowski, A. and Ellis, J.S. (2012) Two implant retained overdentures – a review of the literature supporting the Mcgill and York consensus statements. *J Dent*, **40**, 22–34.

Treasure, P. (1992) The copy denture technique. *N Z Dent J*, **88**, 56–59.

Tyrovolas, S., Koyanagi, A., Panagiotakos, D.B. *et al.* (2016) Population prevalence of edentulism and its association with depression and self-rated health. *Sci Rep*, **6**, 37083.

10

Deep Overbite

10.1 Definition and Prevalence

Deep overbite or deep bite can be defined as the excessive vertical overlap of the mandibular incisor teeth by the maxillary incisor teeth when the mandible is in centric occlusion (Naini *et al.*, 2006). The average overbite depth is 2–4 mm.

The prevalence of deep bite varies among different populations and the reported figures are approximately 8–20% (Proffit *et al.*, 1998).

10.2 Aetiology

Increased overbite is often part of another malocclusion (such as Class II Division II) and can be due to the following reasons (Nielsen, 1991; Sreedhar and Baratam, 2009).

- Hereditary and genetic factors
- Skeletal factors such as discrepancy in horizontal and vertical growth of mandibular and maxillary arches
- Dental factors such as wear or loss of posterior teeth, overeruption or drifting of the anterior teeth
- Muscular factors such as strong muscles of mastication causing molar intrusion
- Habits such as lip sucking and lateral tongue thrust

10.3 Classification

Deep bite can be classified based on its origin (dental or skeletal), dentition (primary, mixed or permanent dentition), and its extent.

Akerly (1977) classified traumatic overbite into four categories.

- Type I: The palatal mucosa is at risk of trauma from the incisal edge of the mandibular incisor teeth.
- Type II: The maxillary palatal marginal gingiva is at risk of trauma from the incisal edge of the mandibular incisor teeth.
- Type III: Direct trauma to the palatal soft tissue of the maxillary incisor teeth, or to the labial mucosa of the mandibular incisor teeth, or both simultaneously.
- Type IV: The mandibular incisor teeth cause progressive attrition of the palatal surfaces of the opposing maxillary incisor teeth.

The factors implicated in the progression of an asymptomatic deep overbite to a traumatic relationship may include loss of posterior support, periodontitis and attachment loss, and iatrogenic damage by orthodontic or restorative treatment (Beddis *et al.*, 2014).

10.4 Treatment Options

Asymptomatic deep bite can often be accepted by the patient and monitored. However, the patient may seek treatment to reduce the trauma caused by the increased overbite, restore function and improve aesthetics. Different treatment modalities are discussed below.

10.4.1 Orthodontic Treatment

Orthodontic treatment is the preferred management option in growing young patients and it can be recommended for the correction of deep overbite in adults as well. It involves the intrusion of the anterior teeth only or in combination with the extrusion of the posterior teeth or proclination of the labial segments (Nanda, 1997).

Incisor intrusion is indicated where there is a large incisor–stomion distance which is often associated with a gummy smile. Incisor intrusion is also favourable when there is a large vertical facial height and inadequate or normal free-way space present. A maxillary anterior bite plane is a commonly used appliance for intrusion of the

Diseases and Conditions in Dentistry: An Evidence-Based Reference, First Edition. Keyvan Moharamzadeh.

Companion website: www.wiley.com/go/moharamzadeh/diseases

mandibular incisor teeth. A high-pull headgear can be useful for intruding the maxillary incisor teeth in extreme deep bite cases.

Extrusion of the posterior teeth is indicated where there is short vertical height with no interlabial gap, normal incisor–stomion distance and adequate free-way space. Functional appliances can reduce the overbite by preventing mandibular incisor overeruption and allowing eruption of the posterior teeth. Fixed orthodontic appliances can be used for both extrusion of the posterior teeth and intrusion of the anterior teeth.

10.4.2 Orthognathic Surgery

Orthognathic surgery in combination with orthodontic treatment can be a viable treatment option in adult patients with large skeletal discrepancy and decreased lower facial height after growth completion (Bell *et al.*, 1984). Le Fort I maxillary osteotomy can correct the deep bite due to vertical maxillary excess by moving the maxilla upward. Mandibular sagittal-split ramus osteotomy can rotate the mandible forward and down to correct the skeletal deep bite in patients with short face. Segmental osteotomy can also be considered in certain cases to correct localised alveolar discrepancies.

10.4.3 Prosthodontic and Restorative Treatment

Restorative treatment including fixed restorations and removable dentures can be a preferred approach for the manage'ment of deep overbite in many patients (Beddis *et al.*, 2014; Cotter and O'Shea, 2002).

Preventive treatment, including oral hygiene education, management of caries, periodontal disease and endodontic conditions, must be carried out prior to complex restorative rehabilitation.

Preparation of clinical photographs, aesthetic assessment, articulated study models, occlusal analysis and diagnostic wax-up are essential steps in restorative treatment planning.

Restorative options for the management of deep overbite are discussed below.

- The anterior Dahl approach can be adopted to reduce a deep overbite. The palatal surfaces of the maxillary anterior teeth can be augmented at an increased vertical dimension (VD) using direct or indirect restorations to provide occlusion with the mandibular anterior teeth. This will result in disclusion of the posterior teeth which will potentially further erupt over time and re-establish the posterior occlusion. The Dahl approach is discussed in detail in Chapter 50.
- Posterior occlusal onlays or crowns placed at increased VD can also reduce the anterior overbite. This option would be preferred if the posterior teeth are worn and require restorations. Providing an anterior bite plane or palatal augmentation of the upper anterior teeth can prevent the overeruption of the lower anterior teeth.
- A removable prosthesis can be indicated when there are missing posterior teeth resulting in overclosure and anterior deep bite. An overlay denture covering the occlusal surfaces of the posterior teeth at an increased VD can be constructed to reduce the overbite. Incorporating an anterior bite-plane to the denture would prevent the overeruption of the mandibular incisor teeth and soft tissue trauma.
- A combination of fixed and removable approaches can also be used in partially dentate patients with deep overbite. This includes restoration of the posterior abutment teeth at an increased VD with milled crowns incorporating the partial denture design features (such as rest seats, guide planes and undercuts) and subsequent fabrication of a cobalt-chromium removable partial denture with an anterior bite plane. The use of metal occlusal surfaces on prosthetic teeth can increase the wear resistance of the posterior teeth in these combination cases.

Case Study

A 37-year-old male patient presented with worn upper and lower anterior teeth, deep overbite and painful bleeding gums. The patient was medically fit and well, a non-smoker and a regular dentist attender (every 6 months).

The patient reported a positive history of bruxism and grinding his teeth at night. There was no history of GI disease or vomiting and no contributory dietary factors such as excessive acidic or carbonated drinks.

The patient's oral hygiene was poor and the basic periodontal exam (BPE) scores were 2 in all quadrants.

The preoperative clinical photographs are shown in Figures 10.1 and 10.2.

Electric pulp testing showed the worn anterior teeth were all vital and there was no obvious periapical pathology on radiographic examination. The mandibular anterior teeth had short roots.

Diagnoses

- Gingivitis
- Localised anterior moderate to advanced tooth surface loss, mainly attrition due to bruxism
- Failed restorations on UR2 and UL2

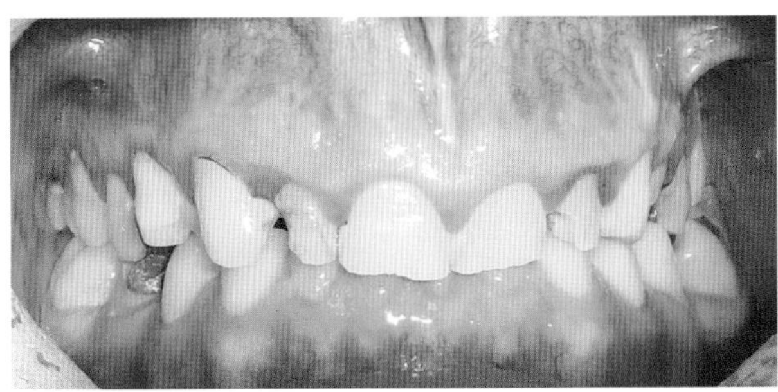

Figure 10.1 Preoperative clinical photograph in centric occlusion showing gingival inflammation, deep overbite and worn upper anterior teeth.

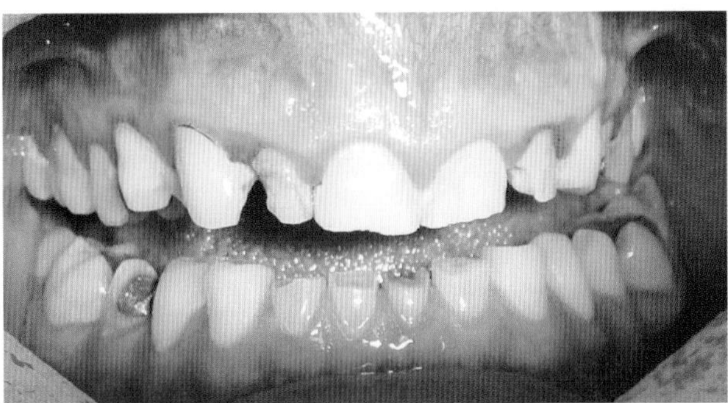

Figure 10.2 Partially open-mouth preoperative photograph showing the attrition of the mandibular anterior teeth with loss of greater than 50% of the clinical crown height.

Treatment Factors

Due to the patient's poor plaque control and the presence of gingival inflammation, oral hygiene education and periodontal treatment were essential prior to any definitive restorative treatment.

Since the posterior molar teeth were not worn and the tooth wear was only localised to the anterior teeth, adopting an anterior Dahl approach would be a suitable management option to restore the worn anterior teeth and reduce the overbite.

Direct restorations with composites were preferred over indirect techniques and crowns for the restorations of the worn teeth for the following reasons:

- presence of sufficient enamel for bonding
- reversible and conservative nature of treatment with direct composites
- presence of short roots which contraindicated surgical crown-lengthening procedures
- risk of damage to the pulp with indirect techniques requiring significant preparation of the teeth.

Treatment Procedures

1) Oral hygiene education, patient motivation and non-surgical periodontal treatment.
2) Reassessment in 3 months showed significant improvement in periodontal condition and resolution of gingival inflammation and bleeding.
3) Impressions, bite registration at retruded contact position (RCP), face-bow transfer and preparation of articulated study models for occlusal analysis was an important step in restorative treatment planning.
4) Diagnostic wax-up of the worn anterior teeth to ideal shape and height at a VD increased by 2 mm to provide occlusal contacts and reduce the overbite (anterior Dahl concept). Diagnostic wax-up enabled visualisation of the final outcome at an early stage by intraoral rehearsal (wax-up trial) using temporary crown material (Protemp).
5) Composite build-up of the worn maxillary and mandibular anterior teeth using a palatal and lingual sectional silicone putty index made over the diagnostic wax-up to enable restoration of the palatal and lingual surfaces of the teeth according to the wax-up.
6) Review of the patient in 3 months showed satisfactory re-establishment of the posterior occlusal contacts.
7) Fabrication and fitting of an upper hard stabilising (Michigan-type) splint to protect the restorations long term as the patient had bruxism.
8) Review and maintenance.

Postoperative clinical photographs are shown in Figures 10.3 and 10.4.

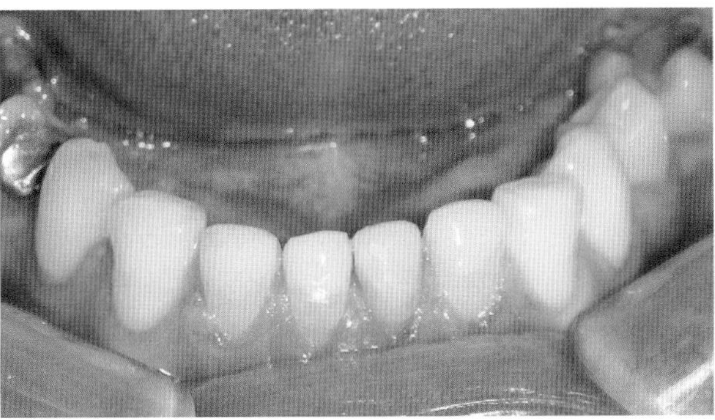

Figure 10.3 Postoperative photograph of the mandibular anterior teeth following composite restorations.

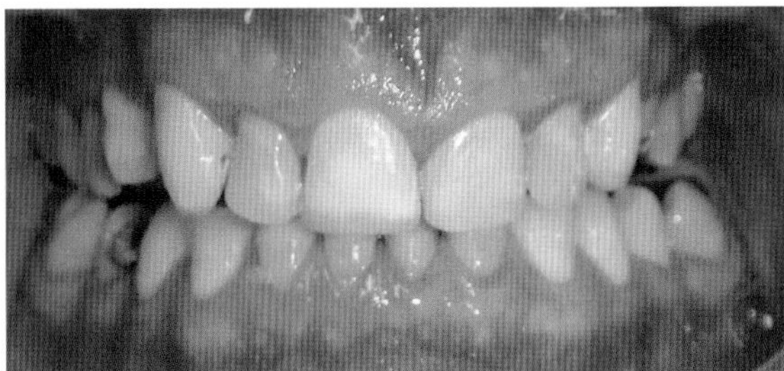

Figure 10.4 Postoperative photograph of the occlusion showing reduced overbite following build-up of the anterior teeth.

References

Akerly, W.B. (1977) Prosthodontic treatment of traumatic overlap of the anterior teeth. *J Prosthet Dent*, **38**, 26–34.

Beddis, H.P., Durey, K., Alhilou, A. and Chan, M.F. (2014) The restorative management of the deep overbite. *Br Dent J*, **217**, 509–515.

Bell, W.H., Jacobs, J.D. and Legan, H.L. (1984) Treatment of class II deep bite by orthodontic and surgical means. *Am J Orthod*, **85**, 1–20.

Cotter, S. and O'Shea, D. (2002) Traumatic overbite: a restorative solution. *Dent Update*, **29**, 136–140.

Naini, F.B., Gill, D.S., Sharma, A. and Tredwin, C. (2006) The aetiology, diagnosis and management of deep overbite. *Dent Update*, **33**, 326–328, 330–332, 334–336.

Nanda, R. (1997) Correction of deep overbite in adults. *Dent Clin North Am*, **41**, 67–87.

Nielsen, I.L. (1991) Vertical malocclusions: etiology, development, diagnosis and some aspects of treatment. *Angle Orthod*, **61**, 247–260.

Proffit, W.R., Fields, H.W. Jr and Moray, L.J. (1998) Prevalence of malocclusion and orthodontic treatment need in the United States: estimates from the NHANES III survey. *Int J Adult Orthodon Orthognath Surg*, **13**, 97–106.

Sreedhar, C. and Baratam, S. (2009) Deep overbite – a review. *Ann Essences Dent*, **1**, 8–25.

11

Dens Invaginatus

Badr Alghaithi - Case study

11.1 Definition and Terminology

Dens invaginatus is a developmental malformation that occurs during tooth development prior to calcification due to an infolding of the enamel organ into the dental papilla. The affected teeth show a deep invagination of the enamel and dentine starting from the crown and sometimes extending deep into the root (Hulsmann, 1997).

Other terminology used for this dental anomaly include dens in dente, dentoid in dente, dilated gestant odontome, dilated composite odontome, invaginated odontome, tooth inclusion and dens telescope.

11.2 Aetiology and Prevalence

The aetiology of this malformation is not completely understood and several theories have been proposed, including growth pressure on the enamel organ, localised growth failure or rapid proliferation of the internal enamel epithelium, distortion of the enamel organ, fusion of two tooth germs, infection and trauma (Alani and Bishop, 2008; Hulsmann, 1997).

The prevalence of dens invaginatus can be variable, ranging from 0.3% to 10%, most commonly affecting the permanent maxillary lateral incisors, followed by the maxillary central incisors, premolars, canines and less frequently the molars. Bilateral conditions have been reported in 43% of cases (Gallacher *et al.*, 2016; Ruprecht *et al.*, 1986).

11.3 Classification

The most commonly used classification system for dens invaginatus lesions is Oehler's classification (Oehlers, 1957) which described three forms for the anomaly of coronal invaginations (Figure 11.1).

- *Type I invagination* occurs within the limits of the crown and does not extend beyond the cementoenamel junction (CEJ).
- *Type II invagination* extends deeper into the root beyond the CEJ but does not communicate with the periodontal ligament (PDL) and may or may not involve the pulp.
- *Type III A invagination* goes through the root and opens laterally into the PDL space, forming a second foramen, often without communicating with the pulp. Periodontal attachment breakdown can lead to the development of peri-invagination periodontitis.
- *Type III B invagination* extends through the root all the way down to the apex as a separate duct without involving the pulp canal and opens through an apical foramen into the PDL.

Other classification systems include Hallet's first classification in 1953 and Schulze and Brand's detailed classification of dens invaginatus (Schulze and Brand, 1972).

11.4 Clinical Examination and Investigations

Dens invaginatus can be difficult to detect during routine dental examination, especially if the tooth is asymptomatic. Only a small palatal pit or slightly raised cingulum may be visible on visual-tactile examination. However, if the undiagnosed teeth are left untreated, caries can develop and progress from the invagination opening and may subsequently expose the pulp, leading to pulpal and periradicular disease (Bishop and Alani, 2008).

The following investigations are helpful in diagnosis of dens invaginatus and would facilitate further management of this condition.

Diseases and Conditions in Dentistry: An Evidence-Based Reference, First Edition. Keyvan Moharamzadeh.

Companion website: www.wiley.com/go/moharamzadeh/diseases

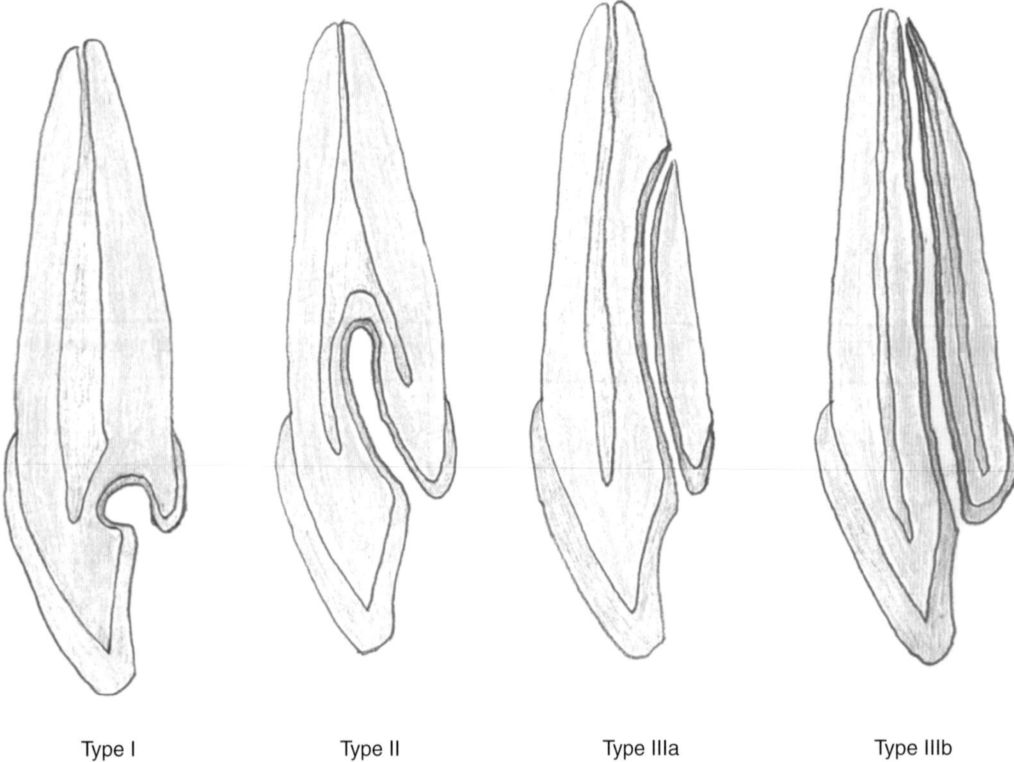

Figure 11.1 Different types of dens invaginatus according to Oehler's classification.

- Tooth vitality (sensibility) testing would be useful to determine if the lesion is related to pulpal necrosis.
- Percussion testing can indicate periapical or periodontal involvement.
- Periodontal probing can identify the presence of associated periodontal pockets.
- Periapical radiograph is an important diagnostic tool to further investigate the suspected teeth to identify the invagination and also to assess the status of the periodontal bone and periapical tissues. A second periapical radiograph with a different horizontal angulation can provide additional information about the depth and type of the lesion.
- Cone beam computed tomography (CBCT) can provide a detailed three-dimensional (3D) image of the lesion and can be helpful in confirming the morphology of the invagination, its relationship with the pulp canal and the periradicular tissues and the proximity of the tooth to the adjacent anatomical structures as well as the bone volume around the tooth (Agrawal *et al.*, 2016; Vier-Pelisser *et al.*, 2012).

11.5 Treatment Considerations

The preferred treatment option for teeth with dens invaginatus depends on the following prognostic factors.

- Type and extent of the invagination and the root canal morphology.
- Vital or non-vital status of the pulp.
- Presence or absence of associated periodontal lesions.
- Restorability of the tooth, as non-restorable teeth would require extraction.

Treatment recommendations for restorable teeth with different types of dens invaginatus are summarised in Table 11.1.

Table 11.1 Treatment recommendations for teeth with different types of dens invaginatus.

Type	Recommendation
Type I (vital)	Sealing of the invagination with acid-etched flowable resin or fissure sealant to prevent the development of caries
Type I (non-vital)	Root canal treatment (RCT) and incorporation of the invagination into the access cavity (Schmitz *et al.*, 2010)
Type II (vital)	Prophylactic access of the invagination entrance using rotary or ultrasonic instruments under appropriate magnification to fully expose the invagination, debridement and then obturation of the invagination using mineral trioxide aggregate (MTA), biodentine or calcium hydroxide cement (indirect pulp capping) and sealing the access cavity with composite resin. The tooth will then need to be monitored (Alani and Bishop, 2009)
Type II (non-vital)	RCT and incorporation of the invagination into the access cavity
Type IIIa (vital)	Sealing of the invagination with acid-etched flowable resin or fissure sealant
Type IIIa (non-vital)	Endodontic treatment of both pulp canal and the invagination. The pulp canal can be prepared and debrided using conventional endodontic instruments and obturated with thermosplasticised gutta percha to achieve 3D obturation. The enamel-lined invagination will need to be prepared using ultrasonic tips under magnification and obturation with MTA as it communicates with the PDL (Bishop and Alani, 2008)
Type IIIa with associated periodontal defect	Endodontic treatment of the infected invagination and management of the periodontal defect which may require surgical assessment and regenerative procedures if there is an intrabony defect (Chaniotis *et al.*, 2008; Falcao *et al.*, 2012)
Type IIIb (vital)	Sealing of the invagination with acid-etched flowable resin or fissure sealant
Type IIIb (non-vital)	Endodontic treatment of both pulp canal and invagination as described above in non-vital type IIIa cases. The two canals can often be combined and prepared as a single merged canal and obturated with an MTA plug at the open apex, backfilled with thermosplasticised gutta percha (Silberman *et al.*, 2006). Management of teeth with open apices is discussed in Chapter 34
Complex anatomy and failed RCT	Teeth with complex anatomy that are not amenable to non-surgical endodontic treatment or failed previous non-surgical treatment attempts may require surgical endodontic treatment (Ozcakir Tomruk *et al.*, 2008) or extraction

Case Study

A 37-year-old male patient was referred by the dentist for endodontic treatment of non-vital UR2.

The patient was asymptomatic at the time of examination and reported no history of trauma and the tooth had no previous treatment. The patient was medically fit and well.

Clinical examination of UR2 showed the tooth was slightly tender to percussion and there was no associated swelling or sinus tract. The tooth was not mobile and there were no deep periodontal pockets associated with the tooth.

Electric pulp testing of UR2 gave a negative response.

Radiographic examination (Figure 11.2) showed that UR2 had a possible dens invaginatus malformation with a wide canal in the mid and apical thirds. There was also an open apex and a periapical radiolucency associated with the tooth.

The diagnoses were:

- non-vital UR2 with associated chronic apical periodontitis
- dens invaginatus (type II) and an open apex.

The prognosis for the tooth was guarded due to the depth of invagination and open apex.

The treatment strategy included root canal treatment of UR2 using microscope magnification and ultrasonic endodontic tips to incorporate the invagination into the access

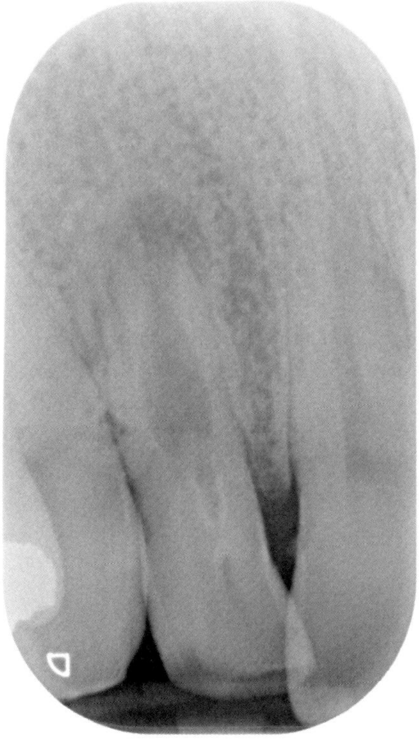

Figure 11.2 Preoperative periapical radiograph showing Oehler's type II dens invaginatus, open apex and periapical radiolucency.

cavity, thorough debridement of the root canal, obturation of the apical part of the canal with an MTA plug and backfilling the root canal with warm gutta percha using the Obtura system. The postoperative radiograph is shown in Figure 11.3.

The patient remained asymptomatic throughout and after treatment. He was not available to obtain a 9-month follow-up radiograph.

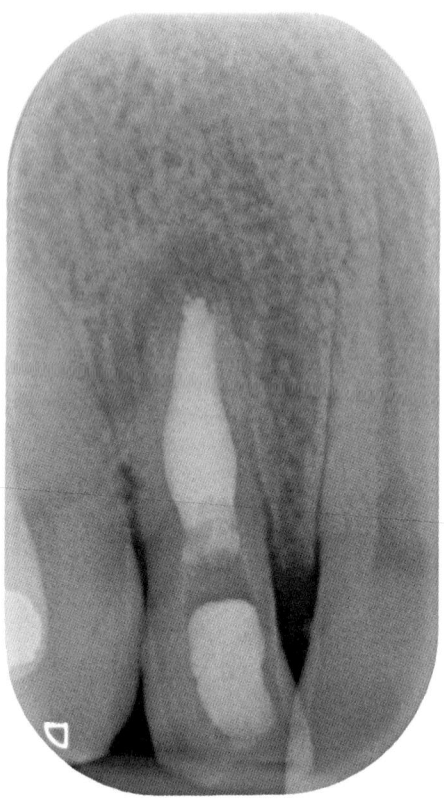

Figure 11.3 Postoperative periapical radiograph of UR2.

References

Agrawal, P.K., Wankhade, J. and Warhadpande, M. (2016) A rare case of type III dens invaginatus in a mandibular second premolar and its nonsurgical endodontic management by using cone-beam computed tomography: a case report. *J Endod*, **42**, 669–672.

Alani, A. and Bishop, K. (2008) Dens invaginatus. Part 1: Classification, prevalence and aetiology. *Int Endod J*, **41**, 1123–1136.

Alani, A. and Bishop, K. (2009) The use of MTA in the modern management of teeth affected by dens invaginatus. *Int Dent J*, **59**, 343–348.

Bishop, K. and Alani, A. (2008) Dens invaginatus. Part 2: Clinical, radiographic features and management options. *Int Endod J*, **41**, 1137–1154.

Chaniotis, A.M., Tzanetakis, G.N., Kontakiotis, E.G. and Tosios, K.I. (2008) Combined endodontic and surgical management of a mandibular lateral incisor with a rare type of dens invaginatus. *J Endod*, **34**, 1255–1260.

Falcao L.S., de Freitas, P.S., Marreiro R.O. and Garrido, A.D. (2012) Management of dens invaginatus type III with large periradicular lesion. *J Contemp Dent Pract*, **13**, 119–124.

Gallacher, A., Ali, R. and Bhakta, S. (2016) Dens invaginatus: diagnosis and management strategies. *Br Dent J*, **221**, 383–387.

Hulsmann, M. (1997) Dens invaginatus: aetiology, classification, prevalence, diagnosis, and treatment considerations. *Int Endod J*, **30**, 79–90.

Oehlers, F.A. (1957) Dens invaginatus (dilated composite odontome). I. Variations of the invagination process and associated anterior crown forms. *Oral Surg Oral Med Oral Pathol*, **10**, 1204–1218.

Ozcakir Tomruk, C., Tanalp, J., Yurdaguven, H. and Ersev, H. (2008) Endodontic and surgical management of a maxillary lateral incisor with type III dens invaginatus: a 12-month follow-up. *Oral Surg Oral Med Oral Pathol Oral Radiol Endod*, **106**, E84–87.

Ruprecht, A., Batniji, S., Sastry, K.A. and El-Neweihi, E. (1986) The incidence of dental invagination. *J Pedod*, **10**, 265–272.

Schmitz, M.S., Montagner, F., Flores, C.B., Morari, V.H., Quesada, G.A. and Gomes, B.P. (2010) Management of dens invaginatus type I and open apex: report of three cases. *J Endod*, **36**, 1079–1085.

Schulze, C. and Brand, E. (1972) [Dens Invaginatus (Dens In Dente)]. *Zwr*, **81**, 699–703.

Silberman, A., Cohenca, N. and Simon, J.H. (2006) Anatomical redesign for the treatment of dens invaginatus type III with open apexes: a literature review and case presentation. *J Am Dent Assoc*, **137**, 180–185.

Vier-Pelisser, F.V., Pelisser, A., Recuero, L.C., So, M.V., Borba, M.G. and Figueiredo, J.A. (2012) Use of cone beam computed tomography in the diagnosis, planning and follow up of a type III dens invaginatus case. *Int Endod J*, **45**, 198–208.

12

Dentine Hypersensitivity

12.1 Definition

Dentine hypersensitivity (DHS) can be defined as a transient sharp pain which arises from the exposed tooth dentine in response to different stimuli such as cold, heat, tactile or osmotic pressure, surface water evaporation, and chemical agents in the absence of any other dental disease or pathology (Addy, 1990).

12.2 Prevalence

Dentine hypersensitivity can affect 10–20% of adults at any age but the highest prevalence is among people aged 30–40 years (Flynn *et al.*, 1985). The most frequently affected teeth are the canines and first premolars, followed by incisors and second premolars. Buccal cervical regions are affected in 90% of cases (Addy *et al.*, 1987).

12.3 Aetiology and Pathogenesis

The UK and Ireland Dentine Hypersensitivity Expert Forum (Gillam *et al.*, 2013) identified three major categories of diseases and conditions associated with DHS.

- Gingival recession caused by mechanical trauma
- Tooth wear lesions
- Periodontal disease and periodontal treatment

Tooth whitening has also been associated with an increased risk of DHS. Mild to moderate transient dentine sensitivity has been reported in 15–65% of patients using 10% carbamide peroxide (Albanai *et al.*, 2015).

Proposed mechanisms of DHS include exposure of dentinal tubules, fluid movement and hydrodynamic forces (the most widely accepted theory) (Braennstroem and Astroem, 1964), direct innervation theory (Irvine, 1988), peripheral sensitisation of pulpal nociceptors and odontoblast receptors (Magloire, 2011) and exacerbation by bacteria-induced pulpal inflammation (Brannstrom, 1992).

In patients with gingival recession, the cementum covering the surface of the exposed root dentine can be easily removed by physical forces or chemical agents, leading to exposure of the underlying dentinal tubules and therefore an increase in the risk of development of DHS (Gillam *et al.*, 2013).

Sixteen percent of patients develop DHS following non-surgical periodontal treatment which peaks during the first week and then often subsides; 26% of patients develop sensitivity 6 months to 5 years after surgical treatment (Draenert *et al.*, 2013).

Different individuals may experience different levels of DHS. These variations can be due to patients' pain perception, local factors and dietary factors. Foods and drinks with high acidity can cause significant tooth surface loss and erosion, particularly when combined with tooth brushing (Addy, 2005).

12.4 History and Examination

Relevant aspects of the patient's history with regard to DHS include the nature of sensitivity, dietary factors, tooth-brushing technique, any previous periodontal treatment and other dental treatments, including tooth whitening.

It is important to rule out other conditions such as caries, failed restorations, enamel/dentine fracture, cracked tooth syndrome, pulpal disease and gingivitis.

Air burst test and dentine scratch test using a sharp probe are two simple diagnostic tests for DHS (Kleinberg *et al.*, 1990).

Diseases and Conditions in Dentistry: An Evidence-Based Reference, First Edition. Keyvan Moharamzadeh.

Companion website: www.wiley.com/go/moharamzadeh/diseases

12.5 Management

The aim of management is to eliminate the underlying conditions and predisposing factors and thus reduce the patient's symptoms. The treatment strategy should be tailored to the relevant aetiological factors in each patient. Other causes of dental pain such as caries, tooth cracks, fractures and failed restorations must be identified and treated as soon as possible.

12.5.1 Management of DHS in Patients with Gingival Recession and/or Periodontal Disease

The treatment strategy for this group of patients includes the following aspects (Gillam *et al.*, 2013; Miglani *et al.*, 2010).

- Patient education and demonstration of the areas of recession.
- Oral hygiene instructions and tooth-brushing advice to avoid aggressive mechanical brushing, including advice against the use of excessive force, hard toothbrush and abrasive toothpaste.
- Single-tufted toothbrushes are recommended for cleaning the recession areas.
- Dietary advice to reduce excessive consumption of acidic foods and drinks.
- Treatment of any inflammatory periodontal disease as described in Chapters 1 and 6.
- Advice on 'at-home' desensitising therapy, including the use of desensitising toothpastes, mouthwashes and chewing gums which often contain agents such as potassium salts, sodium fluoride, sodium monofluorophosphate, stannous fluoride and strontium chloride.
- Application of in-office desensitising agents such as 2.26% sodium fluoride varnish, potassium oxalate gel or adhesive resin tubule sealants, if necessary (da Rosa *et al.*, 2013).
- Regular review and maintenance.

The literature suggests that periodontal soft tissue grafting and surgical root coverage procedures may also reduce cervical DHS. However, the level of evidence is not sufficient to be conclusive (Douglas de Oliveira *et al.*, 2013).

Lasers have also been shown to be effective in sealing dentine tubules and reducing hypersensitivity (Sgolastra *et al.*, 2013).

12.5.2 Management of DHS in Patients with Tooth Surface Loss

Treatment for this group of patients includes the following aspects (Carvalho *et al.*, 2016; Gillam *et al.*, 2013; Miglani *et al.*, 2010).

- Thorough examination, diagnosis and recording of the extent and severity of the wear.
- Identifying and addressing the aetiological factors of tooth wear (see Chapter 50).
- Preventive measures including oral hygiene education, advice against the use of hard toothbrushes, excessive force and abrasive toothpastes, brushing at least 2 hours after acidic drinks and advice on reducing dietary acid intake.
- Appropriate referral to a medical practitioner if there is evidence of gastric acid reflux disease or vomiting.
- Application of 'at-home' and 'in-office' desensitising agents as described above.
- Conservative restorative management of worn teeth with direct adhesive composite restorations if indicated (see Chapter 50) often leads to further reduction and resolution of sensitivity.
- Regular review and maintenance.

In extreme cases where intolerable severe sensitivity persists despite provision of all the treatment modalities above, root canal treatment of the affected tooth may be indicated to alleviate the patient's symptoms.

Case Study

A 25-year-old female patient was referred by her general dental practitioner and presented with generalised sensitivity to cold and worn upper and lower teeth.

The patient reported a history of previous vomiting and gastrointestinal acid reflux disease which had been recently treated by medication. She also reported excessive intake of carbonated drinks.

The patient was not aware of any parafunctional habits such as bruxism or clenching. She used a hard toothbrush with scrub technique to brush her teeth.

The preoperative clinical photographs are shown in Figure 12.1.

Sensibility testing with an electric pulp tester showed a positive response from all the teeth. Exposed areas of dentine in the cervical region of the teeth with gingival recession were sensitive to cold air burst and scratching with a sharp probe.

Based on the history and the above clinical features, the following diagnoses were made.

- Generalised dentine hypersensitivity
- Generalised moderate to advanced tooth wear mainly due to erosion
- Generalised mild gingival recession

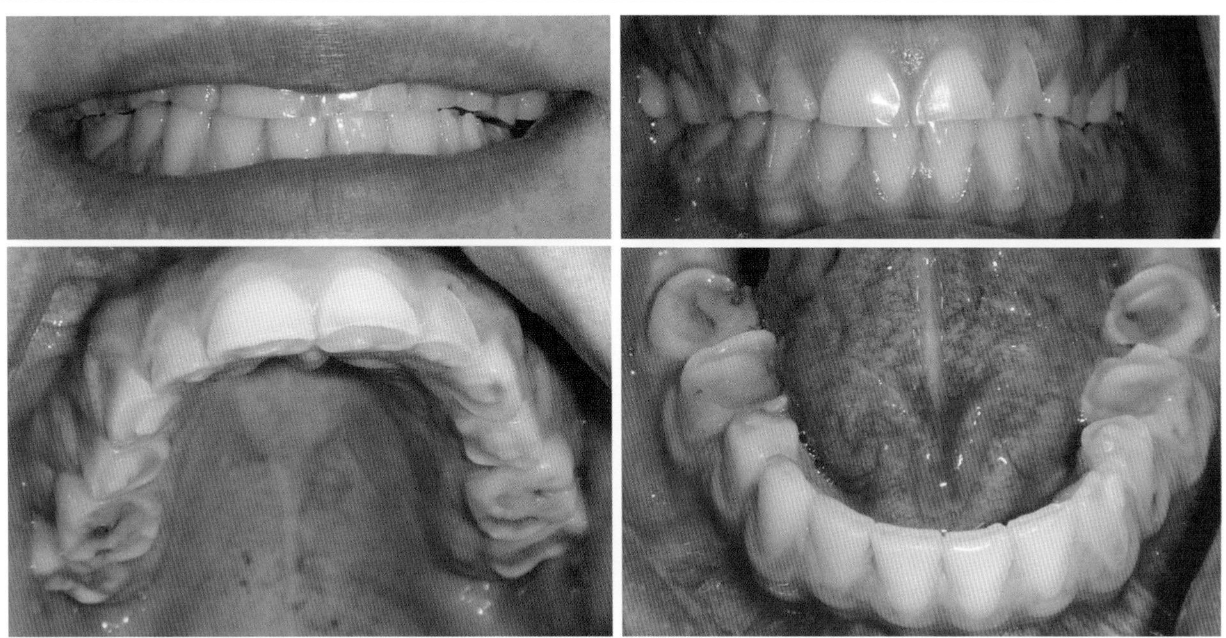

Figure 12.1 Preoperative clinical photographs showing generalised moderate to severe tooth wear with loss of enamel and dentine affecting most of the surfaces of the teeth. The wear is more pronounced in the palatal aspect of the maxillary teeth and buccal and occlusal surfaces of the mandibular posterior teeth. Cupping and outstanding restorations are consistent with the erosive pattern of tooth wear. Mild gingival recession is also visible on the buccal aspects of a number of teeth.

The prognosis for the restoration of the worn teeth with direct adhesive composite restorative material was good as there was plenty of enamel present for bonding and the patient was well motivated.

The treatment procedures are listed below.

1) Preventive measures including oral hygiene instructions, advice on atraumatic tooth-brushing technique with a medium toothbrush and the use of a single-tufted toothbrush in the areas with gingival recession.
2) Diet analysis and dietary advice to reduce the consumption of carbonated and acidic drinks and food.
3) Prescription of desensitising toothpaste and fluoride mouthwash.
4) The patient was advised to continue visiting her general medical practitioner regarding control of the GI disease.
5) Preparation of articulated study models, occlusal analysis and diagnostic wax-up of the worn teeth at a vertical dimension (VD) increased by 2 mm.
6) Direct composite build-ups of UR1, 2, 3, 4, 6, UL1, 2, 3, 4, 6, LR4, 6, 7 and LL3, 4, 6, 7 using the diagnostic wax-up as a guide to fabricate a palatal silicone stent to facilitate the build-ups of the maxillary anterior teeth and a clear stent for the posterior teeth.
7) Application of 'in-office' adhesive resin sealant varnish on the exposed root surfaces with residual sensitivity.
8) Fabrication and fitting of an upper occlusal splint to protect the restorations.
9) Review and long-term maintenance.

The patient's postoperative photographs are shown in Figure 12.2. The patient was very satisfied with the outcome of treatment.

Learning points in this clinical case included the following.

- Importance of effective communication with the patient, information gathering and careful analysis of the patient's history.
- Efficient prevention and management of hypersensitivity using different treatment modalities as described above.
- Appropriate treatment planning, including the use of articulated study models for occlusal analysis, and photographs with smile line for aesthetic analysis.
- Staging the rehabilitation by restoration of the anterior teeth first to achieve canine guidance and evaluate posterior space followed by restoration of the posterior teeth.
- Adhesive technique including appropriate isolation, moisture control and bonding technique.

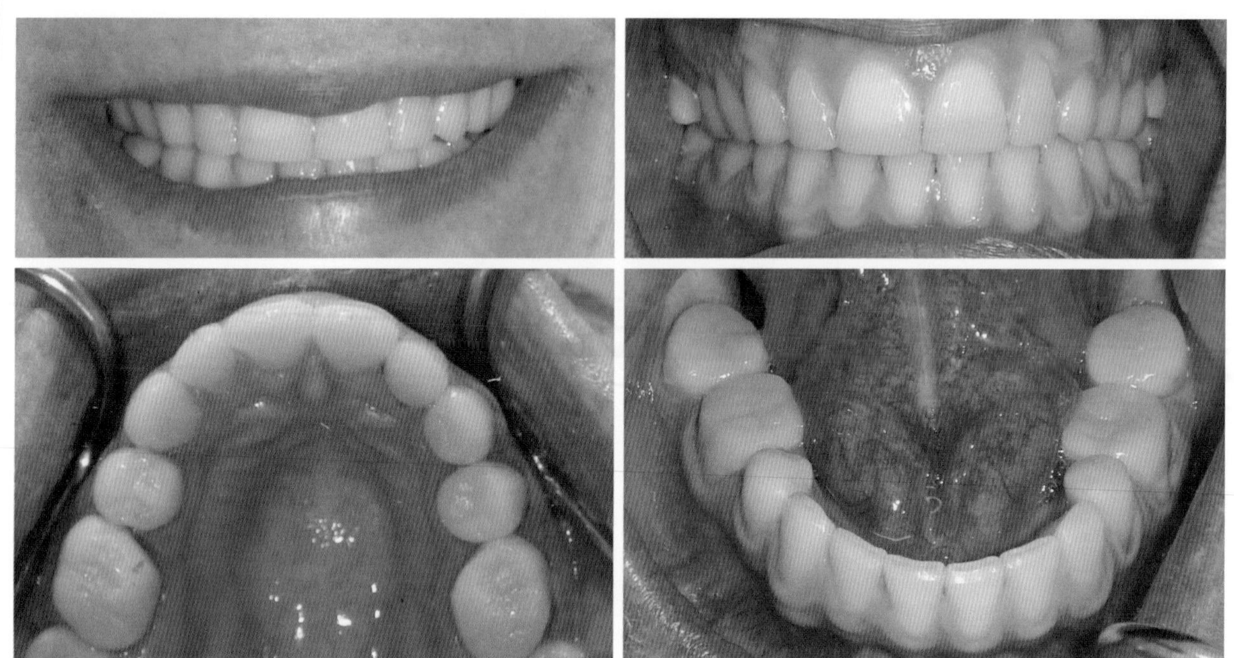

Figure 12.2 Postoperative clinical photographs showing direct composite restorations with reorganised occlusion at an increased VD.

References

Addy, M. (1990) Etiology and clinical implications of dentine hypersensitivity. *Dent Clin North Am*, **34**, 503–514.

Addy, M. (2005) Tooth brushing, tooth wear and dentine hypersensitivity – are they associated? *Int Dent J*, **55**, 261–267.

Addy, M., Mostafa, P. and Newcombe, R.G. (1987) Dentine hypersensitivity: the distribution of recession, sensitivity and plaque. *J Dent*, **15**, 242–248.

Albanai, S.R., Gillam, D.G. and Taylor, P.D. (2015) An overview on the effects of 10% and 15% carbamide peroxide and its relationship to dentine sensitivity. *Eur J Prosthodont Restor Dent*, **23**, 50–55.

Braennstroem, M. and Astroem, A. (1964) A study on the mechanism of pain elicited from the dentin. *J Dent Res*, **43**, 619–625.

Brannstrom, M. (1992) Etiology of dentin hypersensitivity. *Proc Finn Dent Soc*, **88**(Suppl 1), 7–13.

Carvalho, T.S., Colon, P., Ganss, C. *et al.* (2016) Consensus report of the European Federation of Conservative Dentistry: erosive tooth wear diagnosis and management. *Swiss Dent J*, **126**, 342–346.

da Rosa, W.L., Lund, R.G., Piva, E. and da Silva, A.F. (2013) The effectiveness of current dentin desensitizing agents used to treat dental hypersensitivity: a systematic review. *Quintessence Int*, **44**, 535–346.

Douglas de Oliveira, D.W., Oliveira-Ferreira, F., Flecha, O.D. and Goncalves, P.F. (2013) Is surgical root coverage effective for the treatment of cervical dentin hypersensitivity? A systematic review. *J Periodontol*, **84**, 295–306.

Draenert, M E., Jakob, M., Kunzelmann, K.H. and Hickel, R. (2013) The prevalence of tooth hypersensitivity following periodontal therapy with special reference to root scaling. A systematic review of the literature. *Am J Dent*, **26**, 21–27.

Flynn, J., Galloway, R. and Orchardson, R. (1985) The incidence of 'hypersensitive' teeth in the west of Scotland. *J Dent*, **13**, 230–236.

Gillam, D., Chesters, R., Attrill, D. *et al.* (2013) Dentine hypersensitivity – guidelines for the management of a common oral health problem. *Dent Update*, **40**, 514–516, 518–520, 523–524.

Irvine, J.H. (1988) Root surface sensitivity: a review of aetiology and management. *J N Z Soc Periodontol*, **66**, 15–18.

Kleinberg, I., Kaufman, H.W. and Confessore, F. (1990) Methods of measuring tooth hypersensitivity. *Dent Clin North Am*, **34**, 515–529.

Magloire, H. (2011) Odontoblast and dentin thermal sensitivity. *Pain*, **152**, 2191–2192.

Miglani, S., Aggarwal, V. and Ahuja, B. (2010) Dentin hypersensitivity: recent trends in management. *J Conserv Dent*, **13**, 218–224.

Sgolastra, F., Petrucci, A., Severino, M., Gatto, R. and Monaco, A. (2013) Lasers for the treatment of dentin hypersensitivity: a meta-analysis. *J Dent Res*, **92**, 492–499.

13

Dentinogenesis Imperfecta and Dentine Dysplasia

Zaid Ali - Case study

13.1 Definition

Dentinogenesis imperfecta (DGI) and dentine dysplasia (DD) include a group of hereditary genetic (autosomal dominant) disorders affecting dentine formation and are characterised by abnormal dentine structure in primary teeth or both primary and secondary dentitions (Kim and Simmer, 2007).

13.2 Classification and Clinical Features

Shields *et al.* (1973) classified DGI into three types (I, II and III) and DD into two types (radicular type I and coronal type II).

Dentinogenesis imperfecta type I is characterised by the following clinical and radiographic features (Barron *et al.*, 2008; Chetty *et al.*, 2016; Shields *et al.*, 1973; Witkop, 1988).

- Osteogenesis imperfecta including bone fragility and deformity, blue sclera, hearing loss and short stature (Levin, 1981).
- Amber translucent teeth (opalescent teeth).
- Attrition is often present.
- Short and constricted roots.
- Variable degree of pulp canal obliteration due to dentine hypertrophy.
- Affects both primary and permanent dentition.

Dentinogenesis imperfecta type II is characterised by the following features (Barron *et al.*, 2008; Shields *et al.*, 1973).

- Amber translucent teeth with bluish or brown colour.
- Attrition due to defects in the underlying dentine which leads to enamel detachment. Otherwise, the enamel has normal thickness and radiopacity before wear.
- Bulbous crowns with cervical constriction.
- Short and constricted roots.
- Pulp canal obliteration affecting both primary and permanent dentition.

Dentinogenesis imperfecta type III (brandy wine isolate) is characterised by the following features (Barron *et al.*, 2008; Shields *et al.*, 1973).

- Shell teeth (hollow teeth) due to dentine hypotrophy.
- Pulp exposures.
- Periapical radiolucencies.
- Teeth show variable degrees of clinical features seen in DGI type I and II, affecting both primary and permanent dentition.

Teeth affected by dentine dysplasia type I often have normal clinical presentation and are mainly characterised by the following radiographic features (Mk *et al.*, 1991).

- Sharp conical short roots or rootless teeth.
- Periapical radiolucencies.
- Total pulp canal obliteration affecting the primary teeth.
- Partial pulp space obliteration with crescent-shaped remaining pulp chamber in permanent dentition.

Dentine dysplasia type II is characterised by the following features (Mk *et al.*, 1991).

- Similar features to DGI type II in primary dentition with variable expression.
- Thistle tubed pulp chamber or pulp stones in the permanent dentition in some cases, otherwise permanent teeth are unaffected.

13.3 Aetiology and Pathogenesis

Genetic studies indicate that mutations in the genes encoding collagen type 1, including COL1A1 and COL1A2, are the main aetiological factors in the development of DGI type I which explains its association

Diseases and Conditions in Dentistry: An Evidence-Based Reference, First Edition. Keyvan Moharamzadeh.

Companion website: www.wiley.com/go/moharamzadeh/diseases

with osteogenesis imperfecta (Forlino and Marini, 2016; Pallos *et al.*, 2001).

Dentinogenesis imperfecta types II and III and DD type II are mainly caused by mutations in the genes encoding dentine sialophosphoprotein (DSPP) which are involved in the process of dentinogenesis (MacDougall *et al.*, 1997, 2006).

Histological examination shows the dentine is similarly affected in the three types of DGI, exhibiting a layer of normal mantle dentin with an irregular texture of dentinal matrix, reduced number of dentine tubules, presence of areas of atubular dentine and other areas with an abnormal structure of dentine tubules. The loss of enamel is not a result of abnormal dentin–enamel junction but is rather believed to be due to a weakness within the dentin itself (Salvolini *et al.*, 1999).

13.4 Epidemiology

The incidence of DGI is 1 in 6000 to 1 in 8000 and the incidence of DD is 1 in 100 000 (Barron *et al.*, 2008).

Dentinogenesis imperfecta (type I) has been reported in approximately 50% of patients suffering from osteogenesis imperfecta. The incidence of osteogenesis imperfecta is 6–20 in 100 000 children (Malmgren and Norgren, 2002).

13.5 Differential Diagnoses

Other developmental defects of enamel or dentine resembling the appearance of DGI-affected teeth include amelogenesis imperfecta, tetracycline-induced discolouration of teeth, dental defects associated with dermatological conditions such as ectodermal dysplasia and congenital erythropoietic porphyria, enamel defects seen in vitamin D deficiency-related conditions and rickets disease (Seow, 2014). Thorough history taking, as described below, clinical and radiographic examination are essential to rule out these conditions and reach an accurate diagnosis.

13.6 Relevant History and Special Investigations

Below is a list of relevant information and investigations that would assist the diagnosis of DGI and DD (Dhaliwal and McKaig, 2010).

- Medical history to identify symptoms related to syndromes such as osteogenesis imperfecta (bone weakness and fractures, hearing loss, sclera colour and short stature) and Ehlers–Danlos syndrome (joint flexibility).
- Family history of developmental dental disorders, including a pedigree diagram. Genetic counselling and genetic testing would further confirm the diagnosis.
- Dental history and questions regarding involvement of the primary teeth and history of tooth wear, abscesses, tooth mobility and early tooth loss and any other previous dental treatments.
- Radiographs of the affected teeth to assess the presence of pulp canal obliteration and periapical radiolucencies as seen in DGI and DD cases.

13.7 Treatment Considerations

The aims of treatment are to eliminate pain and infection, protect the teeth from further breakdown, restore function and improve aesthetics.

A multidisciplinary team approach, including paediatric dentists, orthodontists, oral and maxillofacial surgeons, restorative dentists and general dental practitioners, is the best way to manage this group of patients.

Depending on the age of the patient, presenting complaint and severity of the disease different treatment considerations are indicated.

13.7.1 Primary Dentition

Preventive measures to reduce the risk of development of caries and periodontal disease is an integral part of dental care for all children with developmental dental defects (Sapir and Shapira, 2007).

In order to prevent wear of the primary molar teeth, stainless steel crowns can be used. This will also maintain the patient's occlusal vertical dimension (VD) and protect the anterior teeth from heavy occlusal forces. The aesthetics of the anterior teeth can be improved by direct composite additions (Sapir and Shapira, 2001).

If the patient presents late with severe wear of the teeth to gingival level, an overdenture would be the only treatment option. Child adaptation to the denture is often good although regular reviews and denture remakes may be necessary during the child's growth (Esposito and Vergo, 1978; Walter, 1988).

Periapical infections and abscesses associated with DGI-affected primary teeth in young children are best managed by extractions as pulp treatment has a lower success rate due to root canal obliteration in most DGI and DD cases (Seow, 2003).

13.7.2 Permanent Dentition

Preventive care, oral hygiene education, dietary advice and fluoride use must be emphasised during regular dental visits. Permanent teeth must be carefully monitored as soon as they erupt to detect initial signs of tooth wear or caries development. Restoration of the permanent posterior teeth with metal occlusal onlays would protect these teeth from wear and maintain the VD. Conservative approaches using adhesive restorations and minimal tooth preparations in young adults are encouraged to preserve the remaining natural tooth structure (Barron *et al.*, 2008).

Indirect full-coverage crowns can be used in some older patients (Groten, 2009). However, tooth preparation can be challenging due to the presence of significant cervical constrictions and thin roots. Furthermore, worn teeth may require crown lengthening procedures prior to preparations and if the teeth have short roots, they may not be suitable for crown lengthening.

Teeth with periapical pathology and abscess may not be amenable to non-surgical endodontic treatment due to pulp canal obliteration (Pettiette *et al.*, 1998), although successful root canal treatment of some DD-affected teeth has been reported (Ravanshad and Khayat, 2006). Alternatively, surgical endodontic treatment can be indicated if the root length is adequate (Coke *et al.*, 1979), or otherwise the infected tooth can be extracted.

An overdenture is a simple removable option that can be indicated for the rehabilitation of severely worn dentition (Goud and Deshpande, 2011).

A fixed option to replace the missing teeth includes dental implants in adult patients after the completion of growth (Bencharit *et al.*, 2014). Bone grafting and ridge augmentation procedures are often required in these patients due to the presence of an atrophic ridge as a result of developmental defects (Seymour *et al.*, 2012).

Case Study

A 17-year-old female patient was referred by a paediatric dentist for restorative management of dentinogenesis imperfecta.

The patient's main concern at presentation was that the upper left lateral incisor tooth had fractured and she was unhappy with the dark lines on her anterior teeth. She was also aware that some of the build-ups on her other teeth had come off.

The patient had previous orthodontic treatment, including a functional twin-block, to reduce the overjet resulting from a Class 2 skeletal pattern malocclusion, and restoration of teeth by the paediatric dental department to manage signs of wear due to the developmental anomalies and to reduce her anterior open bite.

The patient's clinical photographs prior to orthodontic and paediatric interventions are shown in Figure 13.1 and the clinical photographs at referral to the restorative department are shown in Figure 13.2.

The patient was medically fit and well with no relevant medical history. She also reported a positive familial history of DGI.

Radiographic examination showed no obvious periapical pathology.

Diagnoses

The following diagnoses were made for the patient.

- Dentinogenesis imperfecta type II
- Fractured UL2 with a retained root
- Fracture of composite restorations LL5 and LR45
- Lost gold onlay LL7

Treatment

- Replacement of the failed posterior restorations and onlays
- Replacement of the anterior composites to provide appropriate anterior occlusal guidance and improve appearance
- Implant-supported crown at UL2

The following clinical procedures were undertaken.

1) Prevention, oral hygiene education, scaling and polish.
2) Replacement of the lost and fractured onlays at LL5, LL7, LR4 and LR5 with indirect composite onlays for the premolar teeth and gold onlay for LL7.
3) Preparation of articulated study models and diagnostic wax-up maintaining the existing intercuspal position (ICP) for replacement of the restorations on UR3, UR2, UR1, UL1, UL2 and UL3.
4) Direct adhesive composite restorations of UR1, UR2, UR3, UL1, UL2 and UL3.
5) Direct adhesive composite restorations of LR1, LR2, LR3, LL1, LL2 and LL3.
6) Extraction of the retained UL2 root, immediate implant placement (Narrow Platform NobelActive®, NobelBiocare, Kloten, Switzerland) and defect augmentation with bovine-derived bone graft substitute

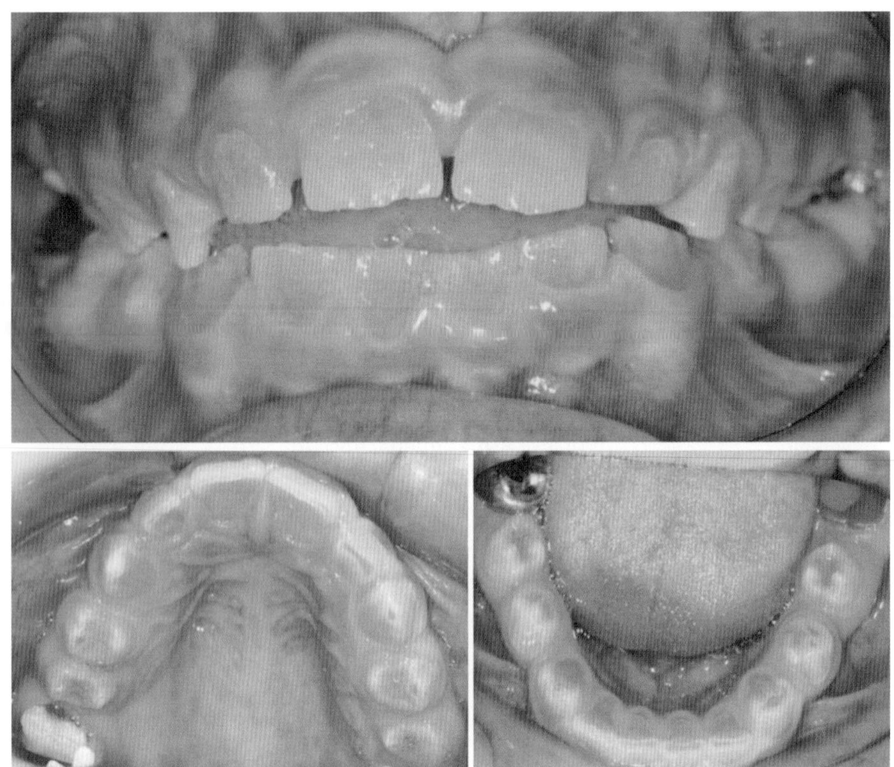

Figure 13.1 Preoperative clinical photographs prior to orthodontic and paediatric treatment showing amber-brownish opalescent teeth with anterior open bite.

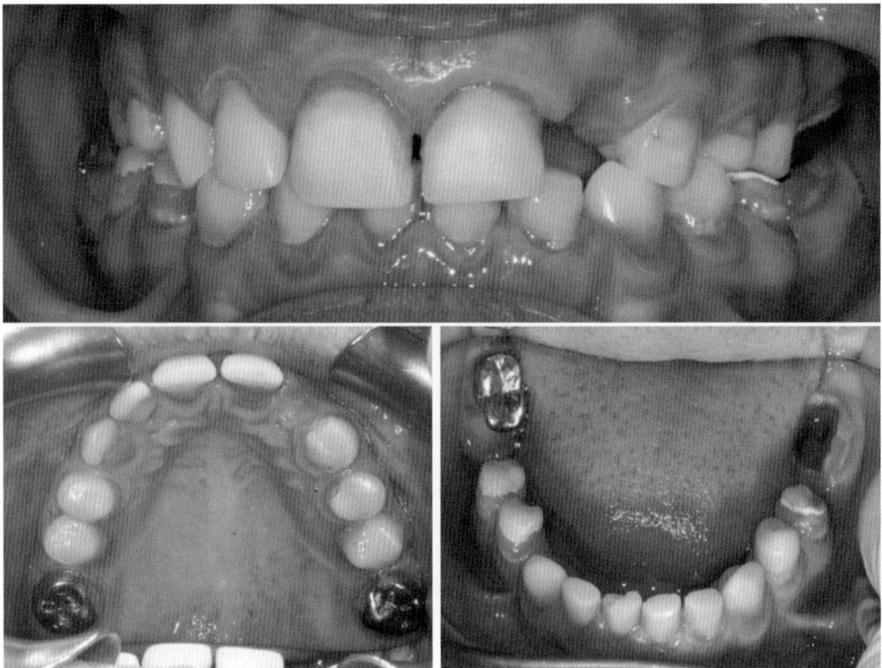

Figure 13.2 Clinical photographs at referral to the restorative department showing old composite restorations with visible margins, gold onlays on some of the posterior molar teeth and multiple failed restorations.

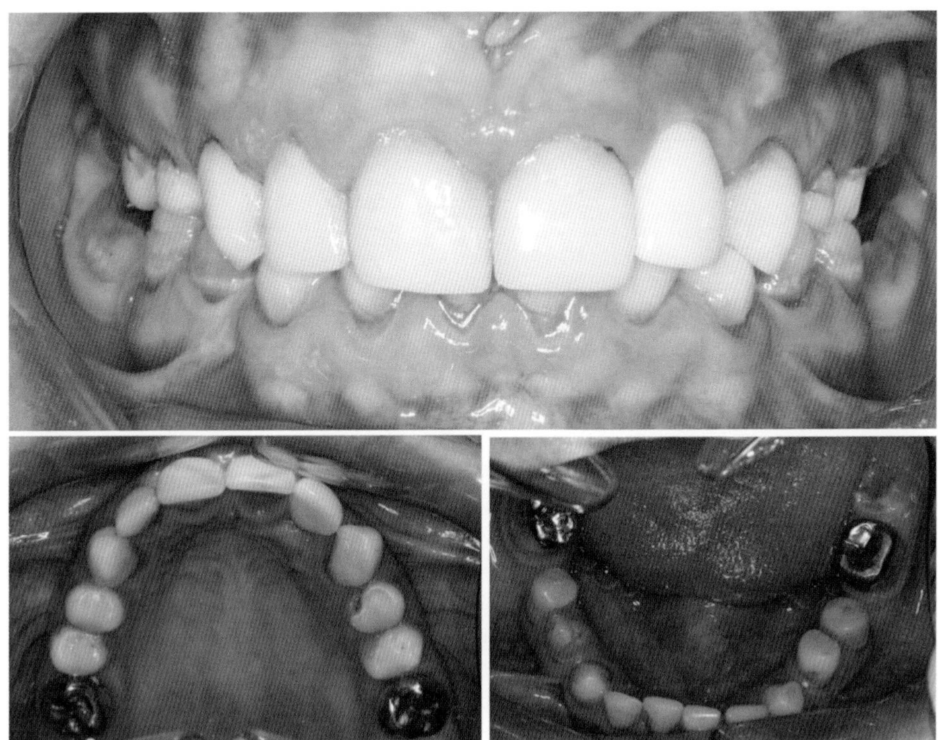

Figure 13.3 Postoperative clinical photographs.

(Bio-Oss®, Geistlich, Wolhusen, Switzerland) and porcine derived sterile resorbable bilayer collagen membrane (Bio-Gide®, Geistlich).

7) Restoration of the implant with a screw-retained all-ceramic crown (Nobel Procera®, NobelBiocare).
8) Review and maintenance.

The patient's postoperative clinical photographs and radiograph are shown in Figures 13.3 and 13.4 respectively.

This was a challenging case and there were a number of learning points.

A more conservative treatment strategy was preferred in this case in contrast to aggressive treatment options to preserve the natural tooth structure and avoid long-term complications associated with complex and invasive treatments.

Early involvement of multidisciplinary planning to ensure tooth positions, preventive and restorative strategies are optimised for the preservation of tooth structure and optimisation of implant sites. This must also be considered alongside an appreciation of the patient journey through orthodontics, paediatrics and restorative specialties. The potential for patient exhaustion with the process should not be underestimated.

The use of angled screw components such as the Nobel Omni Abutment was very helpful to correct the screw emergence up to 25°. Implant planning and placement are discussed in detail in Chapter 26.

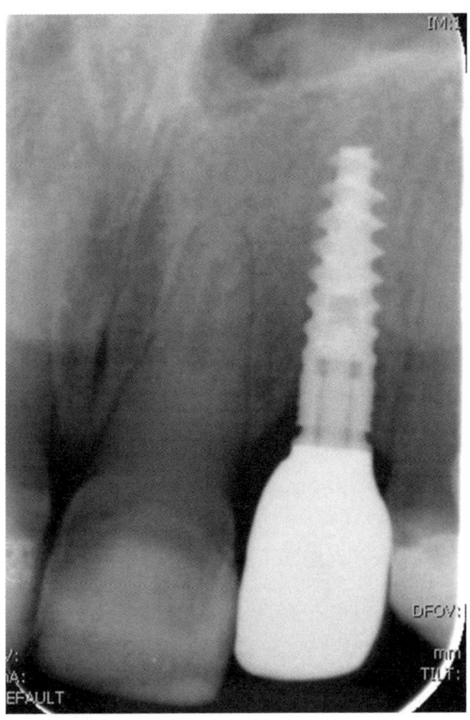

Figure 13.4 Postoperative radiograph of the restored implant UL2.

The patient was very satisfied with the functional and aesthetic outcome of the treatment, though she had to be reminded of the maintenance issues in this case, which include the maintenance of composite restorations, onlays, the implant-retained crown and the management of any future catastrophic failures such as crown fractures of natural teeth which are undermined by dentinogenesis imperfecta.

References

Barron, M.J., McDonnell, S.T., Mackie, I. and Dixon, M.J. (2008) Hereditary dentine disorders: dentinogenesis imperfecta and dentine dysplasia. *Orphanet J Rare Dis*, **3**, 31.

Bencharit, S., Border, M.B., Mack, C.R., Byrd, W.C. and Wright, J.T. (2014) Full-mouth rehabilitation for a patient with dentinogenesis imperfecta: a clinical report. *J Oral Implantol*, **40**, 593–600.

Chetty, M., Roberts, T., Stephen, L.X. and Beighton, P. (2016) Hereditary dentine dysplasias: terminology in the context of osteogenesis imperfecta. *Br Dent J*, **221**, 727–730.

Coke, J.M., del Rosso, G., Remeikis, N. and van Cura, J.E. (1979) Dentinal dysplasia, type I. Report of a case with endodontic therapy. *Oral Surg Oral Med Oral Pathol*, **48**, 262–268.

Dhaliwal, H. and McKaig, S. (2010) Dentinogenesis imperfecta – clinical presentation and management. *Dent Update*, **37**, 364–366, 369–371.

Esposito, S. and Vergo, T.J. Jr (1978) Removable overdentures in the oral rehabilitation of patients with dentinogenesis imperfecta. *J Pedod*, **2**, 304–315.

Forlino, A. and Marini, J.C. (2016) Osteogenesis imperfecta. *Lancet*, **387**, 1657–1671.

Goud, A. and Deshpande, S. (2011) Prosthodontic rehabilitation of dentinogenesis imperfecta. *Contemp Clin Dent*, **2**, 138–141.

Groten, M. (2009) Complex all-ceramic rehabilitation of a young patient with a severely compromised dentition: a case report. *Quintessence Int*, **40**, 19–27.

Kim, J.W. and Simmer, J.P. (2007) Hereditary dentin defects. *J Dent Res*, **86**, 392–399.

Levin, L.S. (1981) The dentition in the osteogenesis imperfecta syndromes. *Clin Orthop Relat Res*, **159**, 64–74.

MacDougall, M., Simmons, D., Luan, X., Gu, T.T. and Dupont, B.R. (1997) Assignment of dentin sialophosphoprotein (DSPP) to the critical DGI2 locus on human chromosome 4 band q21.3 by in situ hybridization. *Cytogenet Cell Genet*, **79**, 121–122.

MacDougall, M., Dong, J. and Acevedo, A.C. (2006) Molecular basis of human dentin diseases. *Am J Med Genet A*, **140**, 2536–2546.

Malmgren, B. and Norgren, S. (2002) Dental aberrations in children and adolescents with osteogenesis imperfecta. *Acta Odontol Scand*, **60**, 65–71.

Mk, O.C., Duncan, W.K. and Perkins, T.M. (1991) Dentin dysplasia: review of the literature and a proposed subclassification based on radiographic findings. *Oral Surg Oral Med Oral Pathol*, **72**, 119–125.

Pallos, D., Hart, P.S., Cortelli, J.R. *et al.* (2001) Novel Col1a1 mutation (G559c) [correction of G599c] associated with mild osteogenesis imperfecta and dentinogenesis imperfecta. *Arch Oral Biol*, **46**, 459–470.

Pettiette, M.T., Wright, J.T. and Trope, M. (1998) Dentinogenesis imperfecta: endodontic implications. Case report. *Oral Surg Oral Med Oral Pathol Oral Radiol Endod*, **86**, 733–737.

Ravanshad, S. and Khayat, A. (2006) Endodontic therapy on a dentition exhibiting multiple periapical radiolucencies associated with dentinal dysplasia type 1. *Aust Endod J*, **32**, 40–42.

Salvolini, E., di Giorgio, R., Caselli, E. and de Florio, L. (1999) [Dentinogenesis imperfecta. Scanning electron microscopic study and microanalysis]. *Minerva Stomatol*, **48**, 87–92.

Sapir, S. and Shapira, J. (2001) Dentinogenesis imperfecta: an early treatment strategy. *Pediatr Dent*, **23**, 232–237.

Sapir, S. and Shapira, J. (2007) Clinical solutions for developmental defects of enamel and dentin in children. *Pediatr Dent*, **29**, 330–336.

Seow, W.K. (2003) Diagnosis and management of unusual dental abscesses in children. *Aust Dent J*, **48**, 156–168.

Seow, W.K. (2014) Developmental defects of enamel and dentine: challenges for basic science research and clinical management. *Aust Dent J*, **59**(Suppl 1), 143–154.

Seymour, D.W., Chan, M.F. and Nixon, P.J. (2012) Dentinogenesis imperfecta: full-mouth rehabilitation using implants and sinus grafts – a case report. *Dent Update*, **39**, 498–500, 503–504.

Shields, E.D., Bixler, D. and El-Kafrawy, A.M. (1973) A proposed classification for heritable human dentine defects with a description of a new entity. *Arch Oral Biol*, **18**, 543–553.

Walter, J.D. (1988) The use of overdentures in patients with dentinogenesis imperfecta. *J Paediatr Dent*, **4**, 17–25.

Witkop, C.J. Jr (1988) Amelogenesis imperfecta, dentinogenesis imperfecta and dentin dysplasia revisited: problems in classification. *J Oral Pathol*, **17**, 547–553.

14

Dentoalveolar Trauma

14.1 Introduction

Dentoalveolar trauma occurs frequently in children and young adults, making up 5% of all injuries. One in four school children has experienced dental trauma and approximately one in three adults has experienced dental trauma involving their permanent teeth (Glendor, 2008).

Traumatic dental injuries can be grouped into the following categories (Andreasen *et al.*, 2007).

- Tooth fractures, including enamel infraction, enamel fracture, enamel-dentine fracture, enamel-dentine-pulp fracture (complicated crown fracture), crown-root fracture without or with pulp involvement and root fracture.
- Luxation injuries, including concussion, subluxation, extrusion, lateral luxation and intrusion.
- Avulsion.
- Alveolar bone fracture.

The most commonly reported type of dental trauma in primary dentition is luxation injury (Flores, 2002). In permanent teeth, the most frequent injuries are crown fractures without pulp exposure, concussions and subluxations (Lauridsen *et al.*, 2012).

Appropriate history taking, clinical and radiographic examination, diagnosis, treatment planning and follow-up are essential steps in the successful management of traumatic dental injuries.

Readers are encouraged to refer to the updated guidelines published by the International Association of Dental Traumatology (IADT) regarding acute management of traumatic dental injuries in primary and permanent teeth based on the best available evidence from the literature and consensus statements produced by a panel of expert professionals (Andersson *et al.*, 2016; DiAngelis *et al.*, 2016; Malmgren *et al.*, 2016).

In this chapter, multidisciplinary strategies for the long-term and late management of some of the adverse conditions caused by dentoalveolar trauma in adult patients are discussed and several relevant clinical cases are presented.

14.2 Displaced and Malpositioned Teeth

Mismanagement of luxation injuries can result in permanent displacement of the traumatised teeth. Altered position of the teeth following periodontal healing can be corrected with orthodontic treatment (Elbay *et al.*, 2014). It is important to ensure that any associated pulpal and periapical disease is controlled and treated prior to applying orthodontic forces to the tooth (Beck *et al.*, 2013; Hamilton and Gutmann, 1999).

Orthodontic space management and restoration of traumatised teeth with composite additions can be a viable conservative treatment option in many cases.

14.3 Loss of Vitality and Discolouration

Pulpal necrosis can occur following dentoalveolar trauma and its risk is dependent on the following factors (Andreasen and Kahler, 2015).

- *Age of the patient and stage of root development*: prognosis for revascularisation is improved in younger patients with incomplete root formation and the risk of pulpal necrosis is higher in teeth with closed apices (Andreasen and Pedersen, 1985).
- *Type of luxation injury*: the risk of pulpal necrosis is increased with the extent of injury (intrusion > lateral luxation > extrusion > subluxation > concussion) (Andreasen, 1970).
- Mobility of the injured tooth at the time of injury (Rock *et al.*, 1974).
- Degree of dislocation (Rock and Grundy, 1981).
- Initial positive reaction to pulp testing (Rock *et al.*, 1974).

Diseases and Conditions in Dentistry: An Evidence-Based Reference, First Edition. Keyvan Moharamzadeh.

Companion website: www.wiley.com/go/moharamzadeh/diseases

- Tenderness to percussion at the time of injury (Arwill *et al.*, 1967).
- Type of reduction procedure (Jacobsen, 1980).
- Fixation type and period (Andreasen *et al.*, 1989; Zachrisson and Jacobsen, 1975).
- Delayed initial treatment (Rock *et al.*, 1974).

Long-term, regular monitoring of the vitality of traumatised teeth is essential for early detection of signs of pulpal necrosis. Endodontic treatment may be indicated for the management of teeth with necrotic pulps at an early stage to prevent the development of periapical infection and associated complications.

Pulp canal obliteration and internal resorption are also observed complications in traumatised teeth (Andreasen and Kahler, 2015; Andreasen *et al.*, 1987) that can further complicate endodontic treatment. Endodontic treatment of non-vital teeth with complete apices is discussed in Chapter 3. Internal resorption is discussed in Chapter 26, and the management options for immature non-vital teeth with open apices are covered in Chapter 34.

Commonly observed discolouration of teeth following dentoalveolar trauma is believed to be due to pulpal haemorrhage (Marin *et al.*, 1997). Treatment strategies for discoloured teeth are discussed in Chapter 15.

14.4 Ankylosis and Root Resorption

Tooth ankylosis and replacement resorption occur most commonly following replantation of avulsed teeth (Andreasen *et al.*, 1995) and traumatic intrusion of the teeth (Tsilingaridis *et al.*, 2016).

Factors affecting the risk of ankylosis in replanted teeth include stage of root development, length of the dry extra-alveolar storage period, immediate replantation, length of the wet period and type of storage medium (Andreasen *et al.*, 1995).

Factors affecting the risk of ankylosis in intruded teeth include the choice of acute treatment, root development stage and degree of intrusion (Tsilingaridis *et al.*, 2016).

Ankylosed traumatised teeth in adult patients can be maintained and restored if necessary as these teeth can survive for a long period of time.

Ankylosis of a traumatised tooth in a young and growing patient can be a challenging condition as the ankylosed tooth will affect alveolar bone growth and development and cause aesthetic problems due to infraocclusion. The decoronation procedure, which involves removal of the crown and leaving the ankylosed root in its alveolar socket *in situ*, has been shown to offer the best and most predictable clinical outcome if performed at an early age, allowing normal alveolar bone growth to accommodate a future implant placement after growth completion (Malmgren *et al.*, 2015; Sigurdsson, 2009).

14.5 Lost Teeth

Traumatised teeth can be lost due to several reasons, including loss of avulsed tooth, loss of significant amount of tooth tissue, making it non-restorable, persistent periodontal or periapical inflammatory disease and advanced root resorption.

14.5.1 Exodontia Considerations

In young and growing patients, it is best to postpone extraction of the teeth with poor prognosis and consider endodontic treatment if possible to prevent periapical infection and preserve the alveolar bone until growth is complete (Alani *et al.*, 2012).

Atraumatic extraction of hopeless teeth is recommended to preserve the alveolar bone. Techniques include the use of special elevators, modified piezo tips and periotomes for dissecting the periodontal ligament and thinning the root walls prior to extraction (Kubilius *et al.*, 2012; Sharma *et al.*, 2015). Socket preservation techniques using bone grafts and membranes have also been shown to be effective in the reduction of bone height remodelling following extraction (Iocca *et al.*, 2017).

14.5.2 Role of Orthodontists

Orthodontic space management following traumatic loss of teeth is an important part of a multidisciplinary team approach. Edentulous spaces can be optimised by correcting the position and angulation of the teeth adjacent to edentulous spaces to achieve the ideal mesiodistal space and root parallelism to allow implant placement. Overerupted teeth in the opposing arch can be intruded by orthodontic treatment or Dahl appliance to provide the ideal space for prosthetic tooth replacement. Otherwise, edentulous spaces can be closed with orthodontic treatment in some cases. Forced eruption of traumatised non-restorable roots can also be used for alveolar bone development (Day *et al.*, 2008).

14.5.3 Autotransplantation

Autotransplantation of premolar teeth to the maxillary anterior region following traumatic tooth loss is a viable treatment option, with a success rate of over 90%

according to Andreasen's studies (Andreasen *et al.*, 1990a,b,c,d). Its advantages include the following.

- The autotrasplanted tooth has bone-inducing capacity and helps alveolar bone development.
- It continues to erupt with the child's growth and allows treatment to be performed at an early age (10–12 years).
- It can be moved by orthodontic treatment if the procedure is successful and the tooth is not ankylosed.

However, it is less predictable than implant treatment and has a number of limitations.

- It is very technique sensitive.
- It requires careful timing in relation to root development. Three-quarters of the root must be developed prior to transplantation.
- The crown of the transplanted tooth requires significant coronal modification to look like an incisor tooth.
- Buccal crowding is not always present to allow removal of a premolar to be used for autotransplantation.

A recent systematic review and meta-analysis (Machado *et al.*, 2016) shows a good survival rate (over 6 years) for autotransplanted teeth (75.3–91%) and a low rate of complications such as ankylosis (4.2–18.2%) and root resorption (3–10%).

14.5.4 Prosthetic Tooth Replacement

Removable partial dentures (RPDs) are simple and quick treatment options to immediately replace missing teeth and restore soft tissue defects with pink acrylic denture base material (Oh and Basho, 2010). RPDs also provide useful information regarding tooth position and the amount of missing soft tissue, which can be used as diagnostic tools in planning for soft or hard tissue augmentation and subsequent implant treatment.

The crowns of avulsed teeth can be used as immediate pontics using an adhesive composite resin splint. Fibre-reinforced resin-bonded bridges are alternative, minimally invasive treatment options for tooth replacement with around a 73.4% survival rate at 4.5 years (van Heumen *et al.*, 2009). Their limitations include the need for greater occlusal clearance to provide space for the retainers and the lack of rigidity which necessitates the use of fixed-fixed bridge design.

Resin-bonded bridges (RBBs) have been used successfully for replacement of missing teeth with satisfactory medium- to long-term survival (Thoma *et al.*, 2017). The RBB is a conservative, fixed and retrievable prosthetic treatment option requiring minimal or even no tooth preparation in some cases. Since this type of bridge relies on bonding to enamel, it is important to choose abutments and retainer design to provide a maximum area of enamel coverage by the retainer to enhance bonding and retention. Thorough assessment of occlusion is important to ensure the pontics are not heavily involved in guidance during mandibular excursive movements (Alani *et al.*, 2012; Durey *et al.*, 2011). Resin-bonded bridges and conventional bridges, which are less conservative tooth replacement options, are further discussed in Chapter 25.

Replacement of missing teeth with dental implants can be considered after growth completion. Major challenges of implant treatment in trauma patients include the lack of adequate bone and soft tissue due to traumatic loss of teeth and associated periodontal structures which may require hard and soft tissue augmentation procedures prior to implant placement (Chesterman *et al.*, 2014; Seymour *et al.*, 2014). Implant treatment of partially dentate patients and management of localised ridge defects are discussed in detail in Chapters 37 and 46 respectively.

Finally, it is important to consider the risk of repeat trauma and its consequences on tooth replacement and maintenance issues when managing this group of patients (Alani *et al.*, 2012).

Case Studies

Case 1

A 25-year-old male patient presented with history of frequent infections and swellings associated with a fractured UR1 caused by a fall accident 4 months earlier. He had received no emergency treatment following the accident.

Clinical and radiographic examinations (Figures 14.1 and 14.2) confirmed the following diagnoses.

- Enamel-dentine fracture
- Horizontal root fracture
- Non-vital coronal fragment with periradicular abscess

Treatment options were discussed with the patient, including (a) attempting initial non-surgical endodontic treatment of the tooth to the root fracture line and restoration of the fractured tooth crown (with a view to surgical removal of the apical root fragment if the non-surgical treatment fails) versus (b) extraction of the tooth and prosthetic replacement.

The patient wanted to keep the tooth and preferred option (a). Therefore the following procedures were undertaken.

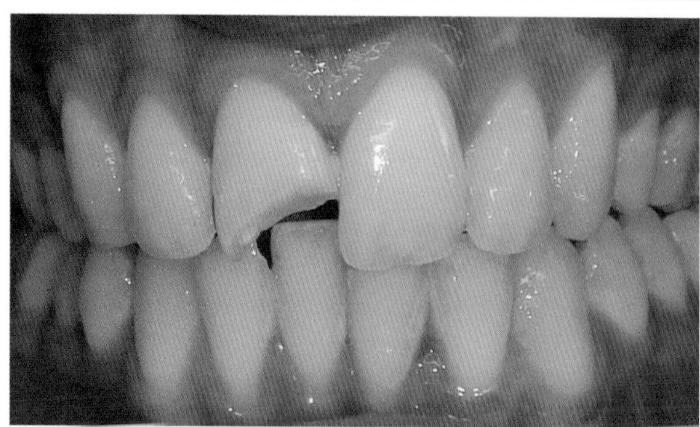

Figure 14.1 Preoperative clinical photograph of the fractured UR1.

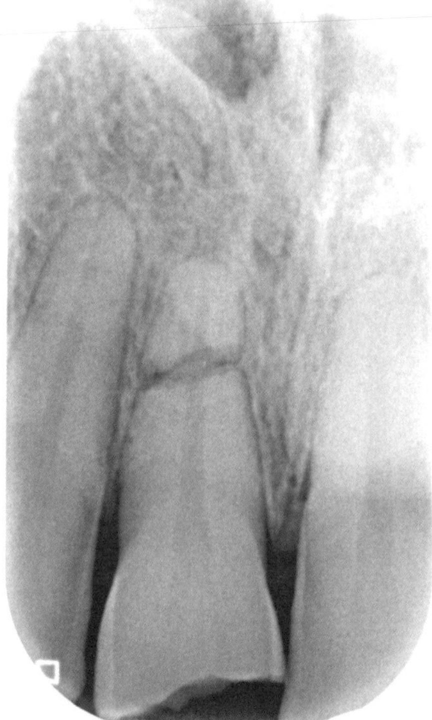

Figure 14.2 Preoperative periapical radiograph showing horizontal root fracture at the apical third of the root with evidence of periradicular radiolucency around the fracture line.

1) Non-surgical endodontic treatment of UR1, preparation and obturation of the root canal up to the fracture line using an MTA plug and back-fill with thermoplasticised gutta percha using the Obtura system (Figure 14.3).
2) Preparation of study model and diagnostic wax-up of UR1 and fabrication of a silicon stent (Figure 14.4) to help direct composite build-up of the fractured tooth.
3) Direct restoration of UR1 using dental composite resin (Figure 14.5).
4) Review.

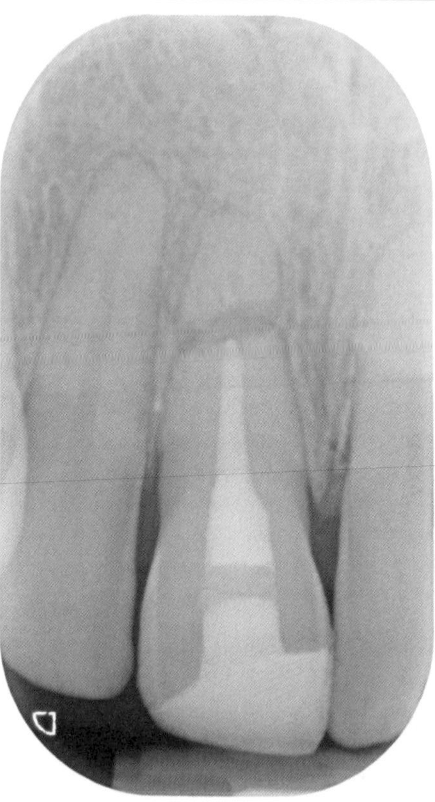

Figure 14.3 Postoperative periapical radiograph of the root-filled tooth (up to the fracture line).

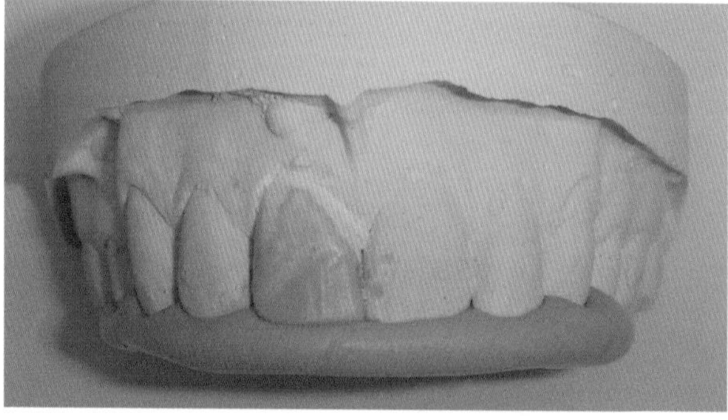

Figure 14.4 Diagnostic wax-up and silicon stent.

The patient's symptoms were completely resolved following the above treatment and he remained asymptomatic. One-year follow-up examination showed evidence of complete healing and the patient was discharged without the need for any further treatment.

Case 2

A 37-year-old male patient presented with missing mandibular anterior teeth due to car accident trauma 1 year earlier.

Clinical examination showed bilateral loss of mandibular incisor and canine teeth (class IV Kennedy) with

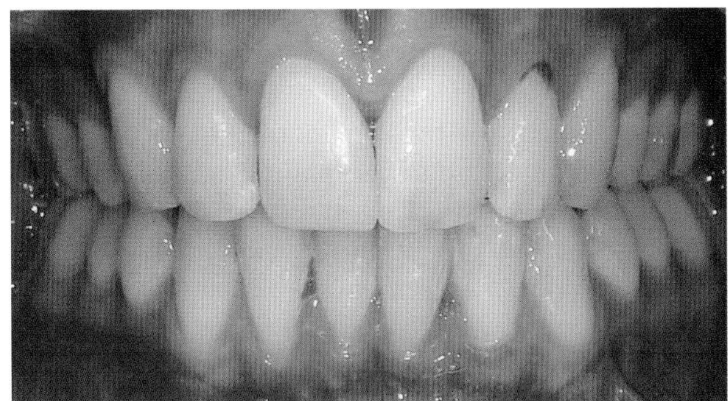

Figure 14.5 Postoperative clinical photograph of the restored tooth.

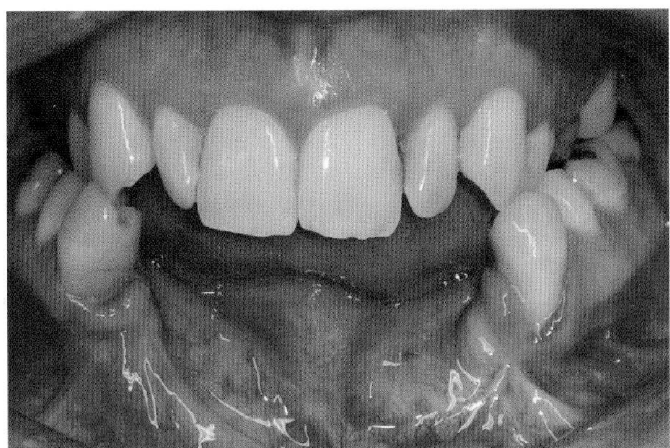

Figure 14.6 Preoperative clinical photograph showing significant loss of hard and soft tissues in the anterior mandible.

significant loss of alveolar bone and soft tissue in the anterior mandible. The patient had skeletal class III malocclusion with bilateral posterior cross-bite (Figure 14.6).

Treatment options were discussed with the patient, including (a) removable partial denture versus (b) bone grafting and dental implants (which would be challenging due to vertical loss of alveolar bone in the mandible, scarring and shortage of soft tissue to cover the bone graft).

The patient did not want bone graft and implants and preferred the removable partial denture option. A cobalt-chromium (Co-Cr) RPD was fabricated and fitted. The metal framework's retentive clasps were placed on the mandibular first molars and embrasure hooks were used for additional retention (Figure 14.7).

Postoperative clinical photographs are shown in Figure 14.8.

This was a relatively simple treatment option to replace the missing hard and soft tissues which obviated the need for complex surgical intervention, including bone graft and implants. However, there were several challenges in this case.

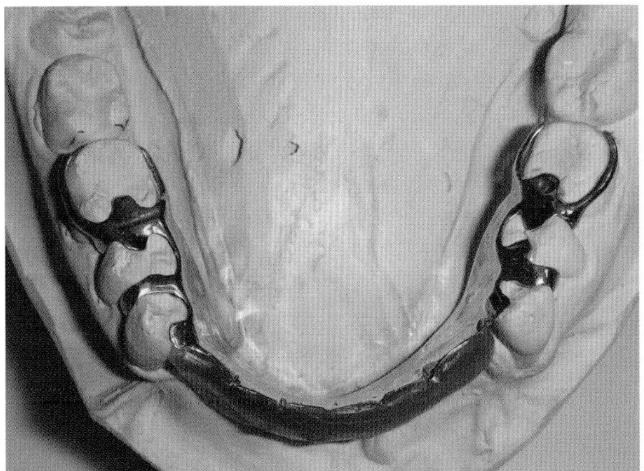

Figure 14.7 Metal framework with appropriate design to incorporate a lingual plate and elements of support (rests), retention (clasps and embrasure hooks), reciprocation (reciprocal arms on molar teeth and framework extension on premolar teeth) and indirect retention (provided by posterior extension of the framework).

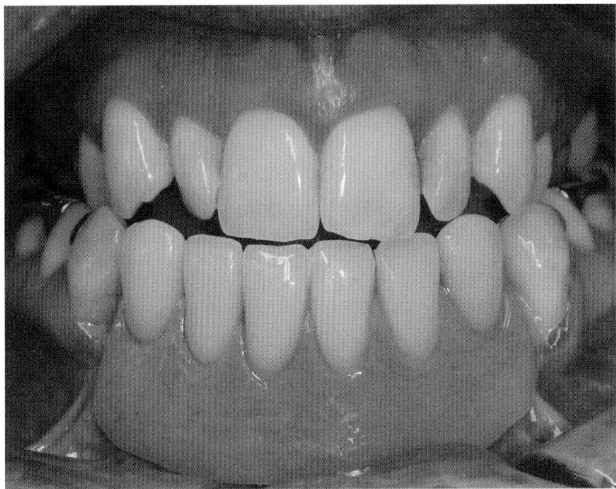

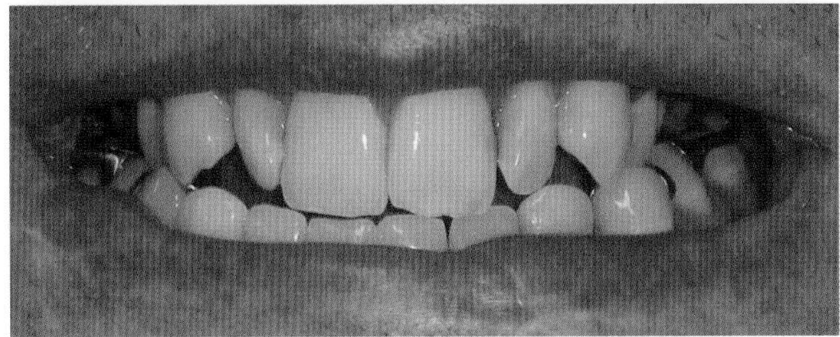

Figure 14.8 Postoperative clinical photographs of the denture occlusion and smile.

The patient had a class III dental and skeletal relationship with posterior cross-bite which complicated the fabrication of the Co-Cr RPD as the anterior teeth had to be placed at an edge-to-edge position. Minimal space was available for the rests due to occlusal interference.

It was also difficult to establish the position of the lingual plate, so an initial wax try-in of the teeth prior to fabrication of the metal framework was necessary.

Survey of the study models showed that the mandibular molar teeth were tilted lingually, and so the lingual arms of the clasps were used as retentive arms to engage appropriate undercuts on the molar teeth.

The shade match was excellent and the patient was very satisfied with the appearance, retention, stability and function of the RPD following minor occlusal adjustments.

Case 3

A 28-year-old male patient presented with missing upper anterior teeth due to trauma 2 years earlier. He was already wearing a removable partial denture and was seeking a fixed prosthetic solution to replace the missing teeth.

The patient had insulin-dependent type 1 diabetes which was moderately controlled. The patient also smoked 10 cigarettes per day.

Clinical examination (Figure 14.9) showed good oral hygiene and healthy soft tissues and periodontium. UR1, UL1 and UL2 were missing but there was only 15 mm mesiodistal space available in the edentulous area. The patient had class II malocclusion with group function in lateral excursions. UR2 was crowded and palatally positioned. There was 3–4 mm overjet and 1–2 mm overbite present in the UR2 and UL3 sites. Both UR2 and UL3 were vital as tested by an electric pulp tester. Both teeth were firm with no increased mobility.

The following treatment options were discussed with the patient, including their risks and benefits.

- Orthodontic treatment to align the crowded teeth prior to prosthetic treatment, but the patient did not want to wear orthodontic appliances.
- Dental implant treatment to replace the missing anterior teeth considering the patient's risk factors, including diabetes and smoking. However, the patient did not want to have surgery and was seeking a simple fixed bridge treatment.
- RBB to replace the missing central incisor teeth. UL3 was a suitable abutment for an RBB but UR2 had a small crown and thick palatal mucosa covering the gingival aspect of the crown, limiting the amount of supragingival enamel available for bonding. The occlusal factors were favourable for an RBB with adequate clearance between the upper and lower anterior teeth.
- The abutment teeth were intact and sound, so a conventional bridge option was discouraged as it would be too destructive and there was a risk of pulp damage and loss of vitality following tooth preparation.

It was decided to replace the missing central incisor teeth with a fixed-fixed RBB using UL3 and UR2 as abutments. Articulated study models and a diagnostic wax-up were initially prepared to assess the occlusion of the pontics and visualise the ideal tooth position and shape prior to bridge fabrication. The patient's existing RPD could not be used as a guide due to incorrect tooth position, midline and guidance.

Electrosurgery was used for palatal gingival trimming of UR2 and UL3 prior to impression taking to increase the area of enamel for retainer bonding (Figure 14.10). The patient's existing RPD was relined chairside using cold-cured acrylic resin to cover the palatal gingival margins following electrosurgery and prevent regrowth of the thick mucosa on the palatal aspect of the abutments.

A fixed-fixed PFM RBB was fabricated as shown in Figure 14.11. The bridge was tried in using calcium hydroxide-based lining material to temporarily fix the bridge in place to assess aesthetics. An opaque cement (Panavia F2.0 opaque, Kuraray America, Inc. New York)

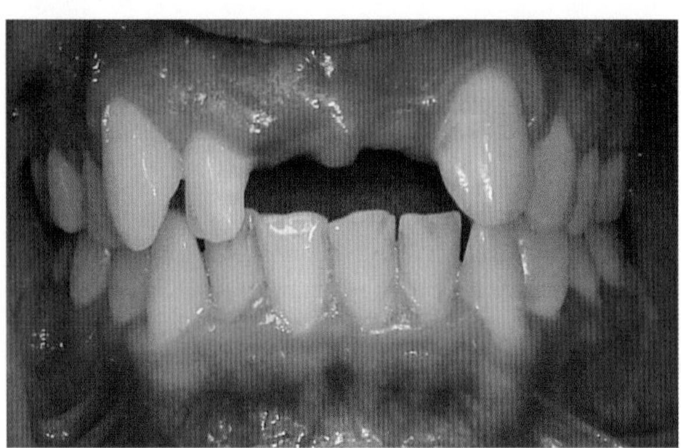

Figure 14.9 Preoperative intraoral clinical photograph.

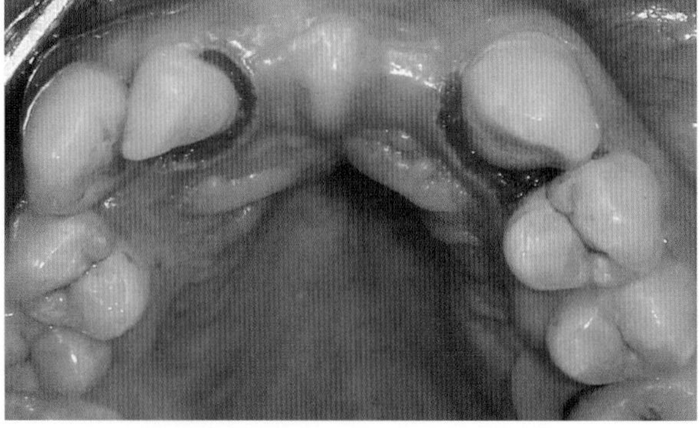

Figure 14.10 Clinical photograph of the palatal aspect of the abutment teeth following electrosurgery showing increased palatal enamel surface area.

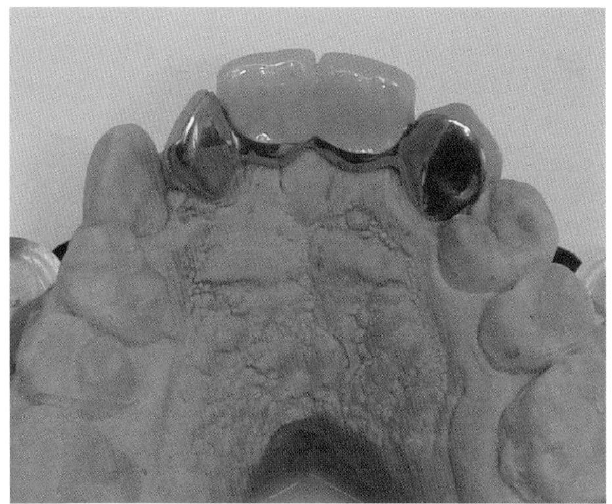

Figure 14.11 PFM fixed-fixed RBB on the stone model.

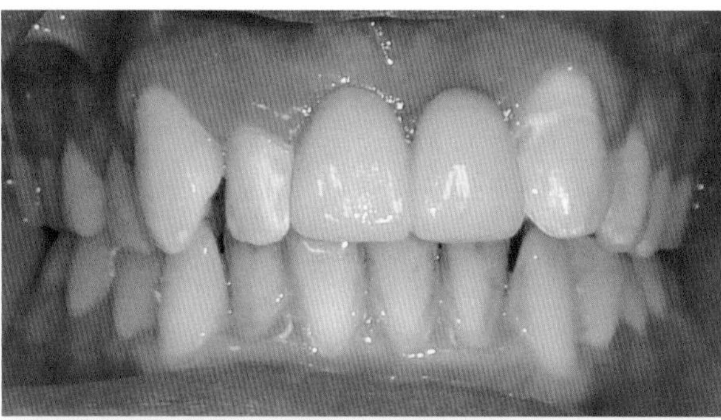

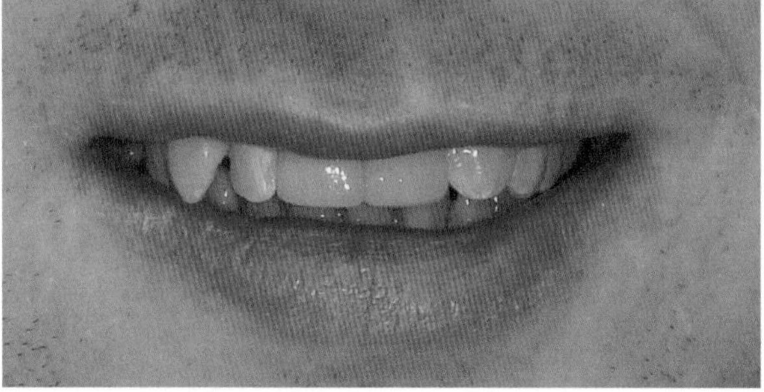

Figure 14.12 Postoperative clinical photographs.

was used to permanently cement the bridge according to the manufacturer's instructions. The patient's postoperative clinical photographs are shown in Figure 14.12. He was satisfied with the outcome of treatment and was discharged to his general dental practitioner for long-term maintenance, which would include monitoring plaque control, smoking cessation, periodontal maintenance and regular assessment of the bridge to detect any possible debond from retainers at an early stage to prevent the risk of caries development.

Case 4

A 20-year-old female patient presented with the loss of multiple maxillary anterior teeth from UR1 to UL3 due to car accident trauma 1 year earlier (Figure 14.13). The patient had also sustained unilateral fracture of the body of the mandible which had been treated with open reduction and internal fixation with two plates (Figure 14.14).

Clinical assessment and cone-beam computed tomography examination showed moderate horizontal and vertical alveolar bone loss in the anterior maxillae. The teeth adjacent to the edentulous space were vital and showed no signs of periodontal or periapical pathology.

The patient was medically fit and well, a non-smoker and had healthy soft tissues and periodontium.

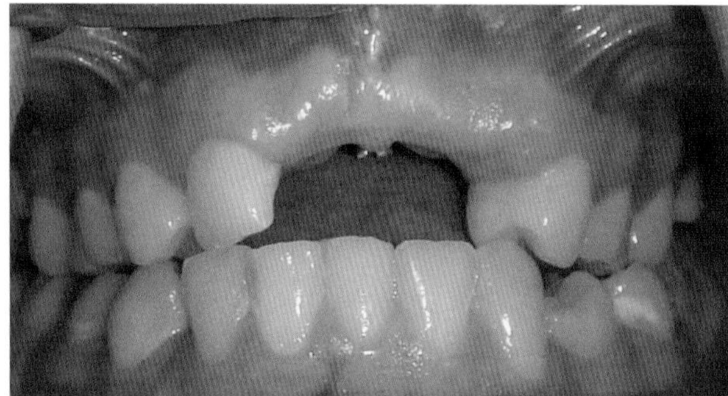

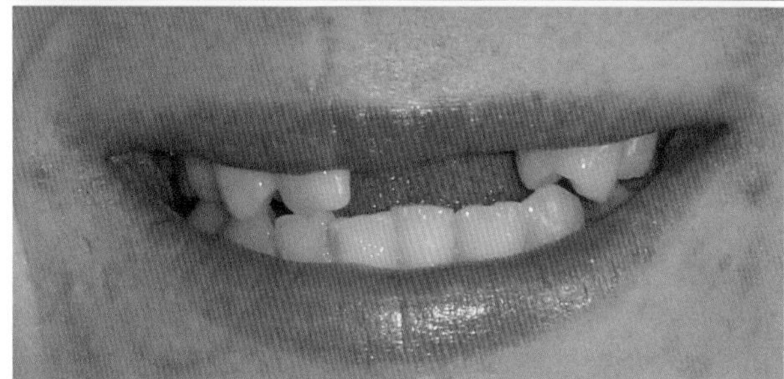

Figure 14.13 Preoperative clinical photographs.

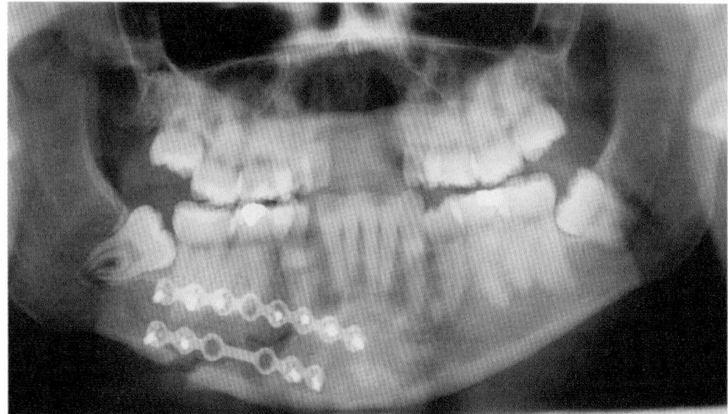

Figure 14.14 Preoperative oral panoramic radiograph.

The patient did not want a removable denture long term and was seeking a fixed predictable solution for replacement of the missing teeth. Since there was a long-span edentulous space, an RBB would not be suitable for this patient as a definitive prosthesis. A conventional bridge was also ruled out as the abutment teeth were intact and there was a high risk of damage to the pulp during tooth preparation in a young patient.

Following discussion of different treatment options, including the risks and benefits, the patient decided to have an implant-retained fixed dental prosthesis.

The challenges for implant treatment included the reduced volume of bone available for implant placement, reduced vertical height of the ridge, loss of soft tissue, drifting of adjacent teeth and midline shift. The patient did not want to have orthodontic treatment to correct the position of the teeth and optimise the space for an implant-retained prosthesis.

Different bone grafting options were discussed with the patient, including autologous block graft harvested from the chin (considering the presence of the plate and screws extending to the anterior mandible) or mandibular ramus versus simultaneous guided bone regeneration (GBR) using bovine-derived bone material and porcine-derived collagen membrane at the time of implant placement. The patient did not want additional bone grafting surgery and preferred implant placement and simultaneous GBR. As she had a low lip line, she was less concerned about the visibility of the margin of the crowns and was happy to replace any residual soft tissue defect with gingival-toned pink porcelain on the margin of the prosthesis.

Articulated study models and a diagnostic wax-up were prepared and tried in to locate the ideal position of the prosthetic teeth and enable fabrication of a surgical stent to guide implant placement (Figure 14.15).

Two implants (Narrow Platform NobelReplace®, Nobel-Biocare, Kloten, Switzerland) were placed in the UR1 and UL2 sites with simultaneous bone augmentation using bovine-derived bone graft substitute (Bio-Oss®, Geistlich, Wolhusen, Switzerland) and porcine-derived sterile resorbable bilayer collagen membrane (Bio-Gide®, Geistlich).

The implants were restored with a fixed-fixed PFM bridge with a hybrid design (screw-retained on UR1 and cement-retained on UL2 with customised milled titanium abutment) incorporating pink porcelain on the gingival and interdental aspect of the bridge to replace the residual soft tissue defects.

Postoperative radiographs are shown in Figure 14.16 and clinical photographs of the fitted implant-retained bridge are shown in Figure 14.17.

The patient was satisfied with the outcome of the treatment.

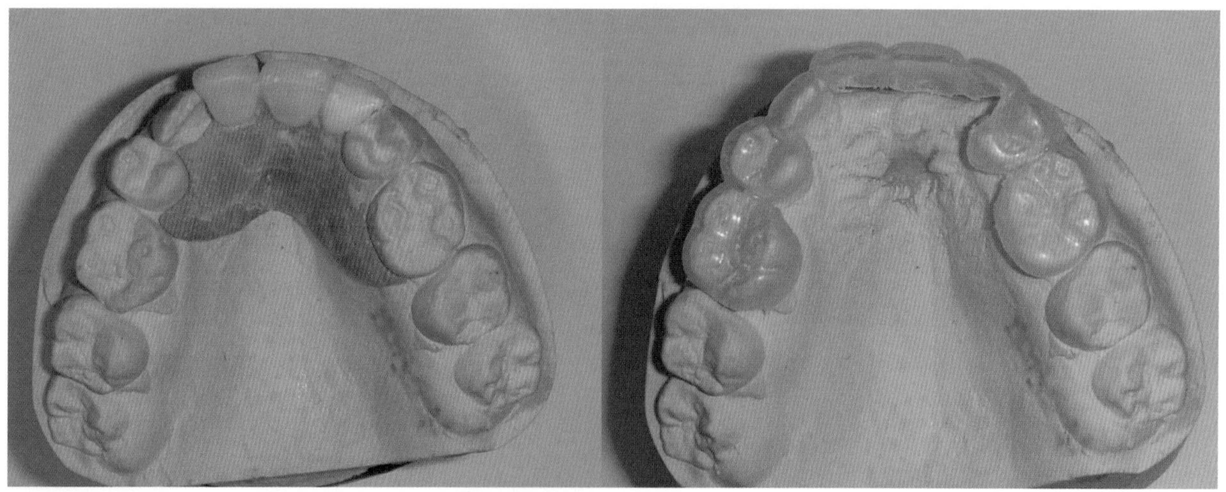

Figure 14.15 Diagnostic wax-up and surgical stent.

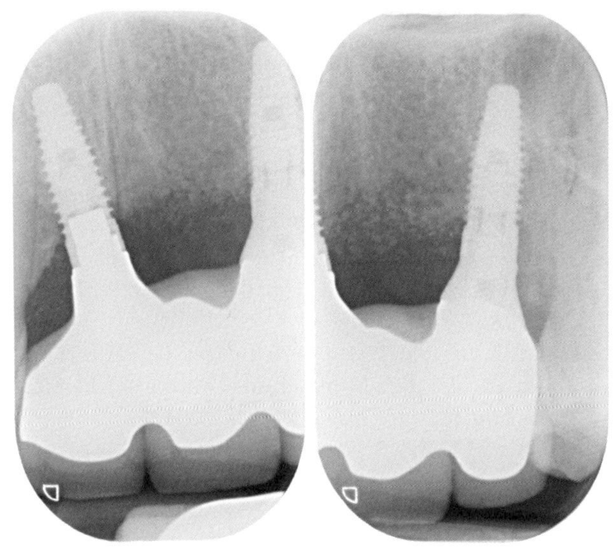

Figure 14.16 Postoperative periapical radiographs of the implants.

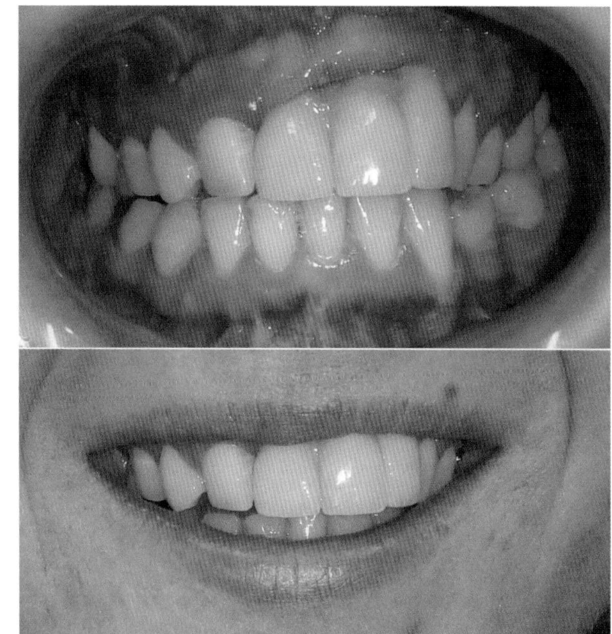

Figure 14.17 Postoperative clinical photographs of the implant-retained bridge and the patient's smile.

References

Alani, A., Austin, R. and Djemal, S. (2012) Contemporary management of tooth replacement in the traumatized dentition. *Dent Traumatol*, **28**, 183–192.

Andersson, L., Andreasen, J.O., Day, P. *et al.* (2016) Guidelines for the management of traumatic dental injuries: 2. Avulsion of permanent teeth. *Pediatr Dent*, **38**, 369–376.

Andreasen, J.O. (1970) Luxation of permanent teeth due to trauma. A clinical and radiographic follow-up study of 189 injured teeth. *Scand J Dent Res*, **78**, 273–286.

Andreasen, F.M. and Kahler, B. (2015) Pulpal response after acute dental injury in the permanent dentition: clinical implications – a review. *J Endod*, **41**, 299–308.

Andreasen, F.M. and Pedersen, B.V. (1985) Prognosis of luxated permanent teeth – the development of pulp necrosis. *Endod Dent Traumatol*, **1**, 207–220.

Andreasen, F.M., Zhijie, Y., Thomsen, B.L. and Andersen, P.K. (1987) Occurrence of pulp canal obliteration after luxation injuries in the permanent dentition. *Endod Dent Traumatol*, **3**, 103–115.

Andreasen, F.M., Andreasen, J.O. and Bayer, T. (1989) Prognosis of root-fractured permanent incisors – prediction of healing modalities. *Endod Dent Traumatol*, **5**, 11–22.

Andreasen, J.O., Paulsen, H.U., Yu, Z., Ahlquist, R., Bayer, T. and Schwartz, O. (1990a) A long-term study of 370 autotransplanted premolars. Part I. Surgical procedures and standardized techniques for monitoring healing. *Eur J Orthod*, **12**, 3–13.

Andreasen, J.O., Paulsen, H.U., Yu, Z. and Bayer, T. (1990b) A long-term study of 370 autotransplanted premolars. Part IV. Root development subsequent to transplantation. *Eur J Orthod*, **12**, 38–50.

Andreasen, J.O., Paulsen, H.U., Yu, Z., Bayer, T. and Schwartz, O. (1990c) A long-term study of 370 autotransplanted premolars. Part II. Tooth survival and pulp healing subsequent to transplantation. *Eur J Orthod*, **12**, 14–24.

Andreasen, J.O., Paulsen, H.U., Yu, Z. and Schwartz, O. (1990d) A long-term study of 370 autotransplanted premolars. Part III. Periodontal healing subsequent to transplantation. *Eur J Orthod*, **12**, 25–37.

Andreasen, J.O., Borum, M.K., Jacobsen, H.L. and Andreasen, F.M. (1995) Replantation of 400 avulsed permanent incisors. 4. Factors related to periodontal ligament healing. *Endod Dent Traumatol*, **11**, 76–89.

Andreasen, J.O., Andreasen, F.M. and L.A. (2007) *Textbook and Color Atlas of Traumatic Injuries to the Teeth*, 4th edn, Wiley-Blackwell, Oxford.

Arwill, T., Henschen, B. and Sundwall-Hagland, I. (1967) The pulpal reaction in traumatized permanent incisors in children aged 9–18. *Odontol Tidskr*, **75**, 130–147.

Beck, V.J., Stacknik, S., Chandler, N.P. and Farella, M. (2013) Orthodontic tooth movement of traumatised or root-canal-treated teeth: a clinical review. *N Z Dent J*, **109**, 6–11.

Chesterman, J., Chauhan, R., Patel, M. and Chan, M.F. (2014) The management of traumatic tooth loss with dental implants: part 1. *Br Dent J*, **217**, 627–633.

Day, P.F., Kindelan, S.A., Spencer, J.R., Kindelan, J.D. and Duggal, M.S. (2008) Dental trauma: part 2. Managing poor prognosis anterior teeth – treatment options for the subsequent space in a growing patient. *J Orthod*, **35**, 143–155.

DiAngelis, A.J., Andreasen, J.O., Ebeleseder, K.A. *et al.* (2016) Guidelines for the management of traumatic dental injuries: 1. Fractures and luxations of permanent teeth. *Pediatr Dent*, **38**, 358–368.

Durey, K.A., Nixon, P.J., Robinson, S. and Chan, M.F. (2011) Resin bonded bridges: techniques for success. *Br Dent J*, **211**, 113–118.

Elbay, U.S., Baysal, A., Elbay, M. and Saridag, S. (2014) Multidisciplinary approach to delayed treatment of traumatic teeth injuries involving extrusive luxation, avulsion and crown fracture. *Oper Dent*, **39**, 566–571.

Flores, M.T. (2002) Traumatic injuries in the primary dentition. *Dent Traumatol*, **18**, 287–298.

Glendor, U. (2008) Epidemiology of traumatic dental injuries – a 12 year review of the literature. *Dent Traumatol*, **24**, 603–611.

Hamilton, R.S. and Gutmann, J.L. (1999) Endodontic-orthodontic relationships: a review of integrated treatment planning challenges. *Int Endod J*, **32**, 343–360.

Iocca, O., Farcomeni, A., Pardinas Lopez, S. and Talib, H.S. (2017) Alveolar ridge preservation after tooth extraction: a bayesian network meta-analysis of grafting materials efficacy on prevention of bone height and width reduction. *J Clin Periodontol*, **44**, 104–114.

Jacobsen, I. (1980) Criteria for diagnosis of pulp necrosis in traumatized permanent incisors. *Scand J Dent Res*, **88**, 306–12.

Kubilius, M., Kubilius, R. and Gleiznys, A. (2012) The preservation of alveolar bone ridge during tooth extraction. *Stomatologija*, **14**, 3–11.

Lauridsen, E., Hermann, N.V., Gerds, T.A., Kreiborg, S. and Andreasen, J.O. (2012) Pattern of traumatic dental injuries in the permanent dentition among children, adolescents, and adults. *Dent Traumatol*, **28**, 358–363.

Machado, L.A., do Nascimento, R.R., Ferreira, D.M., Mattos, C.T. and Vilella, O.V. (2016) Long-term prognosis of tooth autotransplantation: a systematic review and meta-analysis. *Int J Oral Maxillofac Surg*, **45**, 610–617.

Malmgren, B., Tsilingaridis, G. and Malmgren, O. (2015) Long-term follow up of 103 ankylosed permanent incisors surgically treated with decoronation – a retrospective cohort study. *Dent Traumatol*, **31**, 184–189.

Malmgren, B., Andreasen, J.O., Flores, M.T. *et al.* (2016) Guidelines for the management of traumatic dental injuries: 3. Injuries in the primary dentition. *Pediatr Dent*, **38**, 377–385.

Marin, P.D., Bartold, P.M. and Heithersay, G.S. (1997) Tooth discoloration by blood: an in vitro histochemical study. *Endod Dent Traumatol*, **13**, 132–138.

Oh, W.S. and Basho, S. (2010) Esthetic removable partial denture design in replacing maxillary anterior teeth. *Gen Dent*, **58**, E252–256.

Rock, W.P. and Grundy, M.C. (1981) The effect of luxation and subluxation upon the prognosis of traumatized incisor teeth. *J Dent*, **9**, 224–230.

Rock, W.P., Gordon, P.H., Friend, L.A. and Grundy, M.C. (1974) The relationship between trauma and pulp death in incisor teeth. *Br Dent J*, **136**, 236–239.

Seymour, D.W., Patel, M., Carter, L. and Chan, M. (2014) The management of traumatic tooth loss with dental implants: part 2. Severe trauma. *Br Dent J*, **217**, 667–671.

Sharma, S.D., Vidya, B., Alexander, M. and Deshmukh, S. (2015) Periotome as an aid to atraumatic extraction: a comparative double blind randomized controlled trial. *J Maxillofac Oral Surg*, **14**, 611–615.

Sigurdsson, A. (2009) Decoronation as an approach to treat ankylosis in growing children. *Pediatr Dent*, **31**, 123–128.

Thoma, D.S., Sailer, I., Ioannidis, A., Zwahlen, M., Makarov, N. and Pjetursson, B.E. (2017) A systematic review of the survival and complication rates of resin-bonded fixed dental prostheses after a mean observation period of at least 5 years. *Clin Oral Implants Res*, **28**, 1421–1432.

Tsilingaridis, G., Malmgren, B., Andreasen, J.O., Wigen, T.I., Maseng Aas, A.L. and Malmgren, O. (2016) Scandinavian multicenter study on the treatment of 168 patients with 230 intruded permanent teeth – a retrospective cohort study. *Dent Traumatol*, **32**, 353–360.

Van Heumen, C.C., Kreulen, C.M. and Creugers, N.H. (2009) Clinical studies of fiber-reinforced resin-bonded fixed partial dentures: a systematic review. *Eur J Oral Sci*, **117**, 1–6.

Zachrisson, B.U. and Jacobsen, I. (1975) Long-term prognosis of 66 permanent anterior teeth with root fracture. *Scand J Dent Res*, **83**, 345–354.

15

Discolouration

15.1 Introduction

The colour of a tooth can be described by the three-dimensional Munsell colour system, including hue (descriptive name of the colour), value (relative lightness and darkness) and chroma (saturation and strength of the colour).

Tooth discolouration can be classified into intrinsic and extrinsic types (Watts and Addy, 2001).

15.2 Intrinsic Discolouration

Intrinsic discolouration occurs due to changes in the structure or composition of the tooth dentine or enamel. A number of conditions have been associated with intrinsic discolouration of teeth.

15.2.1 Alkaptonuria

Alkaptonuria, or hereditary ochronosis, is caused by deficiency of homogentisic acid oxidase which results in incomplete metabolism of tyrosine and phenylalanine. The excessive deposition of homogentisic acid in collagenous structures affects the permanent dentition by causing a brown discolouration. Other findings include darkening of the skin, sclera pigmentation, joint problems and urine turning black on air exposure (Link, 1973).

15.2.2 Congenital Hyperbilirubinaemia

Elevated serum levels of bilirubin (hyperbilirubinaemia) during dental development can cause permanent green pigmentation in teeth due to bilirubin deposits in dental hard tissues. Hyperbilirubinaemia can occur in paediatric patients following haemolysis associated with several systemic disorders such as acute liver failure, congenital biliary atresia and biliary hypoplasia (Amaral *et al.*, 2008).

15.2.3 Congenital Erythropoietic Porphyria

Congenital erythropoietic porphyria is a rare condition characterised by disruption in the metabolism of porphyrin which leads to its accumulation in various tissues including teeth, urine, bone marrow and red blood cells. The teeth show red to brown discolouration exhibiting red fluorescence under ultraviolet (UV) light (Kooijman and Brand, 2005).

15.2.4 Tetracycline Staining

Yellow to grey-brown discolouration of teeth can be caused by systemic use of tetracyclines during tooth development (both primary and permanent teeth) as deposition of tetracycline can occur within the dentine, enamel and the bone (Sanchez *et al.*, 2004). On examination, exposure to light can change the colour of the teeth from grey to brown or yellow since tetracycline can fluoresce under the UV light. The degree of discolouration depends on the type, dosage and duration of the medication used. Reported prevalence of tetracycline- and minocycline-induced staining varies between 0.4% (Ulvestad *et al.*, 1978) and 9% (Koleoso *et al.*, 2004), depending on the population.

Tetracycline prescription should be avoided from 29 weeks of pregnancy until birth for expecting mothers and from birth up to the age of 12 years for children to prevent incorporation into primary and permanent teeth.

15.2.5 Pulpal Disease

Pulpal haemorrhage following dental traumatic injury can cause discolouration of affected teeth (Marin *et al.*, 1997). The release of red blood cell breakdown products in combination with necrotic pulp tissue byproducts and their penetration into the dentinal tubules can cause variable degrees of discolouration.

The lesions may appear pink initially and progress towards yellow, brown and darker shades with time unless pulpal revascularisation occurs.

Diseases and Conditions in Dentistry: An Evidence-Based Reference, First Edition. Keyvan Moharamzadeh.

Companion website: www.wiley.com/go/moharamzadeh/diseases

Some materials used for endodontic treatment, such as canal irrigants, medicaments and root-filling materials, can also release products that can cause internalised discolouration of the teeth (Ahmed and Abbott, 2012).

15.2.6 Root Resorption

Root resorption can initially present with pink discolouration of the tooth at the cementoenamel junction (CEJ). Internal root resorption is discussed in detail in Chapter 26 and external root resorption in Chapter 17.

15.2.7 Amelogenesis Imperfecta (AI)

Amelogenesis imperfecta-affected teeth can show different degrees of discolouration, depending on the type of AI. The hypoplastic form of AI can present with yellowish-brown thin enamel. In the hypocalcifed form, teeth often become pigmented-dark brown coloured, while the hypomaturation form is characterised by mottled cloudy white or yellow-brown snow-capped teeth (Mehta *et al.*, 2013). AI is covered in detail in Chapter 2.

15.2.8 Dentinogenesis Imperfecta (DI)

Dentinogenesis imperfecta is characterised by amber or grey opalescent teeth (Barron *et al.*, 2008). DI is discussed in detail in Chapter 13.

15.2.9 Fluorosis

Mild fluorosis can exhibit small white streaks or specks in the enamel of affected teeth. In severe fluorosis, the teeth may show dark brown or even black discolouration (Damm and Fantasia, 2001). Fluorosis is further discussed in Chapter 19.

15.2.10 Ageing

Teeth gradually darken with age due to continuous formation of secondary dentine which affects the light transmission properties of the tooth. Age-related tooth wear and attrition can result in the loss of translucent enamel and further expose the yellow underlying dentine. Conservative restorative approaches such as bleaching and bonding have been shown to benefit this group of patients (Kelleher *et al.*, 2011).

15.2.11 Other Conditions Associated with Enamel Defects

Enamel hypoplasia may also occur in a number of other conditions (Pindborg, 1982).

- Nutritional deficiencies such as vitamins A, C and D deficiency.
- Skin diseases such as epidermolysis bullosa, measles and chickenpox.
- Congenital syphilis characterised by screwdriver-shaped anterior teeth (Hutchinson's teeth) and barrel-shaped posterior molar teeth (mulberry molars).
- Hypocalcaemia and pseudohypoparathyroidism.
- Birth injuries and prematurity.
- Local infection or trauma during tooth formation can cause mild brownish discolouration of the enamel to severe pitting and irregularity of the tooth crown (Turner's teeth).
- Syndromes such as Ehlers–Danlos.

15.3 Extrinsic Discolouration

Different classifications have been used to group types and causes of extrinsic discolouration (Prathap *et al.*, 2013).

- Direct staining by adsorption of chromogens present in food and beverages (such as tea and coffee) and tobacco products into the pellicle versus indirect staining due to chemical interaction of the staining agents with the tooth surface.
- Metallic agents including metal salts such as iron (black), copper (green), silver (grey) and tin (golden) versus non-metallic agents including colourants present in food and beverages, tobacco, chlorhexidine and mouthwashes containing quaternary ammonium compounds.

15.4 Treatment Options

Preventive measures to reduce the risk of external staining include the following.

- Dietary advice to reduce exposure of the teeth to food colourants and chromogen-containing beverages.
- Oral hygiene instructions including effective tooth brushing twice a day with an appropriate toothpaste.
- Patients should be warned about the risk of tooth discolouration associated with prolonged use of antiseptic mouthwashes.
- Regular dentist visits, professional tooth cleaning with ultrasonic scalers and polishing with rotary instruments using an abrasive prophylactic paste can further remove extrinsic stains.

Air polishing has also been shown to be an effective and efficient method of removing stains and biofilms from the tooth surface (Cobb *et al.*, 2017). It is important to consider appropriate safety precautions when using this technique (Gutmann, 1998).

Treatment options for teeth with intrinsic discolouration include the following.

- Accepting and monitoring the tooth with no further treatment.
- Tooth bleaching using appropriate tooth-whitening products and techniques (Nixon *et al.*, 2007a).
- Superficial stains, white spots and enamel defects due to hypoplasia, fluorosis and amelogenesis imperfecta can be treated with enamel microabrasion (Nixon *et al.*, 2007b).
- Restorative treatment including labial veneers (direct composite or indirect laboratory constructed composite or porcelain veneers) and crowns.
- Extraction and prosthetic replacement if the tooth has a hopeless prognosis.

15.5 Tooth Bleaching

Depending on the cause of discolouration, the tooth can be whitened from the outside (vital bleaching) or from the inside (non-vital bleaching) using different tooth-whitening products.

15.5.1 Bleaching Techniques

15.5.1.1 Vital Bleaching (External Bleaching)

This technique is used for whitening discoloured vital teeth due to intrinsic discolouration or stubborn extrinsic staining. It involves patient use of a custom-made whitening tray to deliver appropriate bleaching gel to the external surface of the discoloured teeth on a daily basis. A detailed protocol for this technique can be found in the UK National Clinical Guidelines in Paediatric Dentistry (Wray *et al.*, 2001).

15.5.1.2 Non-Vital Bleaching (Internal Bleaching)

This technique is used for whitening discoloured endodontically treated non-vital teeth. It involves placement of an appropriate bleaching agent in the access cavity over the sealed root-filling material. The access cavity can then either be sealed with a temporary restoration over the bleaching agent or left open and the patient instructed to change the bleaching agent in the access cavity regularly until the subsequent appointment (Sulieman, 2005).

15.5.1.3 Inside/Outside Bleaching

Severely discoloured non-vital teeth can be bleached from both inside and outside to enhance the efficiency and speed of the bleaching process. This technique involves placement of an appropriate bleaching agent into the pulp chamber and simultaneous application of a bleaching gel onto the external surface of the tooth using a custom-made whitening tray (Poyser *et al.*, 2004).

15.5.2 Bleaching Products

Tooth-whitening gels and strips are the products most commonly used for tooth bleaching.

15.5.2.1 Whitening Gels

Carbamide peroxide is the active ingredient of most dental bleaching gels. It produces hydrogen peroxide as it reacts with water.

The EU Cosmetic Products Regulations 2012 prohibited the use of products containing or releasing between 0.1% and 6% hydrogen peroxide in children under 18 years of age and concentrations exceeding 6% of hydrogen peroxide remained prohibited for use in adult patients; 6% hydrogen peroxide is equivalent to 18% carbamide peroxide.

Evidence shows that both vital and non-vital tray bleaching using 10% carbamide peroxide can produce excellent clinical outcomes with over 90% success rates. However, shade regression can occur over the first few years which may require retreatment (Burrows, 2009). External bleaching with 10% carbamide peroxide gel can be successfully used long term (up to 3 months) for the treatment of severe tetracycline staining (Tsubura, 2010).

Dahl and Pallesen (2003) reviewed important biological aspects of tooth whitening. Tooth sensitivity is the most common side effect of external tooth whitening, reported in up to 78% of patients (Boushell *et al.*, 2012). The risk of adverse reactions increases with use of high concentrations of above 10% peroxide. It is recommended to avoid using concentrations of over 10% carbamide peroxide for external tooth bleaching (Moharamzadeh, 2016).

Heat and light activation increase the risk of sensitivity during vital bleaching (He *et al.*, 2012). Also, light activation does not have a statistically significant effect on the whitening efficacy of bleaching products containing high concentrations of hydrogen peroxide (Mondelli *et al.*, 2012).

15.5.2.2 Whitening Strips

Whitening strips deliver 6–14% hydrogen peroxide, depending on the product (Moharamzadeh, 2016).

The use of whitening strips containing 6% hydrogen peroxide for 2 weeks can be safe, consistent and as effective as external whitening with bleaching gels (Gerlach *et al.*, 2009). A recent meta-analysis comparing the efficacy and safety of over-the-counter whitening strips versus 10% carbamide peroxide gel tray whitening demonstrated that tooth sensitivity and gingival sensitivity were similar, regardless of the whitening method used. The observed gingival irritation was higher when the 10% carbamide peroxide gel was applied on a tray (Serraglio *et al.*, 2016).

Case Study

A 43-year-old male patient presented with a discoloured UR2. The tooth had previous endodontic treatment 3 years earlier and has been slightly tender to biting in the past year. There was no history of swellings or abscess.

The patient was medically fit and well with no relevant medical history.

Clinical examination showed the soft tissues were normal and there was dark grey discolouration of the cervical aspect of UR2 (Figure 15.1). The tooth was slightly tender to percussion. There were no deep periodontal pockets or mobility associated with UR2.

Radiographic examination showed the presence of suboptimal root filling and a small periapical radiolucency associated with UR2. Based on the clinical and radiographic assessment, a diagnosis of chronic apical periodontitis and internal discolouration of UR2 was made

The treatment strategy included endodontic retreatment of UR2, sealing of the root filling with GIC material below the CEJ level, followed by internal bleaching of UR2 over 2 weeks using 16% carbamide peroxide gel placed in the pulp chamber and sealed by GIC. A non-vital bleaching protocol as described by the UK National Clinical Guidelines in Paediatric Dentistry (Wray *et al.*, 2001) was used in this case, with some modification, including the use of a less concentrated bleaching product to comply with the 2012 legislation on tooth whitening.

As shown in Figure 15.2, there was significant improvement in the shade of the discoloured non-vital tooth following internal bleaching.

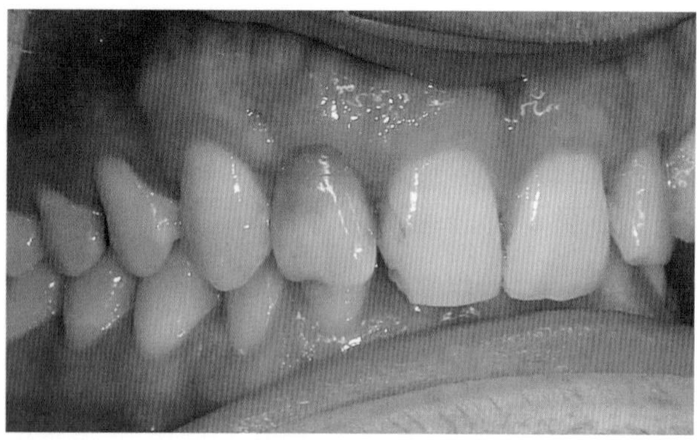

Figure 15.1 Preoperative clinical photograph of the discoloured UR2.

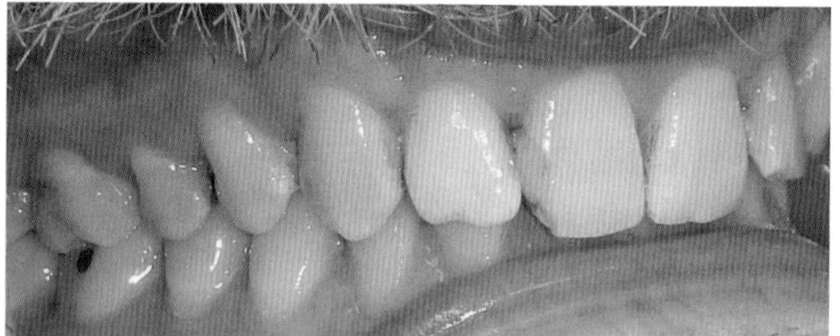

Figure 15.2 Post-bleaching clinical photograph of UR2.

References

Ahmed, H.M. and Abbott, P.V. (2012) Discolouration potential of endodontic procedures and materials: a review. *Int Endod J*, **45**, 883–897.

Amaral, T.H., Guerra C.S., Bombonato-Prado, K.F., Garcia de Paula, E. and de Queiroz, A.M. (2008) Tooth pigmentation caused by bilirubin: a case report and histological evaluation. *Spec Care Dentist*, **28**, 254–257.

Barron, M.J., Mcdonnell, S.T., Mackie, I. and Dixon, M.J. (2008) Hereditary dentine disorders: dentinogenesis imperfecta and dentine dysplasia. *Orphanet J Rare Dis*, **3**, 31.

Boushell, L.W., Ritter, A.V., Garland, G.E. *et al.* (2012) Nightguard vital bleaching: side effects and patient satisfaction 10 to 17 years post-treatment. *J Esthet Restor Dent*, **24**, 211–219.

Burrows, S. (2009) A review of the efficacy of tooth bleaching. *Dent Update*, **36**, 537–538, 541–544, 547–548 passim.

Cobb, C.M., Daubert, D.M., Davis, K. *et al.* (2017) Consensus conference findings on supragingival and subgingival air polishing. *Compend Contin Educ Dent*, **38**, E1–E4.

Dahl, J.E. and Pallesen, U. (2003) Tooth bleaching – a critical review of the biological aspects. *Crit Rev Oral Biol Med*, **14**, 292–304.

Damm, D.D. and Fantasia, J.E. (2001) Diffuse discoloration of teeth. Fluorosis. *Gen Dent*, **49**, 356, 428.

Gerlach, R.W., Barker, M.L., Karpinia, K. and Magnusson, I. (2009) Single site meta-analysis of 6% hydrogen peroxide whitening strip effectiveness and safety over 2 weeks. *J Dent*, **37**, 360–365.

Gutmann, M.E. (1998) Air polishing: a comprehensive review of the literature. *J Dent Hyg*, **72**, 47–56.

He, L.B., Shao, M.Y., Tan, K., Xu, X. and Li, J.Y. (2012) The effects of light on bleaching and tooth sensitivity during in-office vital bleaching: a systematic review and meta-analysis. *J Dent*, **40**, 644–653.

Kelleher, M.G., Djemal, S., Al-Khayatt, A.S. *et al.* (2011) Bleaching and bonding for the older patient. *Dent Update*, **38**, 294–296, 298–300, 302–303.

Koleoso, D.C., Shaba, O.P. and Isiekwe, M.C. (2004) Prevalence of intrinsic tooth discolouration among 11–16 year old Nigerians. *Odontostomatol Trop*, **27**, 35–39.

Kooijman, M.M. and Brand, H.S. (2005) Oral aspects of porphyria. *Int Dent J*, **55**, 61–66.

Link, J. (1973) Discoloration of the teeth in alkaptonuria (ochronosis) and Parkinsonism. *Chronicle*, **36**, 130.

Marin, P.D., Bartold, P.M. and Heithersay, G.S. (1997) Tooth discoloration by blood: an in vitro histochemical study. *Endod Dent Traumatol*, **13**, 132–138.

Mehta, D.N., Shah, J. and Thakkar, B. (2013) Amelogenesis imperfecta: four case reports. *J Nat Sci Biol Med*, **4**, 462–465.

Moharamzadeh, K. (2016) Biocompatibility of oral care products, in *Biocompatibility Of Dental Biomaterials* (ed. R. Shelton), Woodhead Publishing, Cambridge, pp. 113–129.

Mondelli, R.F., Azevedo, J.F., Francisconi, A.C., Almeida, C.M. and Ishikiriama, S.K. (2012) Comparative clinical study of the effectiveness of different dental bleaching methods – two year follow-up. *J Appl Oral Sci*, **20**, 435–443.

Nixon, P.J., Gahan, M., Robinson, S. and Chan, M.F. (2007a) Conservative aesthetic techniques for discoloured teeth: 1. The use of bleaching. *Dent Update*, **34**, 98–100, 103–104, 107.

Nixon, P.J., Robinson, S., Gahan, M. and Chan, M.F. (2007b) Conservative aesthetic techniques for discoloured teeth: 2. Microabrasion and composite. *Dent Update*, **34**, 160–162, 164, 166.

Pindborg, J.J. (1982) Aetiology of developmental enamel defects not related to fluorosis. *Int Dent J*, **32**, 123–134.

Poyser, N.J., Kelleher, M.G. and Briggs, P.F. (2004) Managing discoloured non-vital teeth: the inside/outside bleaching technique. *Dent Update*, **31**, 204–210, 213–214.

Prathap, S., Rajesh, H., Boloor, V.A. and Rao, A.S. (2013) Extrinsic stains and management: a new insight. *J Acad Indus Res*, **1**, 435–442.

Sanchez, A.R., Rogers, R.S. 3rd and Sheridan, P.J. (2004) Tetracycline and other tetracycline-derivative staining of the teeth and oral cavity. *Int J Dermatol*, **43**, 709–715.

Serraglio, C.R., Zanella, L., Dalla-Vecchia, K.B. and Rodrigues-Junior, S.A. (2016) Efficacy and safety of over-the-counter whitening strips as compared to home-whitening with 10 % carbamide peroxide gel – systematic review of RCTs and metanalysis. *Clin Oral Invest*, **20**, 1–14.

Sulieman, M. (2005) An overview of bleaching techniques: 2. Night Guard vital bleaching and non-vital bleaching. *Dent Update*, **32**, 39–40, 42–44, 46.

Tsubura, S. (2010) Clinical evaluation of three months' Nightguard vital bleaching on tetracycline-stained teeth using polanight 10% carbamide gel: 2-year follow-up study. *Odontology*, **98**, 134–138.

Ulvestad, H., Lokken, P. and Mjorud, F. (1978) Discoloration of permanent front teeth in 3,157 Norwegian children due to tetracyclines and other factors. *Scand J Dent Res*, **86**, 147–152.

Watts, A. and Addy, M. (2001) Tooth discolouration and staining: a review of the literature. *Br Dent J*, **190**, 309–316.

Wray, A., Welbury, R. and Faculty of Dental Surgery, RCOS (2001) UK National Clinical Guidelines In Paediatric Dentistry: treatment of intrinsic discoloration in permanent anterior teeth in children and adolescents. *Int J Paediatr Dent*, **11**, 309–315.

16

Ectodermal Dysplasia

16.1 Definition and Prevalence

Ectodermal dysplasia (ED) is a group of approximately 200 rare inherited disorders characterised by abnormalities of the ectodermal structures (Tape and Tye, 1995). ED is estimated to affect 1–7 individuals in every 10 000 live births (Itin and Fistarol, 2004).

16.2 Classification

Several classification systems have been proposed for ED.

- Freire-Maia and Pinheiro's classification based on the clinical features which grouped ED into 11 subtypes (Pinheiro and Freire-Maia, 1994).
- Priolo's classification combining molecular genetics and clinical aspects of ED (Priolo and Lagana, 2001).
- Lamartine proposed a new classification based on the functions of the genes associated with different types of ED (Lamartine, 2003).
- Itin and Fistarol's classification based on the structures affected (Itin and Fistarol, 2004).

Hypohidrotic ectodermal dysplasia (HED) is characterised by abnormalities in skin, hair, nails, teeth and sweat glands. HED can have different modes of inheritance, including autosomal dominant, autosomal recessive and X-linked recessive.

16.3 Aetiology

X-linked HED is the most common type of HED (Nguyen-Nielsen *et al.*, 2013) and is associated with a defect in the ectodysplasin-A gene (Kere *et al.*, 1996).

Some of the ED associated syndromes and genetic conditions include Ellis–van Creveld syndrome, ectrodactyly-ectodermal defects-clefting (EEC) syndrome, Clouston syndrome, ankyloblepharon-ectodermal dysplasia-clefting (AEC syndrome), tooth and nail syndrome, Hay–Wells syndrome, focal dermal hypoplasia (FDH) (Goltz syndrome), Rapp–Hodgkin syndrome, incontinentia pigmenti, Naegeli syndrome, pachyonychia congenital, palmoplantar ectodermal dysplasia, Margarita Island ectodermal dysplasia and ectodermal dysplasia with skin fragility (Freire-Maia and Pinheiro, 1988).

16.4 Diagnosis and Clinical Features

Diagnosis of ED is based on clinical observations combined with the family medical history. Some of the relevant clinical features of ED are listed below (Halai and Stevens, 2015).

- Thin, fragile, sparse and slowly growing hair with very light colour.
- Thick, discoloured, brittle and abnormally shaped fingernails and toenails.
- Lightly pigmented and dry skin prone to rashes or infections.
- Sweat gland abnormalities, hypohidrosis, anhidrosis and risk of overheating particularly during hot weather. It is important for these patients to have access to cooling.
- Reduced lacrimation, photophobia and periorbital pigmentation.
- Facial features such as frontal bossing, depressed nasal bridge and protuberant lips.
- Oral and dental abnormalities including:
  - hypodontia, oligodontial or anodontia (see Chapter 25)
  - microdontia (see Chapter 29)
  - enamel defects and hypoplastic teeth
  - taurodontism
  - underdeveloped alveolar ridge
  - dry mouth.

Diseases and Conditions in Dentistry: An Evidence-Based Reference, First Edition. Keyvan Moharamzadeh.

Companion website: www.wiley.com/go/moharamzadeh/diseases

16.5 Management Considerations

A multidisciplinary team management approach is required involving paediatric dentists, orthodontists, oral and maxillofacial surgeons, restorative dentists, general dental and medical practitioners, dermatologists and psychologists, aiming to address the following aspects of treatment (Hobkirk *et al.*, 2006).

- Child behavioural management
- Prevention of dental disease
- Replacement of the missing teeth and restoration of function
- Improving aesthetics
- Maintaining and restoring the patient's occlusal vertical dimension
- Management of other related medical problems
- Boosting the patient's self-esteem and psychological well-being

16.6 Restorative Treatment

Patients with ED may require the following types of restorative treatments.

16.6.1 Direct Restorations

Direct adhesive composite additions to microdont, hypoplastic and conical teeth is a conservative option for restoring compromised teeth and is highly recommended in young patients with large pulps (Lo Muzio *et al.*, 2005).

16.6.2 Indirect Restorations

Indirect restorations such as posterior onlays can be useful to restore and maintain the occlusal vertical dimension, and anterior veneers or crowns with minimal tooth preparations to improve the aesthetics (Ellis *et al.*, 1992).

16.6.3 Removable Dentures

Removable dentures, including partial dentures, complete dentures and overdentures, are simple and quick options for the replacement of missing multiple teeth and can be used in children as young as 2–3 years old (Bidra *et al.*, 2010; Bonilla *et al.*, 1997). Dentures will often require modifications or replacement as the child grows until they are old enough for a definitive prosthetic treatment (Ladda *et al.*, 2013; Pigno *et al.*, 1996).

16.6.4 Implants

Dental implants can be a definitive treatment option in adolescence after growth completion with a high success rate (Wang *et al.*, 2016; Yap and Klineberg, 2009). Edentulous arches in patients with ED can be rehabilitated with implant-retained fixed prostheses or implant-supported overdentures using conventional or zygomatic implants (Stern *et al.*, 2014; Wu *et al.*, 2015). Due to reduced alveolar ridge development in ED patients, significant numbers of these patients (68%) will require bone augmentation as part of dental implant rehabilitation (Wang *et al.*, 2016).

Implant treatment is fully discussed in Chapter 37 and the considerations of implant treatment in hypodontia patients are outlined in Chapter 25.

Cases of early implant placement in young growing children with severe ED have been reported (Cezaria Triches *et al.*, 2017; Guckes *et al.*, 2002; Kilic *et al.*, 2017; Mankani *et al.*, 2014; Paulus and Martin, 2013). Implant-supported overdenture treatment in patients with anodontia at an early age with regular follow-ups and prosthetic modifications and maintenance has been reported to be a successful alternative approach for aesthetic and functional management of this group of patients (Aydinbelge *et al.*, 2013; Filius *et al.*, 2014; Kilic *et al.*, 2017; Mittal *et al.*, 2015). However, the risks associated with early placement of implants in young growing children include implant movement, reduction of jaw growth and impairment of alveolar ridge development (Cronin *et al.*, 1994).

In an international expert consensus meeting (Klineberg *et al.*, 2013), it was agreed that decision making for this cohort of patients must be based on patient-specific requirements and clinical indications in growing bone, and oral and dental rehabilitation should be minimally invasive and conservative.

Case Study

An 18-year-old female patient was seen in a hypodontia joint clinic and presented with congenital absence of many teeth and retained deciduous teeth.

The patient's family medical history revealed a positive history of ED in her family as well as some abnormalities in skin, hair and nails consistent with features seen in ED.

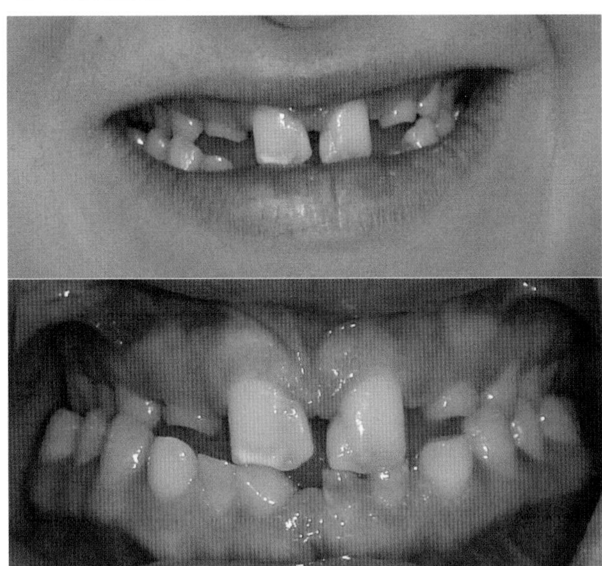

Figure 16.1 Preoperative clinical photograph showing missing teeth, retained primary teeth, enamel hypoplasia, tooth wear and narrow maxillary arch.

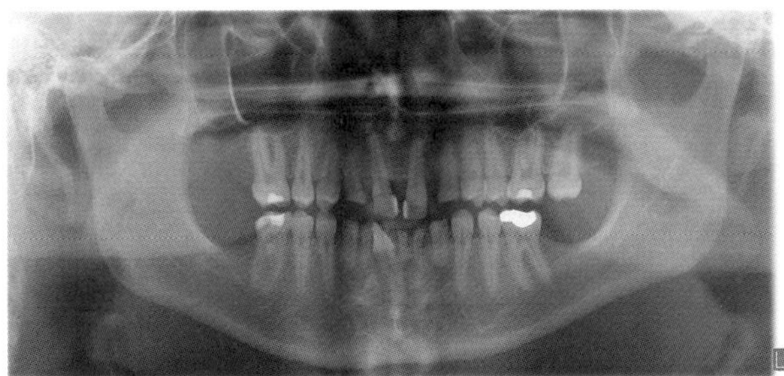

Figure 16.2 Oral panoramic radiograph showing absence of 16 permanent teeth, seven retained primary teeth and an ectopic mandibular canine.

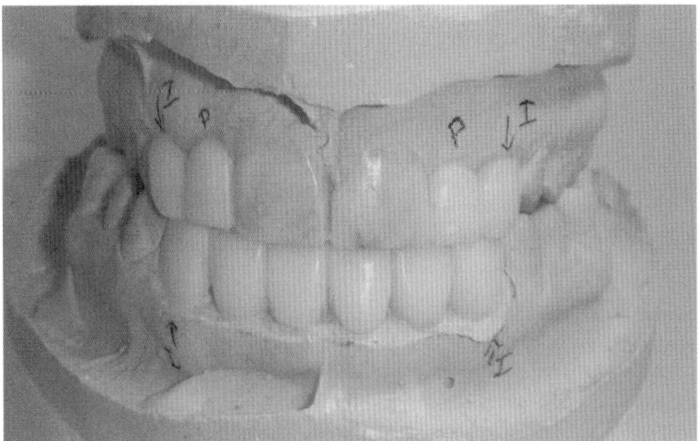

Figure 16.3 Diagnostic wax-up of the teeth to ideal shape and occlusion at an increased vertical dimension.

The patient's preoperative clinical photographs and radiograph are shown in Figures 16.1 and 16.2 respectively.

The diagnoses were as follows.

- Severe hypodontia (oligodontia) in a patient with partial expression of ectodermal dysplasia.
- Retained primary teeth.
- Microdontia and hypoplastic central incisor teeth.
- Tooth wear.
- Ectopic and partially erupted mandibular canine.
- Class III malocclusion and bilateral posterior cross-bite.

After discussion of different multidisciplinary treatment options, the patient did not want orthodontic treatment (to expand the maxillary arch and optimise the edentulous spaces for prosthetic tooth replacement) and preferred restorative-only treatment to replace the missing teeth and improve her aesthetics.

Therefore, the treatment strategy included preventive care, extraction of the retained primary teeth and ectopic mandibular canine tooth, immediate replacement with removable partial dentures (RPDs) and finally definitive replacement of the missing teeth with implant-retained fixed prostheses and maintenance.

The following treatment procedures were undertaken.

1) Oral hygiene instructions and dietary advice.
2) Impressions, bite registration, face-bow record and preparation of articulated study models in duplicates.
3) Removal of the retained primary teeth and ectopic canine tooth from the stone model and diagnostic wax-up of the teeth at an increased vertical dimension (occlusal reorganisation approach) (Figure 16.3).
4) Fabrication of immediate RPDs and surgical stents for immediate implant placement.
5) Extraction of the retained primary teeth and the ectopic mandibular canine tooth under general anaesthesia and placement of immediate implants in UR3, UL3, LR3 and LL3 regions (Figure 16.4).
6) Fitting of immediate temporary RPDs as shown in Figure 16.5.
7) Composite restorations of microdont and hypoplastic UR1, UL1, LR6 and LL6 using a stent made over the diagnostic wax-up to achieve ideal tooth shape and occlusion.
8) Fabrication and fitting of implant-retained provisional fixed bridges for UR3–2, UL3–2 and LL3–LR3 (Figure 16.6).
9) Fabrication and fitting of definitive implant-retained fixed PFM bridges for UR3–UR2 (cantilever design), UL3–UL2 (cantilever design) and LL3–LR3 (fixed-fixed design).

Figure 16.7 shows the final postoperative photograph of the patient's smile. The patient was satisfied with the outcome of the treatment and was discharged back to her general dental practitioner for long-term dental care and maintenance.

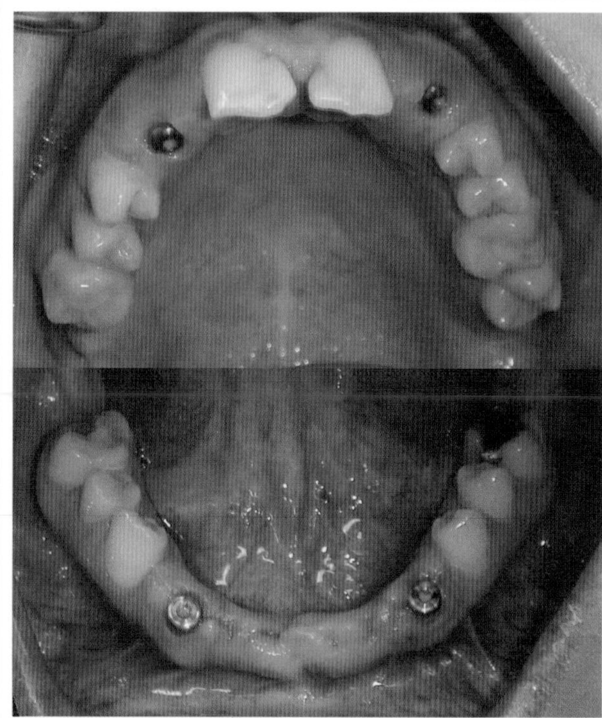

Figure 16.4 Intraoral photographs of the maxillary and mandibular arches following extractions and placement of the implants.

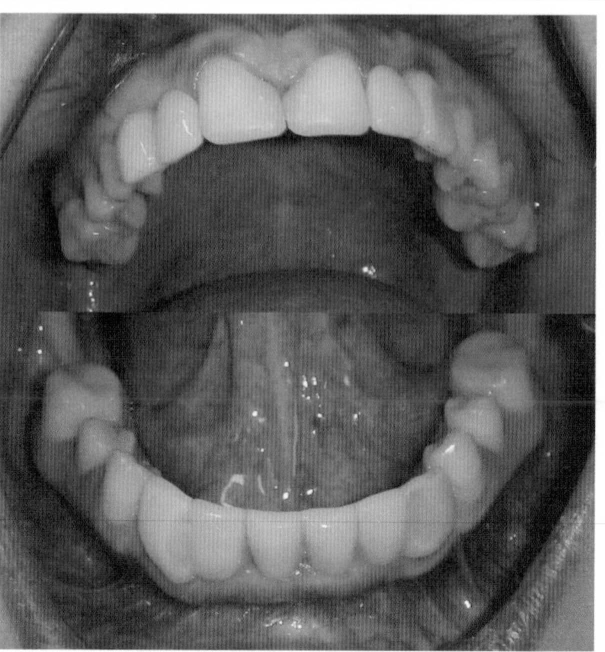

Figure 16.6 Intraoral photographs of the maxillary and mandibular arches following composite build-ups and fitting of provisional implant-retained bridges.

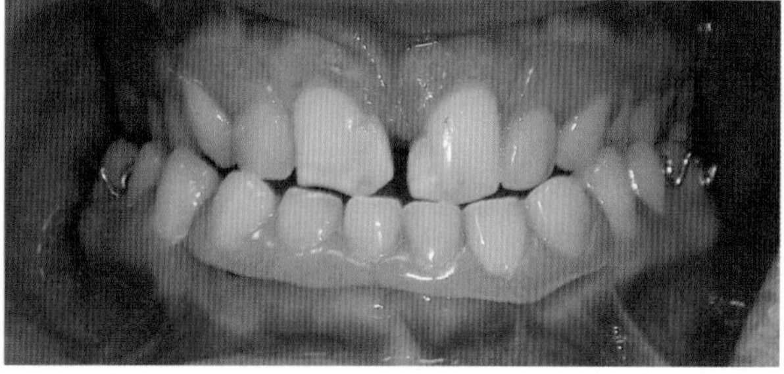

Figure 16.5 Immediate RPDs.

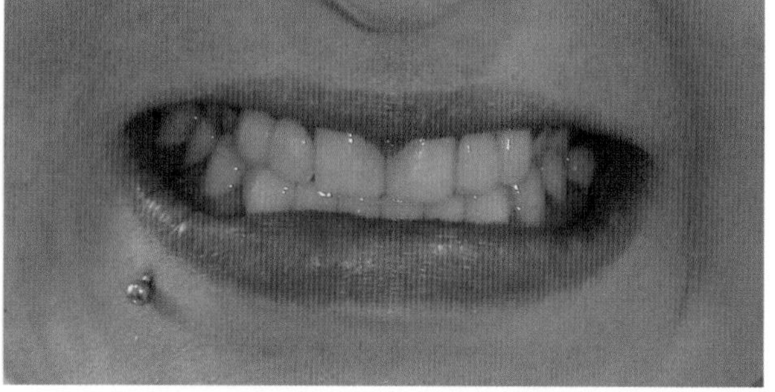

Figure 16.7 Final postoperative smile photograph following fitting of definitive implant-retained bridges.

References

Aydinbelge, M., Gumus, H.O., Sekerci, A.E., Demetoglu, U. and Etoz, O.A. (2013) Implants in children with hypohidrotic ectodermal dysplasia: an alternative approach to esthetic management: case report and review of the literature. *Pediatr Dent*, **35**, 441–446.

Bidra, A.S., Martin, J.W. and Feldman, E. (2010) Complete denture prosthodontics in children with ectodermal dysplasia: review of principles and techniques. *Compend Contin Educ Dent*, **31**, 426–433; quiz 434, 444.

Bonilla, E.D., Guerra, L. and Luna, O. (1997) Overdenture prosthesis for oral rehabilitation of hypohidrotic ectodermal dysplasia: a case report. *Quintessence Int*, **28**, 657–665.

Cezaria Triches, T., Ximenes, M., Oliveira de Souza, J.G., Rodrigues Lopes Pereira Neto, A., Cardoso, A.C. and Bolan, M. (2017) Implant-supported oral rehabilitation in child with ectodermal dysplasia – 4-year follow-up. *Bull Tokyo Dent Coll*, **58**, 49–56.

Cronin, R.J. Jr, Oesterle, L.J. and Ranly, D.M. (1994) Mandibular implants and the growing patient. *Int J Oral Maxillofac Implants*, **9**, 55–62.

Ellis, R.K., Donly, K.J. and Wild, T.W. (1992) Indirect composite resin crowns as an esthetic approach to treating ectodermal dysplasia: a case report. *Quintessence Int*, **23**, 727–729.

Filius, M.A., Vissink, A., Raghoebar, G.M. and Visser, A. (2014) Implant-retained overdentures for young children with severe oligodontia: a series of four cases. *J Oral Maxillofac Surg*, **72**, 1684–1690.

Freire-Maia, N. and Pinheiro, M. (1988) Selected conditions with ectodermal dysplasia. *Birth Defects Orig Artic Ser*, **24**, 109–121.

Guckes, A.D., Scurria, M.S., King, T.S., Mccarthy, G.R. and Brahim, J.S. (2002) Prospective clinical trial of dental implants in persons with ectodermal dysplasia. *J Prosthet Dent*, **88**, 21–25.

Halai, T. and Stevens, C. (2015) Ectodermal dysplasia: a clinical overview for the dental practitioner. *Dent Update*, **42**, 779–780, 783–784, 787–788 passim.

Hobkirk, J.A., Nohl, F., Bergendal, B., Storhaug, K. and Richter, M.K. (2006) The management of ectodermal dysplasia and severe hypodontia. International Conference Statements. *J Oral Rehabil*, **33**, 634–637.

Itin, P.H. and Fistarol, S.K. (2004) Ectodermal dysplasias. *Am J Med Genet C Semin Med Genet*, **131c**, 45–51.

Kere, J., Srivastava, A.K., Montonen, O. *et al.* (1996) X-linked anhidrotic (hypohidrotic) ectodermal dysplasia is caused by mutation in a novel transmembrane protein. *Nat Genet*, **13**, 409–416.

Kilic, S., Altintas, S.H., Yilmaz Altintas, N. *et al.* (2017) Six-year survival of a mini dental implant-retained overdenture in a child with ectodermal dysplasia. *J Prosthodont*, **26**, 70–74.

Klineberg, I., Cameron, A., Hobkirk, J. *et al.* (2013) Rehabilitation of children with ectodermal dysplasia. Part 2: an international consensus meeting. *Int J Oral Maxillofac Implants*, **28**, 1101–1109.

Ladda, R., Gangadhar, S., Kasat, V. and Bhandari, A. (2013) Prosthodontic management of hypohidrotic ectodermal dysplasia with anodontia: a case report in pediatric patient and review of literature. *Ann Med Health Sci Res*, **3**, 277–281.

Lamartine, J. (2003) Towards a new classification of ectodermal dysplasias. *Clin Exp Dermatol*, **28**, 351–355.

Lo Muzio, L., Bucci, P., Carile, F. *et al.* (2005) Prosthetic rehabilitation of a child affected from anhydrotic ectodermal dysplasia: a case report. *J Contemp Dent Pract*, **6**, 120–126.

Mankani, N., Chowdhary, R., Patil, B.A., Nagaraj, E. and Madalli, P. (2014) Osseointegrated dental implants in growing children: a literature review. *J Oral Implantol*, **40**, 627–631.

Mittal, M., Srivastava, D., Kumar, A. and Sharma, P. (2015) Dental management of hypohidrotic ectodermal dysplasia: a report of two cases. *Contemp Clin Dent*, **6**, 414–417.

Nguyen-Nielsen, M., Skovbo, S., Svaneby, D., Pedersen, L. and Fryzek, J. (2013) The prevalence of X-linked hypohidrotic ectodermal dysplasia (XLHED) in Denmark, 1995–2010. *Eur J Med Genet*, **56**, 236–242.

Paulus, C. and Martin, P. (2013) Hypodontia due to ectodermal dysplasia: rehabilitation with very early dental implants. *Rev Stomatol Chir Maxillofac Chir Orale*, **114**, E5–8.

Pigno, M.A., Blackman, R.B., Cronin, R.J. Jr and Cavazos, E. (1996) Prosthodontic management of ectodermal dysplasia: a review of the literature. *J Prosthet Dent*, **76**, 541–545.

Pinheiro, M. and Freire-Maia, N. (1994) Ectodermal dysplasias: a clinical classification and a causal review. *Am J Med Genet*, **53**, 153–162.

Priolo, M. and Lagana, C. (2001) Ectodermal dysplasias: a new clinical-genetic classification. *J Med Genet*, **38**, 579–585.

Stern, J.K., Hansen, T., Frankel, J. and Evian, C. (2014) Implant-supported fixed prosthesis in a hypohidrotic ectodermal dysplasia patient: a case report with 3 years follow-up and review of the literature. *Implant Dent*, **23**, 394–400.

Tape, M.W. and Tye, E. (1995) Ectodermal dysplasia: literature review and a case report. *Compend Contin Educ Dent*, **16**, 524–528.

Wang, Y., He, J., Decker, A.M., Hu, J.C. and Zou, D. (2016) Clinical outcomes of implant therapy in ectodermal dysplasia patients: a systematic review. *Int J Oral Maxillofac Surg*, **45**, 1035–1043.

Wu, Y., Zhang, C., Squarize, C.H. and Zou, D. (2015) Oral rehabilitation of adult edentulous siblings severely lacking alveolar bone due to ectodermal dysplasia: a report of 2 clinical cases and a literature review. *J Oral Maxillofac Surg*, **73**, 1733 E1–12.

Yap, A.K. and Klineberg, I. (2009) Dental implants in patients with ectodermal dysplasia and tooth agenesis: a critical review of the literature. *Int J Prosthodont*, **22**, 268–276.

17

External Root Resorption

17.1 Introduction

Root resorption can be categorised into two main groups: internal root resorption, originating from the pulp space within the tooth (see Chapter 26), and external root resorption originating from the outer surface of the root (Patel and Ford, 2007).

The most widely accepted classification for external root resorption is that described by Andreasen (Andreasen, 1970, 1981).

- Surface resorption, characterised by self-limiting superficial resorption of the cementum and dentine caused by localised and limited injury to the root surface or periodontium due to minor external or occlusal forces.
- Replacement resorption associated with ankylosis, which can be transient or progressive and can lead to total resorption of the root and tooth loss. This type of resorption occurs most commonly following replantation of avulsed teeth (Andreasen *et al.*, 1995) and traumatic intrusion of the teeth (Tsilingaridis *et al.*, 2016) (see Chapter 14).
- Inflammatory root resorption, which is associated with persistent inflammation of the periodontium adjacent to the site of resorption. Inflammatory root resorption can be further subdivided into:
  - external inflammatory root resorption, which can be sterile (due to pressure from orthodontic treatment or an impacted tooth) or infective (associated with trauma or pulpal necrosis)
  - peripheral inflammatory root resorption (also called invasive cervical resorption), which is discussed in this chapter.

17.2 Aetiology and Pathogenesis

Pathological root resorption is believed to be caused by specific clastic cell activity (Heithersay, 1994) which can be triggered by various predisposing factors (Darcey and Qualtrough, 2013a).

- Pulpal disease
- Periodontal infection
- Trauma
- Orthodontic tooth movement
- Pressure from an unerupted tooth or tumour adjacent to the root
- Ankylosis of the tooth
- Periodontal surgery
- Intracoronal tooth bleaching
- Rise in temperature caused by ultrasonic devices and heated endodontic instruments
- Viral infections such as feline herpes virus and shingles
- Systemic disease such as hyperparathyroidism, calcinosis, Paget's disease and Gaucher's disease

There are also rare cases of root resorption with unknown cause that are labelled 'idiopathic'.

17.3 External Invasive Cervical Root Resorption

Invasive cervical resorption (or peripheral inflammatory resorption) often occurs at the cervical region of the root below the epithelial attachment and may present as a subsurface pink lesion due to vascular granulation tissue within the resorption cavity. The tooth may be initially vital and asymptomatic but progressive lesions can cause pulpal exposure and ultimately lead to necrosis of the pulp.

Invasive cervical root resorption is more common in patients aged between 21 and 30 years and occurs more frequently in females (59.04%) than males (Opacic-Galic and Zivkovic, 2004).

Invasive cervical resorption lesions have been classified by Heithersay (1999b) into four subgroups.

- Class 1: small and shallow resorptive lesion near the cervical region of the tooth.

Diseases and Conditions in Dentistry: An Evidence-Based Reference, First Edition. Keyvan Moharamzadeh.

Companion website: www.wiley.com/go/moharamzadeh/diseases

- Class 2: deeper lesion close to the pulp chamber but confined to the coronal dentine.
- Class 3: larger resorptive lesion which extends into the coronal third of the root.
- Class 4: extensive lesion spreading beyond the coronal third of the root.

Patel *et al.* (2017) recently proposed a new three-dimensional classification system for external cervical resorption lesions, taking into account the following three parameters.

- Height of the lesion: (1) at the level of cementoenamel junction or supracrestal, (2) extending into the coronal third of the root and subcrestal, (3) extending into the mid-third of the root, and (4) extending into the apical third of the root.
- Circumferential spread of the lesion: (a): ≤90°, (b) ≤180°, (c) ≤270°, and (d) >270°.
- Proximity of the lesion to the root canal: (d) confined to dentine and (p) probable pulpal involvement.

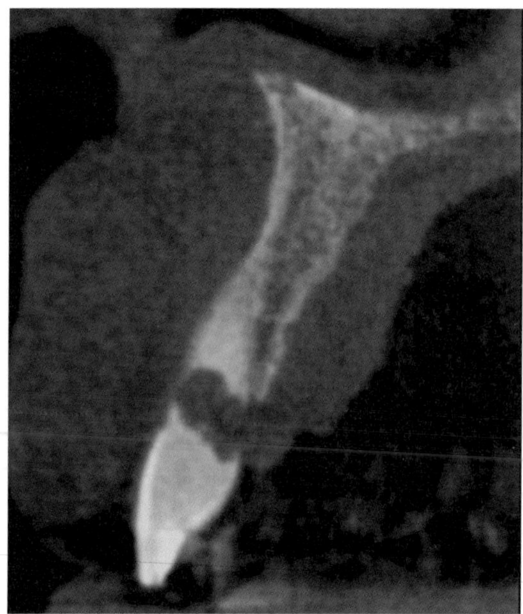

Figure 17.1 CBCT sagittal cross-sectional image of a maxillary central incisor tooth with external cervical resorption showing the extent of the invasive lesion. This tooth had a hopeless prognosis and was not amenable to repair due to the large size of the lesion splitting the tooth into two halves. The tooth was eventually extracted and replaced with a resin-bonded bridge.

17.4 History and Examination

It is important to obtain an accurate and thorough history to identify any potential risk factors associated with root resorption, as described above.

Clinical examination of the teeth with suspected resorptive lesions should include assessment of discolouration, existing restorations, periodontal examination, mobility, percussion testing and sensibility testing.

Radiographic examination should include one or two periapical radiographs with different angulations. Cone beam computed tomography (CBCT) (Figure 17.1) can be very useful in cases where an accurate diagnosis cannot be reached or when the location and extent of the lesions cannot be determined precisely using conventional radiographs (ESE *et al.*, 2014; EU, 2012; Patel *et al.*, 2009). CBCT also provides useful information regarding tooth location and the extent of root resorption caused by impacted teeth (Jawad *et al.*, 2016).

17.5 Differential Diagnosis

Clinical and radiographic features of different types of external root resorption and other similar lesions relevant to the differential diagnosis are summarised in Table 17.1.

17.6 Treatment Considerations

The aim of management is prevention and addressing the risk factors and cause of resorption. Treatment includes appropriate management of trauma, elimination of associated infections, deactivation and removal of hyperplastic resorptive lesions, restoration of the coronal root defect and establishment of periodontal health (Heithersay, 2007).

The external resorption process caused by pressure from an ectopic tooth or orthodontic treatment can be stopped by removal of the unerupted tooth or reduction of orthodontic force in the absence of any infection. However, the long-term prognosis of the resorbed tooth must be determined since an alternative option would be the extraction of the resorbed tooth, surgical exposure, orthodontic treatment of the impacted tooth and space management (Mittal *et al.*, 2012).

Management options for ankylosed teeth with replacement resorption are discussed in Chapter 14.

Teeth with external invasive cervical resorption can be treated non-surgically or surgically to deactivate and remove the resorptive lesion (Darcey and Qualtrough, 2013b) as described below.

17.6.1 Non-Surgical Management

Non-surgical treatment involves topical application of an aqueous solution of 90% trichloracetic acid for 2–3 minutes to the resorptive tissue, followed by curettage, endodontic treatment (if the tooth is non-vital) and restoration of the cavity with glass-ionomer cement (GIC). Adjunctive

Table 17.1 Clinical and radiographic features of different types of root resorption and other similar lesions (Darcey and Qualtrough, 2013b; Gartner *et al.*, 1976; Heithersay, 1999a; Patel *et al.*, 2010).

Condition	Clinical features	Radiographic features
External (invasive) cervical resorption	• Asymptomatic pink lesion on cervical aspect of the tooth • Initially vital tooth but may become non-vital as the lesion advances • Periodontal pocket and bleeding on probing • Sharp margins and hard cavity floor	• Cervical radiolucency with irregular margins • Periodontal bone loss may be present • The original shape of the root canal is often intact and visible
External inflammatory resorption (sterile)	• Teeth are often vital unless there is a concomitant pulpal disease or traumatic injury	• Evidence of causative factors such as impacted tooth or bony pathology • Shortening and blunting of the root end
External inflammatory resorption (infected)	• Teeth are non-vital due to pulpal necrosis • Teeth maybe discoloured	• Irregular resorption concavities on the root surface with a corresponding periapical or lateral bone radiolucency
External replacement resorption	• Evidence of tooth ankylosis such as lack of mobility, metallic sound on percussion and possible infraocclusion	• Loss of lamina dura visible in proximal lesions • Moth-eaten appearance of root and replacement with bone
Internal inflammatory resorption	• May present as a pink or dark red coronal lesion located centrally. • Initially the pulp may be partially vital, resembling symptoms of pulpitis, whereas complete pulp necrosis can develop symptoms of apical periodontitis	• Uniform enlarged area of the root canal • Smooth, sharp and clearly defined margins of the lesion • The canal is not present in the area of the lesion
Internal replacement resorption	• Teeth may be discoloured • The pulp may be vital or necrotic depending on the stage of disease progression	• Irregular enlargement of the pulp canal with evidence of obliteration or replacement with a mixed radiolucent and opaque areas • Absence of the radiopaque line of demarcation between the root canal and the image of resorption in dentine
Dental caries	• Symptoms vary depending on the extent of the caries and pulpal involvement • Presence of carious tissue in the lesion with softer margins of the cavity compared to resorption defects • Less bleeding on probing into the carious lesion	• Located more coronal than the resorption lesions • Less irregular margins of the lesion • Smoother and less defined lesion

orthodontic extrusion combined with gingivoplasty can also be employed in some advanced lesions to facilitate access to the cavity.

Using this approach, Heithersay (1999c) showed that the success rate for treatment of class 1 and class 2 lesions was 100%. In class 3 lesions, favourable outcome was achieved in 77.8% of cases and only 12.5% of teeth with class 4 lesions remained clinically sound and free of resorption following non-surgical treatment.

17.6.2 Surgical Management

Surgical treatment involves elevation of a full-thickness periodontal flap, curettage of the resorption cavity and restoration of the defect with GIC, composite, mineral trioxide aggregate (MTA) (Baratto-Filho *et al.*, 2005; Kqiku *et al.*, 2012; Park and Lee, 2008) or Biodentine® (Septodont, Lancaster, PA) (Baranwal, 2016) and repositioning the flap to its original position.

The chance of periodontal reattachment is high with the use of MTA (Bartols *et al.*, 2017) but its disadvantages include the potential for washout and discolouration of teeth. Alternatively, an apically repositioned flap can be used to place the gingival margin at the base of the resorption defect. However, this can be aesthetically unacceptable on the labial aspect of the anterior teeth and orthodontic extrusion can be used to improve the gingival margin's symmetry.

Periodontal regenerative approaches, including the use of guided tissue regeneration (GTR) membranes in combination with bone graft materials and bioactive agents, have been employed to treat periodontal bony defects associated with external cervical resorption and promote the ingrowth of periodontal ligament cells and periodontal healing (Johns *et al.*, 2013; Rankow and Krasner, 1996).

17.6.3 Endodontic Treatment

Regardless of the type of resorption, if there is pulpal involvement (irreversible pulpitis or necrotic pulp), root canal treatment would be indicated for restorable teeth to eliminate any potential endodontic infection and prevent further inflammatory resorption and associated symptoms.

Endodontic treatment of teeth with apical periodontitis and closed apices has been discussed in Chapter 3. Treatment options for non-vital immature teeth with open apices are discussed in Chapter 34 and the management of root perforations is covered in Chapter 39.

Case Study

A 56-year-old male patient presented with occasional discomfort associated with UR2. He reported a positive history of trauma to the upper anterior teeth. The upper central incisor teeth had been replaced with implant-retained single crowns many years earlier.

Clinical examination showed presence of gingival inflammation in the upper anterior region. UR2 was unrestored and had a normal shade. There was a 6 mm periodontal pocket on the mesial aspect of the tooth with profuse bleeding on probing. Sharp subgingival cavity margins could be felt upon probing on the mesial aspect of the tooth. Five mm deep pockets and bleeding on probing were also noticed on examination of the adjacent implant. UR2 showed positive response to electric pulp testing. There was no increased mobility and the tooth was not tender to percussion. There was no labial swelling or sinus tract.

Radiographic examination (Figure 17.2) showed the presence of a cervical radiolucency with irregular margins on the mesial aspect of UR2 with mild periodontal bone loss. There was no obvious periapical pathology and the original shape of the root canal was intact and visible. Mild bone loss was also noticed on the adjacent implant.

Based on the clinical and radiographic findings, the following diagnoses were made:

- external cervical resorption UR2 (vital tooth)
- peri-implantitis UR1 (mild).

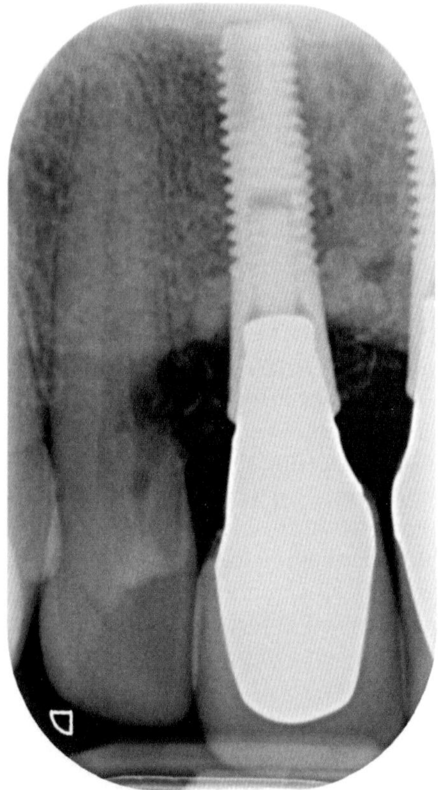

Figure 17.2 Preoperative periapical radiograph showing resorption cavity on the mesial aspect of UR2 and mild periodontal and peri-implant bone loss at UR1–2.

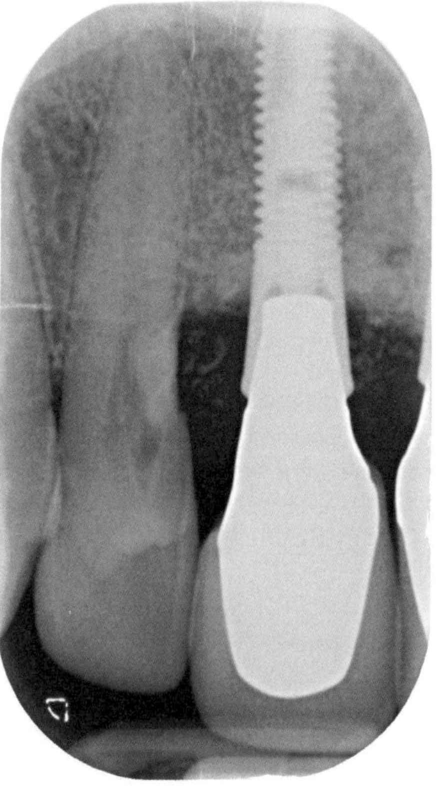

Figure 17.3 Periapical radiograph at 1-year follow-up.

The treatment strategy included the following aspects.

1) Oral hygiene instructions including modified Bass brushing and interdental cleaning.
2) Initial non-surgical periodontal and peri-implant debridement using an ultrasonic scaler under local anaesthesia to reduce bacterial deposits and associated inflammation and bleeding.
3) Surgical treatment including elevation of a full-thickness periodontal flap UR2 to UL1, curettage of the resorption cavity on the mesial aspect of UR2, placement of an MTA base close to the pulp canal and restoration of the defect with GIC. Removal of peri-implant granulation tissue and thorough debridement of the implant surface with ultrasonic tip were also carried out. The flap was then repositioned and sutured to its original position.
4) Review, monitoring the vitality of UR2, and maintenance.

The patient remained asymptomatic following treatment and periodontal reassessment after 3 months showed significant improvement and reduction in pocket depth and bleeding. Monitoring of UR2 after treatment with regular electric pulp testing (every 3 months) also showed that the tooth remained vital in the long term.

Radiographic examination (Figure 17.3) after 12 months showed a well-sealed restoration, absence of resorption or any signs of periapical or periodontal pathology. Periodontal/peri-implant bone levels remained unchanged. These findings indicated a successful outcome for the treatment of both external cervical resorption (UR2) and peri-implant disease (UR1).

References

Andreasen, J.O. (1970) Luxation of permanent teeth due to trauma. A clinical and radiographic follow-up study of 189 injured teeth. *Scand J Dent Res*, **78**, 273–286.

Andreasen, J.O. (1981) Relationship between cell damage in the periodontal ligament after replantation and subsequent development of root resorption. A time-related study in monkeys. *Acta Odontol Scand*, **39**, 15–25.

Andreasen, J.O., Borum, M.K., Jacobsen, H.L. and Andreasen, F.M. (1995) Replantation of 400 avulsed permanent incisors. 4. Factors related to periodontal ligament healing. *Endod Dent Traumatol*, **11**, 76–89.

Baranwal, A.K. (2016) Management of external invasive cervical resorption of tooth with biodentine: a case report. *J Conserv Dent*, **19**, 296–299.

Baratto-Filho, F., Limongi, O., Araujo C.J., Neto, M.D., Maia, S.M. and Santana, D. (2005) Treatment of invasive cervical resorption with MTA: case report. *Aust Endod J*, **31**, 76–80.

Bartols, A.D., Roussa, E., Walther, W. and Dorfer, C.E. (2017) First evidence for regeneration of the periodontium to mineral trioxide aggregate in human teeth. *J Endod*, **5**, 715–722.

Darcey, J. and Qualtrough, A. (2013a) Resorption: Part 1. Pathology, classification and aetiology. *Br Dent J*, **214**, 439–451.

Darcey, J. and Qualtrough, A. (2013b) Resorption: Part 2. Diagnosis and management. *Br Dent J*, **214**, 493–509.

ESE, Patel, S., Durack, C., Abella, F. *et al.* (2014) European Society of Endodontology Position Statement: the use of CBCT in endodontics. *Int Endod J*, **47**, 502–504.

EU (2012) *European Commission Radiation Protection No 172: Cone Beam CT for Dental and Maxillofacial Radiology Evidence-Based Guidelines*. European Union, Brussels.

Gartner, A.H., Mack, T., Somerlott, R.G. and Walsh, L.C. (1976) Differential diagnosis of internal and external root resorption. *J Endod*, **2**, 329–334.

Heithersay, G.S. (1994) External root resorption. *Ann R Australas Coll Dent Surg*, **12**, 46–59.

Heithersay, G.S. (1999a) Clinical, radiologic, and histopathologic features of invasive cervical resorption. *Quintessence Int*, **30**, 27–37.

Heithersay, G.S. (1999b) Invasive cervical resorption: an analysis of potential predisposing factors. *Quintessence Int*, **30**, 83–95.

Heithersay, G.S. (1999c) Treatment of invasive cervical resorption: an analysis of results using topical application of trichloracetic acid, curettage, and restoration. *Quintessence Int*, **30**, 96–110.

Heithersay, G.S. (2007) Management of tooth resorption. *Aust Dent J*, **52**, S105–121.

Jawad, Z., Carmichael, F., Houghton, N. and Bates, C. (2016) A review of cone beam computed tomography for the diagnosis of root resorption associated with impacted canines, introducing an innovative root resorption scale. *Oral Surg Oral Med Oral Pathol Oral Radiol*, **122**, 765–771.

Johns, D.A., Shivashankar, V.Y., Maroli, R.K. and Joseph, R. (2013) Invasive cervical root resorption: engineering the lost tissue by regeneration. *Contemp Clin Dent*, **4**, 536–539.

Kqiku, L., Ebeleseder, K.A. and Glockner, K. (2012) Treatment of invasive cervical resorption with sandwich technique using mineral trioxide aggregate: a case report. *Oper Dent*, **37**, 98–106.

Mittal, M., Murray, A. and Sandler, J. (2012) Impacted maxillary canines – a perennial problem. *Dent Update*, **39**, 487–488, 491–492, 495–497.

Opacic-Galic, V. and Zivkovic, S. (2004) [Frequency of the external resorptions of tooth roots]. *Srp Arh Celok Lek*, **132**, 152–156.

Park, J.B. and Lee, J.H. (2008) Use of mineral trioxide aggregrate in the non-surgical repair of perforating invasive cervical resorption. *Med Oral Patol Oral Cir Bucal*, **13**, E678–680.

Patel, S. and Ford, T.P. (2007) Is the resorption external or internal? *Dent Update*, **34**, 218–220, 222, 224–226, 229.

Patel, S., Kanagasingam, S. and Pitt Ford, T. (2009) External cervical resorption: a review. *J Endod*, **35**, 616–625.

Patel, S., Ricucci, D., Durak, C. and Tay, F. (2010) Internal root resorption: a review. *J Endod*, **36**, 1107–1121.

Patel, S., Foschi, F., Mannocci, F. and Patel, K. (2017) External cervical resorption: a three-dimensional classification. *Int Endod J* 26 July (epub ahead of print).

Rankow, H.J. and Krasner, P.R. (1996) Endodontic applications of guided tissue regeneration in endodontic surgery. *J Endod*, **22**, 34–43.

Tsilingaridis, G., Malmgren, B., Andreasen, J.O., Wigen, T.I., Maseng Aas, A.L. and Malmgren, O. (2016) Scandinavian multicenter study on the treatment of 168 patients with 230 intruded permanent teeth – a retrospective cohort study. *Dent Traumatol*, **32**, 353–360.

18

Failed Restoration and Compromised Tooth

18.1 Introduction

Dental restorations can be divided into two main categories: (1) direct restorations, including amalgam, composite, glass-ionomer cement (GIC) and compomers, and (2) indirect restorations, including full-coverage crowns, partial-coverage crowns, inlays, onlays and veneers. This chapter discusses the evidence from the literature on clinical performance and survival of different types of restorations for single teeth, including those on root-treated teeth.

18.2 Direct Restorations

Direct restorations are simple and conservative treatment options for restoring lost tooth structure without the need for extensive tooth tissue removal which is often required as part of the preparation for indirect restorations. A large number of clinical studies have been conducted to assess the longevity and survival of different types of direct restorative materials. The highest quality of evidence, including the latest systematic reviews of these clinical studies, is discussed below.

18.2.1 Amalgam Restorations

Dental amalgam has been one of the most popular dental materials for the restoration of tooth structure in posterior teeth for many years. However, the Minamata Convention in 2013 called for a global phase-down of amalgam use, due to the biological and environmental effects of mercury in amalgam (Larson, 2014). Following a significant debate by the British Society of Prosthodontics on the implications of this issue, many clinicians felt that even in the event of a complete phase-down, amalgam should remain available for clinicians to choose in certain clinical circumstances, especially when moisture control is challenging for restoration of posterior teeth (Austin *et al.*, 2016).

According to systematic reviews, the amalgam survival rate ranges from 76.3% to 100%. The mean annual failure rate for amalgam restorations is 1.7%, which includes fracture of restoration or tooth, secondary caries, pulpal disease and loss of restoration (Alhareky and Tavares, 2016; Moraschini *et al.*, 2015). High copper amalgam restorations have shown significantly better survival rates and lower failure incidence in terms of secondary caries and bulk fracture compared to composite restorations (Rasines Alcaraz *et al.*, 2014).

18.2.2 Composite Restorations

Dental composites are now widely accepted restorative materials for both anterior and posterior teeth. Their advantages include aesthetics, conservative cavity preparation, adhesive bond to the tooth and ability to reinforce weaken tooth structure. The limitations of composite resins incude polymerisation shrinkage, potential for micro-leakage, sensitivity following placement, marginal discolouration and high cost. Composite restorations are also technique sensitive and require effective isolation and moisture control.

Important prognostic factors affecting the performance of dental composite resins include (Bohaty *et al.*, 2013):

- patient factors such as caries risk and parafunctional habits
- tooth parameters, including tooth position, vitality, number of restored surfaces, preparation design, cavity size and type
- matrix and wedge utilisation
- method of isolation
- acid etching protocol and enamel and dentine bonding method
- type and composition of the composite resin material
- polymerisation shrinkage.

Systematic reviews and meta-analyses have shown 5–10-year survival rates for posterior composite resin restorations around 80–90%, according to different studies.

Diseases and Conditions in Dentistry: An Evidence-Based Reference, First Edition. Keyvan Moharamzadeh.

Companion website: www.wiley.com/go/moharamzadeh/diseases

The mean annual failure rates were 1.46% (±1.74%) for short-term studies and 1.97% (±1.53%) for long-term studies; the main reasons for the failure of restorations were bulk fractures, which were higher in large restorations, and secondary caries development, which was significantly higher in high caries-risk patients (Beck *et al.*, 2015; Heintze and Rousson, 2012; Opdam *et al.*, 2014). In load-bearing situations, conventional composites have the highest probability of survival, whereas siloranes are the least suitable (Schwendicke *et al.*, 2016). Ormocer-based restorative materials also have significantly lower survival rates than other conventional composites after 3 years (Monsarrat *et al.*, 2017). Restorations with hybrid and microfilled composite resins placed using the enamel-etching technique under appropriate rubber dam isolation showed the best overall performance and longevity similar to amalgam restorations (Heintze and Rousson, 2012).

The Academy of Operative Dentistry (European Section) has published useful evidence-based guidance on posterior composite restorations including indications, contraindications and certain aspects of composite placement techniques in posterior teeth (Lynch *et al.*, 2014).

Regarding anterior composite restorations, survival rates vary from 53.4% to 100% according to a systematic review by Demarco *et al.* (2015). Class III restorations have lower annual failure rates than class IV and V anterior composite restorations. Important survival factors included adhesive technique, type of composite resin, risk of retreatment and time required to complete the restoration. The most common reason for failure was tooth or restoration fracture. Aesthetic failures were more frequent when the restorations were placed for aesthetic reasons.

Survival of direct composite restorations specifically in tooth wear patients is discussed in Chapter 50.

18.2.3 GIC, Resin-Modified GIC and Compomers

Glass-ionomer cements are tooth-coloured bulk placement, intrinsically adhesive (Czarnecka *et al.*, 2007) restorative materials with several other favourable properties, including biocompatibility (Rodriguez *et al.*, 2013), fluoride release (Mickenautsch *et al.*, 2011) and a coefficient of thermal expansion compatible with tooth tissues (Sidhu *et al.*, 2004). However, due to their low flexural strength and wear resistance (van Noort, 2013), GIC restorations have poor long-term survival rates (Goldstein, 2010) and are mainly used as temporary restorations in load-bearing surfaces.

Resin matrix has been incorporated in resin-modified GICs and compomers to improve the mechanical properties. Resin-modified GIC restorations have the highest chance of survival in class V cervical lesions. Compomers and composites placed using two-step self-etch bonding agents and three-step etch-and-rinse adhesives have been ranked next. Restorations placed with two-step etch-and-rinse or one-step self-etch adhesives have shown the weakest performance (Schwendicke *et al.*, 2016).

In class I and II cavities, restorations with compomers have a significantly lower survival compared to composite restorations. The main reasons for replacement were bulk fractures and caries adjacent to restorations (Heintze and Rousson, 2012).

18.3 Indirect Restorations

Indirect fixed restorations, including different types of crowns, inlays, onlays and partial-coverage veneers, can be indicated for the following reasons (Rosenstiel *et al.*, 2015).

- Restoring and protecting broken-down or root-treated teeth.
- Trauma (see Chapter 14).
- Tooth wear (see Chapter 50).
- Hypoplastic teeth with atypical shape often seen in developmental disorders (see Chapters 2 and 13).
- To alter and correct occlusion (see Chapter 31).
- To accommodate a removable prosthesis, e.g. creating ideal abutments for removable partial denture (see Chapter 38).
- Restoring missing function due to open bite (see Chapter 35).
- Improving aesthetics.

Indirect restorations are generally less conservative than direct restorations as heavier tooth preparations are often required for indirect restorations and some of the consequences of failure of indirect restorations (e.g. loss of tooth vitality, crown fracture) (Goodacre *et al.*, 2003) can be more catastrophic and irreversible compared to those of direct restorations (e.g. fracture of restoration and staining) which are reversible and amenable to repair.

The evidence for survival of different types of indirect restorations is discussed below.

18.3.1 Crowns

Crowns are indirect extracoronal restorations which are used widely to replace the missing tooth structure and restore anatomy. Restoration of a tooth with a crown often requires preparing the tooth (Goodacre *et al.*, 2001) and removal of a considerable amount of tooth tissue which carries a significant risk of damage to the pulp. Crowns are contraindicated where there are other more conservative restorative options available, and also in patients with poor oral hygiene and active periodontal disease as well as very broken-down, non-restorable teeth with deep subgingival caries.

Crowns used as definitive restorations can be classified into metal-ceramic or porcelain fused to metal (PFM), all-ceramic and gold crowns.

18.3.1.1 Porcelain Fused to Metal (PFM) Crowns

A systematic review and meta-analysis of 17 studies on 4663 PFM crowns indicated that the estimated survival rate was 94.7% after 5 years (Sailer *et al.*, 2015). A similar survival figure (95.6%) was reported in a previous systematic review by the same group (Pjetursson *et al.*, 2007).

The main reported biological complications associated with PFM crowns include:

- loss of tooth vitality, which was the most frequent biological complication (5-year complication rate 1.8%)
- abutment tooth fracture (5-year complication rate 1.2%)
- secondary caries, reported for 1% of PFM crowns.

The main reported technical complications associated with PFM crowns include:

- ceramic chipping, the most frequent technical complication (cumulative 5-year event rate: 2.6%).
- marginal discolouration (1.8% at 5 years)
- loss of retention (0.6% at 5 years).

18.3.1.2 All-Ceramic Crowns

All-ceramic crowns offer the potential for improved aesthetics compared to conventional metal-ceramic crowns (Mizrahi, 2011).

Survival rates of all-ceramic crowns differ by type of ceramic used, fabrication method and clinical indication (Land and Hopp, 2010; Wang *et al.*, 2012).

All-ceramic crowns have overall estimated 5-year survival rates ranging between 90.7% and 96.6% (Sailer *et al.*, 2015). Estimated 5-year survival rates for different types of all-ceramic restorations based on Sailer's meta-analysis are listed below.

- Feldspathic or silica-based ceramics (10 studies): 90.7%
- Leucite/lithium-disilicate reinforced glass ceramics (10 studies): 96.6%
- Glass-infiltrated alumina (15 studies): 94.6%
- Densely sintered alumina (8 studies): 96.0%
- Densely sintered zirconia (8 studies): 93.8% (Sailer *et al.*, 2016)

Feldspathic or silica-based ceramic crowns showed significantly lower survival rates on the posterior teeth (87.8%) than the anterior teeth (94.6%).

In terms of biological complications, loss of tooth vitality was less common for leucite or lithium-disilicate reinforced glass ceramics and glass-infiltrated alumina crowns compared to PFM crowns. Most all-ceramic crowns showed similar 5-year caries rates to PFM crowns. Zirconia-based crowns had significantly less secondary caries, and glass-infiltrated ceramic crowns had higher caries rates. Abutment tooth fracture was also less common in all-ceramic crowns compared to PFM crowns.

The main reported technical complications associated with all-ceramic crowns included:

- ceramic framework fracture: 6.7% for feldspathic/silica-based ceramics, 2.3% for leucite or lithium-disilicate reinforced glass ceramics, and 0.4% for zirconia-based single crowns at 5 years
- loss of retention, which was more common in zirconia-based crowns (4.7%) than other all-ceramic crowns and PFM crowns
- ceramic veneer chipping, which was more common with alumina and zirconia (1.2% at 5 years).

These findings are in agreement with previous systematic reviews on survival of all-ceramic crowns (Al-Amleh *et al.*, 2010; Pjetursson *et al.*, 2007; Wang *et al.*, 2012).

18.3.1.3 Full Gold Crowns (FGG)

It is widely accepted that cast gold restorations can provide extremely predictable and long-term restorative service. In a retrospective clinical study, long-term (up to 52 years) survival of 1314 cast gold restorations was evaluated by Donovan *et al.* (2004). The reported survival rates included 97% at 9 years, 90.3% at 20 years, 94.9% at 25 years, 98% at 29 years, 96.9% at 39 years and 94.1% at over 40 years.

18.3.2 Inlays and Onlays

Inlays and onlays are alternative indirect adhesive restorations used for restoring compromised posterior teeth (Satterthwaite, 2006) and can be made of cast gold, ceramic or composite materials.

Indirect inlays and onlays often require more tooth tissue removal during preparation than direct restorations. However, as indirect restorations are made in the laboratory, better anatomical form, occlusal morphology and contact points can be achieved.

Posterior onlays can be indicated for restoration and protection of root-treated teeth or compromised posterior dentition in patients with developmental dental disorders such as amelogenesis imperfecta or dentinogenesis imperfecta. Onlays are also indicated for restoration of posterior teeth with tooth wear mainly affecting the occlusal surfaces, and for the restorative management of posterior open bite or increased anterior overbite in combination with potential orthodontic treatment.

Onlays are more conservative than full-coverage crowns as they often require minimal tooth tissue removal during preparation.

A systematic review by Goldstein (2010) included studies on survival of different types of inlays and onlays and reported the following annual failure rates (AFR).

- Composite inlays and onlays (20 studies): 2.9%
- Laboratory-fabricated ceramic inlays and onlays (36 studies): 1.9%
- CAD-CAM ceramic inlays and onlays (20 studies): 1.7%
- Cast gold inlays and onlays (19 studies): 1.4%

The main reasons for failure were secondary caries, fracture, marginal deficiencies, wear and postoperative sensitivity.

18.3.3 Veneers

Indirect labial veneers are generally used to improve the appearance of compromised tooth in the aesthetic zone. Reasons include improving the colour of discoloured teeth, addressing enamel defects, fractures, wear, correcting the shape or position of teeth and management of spacing between teeth.

Contraindications to labial veneers include heavily broken-down teeth with significant loss of coronal tooth tissue, bruxism and edge-to-edge occlusion.

Indirect veneers are less conservative than direct composite restorations but are more conservative than full-coverage crowns as they only involve minimal preparation of the labial aspect of the teeth.

Composite veneers are often used as provisional or short-term treatment options and in some cases they can be used as low-cost alternative definitive options (Gresnigt *et al.*, 2013) compared to porcelain veneers which are used as definitive high-cost long-term aesthetic treatment.

A systematic review by Layton *et al.* (2012), including qualitative analysis of 11 studies and meta-analysis of six studies, showed that estimated cumulative survival rates for feldspathic porcelain veneers were 95.7% at 5 years and ranged from 64% to 95% at 10 years. Enamel bonding may increase the 10-year survival rate of feldspathic porcelain veneers to 95.6%.

In a different systematic review of survival of non-feldspathic porcelains by the same group (Layton and Clarke, 2013), it was shown that the pooled estimate survival rates for Empress veneers were 92.4% at 5 years and 66–94% at 10 years.

The main reasons for failure of indirect veneer restorations include fractures and marginal defects. The incidence of secondary caries is also increased in high-risk patients and locations (Peumans *et al.*, 2004).

18.4 Restoration of Root-Treated Teeth

Eliyas *et al.* (2015) comprehensively discussed the important considerations of restoration of root canal-treated teeth, including evidence-based clinical recommendations for how to restore root-treated teeth and maintain coronal seal and tooth integrity during and after endodontic treatment in different situations.

Further evidence on the performance of restorations on root treated teeth is highlighted below.

Success rates of prosthetic restorations on endodontically treated teeth based on a meta-analysis (Ploumaki *et al.*, 2013) of clinical studies with a follow-up period of at least 6 years are as follows.

- Single crowns (4 studies): 94% for teeth without post, and 92% for teeth with posts.
- Fixed bridges (4 studies): 79%.
- Removable partial denture abutment (1 study): 66%.
- Single crowns on cast post and cores: 93%.
- Single crowns on prefabricated posts: 94%.

The most common reason for failure was post loosening.

It has been shown that resin core restorations luted with adhesive resin cement have significantly higher survival rates than cast metal cores. Apart from the type of core material, other risk factors for core failure have included sex (male), inadequate remaining coronal tooth tissue (ferrule effect) and higher age at core insertion (Hikasa *et al.*, 2010).

In terms of the types of posts, the following significant results have been reported according to a systematic review (Theodosopoulou and Chochlidakis, 2009).

- Carbon fibre in resin matrix posts performs significantly better than precious alloy cast posts (number needed to treat (NNT) = 8.30).
- Tapered gold alloy cast posts perform better than ParaPost gold alloy cast posts (NNT = 13.15).
- Glass fibre posts perform significantly better than metal screw posts (NNT = 5.46), but worse than titanium posts (NNT = -21.73).
- Carbon fibre posts perform significantly worse than gold alloy cast posts (NNT = -5.81).

Advances in adhesive technology and development of new and improved materials have enabled successful direct restoration of root-treated posterior teeth in a more conservative, faster and less expensive manner compared to classic indirect crowns supported by radicular metal posts, which have been criticised for their invasiveness (Rocca and Krejci, 2013). Furthermore, there is not sufficient evidence to confirm the superiority of crowns over conventional restorations for restoring root-filled teeth (McReynolds and Duane, 2016; Sequeira-Byron *et al.*, 2015). Therefore, until further evidence becomes available, clinicians should also take into account their own clinical experience, the individual circumstances and patient preferences when deciding how to restore root-filled teeth.

Case Study

A 75-year-old male patient referred by his GDP presented with broken teeth, failed restorations, crowns, poor aesthetics and difficulty eating.

The patient reported loss of multiple posterior teeth over many years and gradual wear and fracture of anterior teeth and failure of restorations and crowns long term. He was not aware of any parafunctional habits and had a normal diet.

The GDP was unable to restore the teeth due to the complexity of treatment and the patient's strong cough reflex and inability to tolerate water spray in his mouth.

The relevant medical history included chronic cough. There was no history of acid reflux disease or vomiting.

The patient's preoperative clinical photographs and radiograph are shown in Figures 18.1 and 18.2.

Periodontal examination showed good oral hygiene, mild generalised gingival recession and the BPE scores were 1 in all quadrants. Sensibility testing with an electric pulp tester revealed non-vital LR4 and LL7.

Based on the clinical and radiographic findings, the following diagnoses were made.

- Generalised moderate-severe tooth surface loss, mainly due to attrition
- Loss of posterior support and reduced occlusal vertical dimension (OVD)
- Caries LR3, LR4, LL3, LL7
- Failed restorations LL4, LR4
- Failed crowns UL3, LL2
- Retained UL2 root
- Chronic apical periodontitis LR3, LR4 and LL3

Important prognostic factors included the following.

- Patient's inability to tolerate water spray in the mouth.
- Due to a strong cough reflex, the patient had to sit up and cough every 5–10 minutes.
- Patient did not want any type of removable denture.
- Some teeth had sufficient remaining tooth structure and enamel present for bonding, but some (UL1 and LL3) had lost significant amounts of coronal tooth tissue.
- LL7 had deep subgingival caries and was non-restorable but the patient wanted to keep the tooth and extract it later, since he wasn't having any problems with it .

The following treatment options were discussed with the patient.

- Extractions and replacement of teeth with dentures.
- Reduction of the teeth and treatment with overdentures.
- Attempting to save the remaining teeth by endodontic treatment and restoration of the teeth and replacement of all the missing teeth with removable partial dentures or implants.

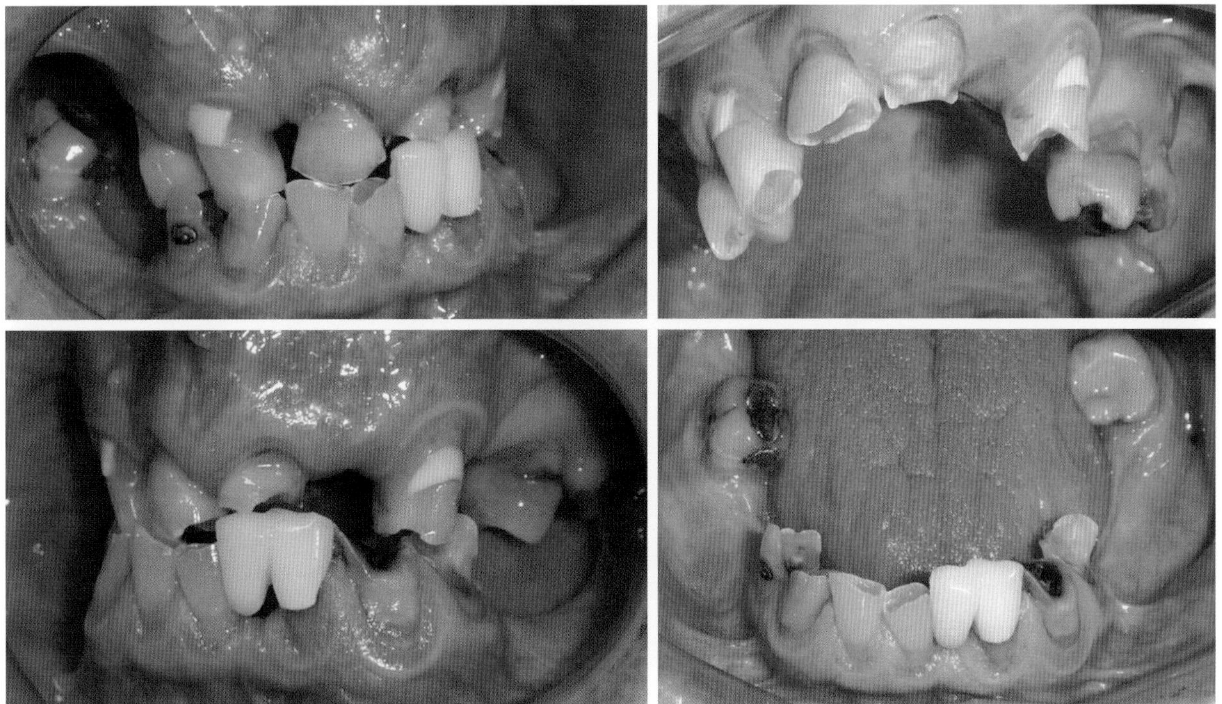

Figure 18.1 Preoperative clinical photographs showing loss of posterior support, generalised moderate-severe toothwear, caries, fractured restorations and failed crowns.

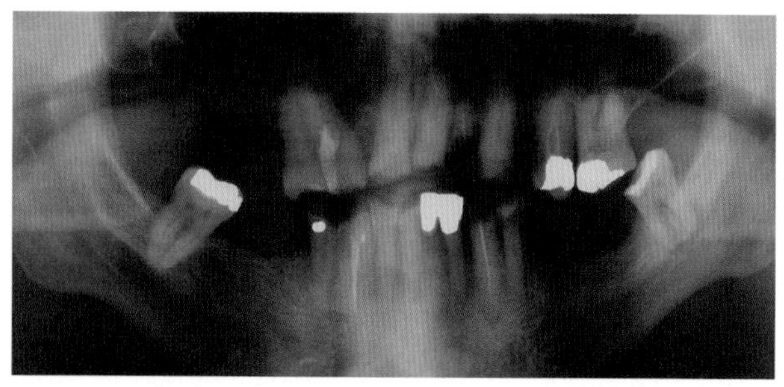

Figure 18.2 Preoperative panoramic radiograph of the patient showing a retained root (UL2), previously root-treated LR3, LL3 with periapical radiolucencies, root-treated UL5 with no obvious apical pathology and periapical radiolucency on LL7.

and premolars with fixed or cantilever bridges and accepting a shortened dental arch.

Treatment agreed with the patient is outlined below.

1) Preventive care, oral hygiene instructions and stabilisation of caries.
2) Endodontic retreatment of LL3 and LR3 and root canal treatment of LR4 (Figure 18.3).
3) Surgical removal of UL2 root under local anaesthesia and crown-lengthening surgery of UL1.
4) Diagnostic wax-up of teeth at an increased vertical dimension (Figure 18.4).
5) Composite build-up of worn anterior teeth (Figure 18.5) using a stent made of silicone putty over diagnostic wax-up.
6) Preparation of teeth for indirect restorations (Figure 18.6).
7) Single crown on UR1.

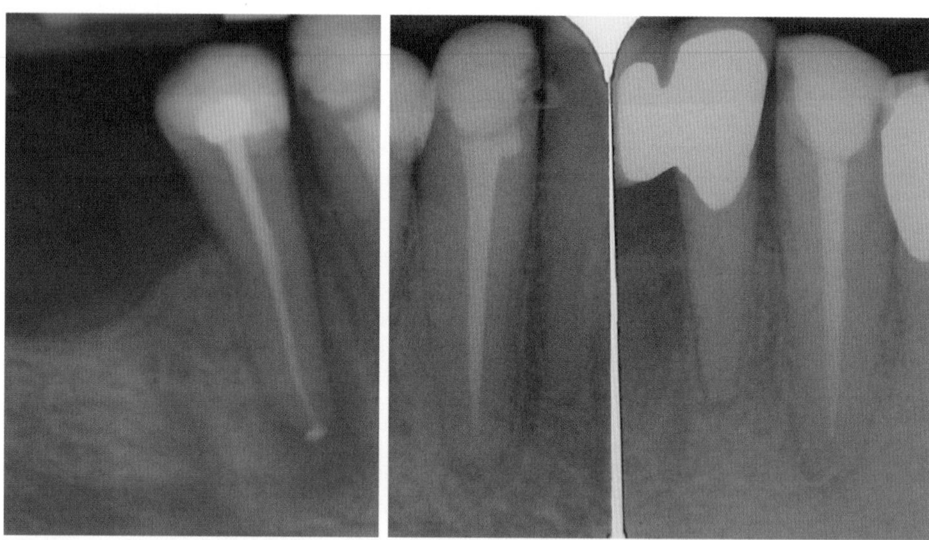

Figure 18.3 Immediate postoperative periapical radiograph of LR4 following root canal treatment and 9 months follow-up radiographs of LR3 and LL3 following endodontic retreatment.

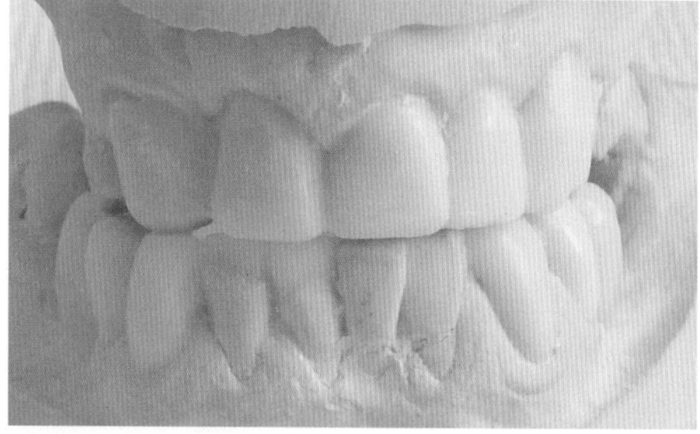

Figure 18.4 Diagnostic wax-up of the teeth to ideal shape and height at an increased OVD.

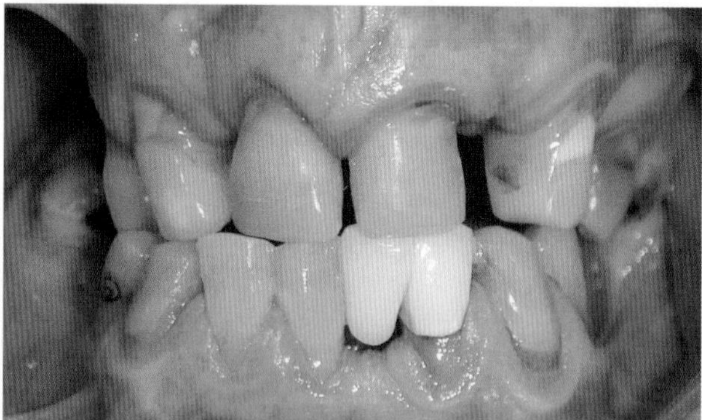

Figure 18.5 Clinical photograph following composite build-up of worn anterior teeth.

- Attempting to save the remaining teeth, endodontic treatment, restoration of the teeth with direct composites and crowns and replacing the missing anterior teeth

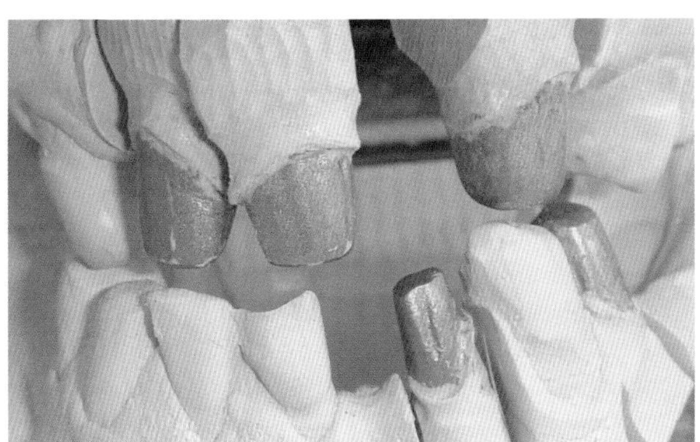

Figure 18.6 Photograph of the prepared teeth on the stone model.

8) A cantilever 4-unit PFM bridge to replace UL2 and UL4 using UL1 and UL3 as abutments.
9) Cantilever 2-unit PFM bridge to replace LL5 using LL4 as abutment.
10) Replacement of cantilever PFM bridge LL1–2.
11) Fitting of the bridges (Figure 18.7) and postoperative instructions.
12) Review and maintenance of the shortened dental arch.

This was a very challenging case due to its complexity and the patient's strong cough reflex. Using rubber dam isolation and treating the patient in an upright position helped to reduce the reflex significantly. Diagnostic wax-up and fabrication of a silicone stent were very helpful for composite build-up of the teeth.

It was interesting to see how by increasing the vertical dimension, the patient's occlusion shifted from a class III to a class I incisor relationship.

Shade selection was another challenge due to severe discolouration of the remaining teeth. The use of external staining resulted in a satisfactory shade match.

Difficulty was encountered during removal of gutta-percha (GP) from the root canal of LL3 as the apical part of the canal had been previously overprepared and some of the old GP was extruded from the end of the apex. However, the tooth remained asymptomatic in the long term after treatment and a follow-up radiograph at 9 months (see Figure 18.3) showed evidence of periapical healing.

The patient was very satisfied with the outcome of treatment and was discharged back to his GDP for extraction of non-restorable carious LL7 at the patient's convenience, long-term care and maintenance.

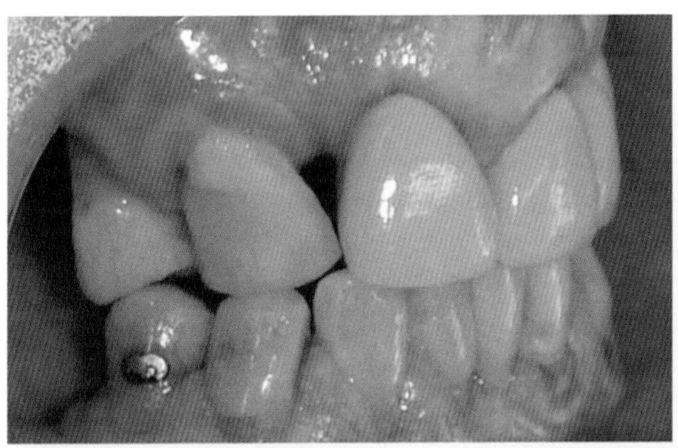

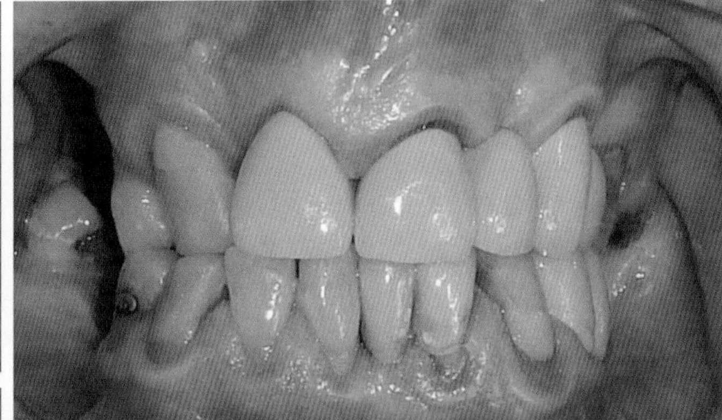

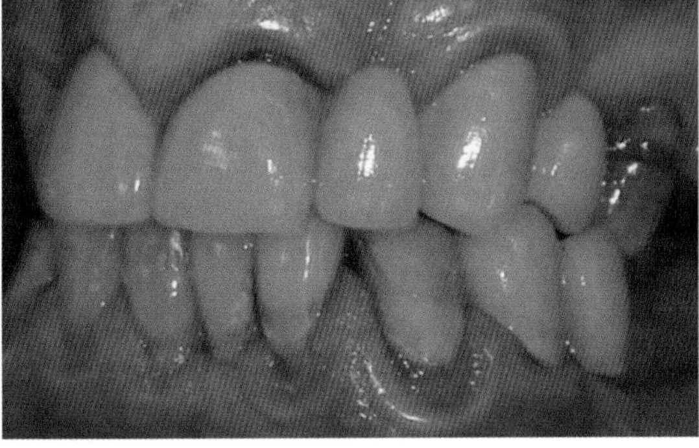

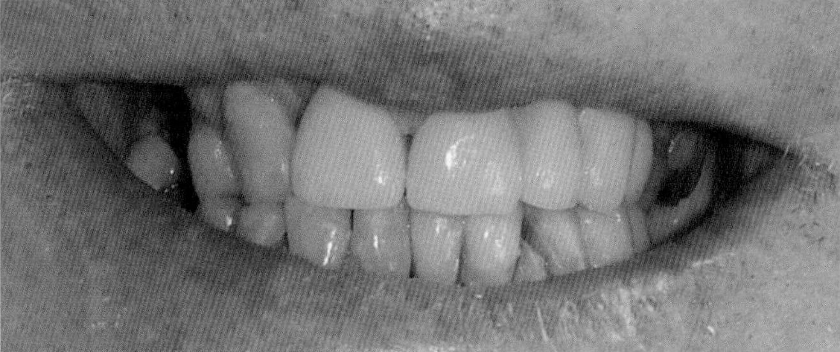

Figure 18.7 Postoperative clinical photographs.

References

Al-Amleh, B., Lyons, K. and Swain, M. (2010) Clinical trials in zirconia: a systematic review. *J Oral Rehabil*, **37**, 641–652.

Alhareky, M. and Tavares, M. (2016) Amalgam vs composite restoration, survival, and secondary caries. *J Evid Based Dent Pract*, **16**, 107–109.

Austin, R., Eliyas, S., Burke, F.J., Taylor, P., Toner, J. and Briggs, P. (2016) British Society of Prosthodontics debate on the implications of the Minamata Convention on mercury to dental amalgam – should our patients be worried? *Dent Update*, **43**, 8–10, 12–14, 16–18.

Beck, F., Lettner, S., Graf, A., Bitriol, B. *et al.* (2015) Survival of direct resin restorations in posterior teeth within a 19-year period (1996–2015): a meta-analysis of prospective studies. *Dent Mater*, **31**, 958–985.

Bohaty, B.S., Ye, Q., Misra, A., Sene, F. and Spencer, P. (2013) Posterior composite restoration update: focus on factors influencing form and function. *Clin Cosmet Invest Dent*, **5**, 33–42.

Czarnecka, B., Deregowska-Nosowicz, P., Limanowska-Shaw, H. and Nicholson, J.W. (2007) Shear bond strengths of glass-ionomer cements to sound and to prepared carious dentine. *J Mater Sci Mater Med*, **18**, 845–849.

Demarco, F.F., Collares, K., Coelho-de-Souza, F.H. *et al.* (2015) Anterior composite restorations: a systematic review on long-term survival and reasons for failure. *Dent Mater*, **31**, 1214–1224.

Donovan, T., Simonsen, R.J., Guertin, G. and Tucker, R.V. (2004) Retrospective clinical evaluation of 1,314 cast gold restorations in service from 1 to 52 years. *J Esthet Restor Dent*, **16**, 194–204.

Eliyas, S., Jalili, J. and Martin, N. (2015) Restoration of the root canal treated tooth. *Br Dent J*, **218**, 53–62.

Goldstein, G.R. (2010) The longevity of direct and indirect posterior restorations is uncertain and may be affected by a number of dentist-, patient-, and material-related factors. *J Evid Based Dent Pract*, **10**, 30–31.

Goodacre, C.J., Campagni, W.V. and Aquilino, S.A. (2001) Tooth preparations for complete crowns: an art form based on scientific principles. *J Prosthet Dent*, **85**, 363–376.

Goodacre, C.J., Bernal, G., Rungcharassaeng, K. and Kan, J.Y. (2003) Clinical complications in fixed prosthodontics. *J Prosthet Dent*, **90**, 31–41.

Gresnigt, M.M., Kalk, W. and Ozcan, M. (2013) Randomized clinical trial of indirect resin composite and ceramic veneers: up to 3-year follow-up. *J Adhes Dent*, **15**, 181–190.

Heintze, S.D. and Rousson, V. (2012) Clinical effectiveness of direct class II restorations – a meta-analysis. *J Adhes Dent*, **14**, 407–431.

Hikasa, T., Matsuka, Y., Mine, A. *et al.* (2010) A 15-year clinical comparative study of the cumulative survival rate of cast metal core and resin core restorations luted with adhesive resin cement. *Int J Prosthodont*, **23**, 397–405.

Land, M.F. and Hopp, C.D. (2010) Survival rates of all-ceramic systems differ by clinical indication and fabrication method. *J Evid Based Dent Pract*, **10**, 37–38.

Larson, H.J. (2014) The Minamata Convention on Mercury: risk in perspective. *Lancet*, **383**, 198–199.

Layton, D.M. and Clarke, M. (2013) A systematic review and meta-analysis of the survival of non-feldspathic porcelain veneers over 5 and 10 years. *Int J Prosthodont*, **26**(2), 111–124.

Layton, D.M., Clarke, M. and Walton, T.R. (2012) A systematic review and meta-analysis of the survival of feldspathic porcelain veneers over 5 and 10 years. *Int J Prosthodont*, **25**, 590–603.

Lynch, C.D., Opdam, N.J., Hickel, R. *et al.* for the Academy of Operative Dentistry European Section (2014) Guidance on posterior resin composites: Academy of Operative Dentistry – European Section. *J Dent*, **42**, 377–383.

McReynolds, D. and Duane, B. (2016) Insufficient evidence on whether to restore root-filled teeth with single crowns or routine fillings. *Evid Based Dent*, **17**, 50–51.

Mickenautsch, S., Mount, G. and Yengopal, V. (2011) Therapeutic effect of glass-ionomers: an overview of evidence. *Aust Dent J*, **56**, 10–15; quiz 103.

Mizrahi, B. (2011) All-ceramic silica/glass-based crowns – clinical protocols. *Br Dent J*, **211**, 257–262.

Monsarrat, P., Garnier, S., Vergnes, J.N., Nasr, K., Grosgogeat, B. and Joniot, S. (2017) Survival of directly placed ormocer-based restorative materials: a systematic review and meta-analysis of clinical trials. *Dent Mater*, **33**, E212–E220.

Moraschini, V., Fai, C.K., Alto, R.M. and dos Santos, G.O. (2015) Amalgam and resin composite longevity of posterior restorations: a systematic review and meta-analysis. *J Dent*, **43**, 1043–1050.

Opdam, N.J., van de Sande, F.H., Bronkhorst, E. *et al.* (2014) Longevity of posterior composite restorations: a systematic review and meta-analysis. *J Dent Res*, **93**, 943–949.

Peumans, M., de Munck, J., Fieuws, S., Lambrechts, P., Vanherle, G. and van Meerbeek, B. (2004) A prospective ten-year clinical trial of porcelain veneers. *J Adhes Dent*, **6**, 65–76.

Pjetursson, B.E., Sailer, I., Zwahlen, M. and Hammerle, C.H. (2007) A systematic review of the survival and complication rates of all-ceramic and metal-ceramic reconstructions after an observation period of at least 3 years. Part I: single crowns. *Clin Oral Implants Res*, **18**(Suppl 3), 73–85.

Ploumaki, A., Bilkhair, A., Tuna, T., Stampf, S. and Strub, J.R. (2013) Success rates of prosthetic restorations on endodontically treated teeth; a systematic review after 6 years. *J Oral Rehabil*, **40**, 618–630.

Rasines Alcaraz, M.G., Veitz-Keenan, A., Sahrmann, P., Schmidlin, P.R., Davis, D. and Iheozor-Ejiofor, Z. (2014) Direct composite resin fillings versus amalgam fillings for permanent or adult posterior teeth. *Cochrane Database Syst Rev*, **3**, CD005620.

Rocca, G.T. and Krejci, I. (2013) Crown and post-free adhesive restorations for endodontically treated posterior teeth: from direct composite to endocrowns. *Eur J Esthet Dent*, **8**, 156–179.

Rodriguez, I.A., Ferrara, C.A., Campos-Sanchez, F., Alaminos, M., Echevarria, J.U. and Campos, A. (2013) An in vitro biocompatibility study of conventional and resin-modified glass ionomer cements. *J Adhes Dent*, **15**, 541–546.

Rosenstiel, S., Land, M. and Fujimoto, J. (2015) *Contemporary Fixed Prosthodontics*, 5th edn, Elsevier, Oxford.

Sailer, I., Makarov, N.A., Thoma, D.S., Zwahlen, M. and Pjetursson, B.E. (2015) All-ceramic or metal-ceramic tooth-supported fixed dental prostheses (FDPS)? A systematic review of the survival and complication rates. Part I: single crowns (SCS). *Dent Mater*, **31**, 603–623.

Sailer, I., Makarov, N.A., Thoma, D.S., Zwahlen, M. and Pjetursson, B.E. (2016) Corrigendum to " All-ceramic or metal-ceramic tooth-supported fixed dental prostheses (FDPS)? A systematic review of the survival and complication rates. Part I: single crowns (SCS)" [Dental Materials 31 (6) (2015) 603-623]. *Dent Mater*, **32**, E389–E390.

Satterthwaite, J.D. (2006) Indirect restorations on teeth with reduced crown height. *Dent Update*, **33**, 210–212, 215–216.

Schwendicke, F., Gostemeyer, G., Blunck, U., Paris, S., Hsu, L.Y. and Tu, Y.K. (2016) Directly placed restorative materials: review and network meta-analysis. *J Dent Res*, **95**, 613–622.

Sequeira-Byron, P., Fedorowicz, Z., Carter, B., Nasser, M. and Alrowaili, E.F. (2015) Single crowns versus conventional fillings for the restoration of root-filled teeth. *Cochrane Database Syst Rev*, **9**, CD009109.

Sidhu, S.K., Carrick, T.E. and Mccabe, J.F. (2004) Temperature mediated coefficient of dimensional change of dental tooth-colored restorative materials. *Dent Mater*, **20**, 435–440.

Theodosopoulou, J.N. and Chochlidakis, K.M. (2009) A systematic review of dowel (post) and core materials and systems. *J Prosthodont*, **18**, 464–472.

Van Noort, R. (2013) Glass-ionomer cements and resin-modified glass-ionomer cements, in *An Introduction to Dental Materials*, 4th edn, Elsevier/Mosby, London, pp. 95–106.

Wang, X., Fan, D., Swain, M.V. and Zhao, K. (2012) A systematic review of all-ceramic crowns: clinical fracture rates in relation to restored tooth type. *Int J Prosthodont*, **25**, 441–450.

19

Fluorosis

19.1 Definition

Dental fluorosis is a developmental disturbance of the enamel layer of the tooth characterised by hypomineralised subsurface enamel caused by exposure to high levels of fluoride during tooth development and presents clinically as enamel opacities (Fejerskov *et al.*, 1990).

19.2 Aetiology and Pathogenesis

Dean (Dean and Elvove, 1936) identified the association between increased fluoride intake and mottled enamel. Sources of fluoride that may cause overexposure include (McGrady *et al.*, 2010):

- dentifrice and fluoridated varnishes and mouthwashes (which young children may swallow)
- public water fluoridation above 1 ppm (responsible for 40% of all fluorosis)
- ingestion of bottled water, foods and beverages containing high levels of fluoride
- inappropriate use of fluoride supplements.

The mechanism of fluorosis has been related to alteration of the enamel mineralisation process caused by a delay in the removal of amelogenins at the early-maturation stage of enamel formation (Den Besten, 1999). The severity of fluorosis is highly dependent on fluoride dose, exposure duration and the age of the child (Aoba and Fejerskov, 2002). The risk of fluoride overexposure occurs between the ages of 3 months and 8 years and the critical period for susceptibility to enamel fluorosis varies between males and females (Evans and Darvell, 1995).

19.3 Prevalence

It has been shown that 40% of the UK population appear to have developmental enamel defects and around 20% have fluorosis characterised by diffused opacities which are mainly mild (Holloway and Ellwood, 1997). One percent of the population in non-fluoridated areas and 3–4% in fluoridated areas have fluorosis with aesthetic concern (Atia and May, 2013).

19.4 Clinical Features and Classifications

Mild fluorosis is often unnoticeable and the enamel contains small areas of white lines or spots. Severe fluorosis, on the other hand, can exhibit diffuse opaque mottling and brown discolouration of enamel with a rough and pitted surface. The brown or black discolouration occurs after eruption of the tooth due to potential internalised extrinsic staining of the porous enamel.

Different classification systems for fluorosis have been introduced (Rozier, 1994). Two of the most widely used fluorosis indices are:

- Dean's Index (Dean, 1934), based on the extent and severity of the enamel defects appearance: normal, questionable, very mild, mild, moderate and severe fluorosis
- Thylstrup and Fejerskov Index (TFI) (Thylstrup and Fejerskov, 1978), based on the biological aspects and clinical appearance and includes scores from 0 (normal enamel) to 9 (severe fluorosis).

19.5 Diagnosis

The differential diagnosis for dental fluorosis includes mild forms of amelogenesis imperfecta (AI) (mainly hypomaturation type), early decalcified carious lesions, molar-incisor hypomineralisation (MIH), other environmental enamel defects and localised enamel hypoplasia due to trauma or infection of the primary teeth (Turner's hypoplasia) (Cutress and Suckling, 1990).

The diagnosis of fluorosis depends on taking an accurate and detailed history and undertaking a thorough

Diseases and Conditions in Dentistry: An Evidence-Based Reference, First Edition. Keyvan Moharamzadeh.

Companion website: www.wiley.com/go/moharamzadeh/diseases

clinical and radiographic examination (Atia and May, 2013). Relevant history includes:

- where the patient lived in childhood, to establish the level of water fluoride
- toothpaste and fluoride supplements used
- the level of parent supervision when tooth brushing in childhood to establish risk of fluoride ingestion
- familial history of developmental dental disorders such as AI.

It is important to assess the symmetry and demarcation of the lesions as dental fluorosis normally presents with bilateral and diffuse opacities that are not well demarcated.

19.6 Treatment Considerations

Tooth bleaching, microabrasion, macroabrasion, conservative adhesive direct composite restorations or indirect porcelain veneers are commonly used for management of enamel opacities, depending on the severity of the defects (Wallace and Deery, 2015). Resin infiltration and sealing the opacity can alter enamel's refractive index, offering a further treatment choice in some cases. However, the use of this technique has some limitations in fluorosis cases and modified techniques have been introduced (Attal *et al.*, 2014).

Mild fluorosis can be treated with conservative options such as vital bleaching and microabrasion (Bertassoni *et al.*, 2008; Higashi *et al.*, 2008). Microabrasion is indicated for superficial surface opacities, and bleaching can whiten the internalised yellow-brown staining. Combination of enamel microabrasion and bleaching has been shown to be more effective than microabrasion alone in aesthetic management of teeth with fluorosis (Celik *et al.*, 2013).

Tooth-bleaching techniques are discussed in detail in Chapter 15.

Enamel microabrasion involves the use of an acidic agent (such as 37% phosphoric acid or 6% hydrochloric acid) combined with an abrasive agent (such as pumice or silica) in the form of gel or paste that can be applied to the enamel surface with repeated mechanical pressure using a rubber cup on a rotatory low-speed handpiece under appropriate rubber dam isolation. Sodium fluoride and amorphous calcium phosphate paste can be applied to the tooth surface following treatment to remineralise the acid-etched enamel surface. The most important prognostic factor for enamel microabrasion is the depth of the enamel defect as deep lesions do not usually respond to microabrasion and often require restorative treatment (Pini *et al.*, 2015).

Macroabrasion involves the use of fine-grit water-cooled diamond abrasives or multi-fluted finishing burs on a high-speed handpiece, lightly swept over the stained area for 5–10 seconds to remove the hypomineralised enamel. Macroabrasion is indicated for the management of enamel defects greater than 0.1–0.3 mm that are not amenable to treatment using conservative microabrasion techniques (Strassler *et al.*, 2011). An initial enamel biopsy using a high-speed diamond bur would be a helpful technique to estimate the depth of the enamel opacities and determine the appropriate treatment modality.

For more severe fluorosis, direct composite restorations (Hoyle *et al.*, 2017) or indirect porcelain veneers (Slaska *et al.*, 2015) may be considered as suitable options in adult patients. Bleaching of the discoloured teeth prior to the placement of restorations may be indicated in severely discoloured cases to reduce the need for the removal of significant amounts of tooth tissue.

Case Study

A 20-year-old female patient was referred by her general dental practitioner (GDP) for management of enamel opacities. The patient was concerned about the appearance of the teeth in terms of colour and white marks on the anterior teeth. Further history taking revealed that she had lived in a region with fluoridated water during her childhood and had used fluoride supplements in the past.

Clinical examination showed the presence of bilateral enamel opacities affecting mainly the incisal third of the maxillary incisor teeth and the cervical aspects of the canines and posterior teeth. Mild yellow-brown staining was also noticed on some of the teeth (Figure 19.1).

Based on the history and clinical presentation, the diagnosis of mild fluorosis was made.

Treatment strategy for this patient included a combination of vital beaching and microabrasion/macroabrasion. The following protocol was used for vital bleaching.

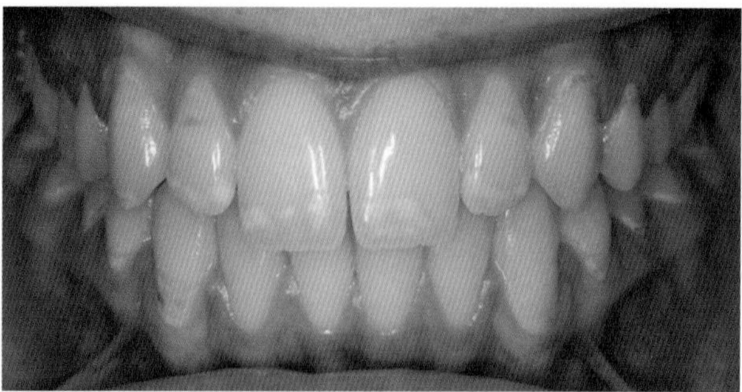

Figure 19.1 Preoperative intraoral clinical photograph showing the extent of the enamel opacities and staining of the teeth.

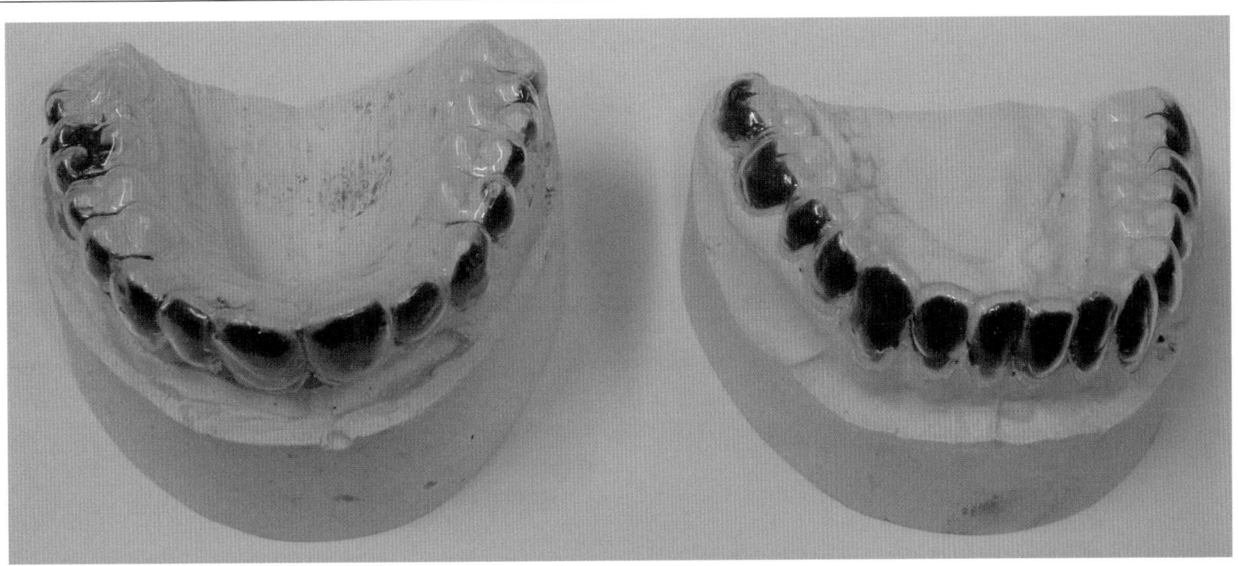

Figure 19.2 Whitening trays on stone models with added wax on the labial aspect of the teeth to provide space for the whitening gel.

1) Informed consent.
2) Advice to avoid smoking and reduce tea/coffee/red wine intake.
3) Alginate impressions.
4) Relieving the labial surfaces of the teeth by approximately 0.5 mm (Figure 19.2) and fabrication of a soft, vacuum-formed whitening tray.
5) Cleaning the teeth with pumice and recording the shade of the teeth.
6) Patient instruction to floss her teeth, apply 10% carbamide peroxide gel into the tray and wear the trays overnight for 1 week.
7) Reassessment after 1 week.

Improvement in the shade of the teeth was noticed after 1 week's vital bleaching with no adverse events (Figure 19.3). However, enamel opacities were still present which necessitated microabrasion. The following protocol was used for enamel microabrasion of the teeth.

1) Rubber dam isolation and application of rubber dam sealer for additional protection.
2) Application of abrasive paste (Opalustre®, Ultradent Inc.) containing 6.6% hydrochloric acid and silicon carbide microparticles over the discoloured areas.
3) Use of a rubber cup on a slow-rate handpiece (500 rpm) and application of medium-to-heavy pressure for 60 seconds at a time.
4) Removal of the paste from the teeth, rinsing, evaluating progress and repeating as necessary.
5) Final rinse and removal of rubber dam.
6) Application of in-office fluoride gel to the enamel for 4 minutes.
7) Review and evaluation of final outcome.

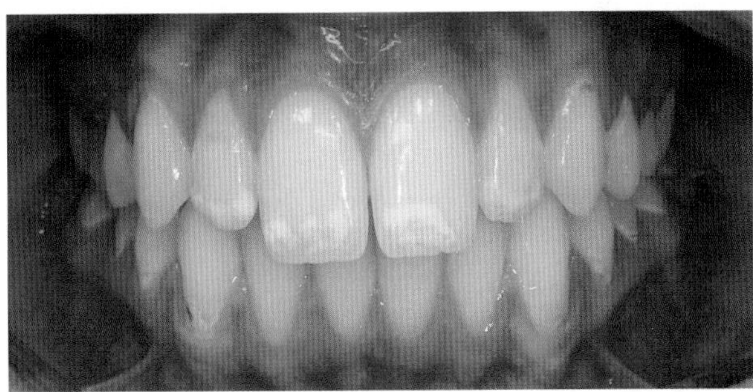

Figure 19.3 Clinical photograph of the teeth following vital bleaching showing whiter shade compared to the preoperative shade with yellow-brown staining.

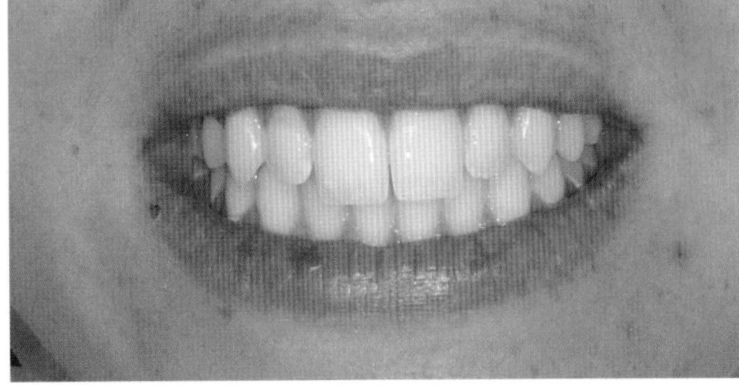

Figure 19.4 Postoperative clinical photographs showing satisfactory outcome and improvement in the shade and aesthetics of the teeth.

Some of the deeper enamel lesions required macroabrasion according to the method described previously in this chapter.

Significant improvement was noticed following the combined treatment and the patient was very satisfied with the appearance of the teeth as shown in Figure 19.4.

References

Aoba, T. and Fejerskov, O. (2002) Dental fluorosis: chemistry and biology. *Crit Rev Oral Biol Med*, **13**, 155–170.

Atia, G.S. and May, J. (2013) Dental fluorosis in the paediatric patient. *Dent Update*, **40**, 836–839.

Attal, J.P., Atlan, A., Denis, M., Vennat, E. and Tirlet, G. (2014) White spots on enamel: treatment protocol by superficial or deep infiltration (Part 2). *Int Orthod*, **12**, 1–31.

Bertassoni, L.E., Martin, J.M., Torno, V., Vieira, S., Rached, R.N. and Mazur, R.F. (2008) In-office dental bleaching and enamel microabrasion for fluorosis treatment. *J Clin Pediatr Dent*, **32**, 185–187.

Celik, E.U., Yildiz, G. and Yazkan, B. (2013) Comparison of enamel microabrasion with a combined approach to the esthetic management of fluorosed teeth. *Oper Dent*, **38**, E134–143.

Cutress, T.W. and Suckling, G.W. (1990) Differential diagnosis of dental fluorosis. *J Dent Res*, **69** Spec No, 714–720; discussion 721.

Dean, H.T. (1934) Classification of mottled enamel diagnosis. *J Am Dent Assoc*, **21**, 1421–1426.

Dean, H.T. and Elvove, E. (1936) Some epidemiological aspects of chronic endemic dental fluorosis. *Am J Public Health Nations Health*, **26**, 567–575.

Den Besten, P.K. (1999) Mechanism and timing of fluoride effects on developing enamel. *J Public Health Dent*, **59**, 247–251.

Evans, R.W. and Darvell, B.W. (1995) Refining the estimate of the critical period for susceptibility to enamel fluorosis in human maxillary central incisors. *J Public Health Dent*, **55**, 238–249.

Fejerskov, O., Manji, F. and Baelum, V. (1990) The nature and mechanisms of dental fluorosis in man. *J Dent Res*, **69** Spec No, 692–700; discussion 721.

Higashi, C., Dall'Agnol, A.L., Hirata, R., Loguercio, A.D. and Reis, A. (2008) Association of enamel microabrasion and bleaching: a case report. *Gen Dent*, **56**, 244–249.

Holloway, P.J. and Ellwood, R.P. (1997) The prevalence, causes and cosmetic importance of dental fluorosis in the United Kingdom: a review. *Community Dent Health*, **14**, 148–155.

Hoyle, P., Webb, L. and Nixon, P. (2017) Severe fluorosis treated by microabrasion and composite veneers. *Dent Update*, **44**, 93–98.

McGrady, M.G., Ellwood, R.P. and Pretty, I.A. (2010) Why fluoride? *Dent Update*, **37**, 595–598, 601–602.

Pini, N.I., Sundfeld-Neto, D., Aguiar, F.H. *et al.* (2015) Enamel microabrasion: an overview of clinical and scientific considerations. *World J Clin Cases*, **3**, 34–41.

Rozier, R.G. (1994) Epidemiologic indices for measuring the clinical manifestations of dental fluorosis: overview and critique. *Adv Dent Res*, **8**, 39–55.

Slaska, B., Liebman, A.I. and Kukleris, D. (2015) Restoration of fluorosis stained teeth: a case study. *Dent Clin North Am*, **59**, 583–591.

Strassler, H.E., Griffin, A. and Maggio, M. (2011) Management of fluorosis macro– and microabrasion. *Dent Today*, **30**, 91–92, 94–96; quiz 97, 90.

Thylstrup, A. and Fejerskov, O. (1978) Clinical appearance of dental fluorosis in permanent teeth in relation to histologic changes. *Community Dent Oral Epidemiol*, **6**, 315–328.

Wallace, A. and Deery, C. (2015) Management of opacities in children and adolescents. *Dent Update*, **42**, 951–954, 957–958.

20

Fractured Endodontic Instrument

20.1 Incidence

The reported incidence of endodontic instrument fracture in the literature varies between 0.25% and 14% (Cheung, 2009). The prevalence of retained fractured instruments within root-treated teeth is estimated to be around 1.6%, mostly stainless steel files (Parashos and Messer, 2006). Approximately 1% of nickel-titanium (NiTi) instruments have been reported to fracture during their first use. There is no difference in the fracture rate of hand versus rotary NiTi instruments but the mode of failure is different (Cheung, 2009).

20.2 Causative Factors and Prevention

Most stainless steel instruments appear to fail by excessive amounts of torque.

There are two mechanisms of fracture for NiTi rotary files: shear (torsional fracture due to plastic deformation) and fatigue (which results in crack propagation) (Cheung, 2009).

Some of the important factors contributing to endodontic instrument failure are summarised below (Cheung, 2009; McGuigan *et al.*, 2013b).

- Operator skill and experience is an important influential factor.
- Instrument size (higher risk of failure with small files).
- Radius of the canal curvature (higher risk in severely curved canals) and type of tooth (molars have higher risk than premolars).
- Instrumentation technique: use of excessive torsional forces on the instrument and use of rotary files in abruptly curved or dilacerated canals can increase the chance of instrument fracture. The use of crown-down technique and establishing an initial glide path (preferably to size 15–20 K-file) prior to rotary instrumentation reduces the risk of fracture.
- Use of torque-controlled motors prevents excessive build-up of stress in the instrument and further reduces the risk of failure.
- Surface condition: presence of cracks on the instrument can cause early failure.
- Repeated usage: files become progressively fatigued with repeated use and the risk of fracture may increase. Therefore, single usage is recommended.
- Rotation rate: there is controversy in the literature on whether the rotation rate has an effect on instrument fracture.
- Effect of sterilisation: there is also contradictory evidence on the effect of sterilisation and heat on the failure rate of endodontic instruments (McGuigan *et al.*, 2013b).

20.3 Impact on Outcome of Endodontic Treatment

Early studies reported significantly poorer outcome of endodontic treatment for teeth containing a broken instrument, especially when the separation occurred in teeth with necrotic pulps. However, recent studies show improved outcome of endodontic treatment for teeth containing separated instruments, with a success rate of 80–86% for teeth with preoperative periapical radiolucency and 92–98% for teeth without periapical radiolucency (McGuigan *et al.*, 2013c; Panitvisai *et al.*, 2010). There was no statistically significant difference between the outcome of treatment for teeth containing broken NiTi and those with stainless steel fragments (Spili *et al.*, 2005). It appears that the cleanliness and asepsis of the root canal is a very important prognostic factor (Cheung, 2009).

Diseases and Conditions in Dentistry: An Evidence-Based Reference, First Edition. Keyvan Moharamzadeh.

Companion website: www.wiley.com/go/moharamzadeh/diseases

20.4 Management Strategies

There are several options for the management of fractured endodontic instruments (Madarati *et al.*, 2013).

- Bypassing fractured instrument: this is a conservative approach and particularly useful when direct access to the fractured instrument is restricted. If successful, it would allow effective chemomechanical debridement of the root canal and also enable the introduction of other instruments such as ultrasonic tips alongside the fragment to facilitate its removal.
- Removal of fractured instrument (non-surgical).
  - The benefits of fragment removal include complete chemomechanical disinfection of the root canal, improved outcome especially in infected canals with apical periodontitis, psychological benefits for the patient and reduced risk of medicolegal action.
  - Preparation of straight-line access to visualise the coronal aspect of the fractured instrument is an essential step when attempting fragment removal. The risks associated with attempting instrument removal where access or visibility is restricted include potential ledge formation, root perforation, excessive canal enlargement and fracture of a second instrument or extrusion of the fragment beyond the apex.
- Leaving the fractured instrument *in situ*: cleaning/shaping and obturation of the root canal to the level of the fragment can be considered if the fractured instrument cannot be bypassed and there is a high risk of iatrogenic errors and damage to the tooth if instrument removal techniques are attempted where the access and visibility are significantly restricted. Disadvantages of leaving the fragment *in situ* include compromised chemomechanical cleansing, uncertain prognosis (especially if there is a pre-existing periapical lesion and the instrument fracture occurs at an early stage of root canal treatment), patient anxiety and risk of medicolegal action.
- Surgical treatment: surgical resection of the portion of the diseased root containing the fractured instrument can be considered if non-surgical treatment options fail to resolve the endodontic infection and associated symptoms and the patient is still interested in further treatment.

The decision making should be based on individual circumstances in terms of patient factors, periodontal and restorative status of the tooth, careful assessment of access and the feasibility, risks and benefits of each treatment option as well as the operator's skill and experience (McGuigan *et al.*, 2013a).

20.5 Factors Affecting Removal of Fractured Instruments

The following factors may have an influence on the removal of separated endodontic instruments (Madarati *et al.*, 2013).

- Tooth factors including tooth type, root canal diameter and cross-sectional shape, curvature degree and the position of the fragment within the root canal. The location of the fragment in relation to the canal curvature is a crucial determinant. When a fragment is positioned coronal to the curve, the chance of successful removal is very high. Success is reduced when the fragment is situated at or beyond the curve. Retrieval becomes extremely unlikely when the breakage occurred beyond the curvature and the coronal end of the fragment cannot be visualised under the operating microscope (Cuje *et al.*, 2010; Ruddle, 2002).
- Fractured instrument factors including type, design and length. NiTi rotary instruments are more difficult to retrieve compared with stainless steel files. K-files are easier to remove than Hedstrom files (Cuje *et al.*, 2010).
- Operator factors include skill, knowledge, experience, training and attitude as well as having access to fragment removal kits and instruments.
- Patient factors include motivation, compliance, attendance, anxiety level, intraoral access and mouth opening.

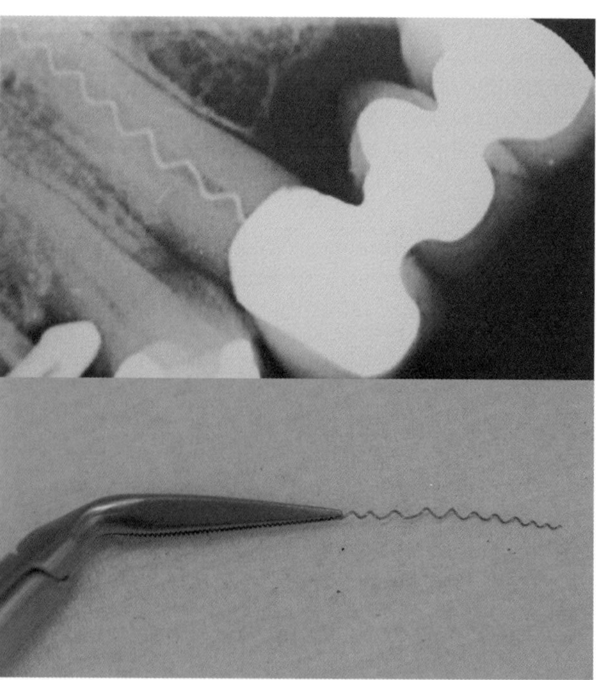

Figure 20.1 The use of Steiglitz forceps (Union Broach, York, PA) for the removal of a fractured spiral instrument from the root canal of an upper right canine tooth supporting a fixed bridge.

20.6 Fragment Removal

It is extremely important to inform the patient about risks, benefits, costs and alternative approaches and to obtain informed consent prior to attempting instrument retrieval . Referral to a specialist colleague can also be considered at this stage.

The fractured instrument's position should be located using periapical radiography and straight-line access to the coronal end of the fragment must be obtained under appropriate microscope magnification. It is often useful to examine the root canal anatomy and consider relieving any present isthmus which may help to release the fractured instrument. It is recommended to attempt to bypass the fragment first. Once bypassed, the fragment may be dislodged using different techniques. Even if removal is not successful, the canal may still be prepared and shaped to its full length to improve the prognosis of treatment. It is crucial to select the right retrieval technique and device to avoid excessive damage to the remaining root structure.

A variety of different devices, techniques and protocols have been developed and used for removal of broken endodontic instruments (Cheung, 2009; Madarati *et al.*, 2013; McGuigan *et al.*, 2013a; Ruddle, 2002). Examples of these methods include mini forceps and pliers (Figure 20.1) (Feldman *et al.*, 1974), wire loops (Roig-Greene, 1983), hypodermic surgical needles (Eleazer and O'Connor, 1999), braiding of endodontic files (Shen *et al.*, 2004), Masserann instruments (Okiji, 2003), tubular extraction devices (Ruddle, 2004a, b), canal finder system (Hulsmann, 1990), ultrasonic instruments (Plotino *et al.*, 2007; Ruddle, 1997), file removal system (Terauchi *et al.*, 2007), softened gutta-percha point (Rahimi and Parashos, 2009), and novel techniques such as laser irradiation (Cvikl *et al.*, 2014) and electrochemical dissolution of the fragment (Ormiga *et al.*, 2015).

Case Study

A 44-year-old female patient was referred by her GDP for treatment of symptomatic root-treated LR6 with a fractured file in its mesio-buccal (MB) root canal.

Clinical and radiographic examination (Figure 20.2) confirmed the diagnoses of chronic apical periodontitis of LR6, fractured file in MB canal, poorly obturated root fillings and distal caries.

Important factors taken into account when deciding about the treatment were as follows.

- Patient motivation and preference: the patient was well motivated and preferred to retain the tooth and attempt instrument removal and endodontic retreatment.
- Restorability of the tooth: the tooth was restorable as there was sufficient supragingival tooth tissue remaining.
- Location of the fractured instrument: the fragment was located within the apical half of the root canal at the root curvature level and it was possible to obtain straight access to the coronal end of the fragment.
- Quality of the previous root filling and presence of periapical lesion: both canals were poorly obturated with underextended root filling and voids and there were pre-existing periapical and furcation radiolucencies.

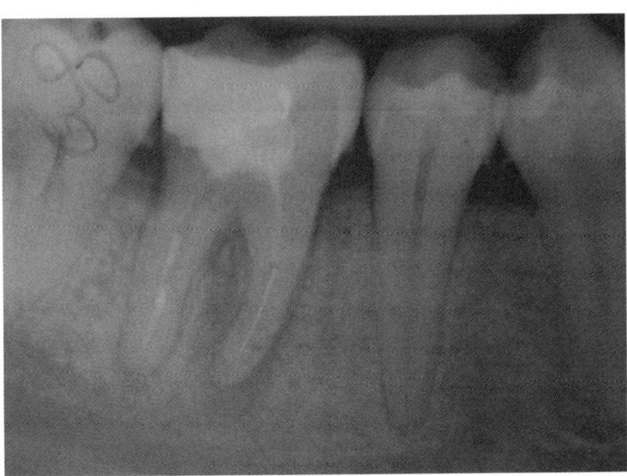

Figure 20.2 Preoperative periapical radiograph of LR6 showing a separated instrument in the mesial root, poorly obturated root fillings, distal caries and periapical radiolucencies associated with the apices of both roots extending to the furcation area.

Endodontic retreatment of the tooth involved the following procedures.

1) Informed consent.
2) Distal caries were removed and the distal wall of the tooth was rebuilt with resin-modified glass-ionomer cement (RM-GIC).
3) Rubber dam isolation.
4) Microscope magnification.
5) Refining the access cavity and orifice preparation using Gates Glidden drills.
6) Removal of the old root-filling material from the canals using rotary instruments in the coronal aspect of the canal and solvent and hand files in deeper parts of the canal.
7) The fractured instrument in the MB canal was identified and straight-line access to its coronal end was achieved after removal of a small amount of dentine using ultrasonic tips.
8) The fragment was bypassed using a curved size 10 K-file and canal lubricant.

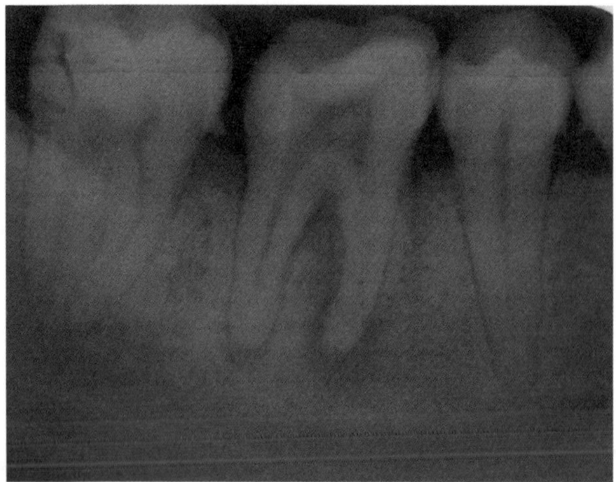

Figure 20.3 Periapical radiograph following fragment retrieval and removal of the old root-filling material.

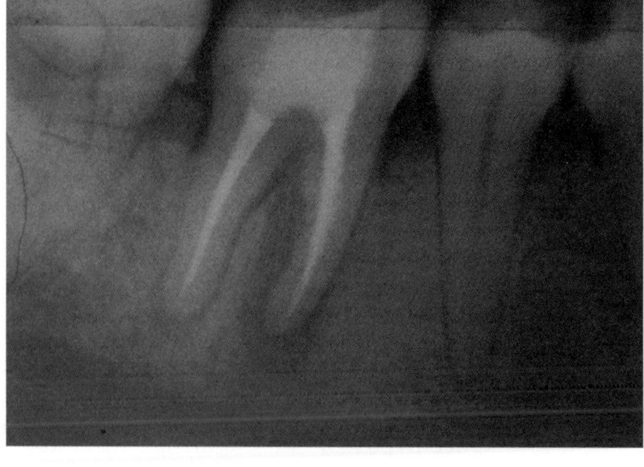

Figure 20.4 Immediate postobturation periapical radiograph showing acceptable obturation.

9) The canal was further prepared and widened using ProTaper files.
10) The fragment was successfully retrieved using a size 20 Hedstrom file with plenty of lubrication and irrigation.
11) A periapical radiograph was taken to confirm complete removal of the fractured instrument and the old root-filling material (Figure 20.3).
12) Working length (WL) determination using an apex locator.
13) Cleaning and shaping of all three canals to WL using ProTaper files and irrigation with hypochlorite solution.
14) Obturation of the canals with Thermafil system.
15) Restoration of the access cavity with RM-GIC and advice to the GDP to provide a definitive restoration if the tooth remains asymptomatic.
16) Immediate postobturation radiograph (Figure 20.4).
17) Review in 9 months with a further follow-up radiograph (Figure 20.5).

Important procedural steps which helped to successfully remove the fractured instrument from the MB canal were:

- adequate access and effective magnification to visualise the broken instrument
- copious amounts of irrigant and lubricant in the canal
- successful bypassing of the fragment
- adequate widening of the canal to allow mobilisation of the fractured instrument
- use of an actively engaging instrument to retrieve the fractured file.

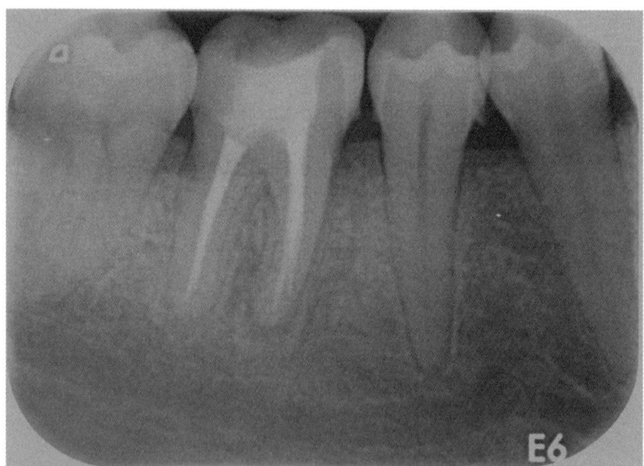

Figure 20.5 Follow-up periapical radiograph 9 months later showing evidence of significant periapical healing and reduction in size of the periapical and furcation radiolucency.

Following the removal of the fractured instrument, the procedure of preparation and obturation of the canals was straightforward.

At 9-month review appointment, the patient had remained asymptomatic and there was evidence of significant periapical healing on radiographic examination. The patient was discharged to her GDP for provision of a definitive restoration for the tooth, routine dental care, periodontal scaling to remove interdental calculus (visible on the radiographs) and maintenance.

References

Cheung, G.S.P. (2009) Instrument fracture: mechanisms, removal of fragments, and clinical outcomes. *Endodont Top*, **16**, 1–26.

Cuje, J., Bargholz, C. and Hulsmann, M. (2010) The outcome of retained instrument removal in a specialist practice. *Int Endod J*, **43**, 545–554.

Cvikl, B., Klimscha, J., Holly, M., Zeitlinger, M., Gruber, R. and Moritz, A. (2014) Removal of fractured endodontic instruments using an Nd:Yag laser. *Quintessence Int*, **45**, 569–575.

Eleazer, P.D. and O'Connor, R.P. (1999) Innovative uses for hypodermic needles in endodontics. *J Endod*, **25**, 190–191.

Feldman, G., Solomon, C., Notaro, P. and Moskowitz, E. (1974) Retrieving broken endodontic instruments. *J Am Dent Assoc*, **88**, 588–591.

Hulsmann, M. (1990) Removal of fractured root canal instruments using the canal finder system. *Dtsch Zahnarztl Z*, **45**, 229–232.

Madarati, A.A., Hunter, M.J. and Dummer, P.M. (2013) Management of intracanal separated instruments. *J Endod*, **39**, 569–581.

McGuigan, M.B., Louca, C. and Duncan, H.F. (2013a) Clinical decision-making after endodontic instrument fracture. *Br Dent J*, **214**, 395–400.

McGuigan, M.B., Louca, C. and Duncan, H.F. (2013b) Endodontic instrument fracture: causes and prevention. *Br Dent J*, **214**, 341–348.

McGuigan, M.B., Louca, C. and Duncan, H.F. (2013c) The impact of fractured endodontic instruments on treatment outcome. *Br Dent J*, **214**, 285–289.

Okiji, T. (2003) Modified usage of the Masserann kit for removing intracanal broken instruments. *J Endod*, **29**, 466–467.

Ormiga, F., Aboud, L.R. and Gomes, J.A. (2015) Electrochemical-induced dissolution of nickel-titanium endodontic instruments with different designs. *Int Endod J*, **48**, 342–350.

Panitvisai, P., Parunnit, P., Sathorn, C. and Messer, H.H. (2010) Impact of a retained instrument on treatment outcome: a systematic review and meta-analysis. *J Endod*, **36**, 775–780.

Parashos, P. and Messer, H.H. (2006) Rotary Niti instrument fracture and its consequences. *J Endod*, **32**, 1031–1043.

Plotino, G., Pameijer, C.H., Grande, N.M. and Somma, F. (2007) Ultrasonics in endodontics: a review of the literature. *J Endod*, **33**, 81–95.

Rahimi, M. and Parashos, P. (2009) A novel technique for the removal of fractured instruments in the apical third of curved root canals. *Int Endod J*, **42**, 264–270.

Roig-Greene, J.L. (1983) The retrieval of foreign objects from root canals: a simple aid. *J Endod*, **9**, 394–397.

Ruddle, C. (1997) Microendodontics. Eliminating intracanal obstructions. *Oral Health*, **87**, 19–21, 23–24.

Ruddle, C.J. (2002) Broken instrument removal. The endodontic challenge. *Dent Today*, **21**, 70–72, 74, 76 passim.

Ruddle, C.J. (2004a) Nonsurgical endodontic retreatment. *J Calif Dent Assoc*, **32**, 474–484.

Ruddle, C. J. (2004b) Nonsurgical retreatment. *J Endod*, **30**, 827–845.

Shen, Y., Peng, B. and Cheung, G.S. (2004) Factors associated with the removal of fractured Niti instruments from root canal systems. *Oral Surg Oral Med Oral Pathol Oral Radiol Endod*, **98**, 605–610.

Spili, P., Parashos, P. and Messer, H.H. (2005) The impact of instrument fracture on outcome of endodontic treatment. *J Endod*, **31**, 845–850.

Terauchi, Y., O'Leary, L., Kikuchi, I. *et al.* (2007) Evaluation of the efficiency of a new file removal system in comparison with two conventional systems. *J Endod*, **33**, 585–588.

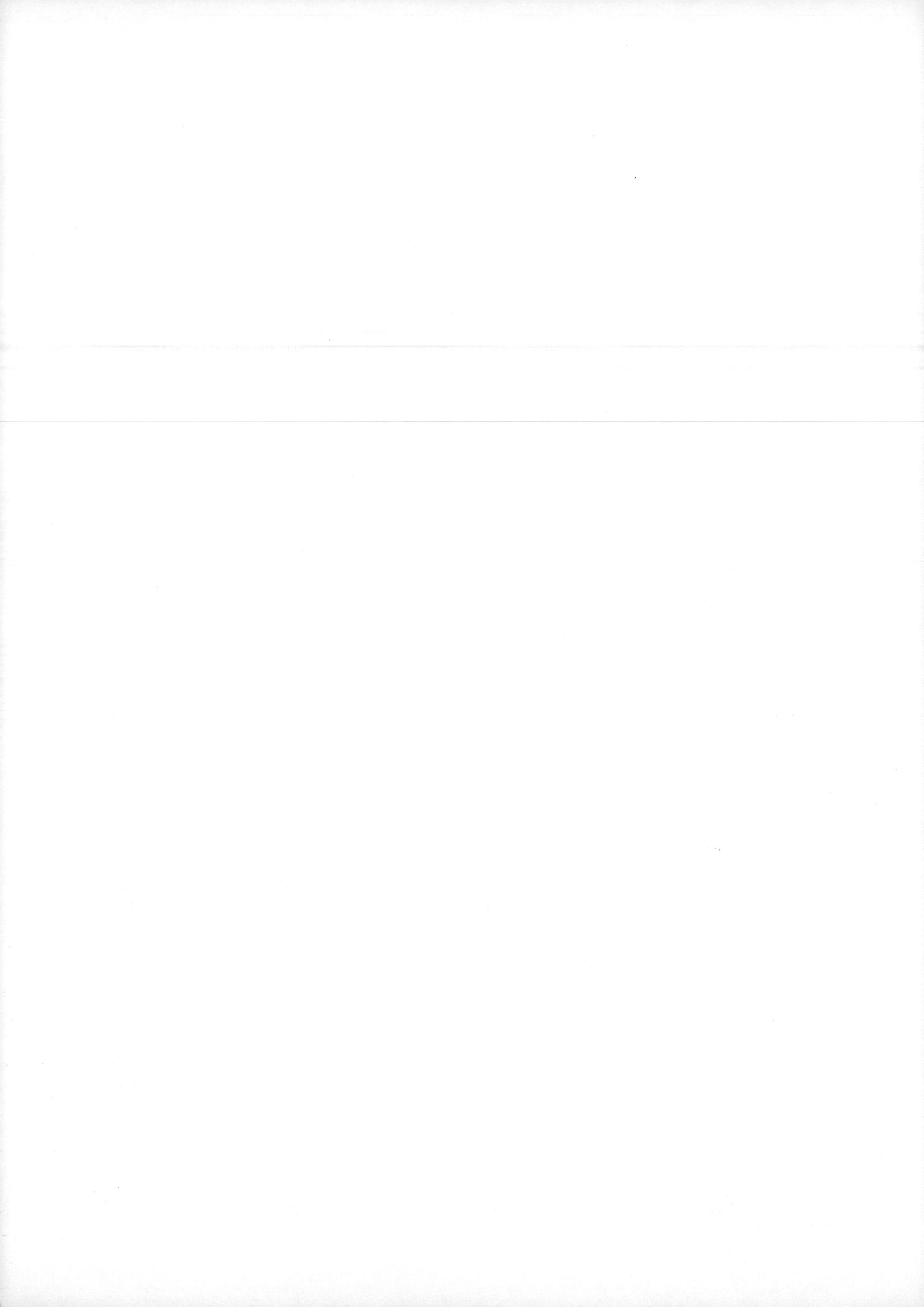

21

Fractured or Failed Post

21.1 Introduction

Posts are used to enhance the retention of cores and restorations on endodontically treated teeth where there is significant loss of coronal tooth tissue. Posts can be classified as active and passive. Active posts are often prefabricated threaded posts that can be either self-threading or pretapped. Passive posts can have a smooth or serrated surface, parallel or tapered shape and can be either prefabricated (such as metal posts, carbon or silica fibre posts and zirconia ceramic posts) or custom made (such as cast posts and cores) (Rollings *et al.*, 2013a).

21.2 Reasons for Failure of Post-Retained Restorations

Evidence on survival of different types of post systems is discussed in Chapter 18.

The most common causes of failure for post-retained restorations are post loosening, root fracture and caries (Goodacre *et al.*, 2003). Other causes include periodontal disease, endodontic failure, root resorption, iatrogenic root perforation, trauma and material failure such as crown or post fracture (Beddis *et al.*, 2014).

21.3 Factors to Consider

Important factors to consider when assessing post-related failures are listed below (Ruddle, 2004).

- The clinician's knowledge, skills, training, experience and access to relevant instruments.
- The position and anatomy of the tooth, including root dimension, length and curvature.
- The length, design, diameter and direction of the post, its coronal extension into the pulp chamber and whether it is integrated with the crown.
- The number and type of posts and cementing agent. Posts bonded with resin cements are more difficult to remove than those cemented with traditional cements.
- Type of core material and the amount of remaining coronal tooth structure.
- The available access and interocclusal space.
- Patient compliance, expectation and the method of temporisation of the tooth.

21.4 Risks of Post Removal

It is crucial to carry out a thorough preoperative assessment and carefully consider the risks, benefits and costs associated with removing the failed or fractured posts. The patient should be fully informed and alternative approaches must be discussed prior to attempting post removal techniques (Dickie and McCrosson, 2014).

Removal of dentine around the post can significantly weaken the root and there is a risk of root perforation or fracture during any phase of retreatment.

In some cases where the risk is too high (e.g. presence of a very large and well-fitted post in a thin root with periapical lesion), it may be wise to consider surgical endodontic retreatment to manage periapical disease. However, surgery should not be performed routinely because of the lack of training and skills for post removal and referral to a specialist for non-surgical retreatment should be considered. Systematic reviews show non-surgical retreatment offers more favourable long-term outcomes than endodontic surgery (Naito, 2010; Torabinejad *et al.*, 2009).

Although a significant number of endodontists have experienced root fracture during attempted post removal (Castrisos and Abbott, 2002), the evidence shows that the incidence of root fracture during post removal is very low (around 0.06%) (Abbott, 2002).

Diseases and Conditions in Dentistry: An Evidence-Based Reference, First Edition. Keyvan Moharamzadeh.

Companion website: www.wiley.com/go/moharamzadeh/diseases

21.5 Post Removal Techniques

Prior to dismantling a post-retained restoration, it is important to discuss the method of tooth temporisation with the patient. This may include fabrication of an immediate removable partial denture.

The first procedural step to remove a post is to remove the coronal restoration and access the pulp chamber under appropriate magnification. The core must then be sectioned and eliminated, preferably using ultrasonic tips under a continuous flow of air into the field. Once the post is fully exposed, a number of post-loosening techniques can be used (Rollings *et al.*, 2013b; Ruddle, 2004).

- Sonic vibration can be used to break weak cements and loosen the posts (Cherukara *et al.*, 2002).
- Ultrasonic energy can be applied by moving a piezo-electric ultrasonic instrument with a large, flat, parallel-sided tip around the post circumferentially and up and down along its exposed length for 10 minutes under water spray to reduce heat (Krell *et al.*, 1986).
- Mechanical options include the following.
  - Masserann kit (Micromega, Besançon, France) which contains trepans of varying sizes to fit closely around the post and cut away the cement lute and loosen the post. It is particularly useful for parallel-sided posts and can be used in conjunction with ultrasonic instruments. Care must be taken not to remove excessive amounts of dentine when using the trepans (Williams and Bjorndal, 1983).
  - The Eggler post remover (Automaton-Vertriebs-Gesellschaft, Germany) has a pair of forceps to grip and withdraw the post and repeller arms anchored on the residual root. It can be used to remove posts in anterior teeth where there is adequate space to accommodate the device. However, care must be taken not to pull the post in a non-axial direction and when there is less than 1 mm of dentine remaining at the apical end of the post (Castrisos *et al.*, 2002).
  - The Gonon (Thomas) Universal Post Remover (UPR) (Thomas, FFDM Pneumat, Bourges, France) is a conservative method of post removal with good success history. It includes a diamond bur and trepans to taper and shape the post head, taps to be placed over the prepared post, washers to be placed over the root face and pliers to apply force and remove the post (Sakkal *et al.*, 1994).
  - The Ruddle Post Removal System (PRS) (SybronEndo, CA, USA) is claimed to be an improved version of the Gonon system and contains a transmetal bur, five trephines with different sizes, five corresponding tubular taps, a torque bar, a selection of rubber bumpers and extracting pliers. It is designed to engage and remove posts with diameter of 0.6 mm or more (Ruddle, 2004).

The choice of post removal technique can be influenced by the type and design of the post. Passive parallel-sided metal posts can be removed using ultrasonic energy, Masserann kit or post pullers. Post pullers should only be used with passive posts and never with active posts, as this is likely to cause a root fracture. The Ruddle PRS can also be used to remove active threaded posts by attaching the tubular tap and rotating in an anticlockwise direction without the use of extracting pliers (Ruddle, 2004). Screwed posts are best unscrewed using a screwdriver or a fine forceps in combination with ultrasonic energy. Masserann kit can also be used if it is not possible to unscrew the screwed posts. Cast posts can be ideally removed using ultrasonic energy and post pullers. Removal of the fibre posts can be challenging and they may need to be drilled out using specific burs or fibre post removal kits by an experienced clinician (Scotti *et al.*, 2013).

Case Studies

Two clinical cases are included in this chapter.

Case 1

The first patient was a 47-year-old lady referred by her GDP for removal of a fractured post in UR1.

The patient was asymptomatic and wanted to retain the tooth and attempt post removal with a view to fabricating a new post crown. Clinical examination showed the crown was loosely attached to the fractured post. Radiographic assessment (Figure 21.1) showed a parallel-sided post in UR1.

Initially, an immediate removable partial denture (RPD) was made to replace UR1 temporarily during treatment and in case the tooth became non-restorable following post removal.

The following clinical steps were carried out to remove the fractured post.

1) Local anaesthesia and tooth isolation.
2) Loose crown was dismantled and removed.
3) Post was exposed 2 mm by dentine removal using an ultrasonic tip.
4) Masserann trepan 18 was selected to fit closely around the post and was used to remove the cement and a small amount of dentine around the post.
5) Ultrasonic vibration was also delivered to the post in a circumferential manner using a water spray.

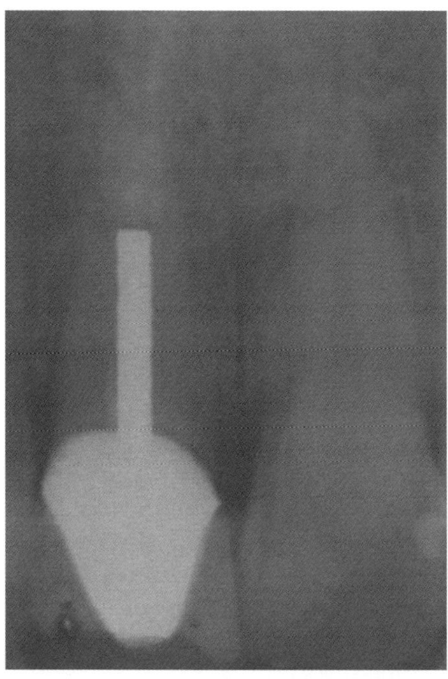

Figure 21.1 Preoperative periapical radiograph of the post crown showing a parallel-sided well-adapted medium to large metal post in the root canal extending to the apical third of the canal with good amount of root dentine remaining on the mesial and distal side of the post.

6) The post was loosened and removed using a fine forceps.
7) The root canal was debrided, dressed and the tooth was temporised and covered by the RPD.
8) A postoperative radiograph was obtained to verify safe and complete post removal (Figure 21.2).
9) The patient was discharged to her GDP for fabrication of a new post crown.

The use of Masserann kit in conjunction with ultrasonic tips was very helpful for removing the fractured post. Use of the trepan and intermittent application of the ultrasonic tip effectively loosened the fractured post and then it could be easily removed.

Case 2

The second patient was a 62-year-old man referred by his GDP with a history of discomfort associated with root-treated UR1 which had a post crown.

Clinical examination showed UR1 was tender to percussion and radiographic assessment (Figure 21.3) showed evidence of periapical radiolucency associated with root-treated UR1 which had a post crown.

Clinical and radiographic examination confirmed the diagnosis of chronic apical periodontitis of post-crowned UR1.

Treatment options discussed with the patient included (a) no treatment, (b) dismantling the post crown and non-surgical endodontic retreatment, or (c) extraction and replacement of the tooth.

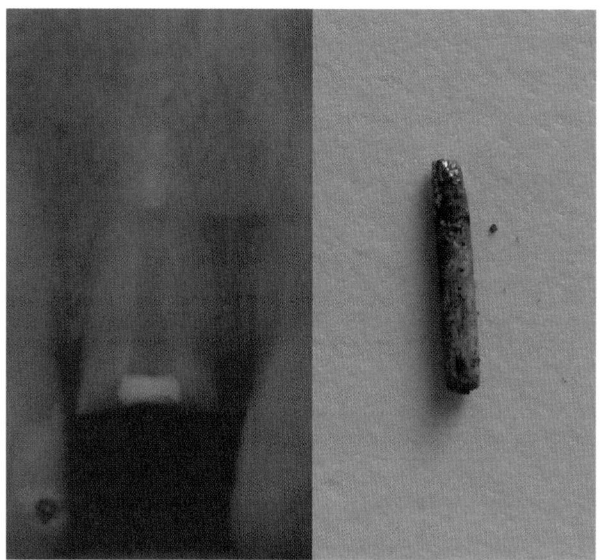

Figure 21.2 Postoperative periapical radiograph and a picture of the removed metal post.

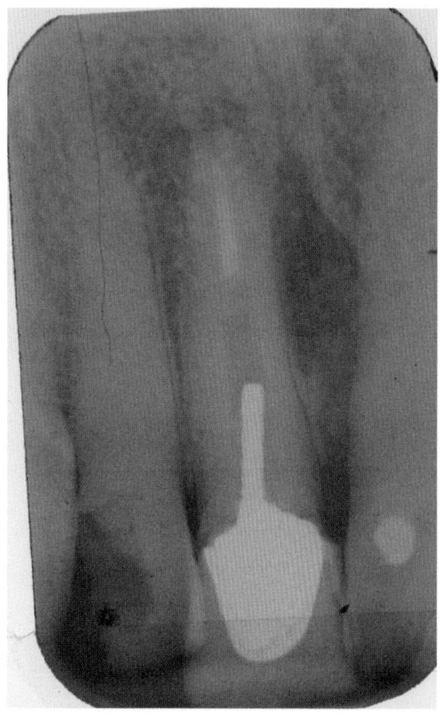

Figure 21.3 Preoperative periapical radiograph showing a parallel-sided short metal post with small diameter and poor adaptation to the root canal walls. Previous root filling appears to be poorly condensed and there is a small periapical radiolucency.

Surgical endodontic treatment was not indicated because the prognosis for dismantling the post crown and non-surgical endodontic retreatment was favourable due to the presence of a small-sized and short post in the canal which would be easier to remove safely than large and well-adapted posts.

The following clinical steps were carried out.

1) A silicone putty index was taken for fabrication of a temporary crown.
2) The crown was sectioned and removed.
3) The cast metal core was reduced using a transmetal bur.
4) Dentine was removed from around the post using an ultrasonic tip under microscope magnification.
5) The post was loosened with ultrasonic vibration and removed using Steiglitz forceps. Figure 21.4 shows the removed post.
6) Endodontic retreatment was carried out.
7) A new post hole was prepared using the Parapost System (Coltene/Whaledent) to accommodate a larger and longer post and the preparation was refined for indirect post crown.
8) An impression was taken using Parapost plastic impression post and silicone impression material.
9) A temporary post crown was made using the silicone putty index, temporary post and Protemp™ temporary crown material (3M ESPE).
10) A new laboratory-made cast post core with a separate crown was fabricated and cemented.
11) A postoperative radiograph was obtained to verify the post crown (Figure 21.5).
12) Postoperative review.

The use of the microscope and ultrasonic tips were very helpful in careful troughing around the post and breaking away the cement. Delivering ultrasonic vibration to the post through the Steiglitz forceps further facilitated loosening of the post.

The Parapost system was very useful in preparing a larger post hole in the canal. Care was taken to avoid weakening the root. The use of plastic impression post and additional silicone impression material resulted in an accurate impression of the post hole and the remaining tooth structure and enabled fabrication of a well-fitting post core and a metal ceramic crown. The patient was satisfied with the outcome of treatment and was discharged back to his GDP for maintenance.

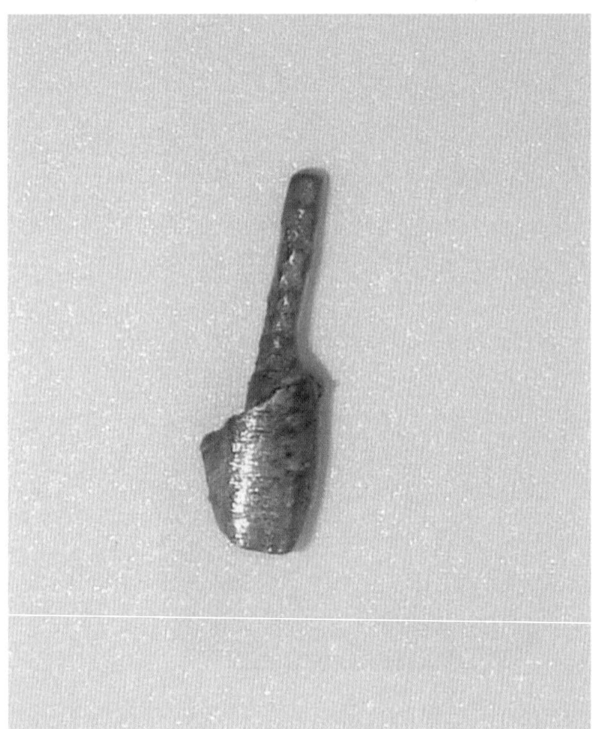

Figure 21.4 Removed metal post with part of the attached core.

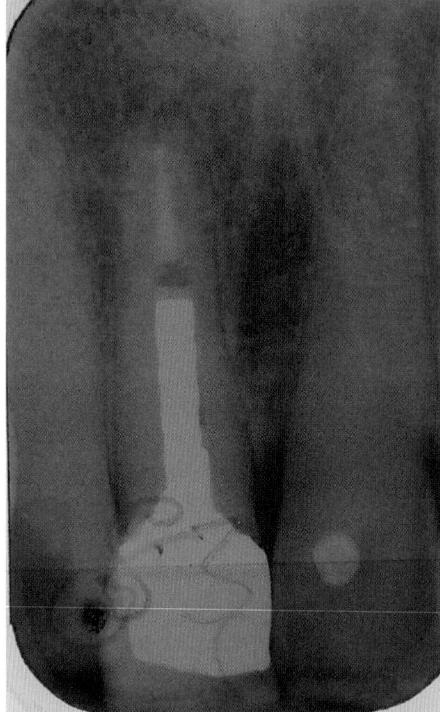

Figure 21.5 Postoperative radiograph of the new post crown.

References

Abbott, P.V. (2002) Incidence of root fractures and methods used for post removal. *Int Endod J*, **35**, 63–67.

Beddis, H.P., Okechukwu, N. and Nattress, B.R. (2014) 'The last post?': assessment of the failing post-retained crown. *Dent Update*, **41**, 386–388, 390–392, 394.

Castrisos, T. and Abbott, P.V. (2002) A survey of methods used for post removal in specialist endodontic practice. *Int Endod J*, **35**, 172–180.

Castrisos, T.V., Palamara, J.E. and Abbott, P.V. (2002) Measurement of strain on tooth roots during post removal with the Eggler post remover. *Int Endod J*, **35**, 337–344.

Cherukara, G.P., Pollock, G.R. and Wright, P.S. (2002) Case report: removal of fractured endodontic posts with a sonic instrument. *Eur J Prosthodont Restor Dent*, **10**, 23–26.

Dickie, J. and McCrosson, J. (2014) Post removal techniques part 1. *Dent Update*, **41**, 490–492, 495–498.

Goodacre, C.J., Bernal, G., Rungcharassaeng, K. and Kan, J.Y. (2003) Clinical complications in fixed prosthodontics. *J Prosthet Dent*, **90**, 31–41.

Krell, K.V., Jordan, R.D., Madison, S. and Aquilino, S. (1986) Using ultrasonic scalers to remove fractured root posts. *J Prosthet Dent*, **55**, 46–49.

Naito, T. (2010) Surgical or nonsurgical treatment for teeth with existing root fillings? *Evid Based Dent*, **11**, 54–55.

Rollings, S., Stevenson, B. and Ricketts, D. (2013a) Posts – when it all goes wrong! Part 1: case assessment and management options. *Dent Update*, **40**, 82–84, 86–88, 90–91.

Rollings, S., Stevenson, B. and Ricketts, D. (2013b) Posts – when it all goes wrong! Part 2: post removal techniques. *Dent Update*, **40**, 166–168, 170–172, 175–178.

Ruddle, C.J. (2004) Nonsurgical retreatment. *J Endod*, **30**, 827–845.

Sakkal, S., Gauthier, G., Milot, P. and Lemian, L. (1994) A clinical appraisal of the Gonon post-pulling system. *J Can Dent Assoc*, **60**, 537–539, 542.

Scotti, N., Bergantin, E., Alovisi, M., Pasqualini, D. and Berutti, E. (2013) Evaluation of a simplified fiber post removal system. *J Endod*, **39**, 1431–1434.

Torabinejad, M., Corr, R., Handysides, R. and Shabahang, S. (2009) Outcomes of nonsurgical retreatment and endodontic surgery: a systematic review. *J Endod*, **35**, 930–937.

Williams, V.D. and Bjorndal, A.M. (1983) The Masserann technique for the removal of fractured posts in endodontically treated teeth. *J Prosthet Dent*, **49**, 46–48.

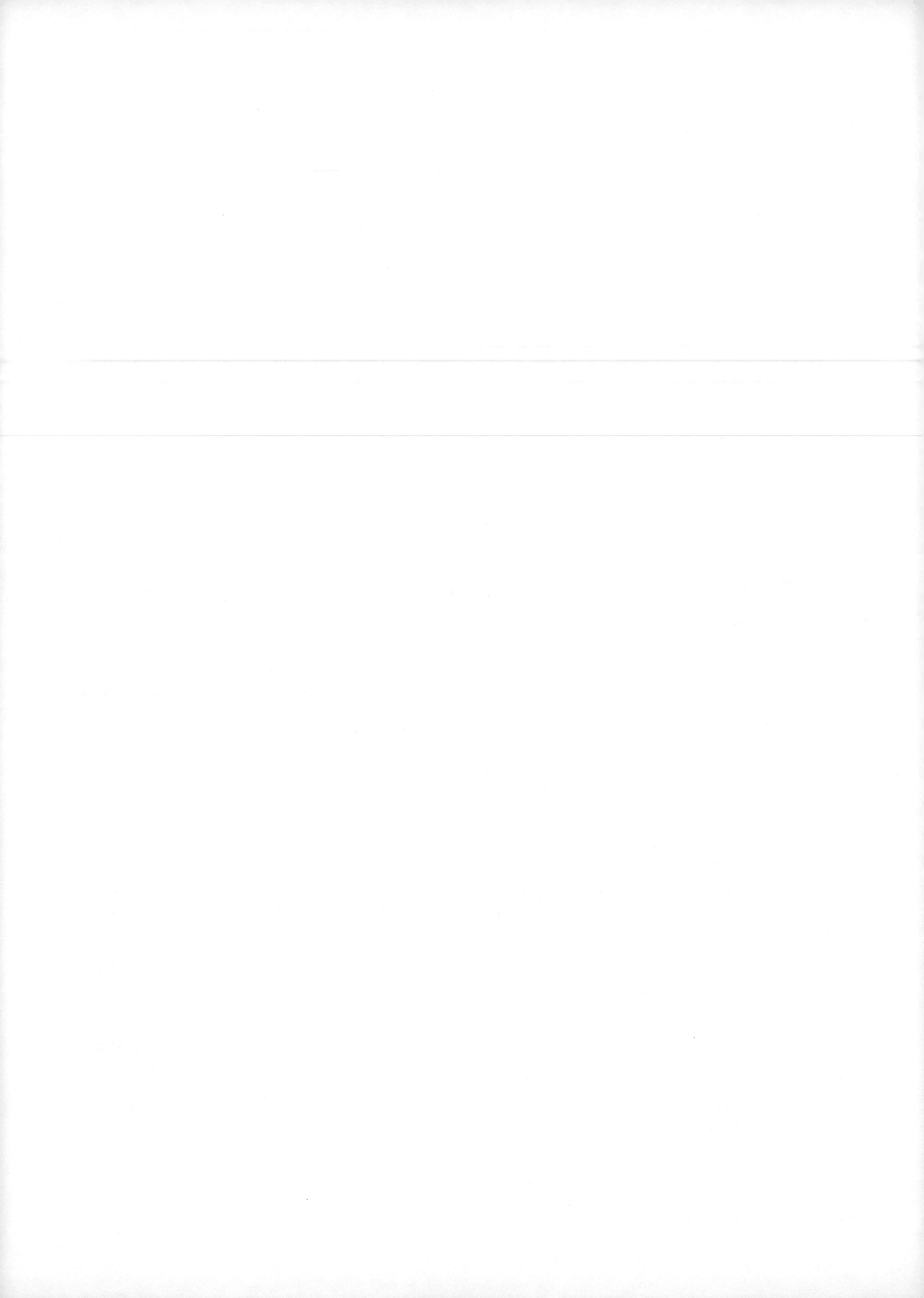

22

Gingival Enlargement and Gingivitis

Yusuf Alzayani - Case study

22.1 Introduction

In 1999, the International Workshop for Classification of Periodontal Disease and Conditions introduced a new category on gingival diseases which was subdivided into two main groups: non-plaque-induced gingival lesions and plaque-induced gingival diseases (Armitage, 1999).

Non-plaque-induced gingival lesions include the following categories (Holmstrup, 1999).

- Gingival diseases of specific bacterial origin
- Gingival diseases of viral origin
- Gingival diseases of fungal origin
- Gingival lesions of genetic origin
- Gingival diseases of systemic origin
- Traumatic lesions
- Foreign body reactions
- Lesions not otherwise specified

Plaque-induced gingival diseases were classified into the following groups (Mariotti, 1999).

- Gingivitis associated with bacterial plaque only
- Gingival diseases modified by systemic factors
- Gingival diseases modified by medications
- Gingival diseases modified by malnutrition

This chapter will focus on the aetiology, diagnosis and management of gingival enlargement which can be plaque induced or non-plaque induced.

22.2 Aetiology and Clinical Features

A number of local or systemic factors and conditions have been associated with gingival enlargement.

- Plaque-induced gingival inflammation or gingivitis (Loe *et al.*, 1965), which is the most common cause of gingival enlargement and is characterised by changes in colour, contour, consistency, bleeding on probing and increase in gingival exudate. Hormonal changes during puberty (Mombelli *et al.*, 1989) and pregnancy (Armitage, 2013) and the use of hormone replacement therapy (Krejci and Bissada, 2002) can increase the level of gingival inflammation and exacerbate plaque-induced gingivitis. Pregnancy-associated epulis or pyogenic granuloma is a pedunculated, fibrogranulomatous lesion which occurs in 0.5–5% of pregnant women due to a combination of vascular response and matrix stimulation by hormones (Jafarzadeh *et al.*, 2006).
- Drug-influenced gingival enlargement that has been related to anticonvulsants (phenytoin and sodium valproate), some immunosuppressant medications (cyclosporine and tacrolimus) and calcium channel blockers (nifedipine, diltiazem, amlodipine, verapamil) (Seymour, 2006). The condition is often more pronounced in the anterior gingivae with an onset within 3 months of medication use, starting from the interdental papillae, and varies between patients. The severity of the lesion is also affected by the patient's plaque control (Hassell and Hefti, 1991; Seymour *et al.*, 1996).
- Hereditary gingival fibromatosis (HGF) which is characterised by diffuse, firm, non-haemorrhagic and non-plaque-related enlargement of gingivae and develops after the eruption of permanent teeth but can also occur in primary dentition with localised or generalised pattern (Coletta and Graner, 2006). HGF is associated with gene mutations (Nibali *et al.*, 2013) and can be accompanied by other syndromes (Nibali *et al.*, 2012). Dental complications include drifting of teeth, diastema, malocclusion, prolonged retention of primary teeth, delayed eruption of teeth and poor access for plaque control (Doufexi *et al.*, 2005).
- Other conditions such as periapical or periodontal abscesses, traumatic gingival lesions, underlying hard tissue abnormalities, neurofibromatosis, orofacial granulomatous diseases, cysts, benign and malignant tumours, leukaemia and metastatic diseases (Beaumont *et al.*, 2017).

Diseases and Conditions in Dentistry: An Evidence-Based Reference, First Edition. Keyvan Moharamzadeh.

Companion website: www.wiley.com/go/moharamzadeh/diseases

22.3 Diagnosis

To reach an accurate diagnosis, it is essential to obtain a comprehensive history and carry out a clinical examination. Relevant history includes:

- onset and progression of periodontal disease and gingival enlargement
- familial history of periodontal disease or gingival enlargement
- patient's oral hygiene methods
- smoking history
- medical history, including medications
- previous periodontal treatment.

Clinical examination must include full periodontal assessment, including probing pocket depth, the position of marginal gingivae and also the base of the pocket in relation to the cementoenamel junction (CEJ) to determine the presence of false pockets due to gingival enlargement rather than true attachment loss. Other periodontal indices such as plaque score, bleeding on probing, mobility and furcation involvement must also be recorded. Assessment of the colour, surface texture, consistency and inflammatory status of the gingivae can be particularly useful to clinically differentiate between plaque-induced inflammatory gingival enlargement and non-plaque-induced diseases.

In some cases, impression taking and preparation of study models can be helpful in recording and 3D analysis of the accurate dimensions of the enlarged gingivae.

22.4 Management

The first stage of the management of gingival enlargement is identifying and addressing the underlying causative factors.

Non-surgical periodontal treatment, including oral hygiene instructions (OHI), supra- and subgingival scaling, reduces the extent of plaque-induced gingival inflammation and enlargement and minimises risk of recurrence (see Chapter 6). Since access for interdental cleaning can be restricted in patients with gingival enlargement, the use of adjunctive antiseptic mouthrinses such as chlorhexidine can be particularly helpful in these patients (Chapple *et al.*, 2015). It is also important to address any other local and systemic risk factors for periodontal disease such as plaque retentive factors, smoking and diabetes, as discussed in detail in Chapter 6.

Underlying medical conditions related to gingival enlargement (e.g. malnutrition, leukaemia, lymphoma and granulomatous diseases) will need to be managed by relevant medical specialists to improve gingival manifestations and reduce the risk of recurrence.

Cysts, tumours and other relevant localised hard or soft tissue pathology will need referral to oral and maxillofacial surgeons for appropriate investigations and management.

In patients with drug-influenced gingival enlargement, liaison with the patient's general medical practitioner or the relevant medical specialist regarding potential change of medication (if possible) can result in significant reduction or even resolution of the enlargement within weeks in some cases if it is combined with proper plaque control and non-surgical periodontal treatment to eliminate the inflammatory component of the lesion (Mavrogiannis *et al.*, 2006b).

Organ-transplanted patients with cyclosporine-related gingival enlargement are often immunosuppressed and may also be taking steroid medications. It is important to consult with the patient's medical specialist regarding the considerations for immunosuppression prior to any surgical treatment. Appropriate preoperative measures for steroid treatment must also be followed according to local policy based on the dosage of the steroid medication (Thomason *et al.*, 1999). The use of adjunctive systemic azithromycin has been shown to have some beneficial effects on the remission of cyclosporine-related gingival enlargement (Clementini *et al.*, 2008; Hirsch *et al.*, 2012). In addition to azithromycin's antimicrobial action, it inhibits cyclosporine-induced gingival proliferation by elevating the reduced metalloproteinase (MMP) activities of fibroblasts (Kim *et al.*, 2008).

Surgical management, including gingivoplasty (Figure 22.1) and gingivectomy (see the case study below) can be indicated after initial non-surgical treatment when the residual gingival enlargement has resulted in compromised function or aesthetics (Chesterman *et al.*, 2017). Excisional biopsy of the enlarged gingivae would enable histological diagnosis of any suspected gingival lesion as well. Surgery may also be indicated in severe cases to remove the bulky gingival tissue, improve access for cleaning and facilitate the patient's plaque control.

Surgical techniques include the following.

- Scalpel gingivectomy is a simple surgical technique that can be used for the removal of the enlarged gingivae where there are suprabony (false) pockets with at least a 3 mm band of keratinised tissue apical to the base of the pockets. The commonly used Goldman's technique involves piercing the gingivae at the level of the base of the pockets, and using the bleeding points as a guide for an external reverse bevel incision (Goldman, 1951).
- Laser gingivectomy provides more precise incision with better haemostasis compared to scalpel gingivectomy and can be useful for resection of highly vascular and friable gingival tissue, especially in patients with bleeding tendencies. It has been shown that laser

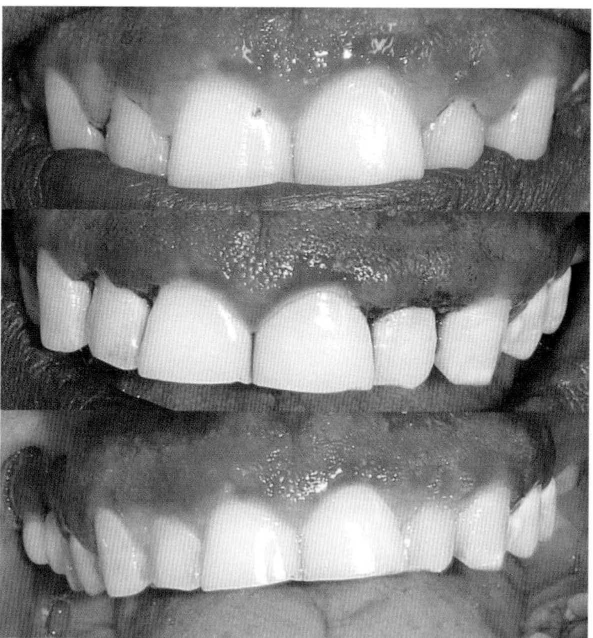

Figure 22.1 (*Top image*) Preoperative photograph of a 27-year-old female patient with mild residual gingival enlargement following pregnancy and non-surgical periodontal treatment. (*Middle image*) Immediate postgingivoplasty photograph using microsurgical instruments to reshape the interdental papillae. (*Bottom image*) One-year postoperative intraoral photograph.

excision results in slightly less postoperative pain and a reduced rate of recurrence (Mavrogiannis *et al.*, 2006a; Sobouti *et al.*, 2014). Its disadvantages include high costs and the need for safety protection (special room and eye protection).

- Electrosurgery also offers improved haemostasis, but its disadvantages include delayed wound healing due to the heat, unpleasant odour and risk of damage to the adjacent soft and hard tissues. Contact with metallic instruments, alveolar bone and restorations in vital teeth should be avoided (Moore, 1995). Electrosurgery devices (particularly monopolar devices) interfere with cardiac pacemakers (especially poorly shielded pacemakers) and their use should be avoided in these patients (Tom, 2016).
- Periodontal flap surgery is indicated when there is periodontal attachment loss in addition to gingival enlargement. It provides access for effective root surface debridement, removal of chronically inflamed granulation tissue, visualisation and treatment of bone defects, and simultaneous debulking and removal of the enlarged gingival tissue with preservation of keratinised gingivae. Periodontal flap surgery is associated with more postoperative pain compared to conventional gingivectomy and similar rate of recurrence (Mavrogiannis *et al.*, 2006a).

Supportive periodontal therapy and maintenance are extremely important to minimise the risk of recurrence of plaque-induced inflammatory disease. In cases where there is recurrence of non-plaque-induced gingival enlargement, repeated surgery may be indicated if the condition becomes severe enough to necessitate further surgical intervention.

Case Study

A 17-year-old male patient was referred by his GDP for management of gingival enlargement. The patient complained of overgrown gums, present for a long time, causing major aesthetic concerns and social embarrassment.

The patient was medically fit and well, a non-smoker and was not taking any medications. There was no family history of gingival or periodontal diseases.

Clinical examination showed firm fibrous gingival enlargement from UR4 to UL4 and LR4 to LL4, mainly on the labial aspect of the teeth as shown in Figure 22.2.

The patient had mild class II div I malocclusion, retained URC and labially erupted UR3. The BPE scores were 3 in all quadrants. Radiographic examination (Figure 22.3) showed that bone levels were at the CEJ level.

Based on the history, clinical and radiographic examination, the following differential diagnoses were made.

- Idiopathic gingival fibromatosis
- Hereditary gingival fibromatosis

The treatment strategy included the following aspects.

- Prevention and OHI.
- Orthodontic consultation lead to the following conclusions.
  - The labially erupting UR3 would continue to improve gradually over the next 3 years.
  - There was insufficient space for UR3 full alignment.
  - Patient was not keen to have orthodontic treatment at this stage.
  - To consider periodontal surgery.
  - To extract URC during or after surgery.
  - To consider orthodontic treatment 6–12 months post surgery.
- Inverse bevel gingivectomy combined with ostectomy and apically repositioned flap UR3–UL3.

The following surgical procedures were carried out.

1) Informed written consent.
2) Local anaesthesia.

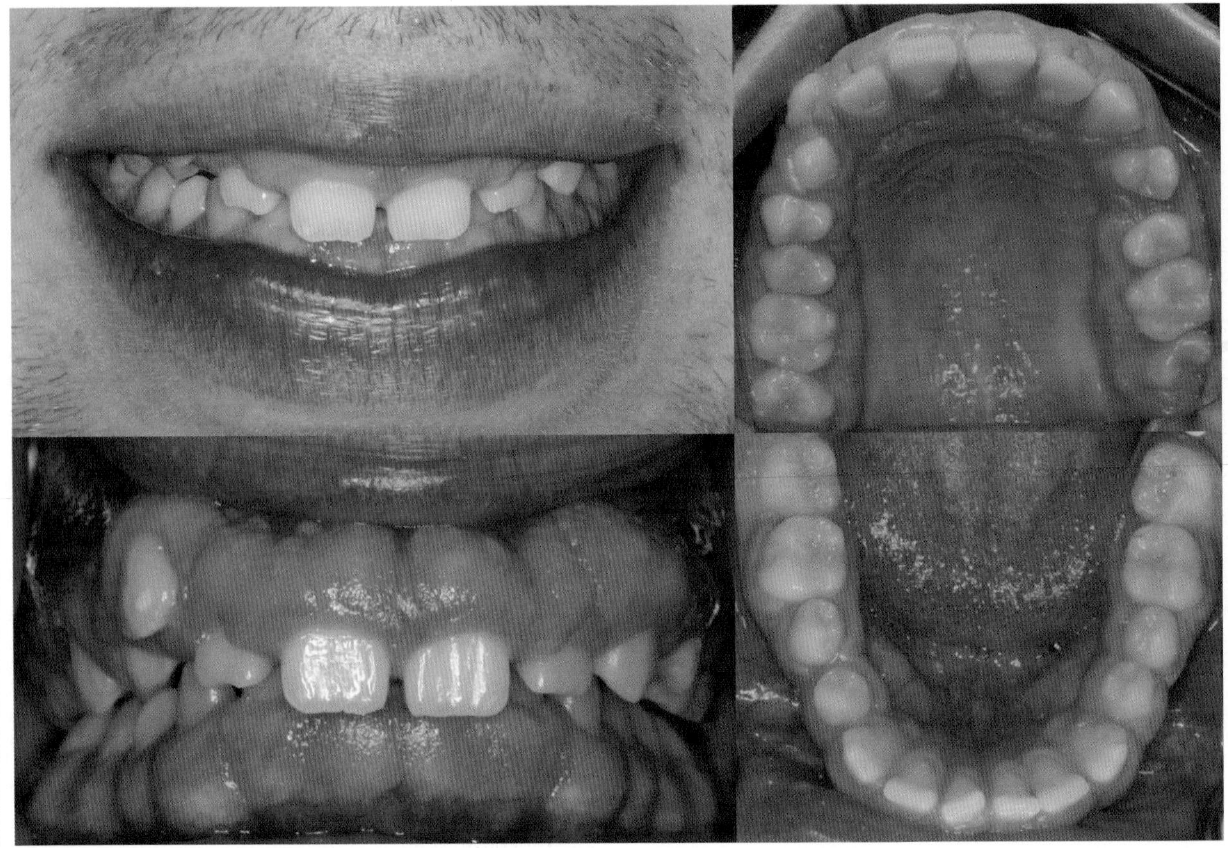

Figure 22.2 Preoperative clinical photographs.

3) Measurement of the width of keratinised gingivae, probing pocket depth and bone sounding in the surgical area (UR2–UL3).
4) Marking the external bleeding points corresponding to the base of the pockets.
5) Outline scalloped incisions, then internal bevel incisions, and then crevicular incisions.
6) Excision of the bulk of enlarged gingival tissues and sending samples for histopathology examination.
7) Undermining and elevation of the buccal flap.
8) Palatal crevicular incisions and elevation of the palatal flap.
9) Removal of interdental tissues and root surface debridement of the exposed root surfaces using an ultrasonic scaler.
10) Ostectomy and bone recontouring to reduce the thickness of the bone and move the bone levels 2–3 mm below the CEJ (Figure 22.4).
11) Flap repositioning, adaptation and suturing (Figure 22.5).
12) Haemostasis and postoperative instructions.
13) Prescription of appropriate analgesia for pain control.
14) Suture removal in 1 week and extraction of the URC.

The patient was reviewed every 3 months to monitor healing, maintain periodontal health and detect any signs of recurrence. Nine-month postoperative photographs are shown in Figure 22.6.

The patient was very satisfied with the outcome of the treatment and was discharged to his GDP for routine dental care and periodontal maintenance.

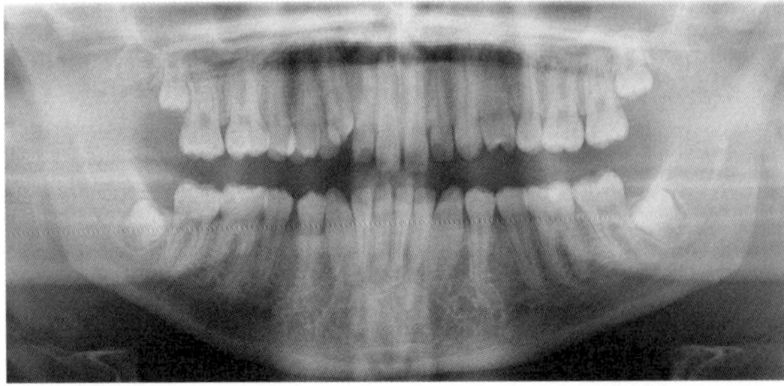

Figure 22.3 Preoperative oral panoramic radiograph.

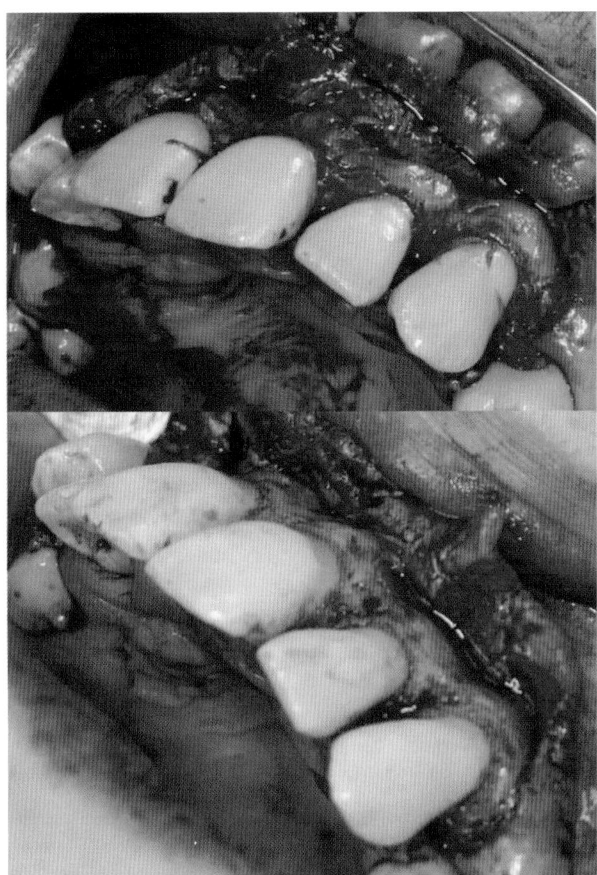

Figure 22.4 Photographs of the surgical site following flap elevation. The upper image shows the presence of thick alveolar bone at the CEJ level of the teeth before ostectomy. The lower image shows the bone has been reduced in thickness and moved 2–3 mm below the CEJ level after ostectomy.

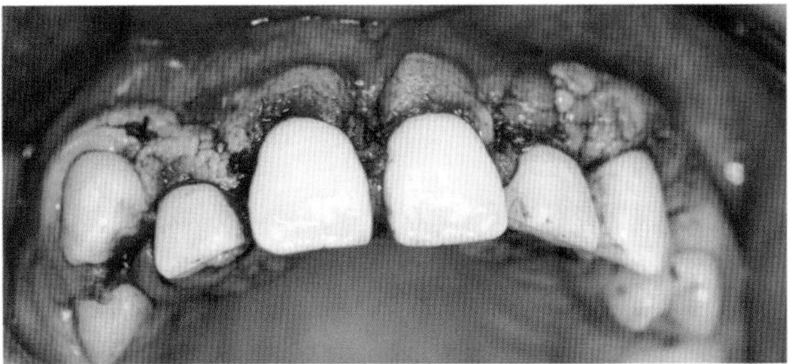

Figure 22.5 Photograph of the apically repositioned and sutured flap.

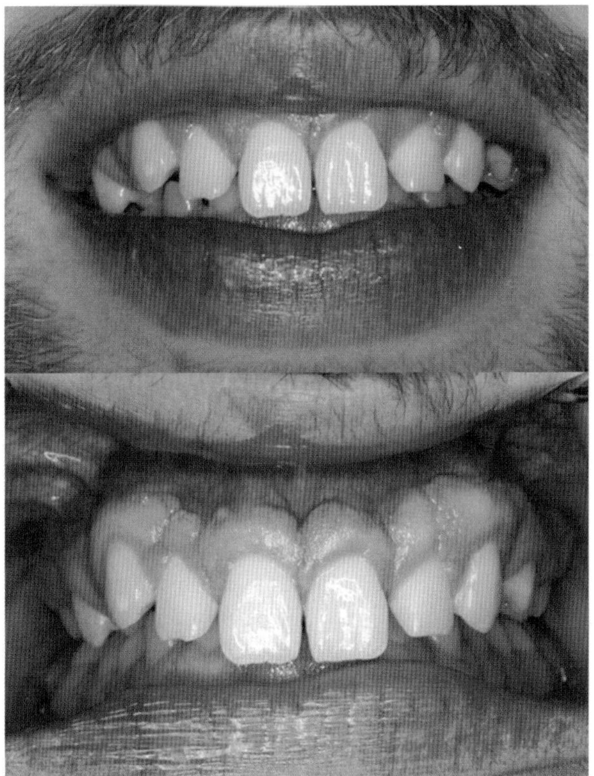

Figure 22.6 Postoperative clinical photographs after 9 months showing significant improvement in aesthetics and gingival contour.

References

Armitage, G.C. (1999) Development of a classification system for periodontal diseases and conditions. *Ann Periodontol*, **4**, 1–6.

Armitage, G.C. (2013) Bi-directional relationship between pregnancy and periodontal disease. *Periodontology 2000*, **61**, 160–176.

Beaumont, J., Chesterman, J., Kellett, M. and Durey, K. (2017) Gingival overgrowth: Part 1: aetiology and clinical diagnosis. *Br Dent J*, **222**, 85–91.

Chapple, I.L., van der Weijden, F., Doerfer, C. *et al.* (2015) Primary prevention of periodontitis: managing gingivitis. *J Clin Periodontol*, **42**(Suppl 16), S71–76.

Chesterman, J., Beaumont, J., Kellett, M. and Durey, K. (2017) Gingival overgrowth: Part 2: management strategies. *Br Dent J*, **222**, 159–165.

Clementini, M., Vittorini, G., Crea, A. *et al.* (2008) Efficacy of AZM therapy in patients with gingival overgrowth induced by cyclosporine A: a systematic review. *BMC Oral Health*, **8**, 34.

Coletta, R.D. and Graner, E. (2006) Hereditary gingival fibromatosis: a systematic review. *J Periodontol*, **77**, 753–764.

Doufexi, A., Mina, M. and Ioannidou, E. (2005) Gingival overgrowth in children: epidemiology, pathogenesis, and complications. A literature review. *J Periodontol*, **76**, 3–10.

Goldman, H.M. (1951) Gingivectomy. *Oral Surg Oral Med Oral Pathol*, **4**, 1136–1157.

Hassell, T.M. and Hefti, A.F. (1991) Drug-induced gingival overgrowth: old problem, new problem. *Crit Rev Oral Biol Med*, **2**, 103–137.

Hirsch, R., Deng, H. and Laohachai, M.N. (2012) Azithromycin in periodontal treatment: more than an antibiotic. *J Periodontal Res*, **47**, 137–148.

Holmstrup, P. (1999) Non-plaque-induced gingival lesions. *Ann Periodontol*, **4**, 20–31.

Jafarzadeh, H., Sanatkhani, M. and Mohtasham, N. (2006) Oral pyogenic granuloma: a review. *J Oral Sci*, **48**, 167–175.

Kim, J.Y., Park, S.H., Cho, K.S. *et al.* (2008) Mechanism of azithromycin treatment on gingival overgrowth. *J Dent Res*, **87**, 1075–1079.

Krejci, C.B. and Bissada, N.F. (2002) Women's health issues and their relationship to periodontitis. *J Am Dent Assoc*, **133**, 323–329.

Loe, H., Theilade, E. and Jensen, S.B. (1965) Experimental gingivitis in man. *J Periodontol*, **36**, 177–187.

Mariotti, A. (1999) Dental plaque-induced gingival diseases. *Ann Periodontol*, **4**, 7–19.

Mavrogiannis, M., Ellis, J.S., Seymour, R.A. and Thomason, J.M. (2006a) The efficacy of three different surgical techniques in the management of drug-induced gingival overgrowth. *J Clin Periodontol*, **33**, 677–682.

Mavrogiannis, M., Ellis, J.S., Thomason, J.M. and Seymour, R.A. (2006b) The management of drug-induced gingival overgrowth. *J Clin Periodontol*, **33**, 434–439.

Mombelli, A., Gusberti, F.A., van Oosten, M.A. and Lang, N.P. (1989) Gingival health and gingivitis development during puberty. a 4-year longitudinal study. *J Clin Periodontol*, **16**, 451–456.

Moore, D.A. (1995) Electrosurgery in dentistry: past and present. *Gen Dent*, **43**, 460–465.

Nibali, L., Brett, P.M., Donos, N. and Griffiths, G.S. (2012) Hereditary gingival hyperplasia associated with amelogenesis imperfecta: a case report. *Quintessence Int*, **43**, 483–489.

Nibali, L., Medlar, A., Stanescu, H., Kleta, R., Darbar, U. and Donos, N. (2013) Linkage analysis confirms heterogeneity of hereditary gingival fibromatosis. *Oral Dis*, **19**, 100–105.

Seymour, R.A. (2006) Effects of medications on the periodontal tissues in health and disease. *Periodontology 2000*, **40**, 120–129.

Seymour, R.A., Thomason, J.M. and Ellis, J.S. (1996) The pathogenesis of drug-induced gingival overgrowth. *J Clin Periodontol*, **23**, 165–175.

Sobouti, F., Rakhshan, V., Chiniforush, N. and Khatami, M. (2014) Effects of laser-assisted cosmetic smile lift gingivectomy on postoperative bleeding and pain in fixed orthodontic patients: a controlled clinical trial. *Prog Orthod*, **15**, 66.

Thomason, J.M., Girdler, N.M., Kendall-Taylor, P., Wastell, H., Weddel, A. and Seymour, R.A. (1999) An investigation into the need for supplementary steroids in organ transplant patients undergoing gingival surgery. a double-blind, split-mouth, cross-over study. *J Clin Periodontol*, **26**, 577–582.

Tom, J. (2016) Management of patients with cardiovascular implantable electronic devices in dental, oral, and maxillofacial surgery. *Anesth Prog*, **63**, 95–104.

23

Gingival Recession

Poyan Barabari and Abdul-Rahman Elmougy - Case study

23.1 Introduction

Gingival recession can be defined as the exposure of root surface due to apical migration of the gingival margin beyond the cementoenamel junction (CEJ) (Wennstrom, 1996).

The architecture of gingivae is related to the contour of the underlying bone crest. There are two basic gingival biotypes: pronounced scalloped (thin) biotype, which is more prone to recession, and flat (thick) biotype, which is less susceptible to recession (Ochsenbein and Ross, 1969). The biological width (BW) of the soft tissue attachments above the bone crest includes the connective tissue attachment (1.06–1.08 mm) and the attached epithelium (0.7–1.4 mm). BW varies from 2.5 mm in healthy gingivae to 1.8 mm in diseased conditions. (Lang and Lindhe, 2015).

The prevalence of gingival recession varies from 30% to 100%, depending on the population (Kassab and Cohen, 2003; Susin *et al.*, 2004), and it increases with age (Serino *et al.*, 1994).

Although gingival recession may go unnoticed by some patients, the following problems can be associated with recession defects.

- Poor gingival appearance, especially if the teeth in the aesthetic zone are affected and the patient has a 'gummy smile'.
- Dentine hypersensitivity due to exposed root surface (see Chapter 12).
- Potential risk of development of root and interproximal caries (Griffin *et al.*, 2004).
- Phonetic disability in some cases of multiple severe recession defects, especially in the anterior maxillae due to air escaping through the interproximal spaces.
- Food impaction in interproximal areas with lost interdental papillae.

Therefore, appropriate diagnosis, prevention and effective management of gingival recession are an essential part of patient dental care.

23.2 Aetiology and Risk Factors

Gingival recession can be directly caused by the following.

- Mechanical trauma such as improper tooth brushing, which is the most common cause of recession in young patients (Baker and Spedding, 2002). It is characterised by clean root surface and wedge-shaped cervical abrasion lesions on the buccal surfaces of the roots. The most important tooth-brushing factors for gingival recession include frequency, duration, the use of horizontal or scrub method, hardness of the bristles and the frequency of toothbrush change (Heasman *et al.*, 2015). Other traumatic causes of gingival recession include traumatic deep bite (class II division II), denture trauma (by poorly designed mucosa-borne 'gum-stripping' dentures) or removable orthodontic appliances, damaging oral habits, foreign body trauma such as lower lip piercing, and iatrogenic damage caused by subgingival restorations breaching the biological width (Patel *et al.*, 2011a).
- Localised plaque-induced inflammatory disease (Sarfati *et al.*, 2010). The affected teeth often have thin or absent labial or buccal alveolar bone and thin gingival biotype. High muscle attachment and frenal pull can also impair plaque control and further exacerbate the problem (Merijohn, 2016).
- Generalised periodontal disease which can affect all surfaces of the teeth, including the interproximal surfaces, resulting in the loss of interdental hard and soft tissues; common in older adults (see Chapter 6).

Placement of restoration margins at subgingival level increases the risk of gingival recession due to mechanical trauma during tooth preparation and microbial plaque retention (Valderhaug, 1980). However, the magnitude of recession can be influenced by the thickness of the marginal gingivae (gingival biotype) and the design of the preparation (Paniz *et al.*, 2016).

Diseases and Conditions in Dentistry: An Evidence-Based Reference, First Edition. Keyvan Moharamzadeh.

Companion website: www.wiley.com/go/moharamzadeh/diseases

Orthodontic tooth movement beyond the envelope of the alveolar bone may result in buccal bone dehiscence and decreased gingival tissue thickness. A thin mucosa can subsequently develop recession in the presence of tooth-brushing trauma or plaque-induced inflammatory disease (Lang and Lindhe, 2015).

23.3 Classification

Gingival recession defects have been classified by Miller (1985) into four categories (Figure 23.1).

- Class I: recession not extending to the mucogingival junction (MGJ) with no loss of interdental bone or papillae.
- Class II: recession extending to or beyond the MGJ with no loss of interdental bone or papillae.
- Class III: recession extending to or beyond the MGJ with loss of interdental bone or papillae coronal to apical extension of recession.
- Class IV: recession extending to or beyond the MGJ with loss of interdental bone or papillae apical to the apical extension of recession.

23.4 Diagnosis

Accurate diagnosis is based on thorough assessment of the patient's periodontal condition, including the patient's main concerns, obtaining complete medical and dental histories, conducting full clinical examination, appropriate radiographic evaluation and any other relevant special investigations such as sensibility testing. General periodontal risk factors (see Chapter 6) and also susceptibility factors and modifiable conditions associated with gingival recession (described above) should be accurately recorded (Merijohn, 2016).

23.5 Prevention and Non-Surgical Management

23.5.1 Monitoring and Maintenance

Mild asymptomatic gingival recession in patients without aesthetic concerns can be accepted and monitored. It is essential to address any potential risk factors and educate the patient to maintain optimal and atraumatic plaque control to prevent further recession. Single-tufted toothbrushes are particularly useful in cleaning the lingual and buccal surfaces of the teeth with gingival recession (Lee and Moon, 2011).

It has been shown that the maintenance of gingival health is independent of the width of keratinised attached gingivae and the presence of a narrow zone of attached gingiva does not necessarily increase the risk of gingival recession (Wennstrom, 1987) unless there are other risk factors present such as subgingival restoration margins (Ericsson and Lindhe, 1984).

Management of teeth with dentine hypersensitivity was discussed thoroughly in Chapter 12.

23.5.2 Adhesive Restorations

The use of adhesive pink porcelain or gingival coloured composite resin restoration is an alternative non-surgical conservative approach to improve aesthetics of teeth with gingival recession (Zalkind and Hochman, 1997). However, the limitations of this technique include difficulty with moisture control and colour match, achieving non-plaque retentive margins and acceptable emergence profile of the restoration.

23.5.3 Gingival Prosthesis

Prosthetic treatment with removable gingival veneers or prosthesis can be indicated for masking recession areas with the loss of interdental papillae (black triangles) in

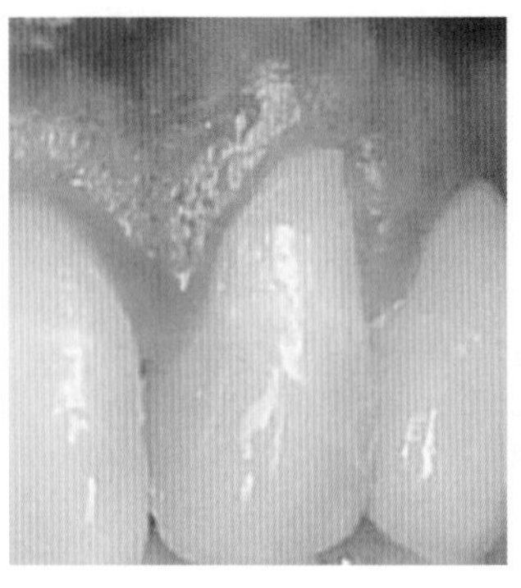
Class I

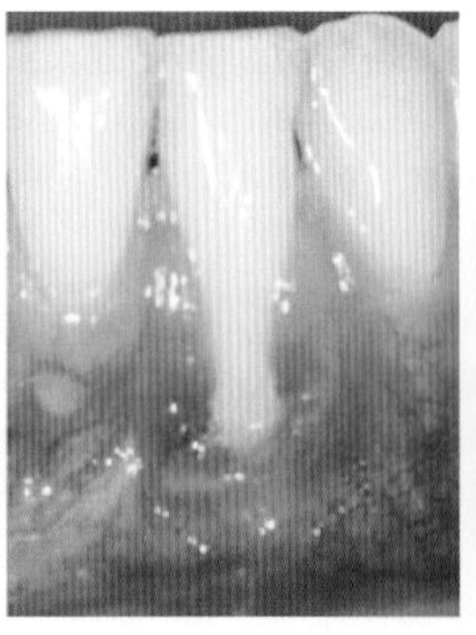
Class II

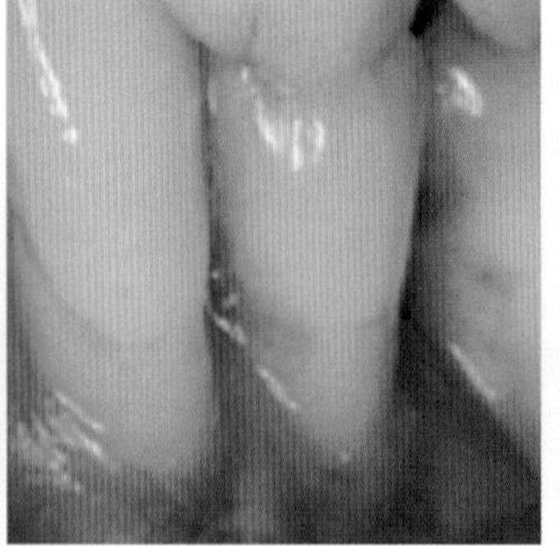
Class III

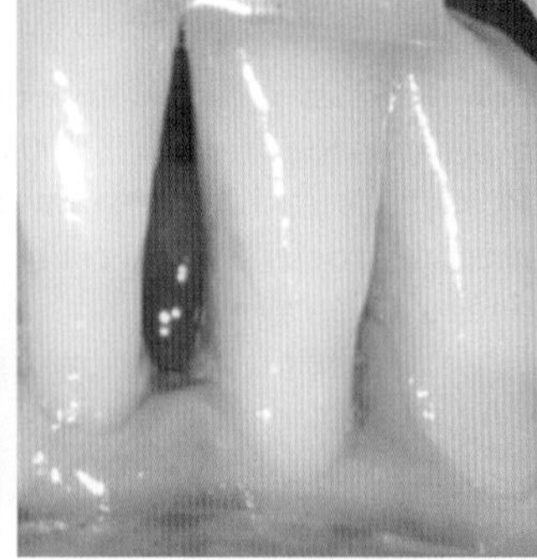
Class IV

Figure 23.1 Clinical photographs of Miller class I–IV gingival recession defects.

the aesthetic zone (Alani *et al.*, 2011). Gingival veneers made of hard acrylic resin or soft silicone-based materials can replace the missing soft tissues, cover the exposed root surfaces and significantly improve the appearance (Figure 23.2). The clinical procedures involve:

1) blocking out the palatal aspect of the embrasure areas using soft wax or silicone putty with separating medium
2) impression taking from the labial aspect of the teeth and the embrasures with silicone or alginate impression material using a special tray
3) shade selection
4) trial, adjustment and final insertion of the gingival prosthesis.

23.5.4 Orthodontic Space Closure

Interdental spaces and black triangles can also be closed with orthodontic treatment which may require interdental stripping to move the contact area further apically (Ziahosseini *et al.*, 2014). The limitations of this approach include the need for wearing orthodontic appliances for a long period of time, high cost and need for strict periodontal maintenance.

23.6 Surgical Treatment

Surgical approaches in mucogingival therapy relevant to gingival recession include gingival augmentation procedures to increase the width of attached keratinised gingivae, root coverage procedures to cover the exposed root surfaces due to gingival recession and interdental papillae reconstruction in the management of black triangles (Prato, 2000).

23.6.1 Gingival Augmentation

The presence of a narrow zone of keratinised gingivae does not necessarily justify surgical intervention. The evidence suggests that a minimum amount of keratinised tissue is not required to prevent attachment loss when optimal plaque control is maintained. However, if plaque control is not optimal, a minimum of 2 mm of keratinised gingivae is needed (Scheyer *et al.*, 2015). Gingival

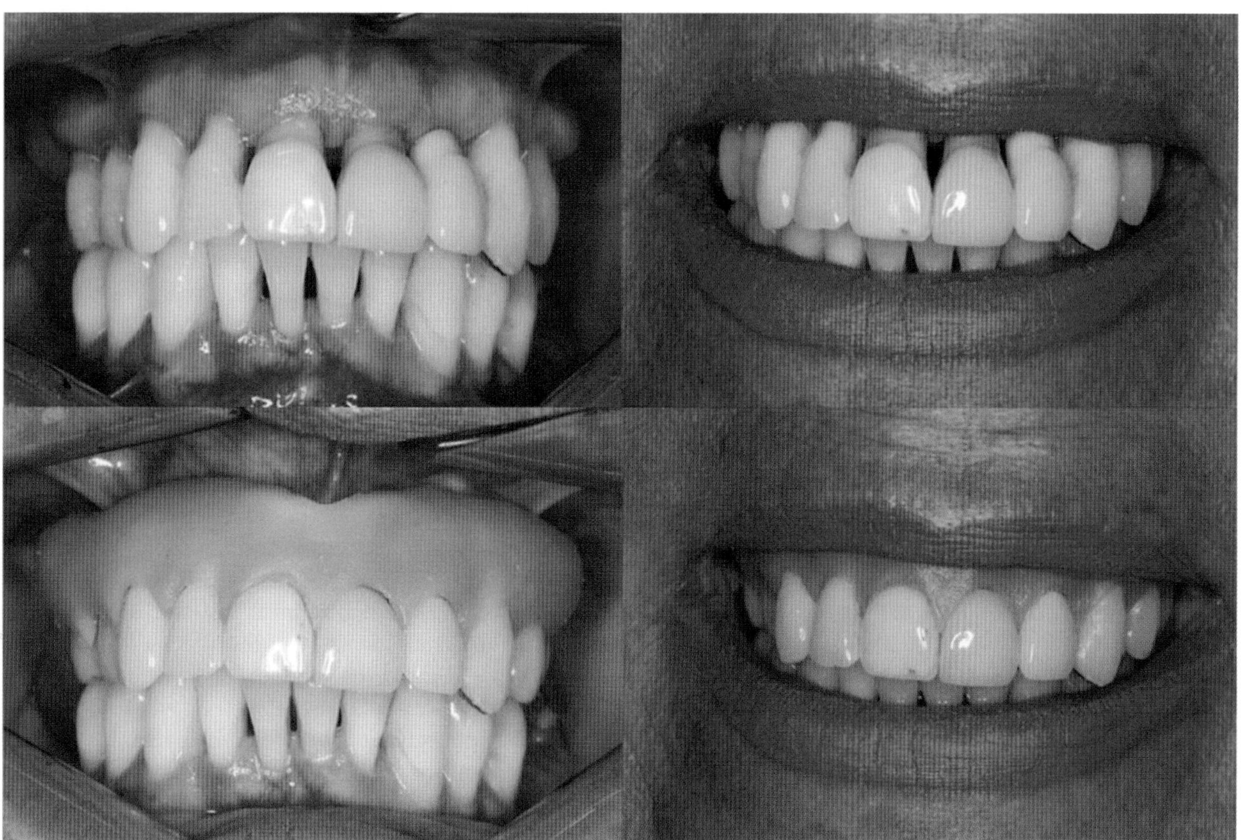

Figure 23.2 Preoperative clinical photographs of a patient with a high smile line and multiple severe gingival recession defects and black triangles in the aesthetic zone following periodontal treatment (*upper panel*) and postoperative photographs after successful treatment with a gingival prosthesis (*lower panel*).

augmentation around natural teeth (Bertl *et al.*, 2017) and implants (Bassetti *et al.*, 2017) may also be indicated in the following circumstances.

- To reduce the patient's discomfort during toothbrushing or chewing due to interfering lining mucosa and to facilitate plaque control (Kim and Neiva, 2015).
- To prevent future gingival recession by increasing the thickness of the gingivae prior to orthodontic treatment that is expected to move the teeth beyond the alveolar envelope, especially in patients with thin gingival biotype (Kloukos *et al.*, 2014).
- To increase the thickness of attached gingiva prior to placement of restorations with subgingival margins (Kim and Neiva, 2015).
- For management of an ectopic tooth erupting close to or in the MGJ.

Different surgical techniques for gingival augmentation are described briefly below. Further details can be found in the relevant periodontology textbook (Lang and Lindhe, 2015).

- Vestibular extension procedures have been used in the past without grafting, including denudation technique, split flap procedure and apically positioned flap. These techniques are not used these days due to associated pain, discomfort and risk of bone resorption and papillae recession.
- Gingival augmentation using pedicle grafts such as a split-thickness, laterally positioned keratinised flap from the adjacent site.
- Free gingival graft (FGG) procedure involves (1) preparation of a periosteal recipient bed free from muscle attachment using sharp dissection, (2) apical displacement of the split-thickness flap and suturing, (3) harvesting a correct size graft from the premolar region in palate, and (4) suturing and stabilising the graft onto the recipient site. The palatal wound can be covered with a surgical plate.
- Soft tissue substitute grafts (STSG), including acellular matrices such as AlloDerm® (LifeCell Corp., Branchburg, NJ, USA), DynaMatrix® (Keystone Dental, Turnpike Burlington, MA, USA), and Mucograft® (Geistlich Pharma, Wolhusen, Switzerland) and tissue-engineered grafts such as CelTx™ or Apligraf® (Organogenesis, Canton, MA, USA) and Dermagraft® (Advanced Tissue Sciences, Inc., La Jolla, CA, USA).

A meta-analysis of eight human clinical trials has shown that FGG yields a significantly larger increase in the width of keratinised tissue (consistently 2 mm or more) compared to STSG. On the other hand, STSGs result in significantly better aesthetics and patient preference (Bertl *et al.*, 2017).

Soft tissue healing includes four phases of haemostasis, inflammation, proliferation and maturation/matrix remodelling (Hammerle *et al.*, 2014). It is important to realise that during the initial phase (0–3 days) of healing, autologous grafts survive with plasmatic circulation and the presence of any blood clot between the graft and the wound bed can hamper this process and result in graft failure. Therefore, close adaptation and stabilisation of the graft to the recipient bed is a critical factor for successful outcome of treatment.

23.6.2 Surgical Root Coverage

Root coverage procedures are indicated to improve aesthetics, reduce sensitivity and facilitate plaque control. It has been shown that untreated gingival recession defects have a high probability of progressing in the long term (Chambrone and Tatakis, 2016).

Complete root coverage can be achieved in Miller class I and class II defects. However, only partial root coverage can be expected in class III defects. Class IV defects have a poor prognosis for root coverage procedures (Chambrone and Tatakis, 2015; Tatakis *et al.*, 2015).

Different types of periodontal soft tissue root coverage procedures are described briefly in the following sections. Details of the individual surgical procedure with useful illustrations can be found in the relevant periodontology textbook (Lang and Lindhe, 2015).

23.6.2.1 Pedicle Soft Tissue Grafts

Pedicle flaps include rotational flaps, advanced flaps and a combination of rotational and advanced flaps (Patel *et al.*, 2011b) as listed below.

- A laterally sliding flap involves preparation of a 3 mm-wide recipient bed at one side of the recession defect as well as apical to the defect by sharp dissection and then rotation (45°) of a submarginal split-thickness flap from the adjacent donor site to cover the defect.
- A double papillae flap involves preparation of two split-thickness flaps containing half of the papillae from both sides of the defect and then approximation and suturing of the flaps over the exposed root surface.
- A coronally advanced (repositioned) flap (CAF) as described by Allen and Miller (1989) consists of two oblique apically diverging incisions, starting from the mesial and distal line angle of the affected tooth coronal to the CEJ and directed apically into the alveolar mucosa. A split-thickness flap is then elevated to protect the underlying bone. Following root surface debridement, periosteal release and de-epithelialising the coronal papillae, the flap is coronally advanced and secured with interrupted sutures. Zucchelli and de Sanctis (2000) introduced a modification of this procedure to treat multiple recession defects. A split-full-split-thickness approach (split-thickness flap mesial

and distal side but full thickness on the labial aspect apical to the receded tissue margin) was used to elevate the flap to maintain the maximum soft tissue thickness above the exposed root.

- A coronally repositioned flap can be used for multiple adjacent recession defects without releasing incisions but oblique submarginal incisions can be made in the interdental areas to prepare surgically created papillae symmetrical to the midline of the surgical field.
- A semi-lunar coronally repositioned flap can be used when there is a shallow recession defect with no deep periodontal pockets (Tarnow, 1986).
- A laterally moved and coronally advanced flap can be used for isolated deep gingival recession defects affecting a lower incisor tooth (Zucchelli *et al.*, 2004).

Pedicle flaps have been combined with guided tissue regeneration (GTR) membranes (Pini-Prato *et al.*, 1992). If a membrane is used, adequate space needs to be provided by flattening the root surface. The membrane is then sutured in place and covered with the flap. Membranes may be useful in cases of large recession defects where there is inadequate free autologous soft tissue graft present for harvesting from the palate (see below) (Chambrone *et al.*, 2010).

Pedicle flaps such as coronallly advanced flaps have also been combined with enamel matrix proteins (e.g. EMD) to improve the clinical outcomes of regeneration (Koop *et al.*, 2012). In this technique, the exposed root surface is first conditioned and then EMD is applied to the root surface. The flap is then coronally advanced and sutured in place (Abbas *et al.*, 2003).

23.6.2.2 Free Soft Tissue Grafts

Free soft tissue grafts include epithelialised FGGs and subepithelial connective tissue (CT) grafts (Patel *et al.*, 2011c).

- The epithelialised FGG developed by Sullivan and Atkins (1968) and modified by Miller (1982) can be used either as a two-stage surgery technique (surgery 1: gingival augmentation to increase the width of keratinised tissue and surgery 2: coronally advanced flap as described above) or as a combined one-stage surgical technique including recipient bed preparation 3–4 mm apical and lateral to the recession defect, harvesting an epithelialised graft (2–3 mm thick) from the palate and suturing the graft at a coronal position to cover the exposed root surface.
- Subepithelial CT grafts can be harvested from the palate or retromolar pad area using the trapdoor surgical approach. A palatal incision is made 3 mm apical to the gingival margin with a length of 6 mm longer than the width of the recession defect measured at the CEJ level. Different grafting techniques are listed below.
  - A CT graft placed between a split-thickness coronally advanced flap and the underlying periosteum at the recipient site (Langer and Langer, 1985).
  - The envelope technique (Raetzke, 1985) involves placement of the CT graft within a split-thickness envelope flap prepared around the recession defect by extending the sulcular incision to the adjacent teeth and undermining the gingivae to create a pouch. A sling suture can be used to advance the tissues coronally (Allen, 1994).
  - The tunnel technique (Zabalegui *et al.*, 1999) is used to treat multiple adjacent recessions by connecting the adjacent envelope recipient beds to create a tunnel flap. A large CT graft is then passed through the tunnel and sutured. In a modified tunnel technique, mucoperiosteal dissection is extended beyond the mucogingival junction and under each papilla and a subpapillary continuous sling suturing method is used to coronally advance the pouch margins over the graft (Allen, 2010).

A subepithelial CT graft is often preferred to epithelialised FGGs for root coverage as it results in a less invasive palatal wound and provides better aesthetics (Cairo *et al.*, 2016). Factors involved in the selection of technique include depth and width of recession, availability of the donor tissue, presence of muscle attachments and aesthetics.

23.6.2.3 Prognostic Factors

Several factors can affect the outcome of root coverage procedures (Lang and Lindhe, 2015; Patel *et al.*, 2011b).

- Patient-related factors including poor plaque control, smoking and tooth-brushing trauma have a negative effect on regeneration.
- Site-related factors, such as dimensions of the recession defect, gingival biotype, the level of interdental periodontal support and root surface condition. Less favourable outcomes are expected for defects larger than 3 mm in width and 5 mm in depth with thin biotype as well as defects with reduced interdental support. It is essential to clean the root surface, remove the cervical restorations and reduce the root prominence if necessary prior to surgery.
- Technique-related factors including flap thickness (Hwang and Wang, 2006) and size, which need to be at least 1 mm for CAF and 2 mm for FGG and cover the whole recipient site; position of the advanced flap, which needs to be at least 2 mm above the CEJ; and flap tension caused by suturing or prominent frenal attachments which need to be removed prior to or during root coverage surgery.
- Surgical complications include pain, excessive bleeding, graft necrosis, membrane exposure and infection (Curtis *et al.*, 1985).

23.6.2.4 Clinical Outcome of Various Root Coverage Procedures

All root coverage procedures can provide significant reduction in recession depth and clinical attachment level gain for Miller class I and II recession-type defects (Chambrone and Tatakis, 2015). There is a large body of evidence to support the use of CAF procedures alone or with CT grafts or EMD for periodontal plastic surgery (Cairo *et al.*, 2014). Subepithelial CT graft-based procedures provide the best outcomes as they result in superior percentages of mean and complete root coverage and significant increase of the width of keratinised tissue (Chambrone and Tatakis, 2015). Clinical guidelines suggest that the best way to surgically treat Miller class I and II single gingival recession defects is using the CAF procedure in combination with CT grafts (Pini-Prato *et al.*, 2014).

For multiple adjacent class I and II gingival recessions, CAF with or without CT grafts may lead to predictable complete root coverage. The use of CT graft appears to improve the long-term stability of the CAF. The use of subepithelial CT graft yields better outcomes than the use of bioabsorbable membranes, acellular dermal matrix or platelet-rich fibrin. Modified coronally advanced tunnel flap in combination with CT graft appears to be a valuable technique for the treatment of Miller class III multiple adjacent gingival recessions (Hofmanner *et al.*, 2012).

23.6.3 Surgical Reconstruction of Interdental Papillae

A classification system for interdental papilla height was developed by Nordland and Tarnow (1998).

- Normal: papilla occupies the entire interdental space.
- Class I: the tip of the papilla is between the CEJ and the contact point.
- Class II: the tip of the papilla is at or apical to the proximal CEJ but coronal to the midbuccal CEJ.
- Class III: the tip of the papilla is at or apical to the midbuccal CEJ.

The distance between the contact point and alveolar bone crest influences the interdental papilla height. Complete papilla is present if this distance is 5 mm or less (Tarnow *et al.*, 1992).

Surgical papillae reconstruction using soft tissue grafts can be indicated when a black triangle is present with the papilla height less than 4 mm and the distance between the contact point and bone crest is 5 mm or less.

Different soft tissue surgical techniques have been developed for papillae reconstruction.

- Beagle (1992) used a pedicle graft procedure for papillae reconstruction. A split-thickness flap is dissected on the palatal aspect of the interdental area, elevated labially, folded and sutured to create the new papilla at the labial part of the interdental area.
- Han and Takei (1996) employed a split-thickness semilunar coronally repositioned papilla approach based on the use of CT graft.
- Azzi *et al.* (1999) used an envelope-type flap for the coverage of CT graft in class IV recession defect to reconstruct the interdental papilla.
- The use of a micronised acellular dermal matrix allograft technique has also been investigated for papilla reconstruction (Geurs *et al.*, 2012).

Other less invasive biological approaches for papilla augmentation include cell transplantation by injecting autologous fibroblasts following papilla priming (McGuire and Scheyer, 2007) and tissue volumising by injection of hyaluronic acid gel into the interdental papilla, which appears to have the potential to be a promising treatment for small defects according to recent short-term studies (Awartani and Tatakis, 2016; Becker *et al.*, 2010; Lee *et al.*, 2016).

Where the distance between the contact point and alveolar bone crest is greater than 5 mm, supracrestal alveolar bone augmentation and papillae reconstruction can be attempted. The technique described by Kotschy and Laky (2006) involved the use of a modified or simplified papilla preservation flap in combination with the application of EMD on root surfaces and the use of bone substitute and GTR membrane to vertically augment the interdental bone.

Simpler non-surgical alternatives would be to modify the tooth crown and lower the contact point to close the black triangle or the use of a gingival prosthesis as previously discussed (Ziahosseini *et al.*, 2014).

23.6.4 Periodontal Microsurgery

Periodontal microsurgical techniques have been developed to enhance visual acuity and improve flap design and soft tissue handling (Cortellini and Tonetti, 2001). Microsurgery is a minimally invasive approach performed using a surgical microscope and adapted instruments and suture materials (Burkhardt and Hurzeler, 2000).

Magnification can also be achieved using loupes which are less technique sensitive, easy to use and cheaper than microscopes. However, they often provide insufficient lighting. Ideal loupes for periodontal microsurgery are adjustable, sealed-prism loupes with high-quality, coated lenses with magnification between 4× and 4.5×. They should be either headband or front frame mounted with a suitable working distance and a large field of view (Lang and Lindhe, 2015).

Microscopes consist of a mounting system, lighting unit and optical components (magnification changer, objective lenses, binocular tubes, eyepieces and lighting unit) and have the following advantages: optimal lighting of the operation area, more ergonomic working posture and freely selectable magnification levels. However, they are expensive and clinicians require appropriate training. Furthermore, their use is difficult when accessing lingual or palatal sites. Common errors include too high magnification, inadequate task sharing and lack of practice (Lang and Lindhe, 2015).

The ideal magnification for periodontal surgery is 10×.

Microsurgical instrument kits contain microsurgical scalpel handles and blades, probes, periosteal elevators, microneedle holders, surgical scissors, tissue pliers and micro-mini curettes.

The recommended suture needle type is a reverse-cutting circular needle (3/8 curvature) with a precision tip. The ideal needle length for papillary sutures in the posterior area is 13–15 mm, for the anterior area 10–12 mm and for buccal releasing incisions 5–8 mm.

The preferred suture size is 6-0 for interdental, 7-0 for buccal and 9-0 for papilla base. Non-resorbable synthetic monofilament suture materials such as polyamide (Ethilon®) or polypropylene (Prolene®) are recommended. However, internal sutures that secure the membranes and soft tissue grafts will have to be resorbable.

One of the clinical benefits of the microsurgical approach is the enhanced ability to obtain and maintain primary closure of the interdental tissues over the barrier membranes (Cortellini and Tonetti, 2001).

It has been shown that the microsurgical technique significantly improves the vascularisation of grafts and the percentages of root coverage in comparison with conventional periodontal surgery (Burkhardt and Lang, 2005).

The use of microsurgical instruments such as new tunnel instruments (tunnelling knife I/II, Hu-Friedy, Rotterdam) has been particularly helpful in the modified microsurgical tunnel technique (MMTT) for treatment of recession defects. Small and specially curved elevators facilitate supraperiosteal undermining split flap preparation of the tunnel, minimise trauma and risk of iatrogenic perforations and ensure a better blood supply for the connective tissue graft (Azaripour *et al.*, 2016; Zuhr *et al.*, 2007).

Case Study

A 23-year-old male patient was referred by his GDP for treatment of gingival recession defect associated with LL1. The patient complained of pain and discomfort when brushing and eating food.

The patient had noticed that the recession started after completion of his orthodontic treatment to align crowded mandibular anterior teeth. The recession started approximately 4 years earlier and progressed more rapidly over the last 18 months to 2 years to the extent seen at presentation (Figure 23.3).

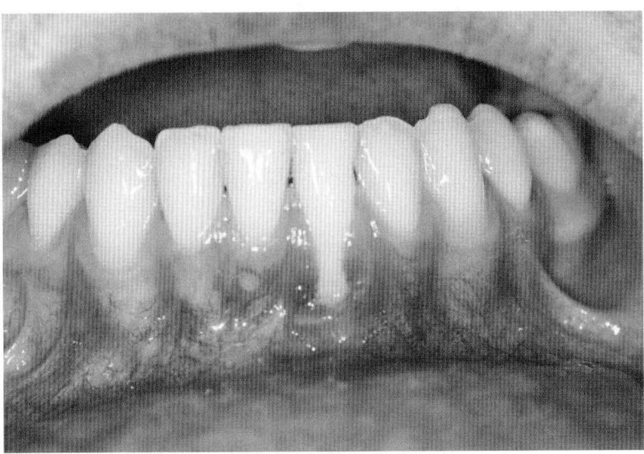

Figure 23.3 Preoperative clinical photograph showing an isolated narrow and deep recession defect associated with LL1 and a thin gingival biotype.

Clinical examination showed the BPE scores were 1 in all quadrants except for the lower anterior sextant, which was 2 due to the presence of calculus on the lingual aspects of the mandibular anterior teeth. Plaque and bleeding on probing were noticed on the gingival margins of LL1.

The diagnosis was Miller class II recession defect associated with LL1.

Following the initial hygienic phase, including oral hygiene education and periodontal scaling, surgical treatment options were discussed with the patient, including risks, benefits and expected outcomes.

It was decided to use a subepithelial CT graft harvested from the palate in combination with an envelope flap technique. The aim was to achieve complete root coverage and increase the width of the keratinised tissue. The surgical procedure is described below.

1) The recipient site was prepared by creating a split-thickness supraperiosteal envelope flap (Figure 23.4). It is important to tunnel laterally and apically to provide adequate space for the CT graft.
2) The root surface was cleaned and its prominence was slightly reduced.
3) The CT graft measuring over a centimetre in length was harvested from the patient's palate (Figure 23.5).
4) The graft was placed within the pouch using a pair of fine forceps.

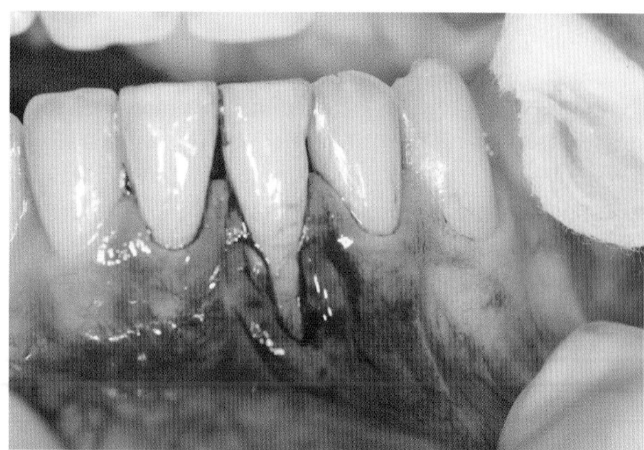

Figure 23.4 Recipient site preparation using the envelope flap technique.

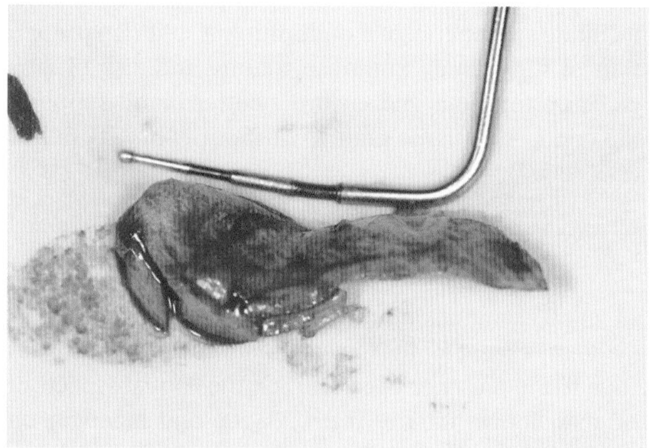

Figure 23.5 CT graft harvested from the palate with sufficient size to extend at least 3 mm beyond the margins of the recession defect to allow sufficient overlap with the recipient connective tissue bed.

5) The graft was secured *in situ* with a Vicryl 5-0 sling suture. An additional suture was placed to approximate the mesial and distal gingival margins over the graft material without tension (Figure 23.6).
6) Postoperative instructions included advising the patient not to brush in the area to begin with and then use a soft brush gently in the area.
7) Suture removal 1 week after surgery (Figure 23.7).
8) Further follow-up and maintenance.

At 6-month review, complete healing of the recipient site with satisfactory outcome for root coverage and an increased band of keratinised tissue was evident (Figure 23.8).

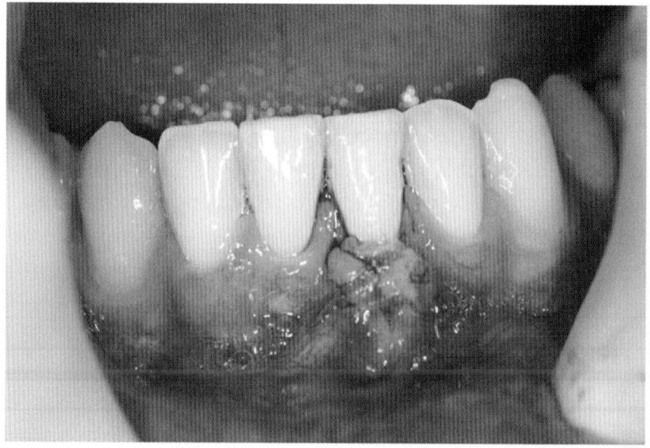

Figure 23.6 Sutured subepithelial CT graft and split-thickness envelope flap covering the root surface.

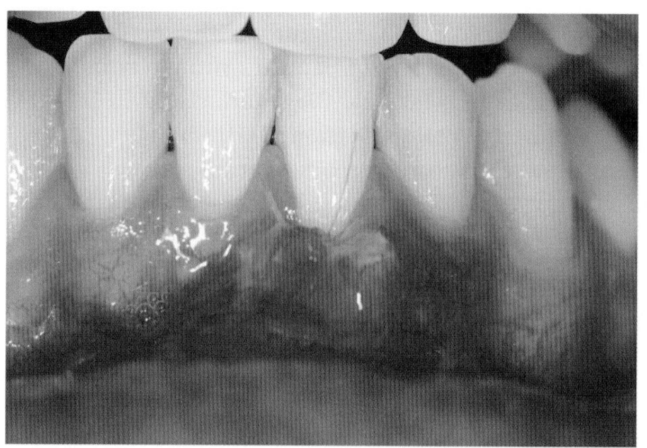

Figure 23.7 One-week postoperative photograph showing the graft with good vascular supply and satisfactory appearance.

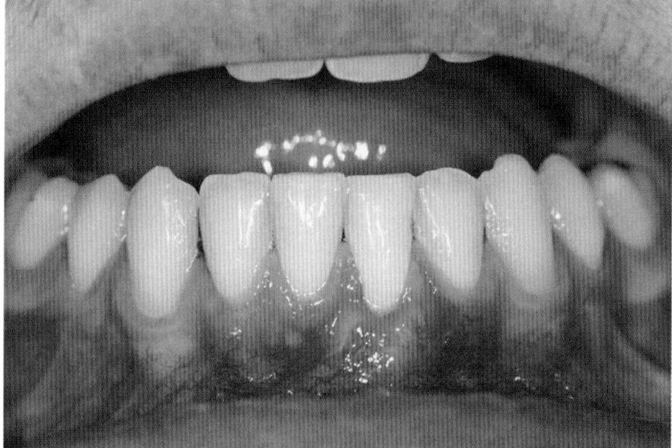

Figure 23.8 Six-month follow-up clinical photograph showing satisfactory root coverage and an increased band of keratinised tissue.

References

Abbas, F., Wennstrom, J., van der Weijden, F., Schneiders, T. and van der Velden, U. (2003) Surgical treatment of gingival recessions using Emdogain gel: clinical procedure and case reports. *Int J Periodontics Restorative Dent*, **23**, 607–613.

Alani, A., Maglad, A. and Nohl, F. (2011) The prosthetic management of gingival aesthetics. *Br Dent J*, **210**, 63–69.

Allen, A.L. (1994) Use of the supraperiosteal envelope in soft tissue grafting for root coverage. I. Rationale and technique. *Int J Periodontics Restorative Dent*, **14**, 216–227.

Allen, E.P. (2010) Subpapillary continuous sling suturing method for soft tissue grafting with the tunneling technique. *Int J Periodontics Restorative Dent*, **30**, 479–485.

Allen, E.P. and Miller, P.D. Jr (1989) Coronal positioning of existing gingiva: short term results in the treatment of shallow marginal tissue recession. *J Periodontol*, **60**, 316–319.

Awartani, F.A. and Tatakis, D.N. (2016) Interdental papilla loss: treatment by hyaluronic acid gel injection: a case series. *Clin Oral Invest*, **20**, 1775–1780.

Azaripour, A., Kissinger, M., Farina, V.S. *et al.* (2016) Root coverage with connective tissue graft associated with coronally advanced flap or tunnel technique: a randomized, double-blind, mono-centre clinical trial. *J Clin Periodontol*, **43**, 1142–1150.

Azzi, R., Etienne, D., Sauvan, J.L. and Miller, P.D. (1999) Root coverage and papilla reconstruction in class iv recession: a case report. *Int J Periodontics Restorative Dent*, **19**, 449–455.

Baker, P. and Spedding, C. (2002) The aetiology of gingival recession. *Dent Update*, **29**, 59–62.

Bassetti, R.G., Stahli, A., Bassetti, M.A. and Sculean, A. (2017) Soft tissue augmentation around osseointegrated and uncovered dental implants: a systematic review. *Clin Oral Invest*, **21**, 53–70.

Beagle, J.R. (1992) Surgical reconstruction of the interdental papilla: case report. *Int J Periodontics Restorative Dent*, **12**, 145–151.

Becker, W., Gabitov, I., Stepanov, M., Kois, J., Smidt, A. and Becker, B.E. (2010) Minimally invasive treatment for papillae deficiencies in the esthetic zone: a pilot study. *Clin Implant Dent Relat Res*, **12**, 1–8.

Bertl, K., Melchard, M., Pandis, N., Muller-Kern, M. and Stavropoulos, A. (2017) Soft tissue substitutes in non-root coverage procedures: a systematic review and meta-analysis. *Clin Oral Invest*, **21**, 505–518.

Burkhardt, R. and Hurzeler, M.B. (2000) Utilization of the surgical microscope for advanced plastic periodontal surgery. *Pract Periodont Aesthet Dent*, **12**, 171–180; quiz 182.

Burkhardt, R. and Lang, N.P. (2005) Coverage of localized gingival recessions: comparison of micro- and macrosurgical techniques. *J Clin Periodontol*, **32**, 287–293.

Cairo, F., Nieri, M. and Pagliaro, U. (2014) Efficacy of periodontal plastic surgery procedures in the treatment of localized facial gingival recessions. A systematic review. *J Clin Periodontol*, **41**(Suppl 15), S44–62.

Cairo, F., Pagliaro, U., Buti, J. *et al.* (2016) Root coverage procedures improve patient aesthetics. a systematic review and Bayesian network meta-analysis. *J Clin Periodontol*, **43**, 965–975.

Chambrone, L. and Tatakis, D.N. (2015) Periodontal soft tissue root coverage procedures: a systematic review from the AAP Regeneration workshop. *J Periodontol*, **86**, S8–51.

Chambrone, L. and Tatakis, D.N. (2016) Long-term outcomes of untreated buccal gingival recessions: a systematic review and meta-analysis. *J Periodontol*, **87**, 796–808.

Chambrone, L., Sukekava, F., Araujo, M.G., Pustiglioni, F.E., Chambrone, L.A. and Lima, L.A. (2010) Root-coverage procedures for the treatment of localized recession-type defects: a Cochrane systematic review. *J Periodontol*, **81**, 452–478.

Cortellini, P. and Tonetti, M.S. (2001) Microsurgical approach to periodontal regeneration. *Initial evaluation in a case cohort. J Periodontol*, **72**, 559–569.

Curtis, J.W. Jr, Mclain, J.B. and Hutchinson, R.A. (1985) The incidence and severity of complications and pain following periodontal surgery. *J Periodontol*, **56**, 597–601.

Ericsson, I. and Lindhe, J. (1984) Recession in sites with inadequate width of the keratinized gingiva. *An experimental study in the dog. J Clin Periodontol*, **11**, 95–103.

Geurs, N.C., Romanos, A.H., Vassilopoulos, P.J. and Reddy, M.S. (2012) Efficacy of micronized acellular dermal graft for use in interproximal papillae regeneration. *Int J Periodontics Restorative Dent*, **32**, 49–58.

Griffin, S.O., Griffin, P.M., Swann, J.L. and Zlobin, N. (2004) Estimating rates of new root caries in older adults. *J Dent Res*, **83**, 634–638.

Hammerle, C.H., Giannobile, W.V. and Working Group 1 of the European Workshop on Periodontology (2014) Biology of soft tissue wound healing and regeneration – Consensus Report of Group 1 of the 10th European Workshop On Periodontology. *J Clin Periodontol*, **41**(Suppl 15), S1–5.

Han, T.J. and Takei, H.H. (1996) Progress in gingival papilla reconstruction. *Periodontology 2000*, **11**, 65–68.

Heasman, P.A., Holliday, R., Bryant, A. and Preshaw, P.M. (2015) Evidence for the occurrence of gingival recession and non-carious cervical lesions as a consequence of traumatic toothbrushing. *J Clin Periodontol*, **42**(Suppl 16), S237–255.

Hofmanner, P., Alessandri, R., Laugisch, O., Aroca, S., Salvi, G.E., Stavropoulos, A. and Sculean, A. (2012) Predictability of surgical techniques used for coverage of multiple adjacent gingival recessions – a systematic review. *Quintessence Int*, **43**, 545–554.

Hwang, D. and Wang, H.L. (2006) Flap thickness as a predictor of root coverage: a systematic review. *J Periodontol*, **77**, 1625–1634.

Kassab, M.M. and Cohen, R.E. (2003) The etiology and prevalence of gingival recession. *J Am Dent Assoc*, **134**, 220–225.

Kim, D.M. and Neiva, R. (2015. Periodontal soft tissue non-root coverage procedures: a systematic review from the AAP Regeneration Workshop. *J Periodontol*, **86**, S56–72.

Kloukos, D., Eliades, T., Sculean, A. and Katsaros, C. (2014) Indication and timing of soft tissue augmentation at maxillary and mandibular incisors in orthodontic patients. A systematic review. *Eur J Orthod*, **36**, 442–449.

Koop, R., Merheb, J. and Quirynen, M. (2012) Periodontal regeneration with enamel matrix derivative in reconstructive periodontal therapy: a systematic review. *J Periodontol*, **83**, 707–720.

Kotschy, P. and Laky, M. (2006) Reconstruction of supracrestal alveolar bone lost as a result of severe chronic periodontitis. five-year outcome: case report. *Int J Periodontics Restorative Dent*, **26**, 425–431.

Lang, N.P. and Lindhe, J. (2015) *Clinical Periodontology and Implant Dentistry*, Wiley-Blackwell, Oxford.

Langer, B. and Langer, L. (1985) Subepithelial connective tissue graft technique for root coverage. *J Periodontol*, **56**, 715–720.

Lee, D.W. and Moon, I.S. (2011) The plaque-removing efficacy of a single-tufted brush on the lingual and buccal surfaces of the molars. *J Periodontal Implant Sci*, **41**, 131–134.

Lee, W.P., Kim, H.J., Yu, S.J. and Kim, B.O. (2016) Six month clinical evaluation of interdental papilla reconstruction with injectable hyaluronic acid gel using an image analysis system. *J Esthet Restor Dent*, **28**, 221–230.

McGuire, M.K. and Scheyer, E.T. (2007) A randomized, double-blind, placebo-controlled study to determine the safety and efficacy of cultured and expanded autologous fibroblast injections for the treatment of interdental papillary insufficiency associated with the papilla priming procedure. *J Periodontol*, **78**, 4–17.

Merijohn, G.K. (2016) Management and prevention of gingival recession. *Periodontology 2000*, **71**, 228–242.

Miller, N.A. (1982) Sutureless gingival grafting. A simplified procedure. *J Clin Periodontol*, **9**, 171–177.

Miller, P.D. Jr (1985) A classification of marginal tissue recession. *Int J Periodontics Restorative Dent*, **5**, 8–13.

Nordland, W.P. and Tarnow, D.P. (1998) A classification system for loss of papillary height. *J Periodontol*, **69**, 1124–1126.

Ochsenbein, C. and Ross, S. (1969) A reevaluation of osseous surgery. *Dent Clin North Am*, **13**, 87–102.

Paniz, G., Nart, J., Gobbato, L., Chierico, A., Lops, D. and Michalakis, K. (2016) Periodontal response to two different subgingival restorative margin designs: a 12-month randomized clinical trial. *Clin Oral Invest*, **20**, 1243–1252.

Patel, M., Nixon, P.J. and Chan, M.F. (2011a) Gingival recession: Part 1. Aetiology and non-surgical management. *Br Dent J*, **211**, 251–254.

Patel, M., Nixon, P.J. and Chan, M.F. (2011b) Gingival recession: Part 2. Surgical management using pedicle grafts. *Br Dent J*, **211**, 315–319.

Patel, M., Nixon, P.J. and Chan, M.F. (2011c) Gingival recession: Part 3. Surgical management using free grafts and guided tissue regeneration. *Br Dent J*, **211**, 353–358.

Pini-Prato, G., Tinti, C., Vincenzi, G., Magnani, C., Cortellini, P. and Clauser, C. (1992) Guided tissue regeneration versus mucogingival surgery in the treatment of human buccal gingival recession. *J Periodontol*, **63**, 919–928.

Pini-Prato, G., Nieri, M., Pagliaro, U. *et al.* for the National Association Of Italian Dentists (2014) Surgical treatment of single gingival recessions: clinical guidelines. *Eur J Oral Implantol*, **7**, 9–43.

Prato, G.P. (2000) Advances in mucogingival surgery. *J Int Acad Periodontol*, **2**, 24–27.

Raetzke, P.B. (1985) Covering localized areas of root exposure employing the 'envelope' technique. *J Periodontol*, **56**, 397–402.

Sarfati, A., Bourgeois, D., Katsahian, S., Mora, F. and Bouchard, P. (2010) Risk assessment for buccal gingival recession defects in an adult population. *J Periodontol*, **81**, 1419–1425.

Scheyer, E.T., Sanz, M., Dibart, S. *et al.* (2015) Periodontal soft tissue non-root coverage procedures: a consensus report from the AAP Regeneration Workshop. *J Periodontol*, **86**, S73–76.

Serino, G., Wennstrom, J.L., Lindhe, J. and Eneroth, L. (1994) The prevalence and distribution of gingival recession in subjects with a high standard of oral hygiene. *J Clin Periodontol*, **21**, 57–63.

Sullivan, H.C. and Atkins, J.H. (1968) Free autogenous gingival grafts. I. Principles of successful grafting. *Periodontics*, **6**, 121–129.

Susin, C., Haas, A.N., Oppermann, R.V., Haugejorden, O. and Albandar, J.M. (2004) Gingival recession: epidemiology and risk indicators in a representative urban Brazilian population. *J Periodontol*, **75**, 1377–1386.

Tarnow, D.P. (1986) Semilunar coronally repositioned flap. *J Clin Periodontol*, **13**, 182–185.

Tarnow, D.P., Magner, A.W. and Fletcher, P. (1992) The effect of the distance from the contact point to the crest of bone on the presence or absence of the interproximal dental papilla. *J Periodontol*, **63**, 995–996.

Tatakis, D.N., Chambrone, L., Allen, E.P. *et al.* (2015) Periodontal soft tissue root coverage procedures: a consensus report from the AAP Regeneration Workshop. *J Periodontol*, **86**, S52–55.

Valderhaug, J. (1980) Periodontal conditions and carious lesions following the insertion of fixed prostheses: a 10-year follow-up study. *Int Dent J*, **30**, 296–304.

Wennstrom, J.L. (1987) Lack of association between width of attached gingiva and development of soft tissue recession. A 5-year longitudinal study. *J Clin Periodontol*, **14**, 181–184.

Wennstrom, J.L. (1996) Mucogingival therapy. *Ann Periodontol*, **1**, 671–701.

Zabalegui, I., Sicilia, A., Cambra, J., Gil, J. and Sanz, M. (1999) Treatment of multiple adjacent gingival recessions with the tunnel subepithelial connective tissue graft: a clinical report. *Int J Periodontics Restorative Dent*, **19**, 199–206.

Zalkind, M. and Hochman, N. (1997) Alternative method of conservative esthetic treatment for gingival recession. *J Prosthet Dent*, **77**, 561–563.

Ziahosseini, P., Hussain, F. and Millar, B.J. (2014) Management of gingival black triangles. *Br Dent J*, **217**, 559–563.

Zucchelli, G. and de Sanctis, M. (2000) Treatment of multiple recession-type defects in patients with esthetic demands. *J Periodontol*, **71**, 1506–1514.

Zucchelli, G., Cesari, C., Amore, C., Montebugnoli, L. and de Sanctis, M. (2004) Laterally moved, coronally advanced flap: a modified surgical approach for isolated recession-type defects. *J Periodontol*, **75**, 1734–1741.

Zuhr, O., Fickl, S., Wachtel, H., Bolz, W. and Hurzeler, M.B. (2007) Covering of gingival recessions with a modified microsurgical tunnel technique: case report. *Int J Periodontics Restorative Dent*, **27**, 457–463.

24

Halitosis

24.1 Terminology

Different terms describing halitosis include breath malodour, oral malodour, *fetor ex ore*, *fetor oris* and bad or foul breath (Lindhe *et al.*, 2008).

24.2 Aetiology

Halitosis is related to intraoral causes in 90% of cases and extraoral causes in 10%.

Intraoral halitosis can be caused by periodontal disease or excessive bacteria (mainly gram-negative) on the tongue degrading and converting both sulfur- and non-sulfur-containing amino acids into volatile and bad-smelling gases (de Geest *et al.*, 2016).

Extraoral halitosis can be caused by the following conditions (Tangerman, 2002; Tangerman and Winkel, 2010).

- Upper respiratory tract infections, such as sinusitis, nasal obstruction, nasolaryngeal abscess and carcinoma of larynx.
- Lower respiratory tract infections such as bronchitis, pneumonia, pulmonary abscess and carcinoma of lungs.
- Other conditions including hiatus hernia, hepatic cirrhosis, diabetic ketoacidosis, uraemia, kidney disease and gastrointestinal diseases.

Halitosis can also have temporary causes such as morning bad breath, dry mouth, hunger, stress and dietary causes, such as eating garlic.

24.3 Epidemiology

Halitosis affects 22–50% of the population and its incidence increases with age (Akaji *et al.*, 2014).

24.4 Classification

Miyazaki (1999) classified halitosis into:

- genuine halitosis which can be physiological or pathological
- pseudo-halitosis, where there is no halitosis but the patient is convinced that they have halitosis
- halitophobia where there is no confirmation of halitosis but this belief persists after therapy.

Tangerman and Winkel's (2010) classification included intraoral and extraoral (subdivided into non-blood-borne and blood-borne) halitosis. Aydin and Harvey-Woodworth (2014) proposed a new classification: type 0 (physiological odour) and type 1–5 (pathological halitosis), described as type 1 (oral), type 2 (airway), type 3 (gastro-oesophageal), type 4 (blood-borne) and type 5 (subjective).

24.5 Diagnosis

Diagnosis is based on accurate and comprehensive history taking and clinical examination as well as carrying out relevant special investigations.

History should contain full medical history, including recent medications, and completion of a halitosis questionnaire about diet, dry mouth, severity of halitosis, mouth breathing, bad taste, smoking, alcohol, oral hygiene and mouthwash use.

Clinical examination should include oral inspection of the tongue (for bacterial coating), soft and hard tissues and periodontal assessment.

Relevant special investigations that may be required for diagnosis of halitosis are as follows.

- Organoleptic measurements for mouth and nose involve the patient closing the mouth for 1 minute and

Diseases and Conditions in Dentistry: An Evidence-Based Reference, First Edition. Keyvan Moharamzadeh.

Companion website: www.wiley.com/go/moharamzadeh/diseases

then exhaling slowly with a distance of 10 cm from the nose of the examiner. Organoleptic scoring scales are: 0 (absence of halitosis), 1 (questionable), 2 (slight), 3 (moderate), 4 (strong) and 5 (severe halitosis) (Yaegaki and Coil, 2000).

- Sulfide monitors such as the Breathtron® (New Cosmos Electric, Osaka, Japan) or Halimeter® (Interscan Corporation, Chatsworth, CA), which measure the levels of sulfur emissions, can be very useful for diagnosis of intraoral halitosis but they are sensitive to alcohol and garlic which must be avoided before the test (Yoneda *et al.*, 2015).
- Gas chromatography (GC) devices such as OralChroma™ (Abilit, Osaka, Japan) and Twin Breasor™ (GC Co., Tokyo, Japan) are the gold standard for detection of different origins of halitosis. Collected air from the patient's mouth is injected into the GC device for analysis (Yoneda *et al.*, 2015).

Intraoral halitosis is characterised by low nose organoleptic score and high mouth score, as well as high hydrogen sulfide (H_2S) and methyl mercaptan levels and low dimethylsulfide level in GC examination.

Extraoral halitosis caused by nose and throat infection is characterised by high nose organoleptic score and low score for mouth.

Extraoral halitosis caused by systemic conditions is characterised by high and similar organoleptic scores for both nose and mouth.

24.6 Management Strategies

Identifying and addressing the cause and type of halitosis is an important aspect of patient management (Seemann *et al.*, 2014).

Patients with pseudo-halitosis and halitophobia would require psychiatrist referral (Coil *et al.*, 2002).

Temporary halitosis often requires no treatment. The use of tongue scrapers and mouthrinses before bed can be useful in reducing morning bad breath.

Patients suffering from xerostomia should be referred to oral medicine specialists for further investigation and treatment of dry mouth.

Extraoral halitosis caused by nose and throat infection would need to be referred to otorhinolaryngology specialists.

Extraoral halitosis caused by systemic conditions should be referred to appropriate medical specialists for treatment of the underlying systemic disease.

Intraoral physiological halitosis caused by tongue coating can be treated by mechanical tongue cleaning using tongue scrapers or tongue brushing with a toothbrush wetted with chlorhexidine mouthrinse or toothpaste. The use of mouthrinses can be effective in reducing oral malodour but their long-term use cannot be recommended due to their side effects (Loesche and Kazor, 2002).

Pathological intraoral halitosis caused by periodontal or peri-implant diseases, dry socket, oral infections and caries will require treatment of the underlying conditions (see Chapters 1, 5, 6, 30, 40, 41, 42 and 43).

Case Study

A 41-year-old female patient referred by her GDP presented with constant bad breath and taste and mobility of a lower front tooth.

The patient did not have any previous periodontal treatment and only had supragingival scaling and polishing by the GDP without local anaesthesia. There was no familial history of periodontal disease.

The patient was medically fit and well, a former smoker and did not drink alcohol. She had a normal diet and there was no history of dry mouth or mouth breathing.

Clinical examination showed presence of plaque and calculus deposits, mainly on the lingual aspect of the mandibular anterior teeth. Bacterial tongue coating was also noticed affecting between one-third and two-thirds of the tongue surface.

The BPE scores were 3 in LL and UL quadrants and 4 in all other quadrants, with generalised 4–9 mm periodontal pockets and bleeding on probing. LR1 was grade III mobile and UL1 had drifted forward as shown in Figure 24.1.

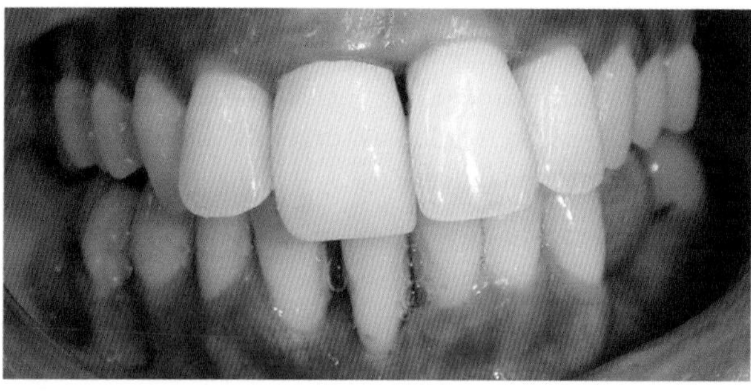

Figure 24.1 Preoperative clinical photograph.

Radiographic examination showed generalised mild to moderate periodontal bone loss and advanced periodontal bone loss associated with LR1.

Organoleptic measurements for mouth and nose gave a high score (4) for mouth and low score (0) for nose, indicating strong intraoral halitosis.

The diagnosis of generalised moderate chronic periodontitis was made. The disease was more advanced in the mandibular incisor region with severe attachment loss on LR1 which had a hopeless prognosis.

The following treatment was provided.

1) Oral hygiene instructions including modified Bass technique and interdental brushing, tongue cleaning with a tongue scraper or toothbrush and the use of chlorhexidine antiseptic mouthrinse.
2) Root surface debridement under local anaesthesia in all sites with deep periodontal pockets equal to or greater than 4 mm.
3) LR1 was extracted and its root was shortened, smoothed, sealed with composite resin and splinted to the adjacent teeth using an adhesive composite fibre splint (Figure 24.2).
4) Periodontal reassessment and retreatment of the sites with residual deep pockets.
5) Supportive periodontal therapy (SPT).

The patient responded very well to non-surgical periodontal treatment and reported significant improvement in symptoms and complete resolution of halitosis following the above treatment. Probing pocket depths and other periodontal indices were significantly reduced at the second reassessment.

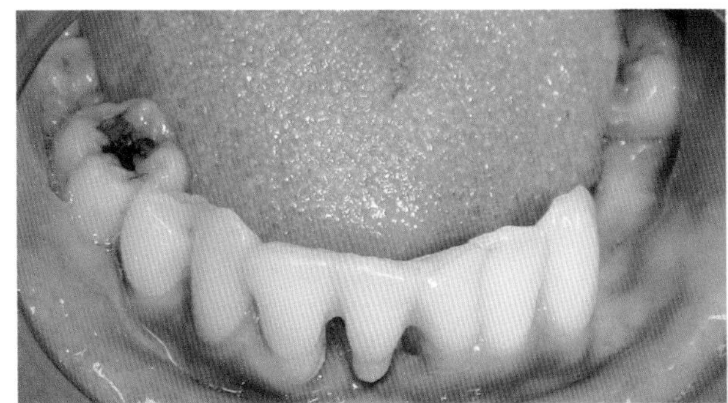

Figure 24.2 Postoperative clinical photograph showing the extracted and splinted LL1.

Orthodontic referral for the alignment of the drifted maxillary incisor teeth was recommended to the patient to address her aesthetic concern since the periodontal health of the teeth was maintained satisfactorily after non-surgical periodontal treatment.

References

Akaji, E.A., Folaranmi, N. and Ashiwaju, O. (2014) Halitosis: a review of the literature on its prevalence, impact and control. *Oral Health Prev Dent*, **12**, 297–304.

Aydin, M. and Harvey-Woodworth, C.N. (2014) Halitosis: a new definition and classification. *Br Dent J*, **217**, E1.

Coil, J.M., Yaegaki, K., Matsuo, T. and Miyazaki, H. (2002) Treatment needs (TN) and practical remedies for halitosis. *Int Dent J*, **52**(Suppl 3), 187–191.

De Geest, S., Laleman, I., Teughels, W., Dekeyser, C. and Quirynen, M. (2016) Periodontal diseases as a source of halitosis: a review of the evidence and treatment approaches for dentists and dental hygienists. *Periodontology 2000*, **71**, 213–227.

Lindhe, J., Lang, N.P. and Karring, T. (2008) *Clinical Periodontology and Implant Dentistry*, 5th edn, Wiley-Blackwell, Oxford.

Loesche, W.J. and Kazor, C. (2002) Microbiology and treatment of halitosis. *Periodontology 2000*, **28**, 256–279.

Miyazaki, H., Arao, M., Okamura, K. *et al.* (1999) Tentative classification of halitosis and its treatment needs. *Niigata Dent J*, **32**, 7–11.

Seemann, R., Conceicao, M.D., Filippi, A. *et al.* (2014) Halitosis management by the general dental practitioner – results of an international consensus workshop. *J Breath Res*, **8**, 017101.

Tangerman, A. (2002) Halitosis in medicine: a review. *Int Dent J*, **52**(Suppl 3), 201–206.

Tangerman, A. and Winkel, E.G. (2010) Extra-oral halitosis: an overview. *J Breath Res*, **4**, 017003.

Yaegaki, K. and Coil, J.M. (2000) Examination, classification, and treatment of halitosis; clinical perspectives. *J Can Dent Assoc*, **66**, 257–261.

Yoneda, M., Suzuki, N., Hirofuji, T. (2015) Current status of the techniques used for halitosis analysis. *Austin Chromatogr*, **2**, 1024.

25

Hypodontia

25.1 Definition and Classification

Hypodontia is defined as developmental absence of teeth (Hobkirk *et al.*, 2012). This condition can be classified based on the number of missing teeth into three categories.

- Hypodontia: missing fewer than six teeth excluding the third molars.
- Oligodontia: missing six or more teeth excluding the third molars.
- Anodontia: missing all the teeth.

Based on the severity, hypodontia can be classified as follows.

- Mild: 1–2 missing teeth excluding the third molars.
- Moderate: 3–5 teeth missing excluding the third molars.
- Severe: six or more teeth missing excluding the third molars.

And based on syndrome association, it can be grouped as follows.

- Isolated hypodontia: not associated with any syndrome.
- Syndromic hypodontia: associated with syndromes.

25.2 Aetiology

Hypodontia is believed to be multifactorial and associated with genetic, epigenetic and environmental factors (Parkin *et al.*, 2009). These factors include:

- conditions and over 150 syndromes such as ectodermal dysplasia, Down's syndrome, cleft lip and palate, Ellis–van Creveld syndrome, hereditary osteodystrophy, toxic epidermal necrolysis, Crouzon's and Albright's syndromes
- increased maternal age, low birth weight, multiple births and rubella infection during embryonic life
- hormonal defects such as hypoparathyroidism
- environmental factors such as radiation exposure, chemotherapy and allergy
- genetic factors, including over 80 genes; mainly Msx1, Pax9, Axin2 and EDA are known to be related to tooth agenesis (Yin and Bian, 2015).

25.3 Epidemiology

The overall prevalence of hypodontia is 6.4%. Prevalence is highest in Africa (13.4%) followed by Europe (7%), Asia (6.3%), Australia (6.3%), North America (5.0%) and Latin America and Caribbean (4.4%) (Khalaf *et al.*, 2014).

Females have a higher prevalence than males (3:2 ratio). Missing third molars occur in 9–30% of the population. The prevalence of missing primary teeth is 0.1–0.9%, with a 1:1 male to female ratio. Permanent anomalies are found in 30–50% of cases with missing primary teeth.

The most commonly missing teeth are the third molars (25–35%), mandibular second premolars (3%), maxillary lateral incisors (2%), maxillary second premolars (<2%) and mandibular incisors (<2%). Maxillary central incisors are the least affected (Bishop *et al.*, 2006).

25.4 Clinical Features

The following clinical features can be seen in hypodontia patients (Hobkirk *et al.*, 2012).

- Missing teeth
- Microdontia
- Conical teeth
- Ectopic eruption
- Retained primary teeth
- Tooth surface loss (TSL)
- Reduced alveolar development
- Increased free way space (FWS) due to TSL and reduced alveolar development

Diseases and Conditions in Dentistry: An Evidence-Based Reference, First Edition. Keyvan Moharamzadeh.

Companion website: www.wiley.com/go/moharamzadeh/diseases

- Delayed eruption of permanent teeth
- Altered craniofacial morphology
- Poor aesthetics
- Spacing
- Reduced oral health-related quality of life

25.5 History and Examination

Relevant history includes:

- medical history to identify possible causes and syndromes
- familial history of hypodontia
- adverse parafunctional habits
- patient's social history, attendance, preference and expectations
- previous dental treatment and access to long-term care and maintenance.

Clinical examination of hypodontia patients should include:

- examination of the soft tissues and gingival biotype
- oral hygiene and periodontal assessment
- caries examination
- tooth size, shape, colour and position, especially in relation to the facial and dental midlines, crowding and spacing
- assessment of retained primary teeth, infraocclusion and ankylosis
- tooth wear and sensitivity assessment
- assessment of colour difference and gingival level mismatch between canines and anterior teeth
- assessment of alveolar bone width and height in edentulous areas
- evaluation of the static occlusal relationship and, in particular, the interocclusal space available in the edentulous regions
- examination of the dynamic occlusal relationship to determine if anterior guidance is present, and whether it can be preserved
- FWS assessment, particularly when restoring the vertical height with overdentures.

25.6 Relevant Investigations

In addition to thorough history taking and clinical examination, the following further information and special investigations may be required in treatment planning of hypodontia patients.

- Clinical photographs with full face, smile line and lip line.
- Oral panoramic (OPT) and lateral cephalometric radiographs.
- Periapical radiographs of the teeth adjacent to the edentulous areas to assess the teeth and their root parallelism.
- Articulated study models to enable occlusal analysis.
- Orthodontic opinion to treat malocclusion and idealise the edentulous spaces and the position of the teeth for subsequent restorative treatment.
- Diagnostic wax-up when planning for restorative-only treatment.
- Kesling diagnostic set-up is recommended to illustrate the feasibility of space opening versus space closure prior to orthodontic treatment. Digital Kesling-type set-up can also be a helpful tool (Sandler *et al.*, 2005).
- Percussion, mobility testing and radiographic examination of infra-occluded (ankylosed) retained primary teeth.
- Cone beam computed tomography (CBCT) scan provides a three-dimensional image to assess the alveolar bone width and height, position of inferior alveolar and mental nerves and maxillary sinus level as part of planning for potential implant treatment (Harris *et al.*, 2012).

25.7 Care Pathway

Patients are usually referred by their general medical (GP) or dental (GDP) practitioners, specialist orthodontists or through tertiary referral from another hospital. These patients often go through an integrated care pathway in multidisciplinary hypodontia clinics (Gill and Barker, 2015; Stevenson *et al.*, 2013).

The hypodontia team may provide only advice for treatment, only orthodontic treatment and advice for restorative treatment or all of the orthodontic and restorative treatment, depending on the circumstances.

In situations where there are in-house resource issues or long patient waiting lists, involvement of the GDPs on an outreach basis as part of a managed clinical network (MCN) can be helpful.

Treatment phases may involve (1) interceptive orthodontic/restorative therapy, (2) definitive orthodontics, (3) intermediate restorative therapy, (4) definitive restorative therapy and (5) long-term maintenance.

25.8 Multidisciplinary Team

The roles of the MDT team involved with the management of hypodontia patients are described below.

- *Orthodontist*: growth modification, treatment of malocclusion, space closure, space opening and optimisation, root parallelism, tooth repositioning, orthodontic management of ectopic or partially erupted teeth, advice to extract primary teeth, and retention (Addy *et al.*, 2006; Lewis *et al.*, 2010).

- *Paediatric dentist*: behavioural management, prevention, treatment of caries, composite build-ups in childhood, resin-bonded bridges (RBB), and overdentures in severe cases (Nunn *et al.*, 2003).
- *Restorative dentist*: advice to the orthodontist on the ultimate locations and sizes of edentulous spaces and intended functional occlusion, restoration of spaces following orthodontic treatment, and advice to the GDP on maintenance (Bishop *et al.*, 2007a; Durey *et al.*, 2014b).
- *Oral and maxillofacial surgeon (OMFS)*: extractions, surgical exposures of ectopic permanent teeth, autotransplantation of teeth, bone grafting and sinus augmentation surgery prior to the placement of dental implants, and orthognathic surgery (Breeze *et al.*, 2017; Durey *et al.*, 2014a).
- Other members of the team include the GDP (shared dental care and maintenance), nurse (first contact), laboratory technician (laboratory support, retainer fabrication), psychologist (psychological well-being), clinical geneticist (genetic counselling), dermatologist (syndrome support) and speech and language therapist (SLT) (Hobkirk *et al.*, 2012).

25.9 Restorative Considerations

Important restorative considerations in the management of hypodontia are listed below (Bishop *et al.*, 2006; Durey *et al.*, 2014b).

- Patient's age, compliance and expectations, including the parent's wishes.
- Previous dental treatment and long-term access to care and maintenance.
- Presence, position and eruptive potential of all unerupted permanent teeth.
- Size, shape and location of all edentulous areas, including ridge morphology.
- Skeletal and existing dental occlusion.
- Predictability of any restorative treatment and its long-term effect on dentition.
- Presence or absence of syndromes.

Further restorative challenges in hypodontia patients include:

- retained primary teeth, wear, antagonist tooth overeruption and tilting of the adjacent teeth
- permanent teeth with atypical shape, spatial relationship, microdontia, ectopic canines and tooth transposition
- atrophic edentulous spaces
- reduced face height.

25.10 Treatment Considerations

25.10.1 Preventive Care

Behavioural management and preventive care, including oral hygiene education, fluoride therapy, fissure sealing and dietary advice, are particularly important in children. Caries and periodontal disease need to be treated first and maintained in the long term. Intermediate restorations can be placed in early adolescents.

25.10.2 Treatment Options for Missing Teeth

Treatment options for the missing teeth include (Addy *et al.*, 2006):

- no treatment and accepting the space
- restorative treatment alone using fixed restorations or removable prostheses
- orthodontic treatment alone to close the space
- combined orthodontic and restorative treatment
- orthodontic treatment and orthognathic surgery with or without restorative treatment.

25.10.3 Missing Maxillary Lateral Incisors

Treatment options specifically for bilateral missing permanent maxillary lateral incisor teeth are listed below (Savarrio and McIntyre, 2005).

- Accepting the space.
- Orthodontic space closure and reshaping (lateralising) the canine tooth.
- Orthodontic space opening to provide ideal spaces for a RBB or dental implant.
- Restorative-only treatment by replacing the missing lateral incisors with RBBs or dental implants.

Treatment of unilateral missing anterior teeth is more challenging due to the asymmetry and space opening is usually preferred in these cases. However, in addition to the above options, an alternative choice for unilateral cases is extraction of the contralateral maxillary lateral incisor tooth (especially if the tooth prognosis is poor), canine reshaping and orthodontic space closure.

25.10.3.1 Space Closure

Space closure is usually preferred in cases with crowding, class II malocclusion, and where the maxillary canine teeth are a good match to the lateral incisor teeth (Savarrio and McIntyre, 2005).

Canine teeth would require reduction of height, width (both buccolingually and mesiodistally) and contour of the tooth and addition of adhesive composite to the incisal edge. There is often a shade mismatch between the canine and incisor teeth and possible need for single tooth bleaching prior to composite restoration.

Gingival contour of the canine tooth is normally more apical compared to the lateral incisor. Canines may need to be extruded to reverse the gingival margin position in relation to the central incisor to appear more like a lateral incisor tooth.

Root prominence of canine teeth can be corrected by palatal root torque.

There are maintenance issues for composite restorations including staining and differential colour changes which would require future replacement.

Regarding occlusal guidance in mandibular excursions, it is best to either continue with canine guidance or change to a group function occlusal scheme. It is important to establish the guidance on the natural permanent teeth. If this is impossible, a group function occlusal scheme to share the occlusal loads would be preferred.

The first maxillary premolar may require the following modifications (Hobkirk *et al.*, 2012).

- Slight mesiopalatal rotation to hide the palatal cusp.
- Buccal torque to increase the root prominence.
- Reduction of the palatal cusp to act like a canine tooth if possible. However, if there is a risk of pulp exposure, intruding the first premolar to move the gingival margin apically and addition of composite to the occlusal surface to make the premolar tooth look like a canine and provide guidance would be recommended.

25.10.3.2 Space Opening

Space opening may be preferred in cases where there is generalised hypodontia, microdontia, spacing, skeletal class III malocclusion and class I with non-extraction lower arch. Patients with a 'toothy smile' can also be suitable for space opening. Large, yellow and bulbous canines with high gingival margin are not desirable for lateralising and space closure. Therefore, space opening is usually more appropriate in these patients (Savarrio and McIntyre, 2005).

Composite resin build-up of microdont teeth can be undertaken before, during or after orthodontic treatment, depending on the availability of space, degree of gingival inflammation and possibility of moisture control. Early build-up of primary teeth or microdont permanent teeth with composites can reduce the spacing, improve the appearance, increase the patient's self-confidence and create rapport with the dental team.

25.10.4 Missing Mandibular Incisor Teeth

A single missing mandibular incisor tooth can be managed by either orthodontic space closure or prosthetic replacement of the missing tooth (see below).

If two mandibular central incisor teeth are missing, it is recommended to close or reduce the space to one unit space to facilitate prosthetic replacement. If all four mandibular incisor teeth are missing, prosthetic replacement of the missing teeth is often the treatment of choice.

25.10.5 Maxillary Midline Diastema

Where there is frenum involvement, frenectomy should be considered.

If the size of the maxillary central incisors is within the acceptable range (0.75/0.85 width to length ratio), orthodontic space closure is preferred. If the central incisors are microdont, composite additions are recommended.

25.10.6 Management of Retained Primary Teeth

Primary teeth can be maintained up to 40–50 years of age if the permanent successor is missing. Delayed root resorption is variable depending on the teeth. Primary canine teeth show the least resorption and primary first molar teeth show the most resorption (Hobkirk *et al.*, 2012).

Benefits of retaining primary teeth include:

- masking the effect of hypodontia
- space maintenance
- maintenance of alveolar bone volume.

Risks of retaining primary teeth include:

- ankylosis and infraocclusion
- tipping of the adjacent teeth and overeruption of the opposing tooth
- impaction, caries development and periodontal disease
- tooth size (Bolton) discrepancy, making it difficult to achieve an ideal class I molar relationship
- retention of large Es complicates subsequent prosthetic tooth replacement due to large size and restricts orthodontic tooth movements even with stripping due to divergent roots.

Assessment of ankyloses can be carried out using the following tests.

- Percussion test which requires at least 20% root surface ankylosis to produce a metallic sound.
- Mobility test which requires at least 10% root surface ankylosis to be detected.
- Periapical radiograph showing an absent periodontal ligament which is a two-dimensional image and may not be precise.
- The most reliable indicator is the development of a vertical step (angular alveolar defect) in the interproximal bone around the infraoccluded molar.

Incidence of ankyosis is the highest in primary molar teeth, ranging from 1.5% to 9.9%. The degree of infraocclusion can be categorised according to the following classification (Brearley and McKibben, 1973).

- *Mild*: the infraoccluded tooth crown is above the contact point of the adjacent tooth and 1 mm below the occlusal plane.
- *Moderate*: the infraoccluded tooth crown is within the contact area.
- *Severe*: the infraoccluded tooth crown is below the contact point.

Risks of removal of an ankylosed primary mandibular molar include difficult removal, risk of mental nerve damage and traumatic alveolar bone loss which would compromise subsequent implant treatment or orthodontic tooth movement.

The following recommendations can be made for the management of infraoccluded primary molars.

- If the tooth is mildly infraoccluded and there is minimal remaining vertical facial growth, it is best to monitor the tooth.
- If the tooth is moderately infraoccluded and is healthy with good root length and there is no tipping of adjacent teeth, it is best to maintain and restore the occlusal surface with composites, gold onlays or preformed metal crowns.
- If the tooth is severely infraoccluded and the adjacent molar tooth is tilting, or if the tooth is carious, it is best to consider extraction of the retained primary tooth and orthodontic space management and/or prosthetic replacement.

25.10.7 Prosthetic Options to Replace the Missing Teeth

Prosthetic options for replacing missing teeth include RBB, conventional bridge, removable partial denture (RPD) or overdenture and implant-retained prosthesis (Bishop *et al.*, 2007a, b; Morgan and Howe, 2003).

25.10.7.1 Resin-bonded Bridge (RBB)

An RBB is a conservative, minimally invasive fixed treatment option for the replacement of missing teeth and is desirable especially in young patients (with intact abutment teeth) who are still growing and too young to receive implant treatment. RBBs provide reliable short- to medium-term longevity for patients with hypodontia (Allen *et al.*, 2016) and can be considered as an acceptable and definitive restoration for many hypodontia patients if provided by experienced clinicians (Garnett *et al.*, 2006).

Important factors to consider when planning for RBB treatment include patient factors such as age, expectations, motivation, compliance, parafunctional habits and access to GDP for maintenance, and site-related factors such as the length of the edentulous space, position and quality of the abutment teeth, occlusion and aesthetics (Durey *et al.*, 2011).

Recommended RBB is a cantilever design for single tooth replacement in most cases. Fixed-fixed design or two separate cantilever bridges can be used when replacing two adjacent missing teeth.

Surgical exposure of the full clinical crown may be necessary in young patients to maximise the enamel surface area for bonding (Elder and Djemal, 2008).

Use of heavily restored abutments should be avoided if possible. Existing restorations should be replaced with composites and minimal or no preparation of the sound abutment teeth is recommended in most cases (Dayanik, 2016).

It is important to ensure that adequate interocclusal space is available or created for the pontic. The dimension of the pontic should be reduced with minimal contacts at the intercuspal position (ICP) and it is recommended to avoid loading the pontic in excursive movements and only load the retainer against the cement.

Extending the retainer to the incisal edges of the anterior abutment teeth will result in grey-out appearance. The use of opaque cements may help to reduce the grey appearance.

The metal retainer should be 0.7 mm thick and extended onto the occlusal surfaces of the posterior abutment teeth to maximise the bonding area if allowed by the patient's aesthetic demands (Durey *et al.*, 2011).

Options to manage a ridge defect in the pontic area include:

- surgical pontic site augmentation
- camouflage with gingival-coloured ceramics
- incorporation of the root contours if the adjacent teeth have recession
- use of removable acrylic denture flanges.

In hypodontia patients who have had orthodontic treatment, orthodontic retention is required after fitting a RBB. Retention can be achieved by either making a new removable orthodontic retainer or incorporating a palatal groove in the RBB framework to allow placement of a fixed wire retainer.

Where a midline diastema has been closed and there is bilateral absence of maxillary lateral incisor teeth, a double cantilever design can be considered. However, there is a risk of debonding from one retainer and caries development or relapse which will require close monitoring and maintenance.

Several studies have investigated the clinical performance and survival of RBBs (Aggstaller *et al.*, 2008;

Creugers, 1991; Djemal *et al.*, 1999; Hussey and Linden, 1996; Kellett *et al.*, 1994; King *et al.*, 2015), fibre-reinforced resin-bonded fixed bridges (van Heumen *et al.*, 2009) and fixed-movable bridges (Botelho and Dyson, 2005).

In a systematic review and meta-analysis by Thoma *et al.* (2017), reporting on 2300 RBBs, the following observations were made.

- Estimated 5-year survival of RBBs was 91.4% and 10-year survival was 82.9%.
- Survival rate was significantly higher for RBBs with zirconia framework compared to RBBs made from other materials.
- Cantilever RBBs had a significantly higher survival rate and a lower debonding rate than RBBs with fixed-fixed design.
- Anterior RBBs had higher survival rate than posterior RBBs.
- The most frequent modes of failure were debonding (15% over 5 years) and chipping of the veneering material (4.1% over 5 years).

25.10.7.2 Conventional Bridge

Full-coverage conventional bridges can be considered in older patients if the abutment teeth are restored and are not suitable for RBBs. However, there is a high risk of pulpal injury during extensive tooth preparations (Mjor and Odont, 2001). Therefore, conservative designs are recommended such as partial coverage, short-span, cantilever, metal surface coverage if aesthetic allows and hygienic pontics.

Root-treated teeth and teeth with post crowns are less desirable abutments for conventional bridges (see Chapter 18).

Tilted abutments can be up-righted by orthodontic treatment prior to bridge preparation.

Many studies have evaluated the clinical performance of conventional bridges (Heintze and Rousson, 2010; Layton, 2011; Pjetursson and Lang, 2008; Raigrodski *et al.*, 2012; Sailer *et al.*, 2007). Pjetursson *et al.* (2015) conducted a meta-analysis of clinical studies on the survival of porcelain fused to metal (PFM) and all-ceramic fixed bridges and reported the following results.

- The estimated 5-year survival rate of PFM bridges were 94.4%.
- The estimated 5-year survival of all ceramic bridges were: 85.9% for reinforced glass ceramic bridges, 86.2%, for glass-infiltrated alumina–based bridges, and 90.1% for densely sintered zirconia bridges (Pjetursson *et al.*, 2017).
- Compared to the PFM bridges, the survival rates were statistically significantly lower for reinforced glass ceramic bridges and the glass-infiltrated alumina bridges.
- Incidence of secondary caries were higher in abutment teeth of densely sintered zirconia bridges compared to PFM bridges.
- Framework fracture rate was higher for reinforced glass ceramic bridges (10.1%) and glass-infiltrated alumina bridges (12.9%) compared to PFM bridges (0.6%) and densely sintered zirconia bridges (1.9%).
- The incidence of ceramic fractures and loss of retention was significantly higher for densely sintered zirconia bridges compared to all other types of bridges.

25.10.7.3 Removable Partial Denture (RPD) and Overdenture

An RPD is a simple and quick option for the replacement of missing teeth in hypodontia patients and can be used as a temporary solution until definitive fixed restorations are placed. However, an RPD can be plaque retentive and would require strict periodontal maintenance. RPD treatment is further discussed in Chapter 38.

Overdentures are indicated for the treatment of severe oligodontia in early and late childhood until the patient is old enough for implant treatment. Overdentures are often well tolerated in oligodontia patients due to the increased FWS. They can restore the reduced lower face height and can also be used as a fluoride tray to prevent the remaining teeth from developing dental caries. Overdentures can also be useful in patients with significant skeletal problems (see Chapter 16).

25.10.7.4 Implant-Retained Prosthesis

Implant treatment is fully discussed in Chapter 37. Important aspects of implant treatment in hypodontia patients are discussed below (Bishop *et al.*, 2007b; Durey *et al.*, 2014a; Holst *et al.*, 2008; Morgan and Howe, 2004).

Implants are usually not suitable for young growing children and there is a risk of damage to the permanent tooth germs as well as the risks of general anaesthesia. Therefore, implant treatment should be delayed until growth is complete. Growth records can be useful to determine growth completion. The most reliable method is to superimpose two lateral-cephalometric radiographs with 6–12 months interval to confirm growth cessation.

General site-related implant requirements are as follows.

- Minimum 6–7 mm mesiodistal space is required to replace a missing lateral incisor or a premolar tooth.
- Root parallelism with adequate space between the roots of the teeth adjacent to the edentulous space is required prior to implant placement.
- Usually 7 mm of interocclusal space is required, although this can be minimised to around 4 mm when fixture head-level impressions and customised abutments are used.
- Implant shoulder should ideally be placed at 3 mm below the level of the labial gingival margin of the

healthy adjacent teeth but not more than 5 mm below the contact point and the interdental papillae must be preserved in the aesthetic zone, especially in patients with high lip line.

- Adequate bone volume is required which can be assessed using different methods: clinical and 2D radiographic examination, CBCT, direct evaluation during surgery, and ridge mapping.
- The implant fixture should have adequate size and length to achieve good primary stability without causing damage to the adjacent anatomical structures.

Oral hygiene education and access to long-term care and maintenance of implants are essential components of care.

25.10.8 General Maintenance Requirements

To prevent relapse, immediate new orthodontic retainers are required following prosthetic replacement of the missing teeth if the patient has had previous orthodontic treatment as the patient's old retainers may not fit. Retainer wear in most cases is recommended for 6 months full-time, followed by 6 months night-only wear and then several nights per week indefinitely. Retainer wear and appropriate oral hygiene instruction require periodic re-emphasis.

Complications of orthodontic treatment also include root resorption, loss of tooth vitality, and gingival recession which may require further treatment.

Restorative maintenance issues include RBB debonding, caries, implant complications and failure of restorations which may require repair, replacement and further treatment.

Regular monitoring is required for occlusal changes, tooth wear, composite restorations, crowns and bridges for debond, periodontal diseases, caries and loss of vitality.

If a RBB fails frequently in a young patient, it is preferred to wear a RPD and not a conventional bridge until the patient is old enough for implant treatment. An RPD will also require appropriate maintenance.

Implant maintenance includes plaque control and regular clinical and radiographic assessment of the implants, bone levels and management of any biological or biomechanical complications (see Chapters 37 and 40).

Case Study

Two clinical cases are presented in this chapter.

Case 1

A 17-year-old male patient presented with missing mandibular central and lateral incisors, maxillary lateral incisors and first premolars following orthodontic treatment which included moving the maxillary canines to the lateral incisor position and leaving the space distal to the canines for prosthetic tooth replacement. The patient preferred fixed bridges.

Preoperative clinical photographs are shown in Figure 25.1.

The diagnoses were severe hypodontia (oligodontia), microdontia, tooth wear and gingival recession on LR4 and LR5.

The treatment strategy included prevention, composite build-up of worn anterior teeth, adhesive bridges to replace the missing teeth, monitoring gingival recession as the patient did not want any surgical treatment, retention and maintenance.

The following treatment procedures were carried out.

1) Preparation of articulated study models, diagnostic wax-up and intraoral rehearsal.
2) Direct composite build-up of maxillary central incisor teeth and reshaping the maxillary canines to resemble lateral incisor teeth.

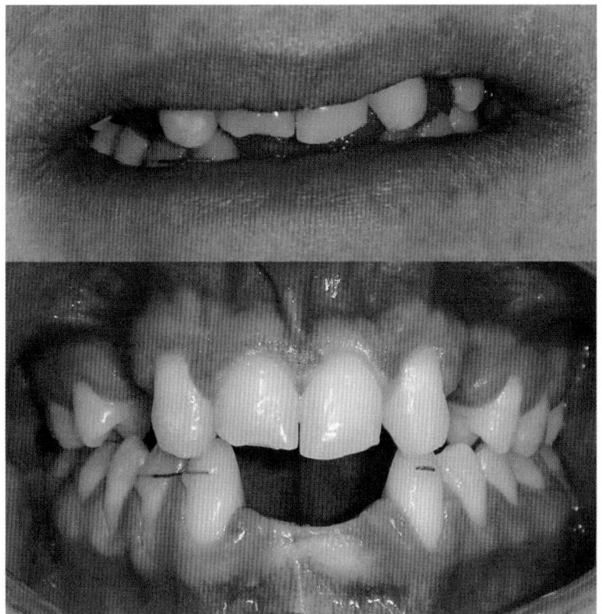

Figure 25.1 Preoperative clinical photographs.

3) Fabrication and cementation of resin-bonded bridges LL2–LR2, UR3–UR2 and UL3–UL2 (Figure 25.2) using Panavia™ F2.0 (Kuraray, New York) cement.

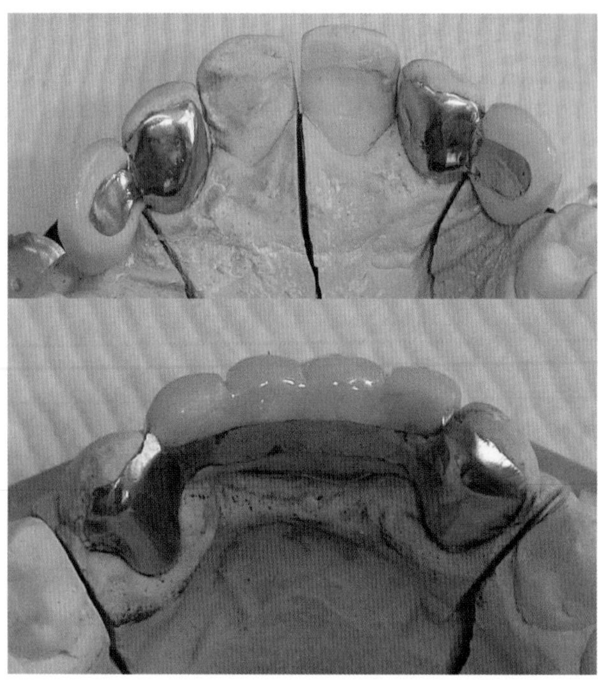

Figure 25.2 Lower fixed-fixed and upper cantilever PFM RBBs on the cast.

4) Fabrication and fitting of immediate upper and lower Essix retainers.
5) Review and maintenance.

The patient's postoperative clinical photographs are shown in Figure 25.3.

There were several important learning points in this case.

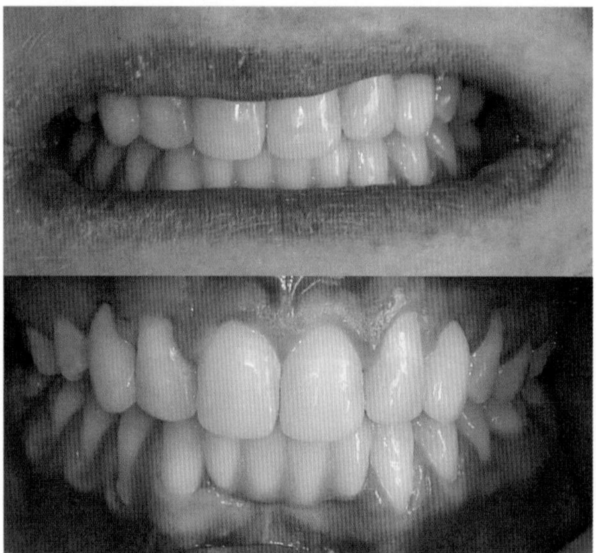

Figure 25.3 Postoperative clinical photographs.

- Composite build-up of worn incisor teeth using a stent made over the diagnostic wax-up significantly improved the appearance of the patient.
- There was inadequate bone available in all edentulous areas and the patient did not want to consider bone grafting and implant surgery. RBBs appeared to be the ideal fixed treatment options for this patient.
- A cantilever RBB design was used in the maxillary arch for single tooth replacement. A fixed-fixed RBB design was used in the anterior mandible with the addition of pink-shade porcelain to the gingival margins of the pontics to replace the missing soft tissue. This design will require careful monitoring of the abutment teeth for possible debond and prevention of secondary caries development. There is limited evidence available on the clinical performance of fixed-fixed RBBs replacing four incisor teeth (see above).
- There was inadequate space for the maxillary first premolars to be replaced. The patient accepted the space distal to the canines and was not prepared to consider further orthodontic treatment. With careful positioning of the canine pontics, the visibility of the spaces distal to the canines was minimised.
- This patient had a thin gingival biotype which could be a contributing factor to the development of inflammatory or traumatic gingival recession following orthodontic treatment. Management of gingival recession defects is discussed in Chapter 23.
- Long-term follow-up of this patient showed a satisfactory outcome and the patient was satisfied with the aesthetics and function.

Case 2

A 21-year-old male patient was referred by an orthodontist for restorative management of congenitally missing teeth. The patient had previous orthodontic treatment to create ideal spaces for prosthetic replacement of the missing maxillary lateral incisors and mandibular premolar teeth. The lack of retainer wear had resulted in some relapse and the patient was not prepared to have any further orthodontic treatment and was seeking a restorative-only solution.

The patient's preoperative clinical photographs and radiograph are shown in Figures 25.4 and 25.5 respectively.

The diagnoses were severe hypodontia (oligodontia), missing UR2, 4, 5, 8, UL2, 4, 5, 8, LR4, 5, 7, 8, LL4, 5, 7, 8, retained primary maxillary lateral incisor teeth, microdontia, tooth wear (attrition of UR1 and UL1), reduced OVD, gingivitis, localised gingival recession LR6 and class III malocclusion with posterior open bite.

The treatment strategy included prevention, composite build-ups on UR1, UR3, UL1, UL3 and UL6, implant-retained single crowns for UR2 and UL2, RBBs to replace LR4, 5 and LL4, and maintenance

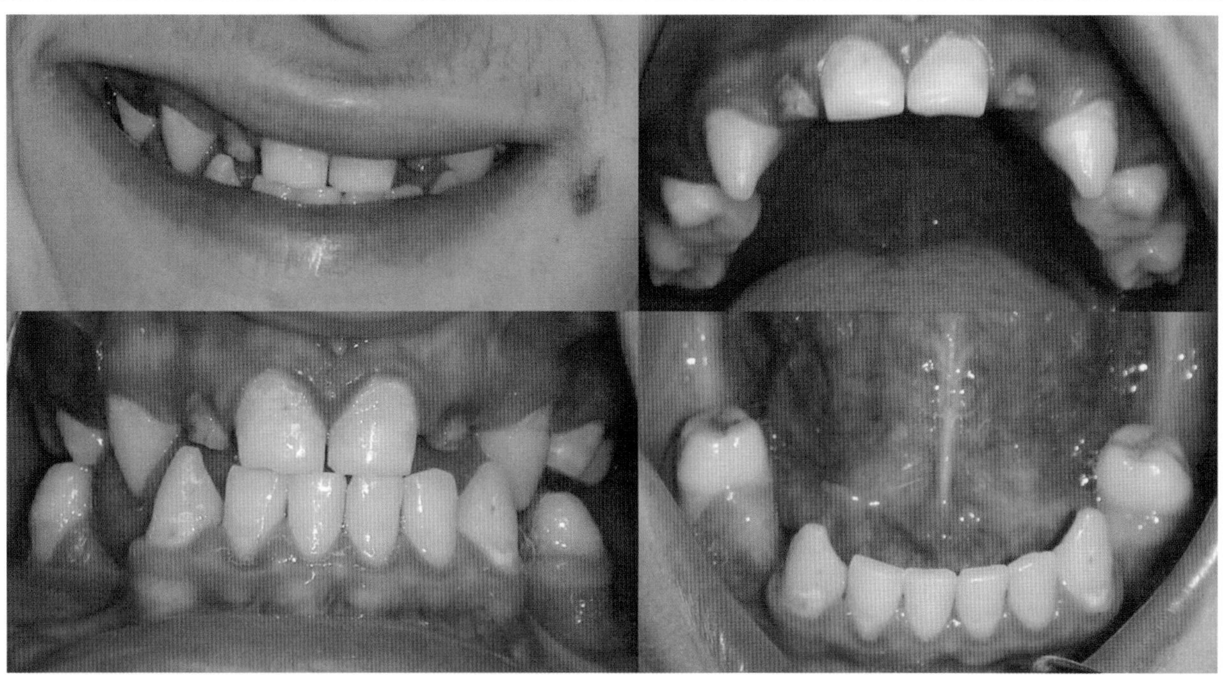

Figure 25.4 Preoperative clinical photographs.

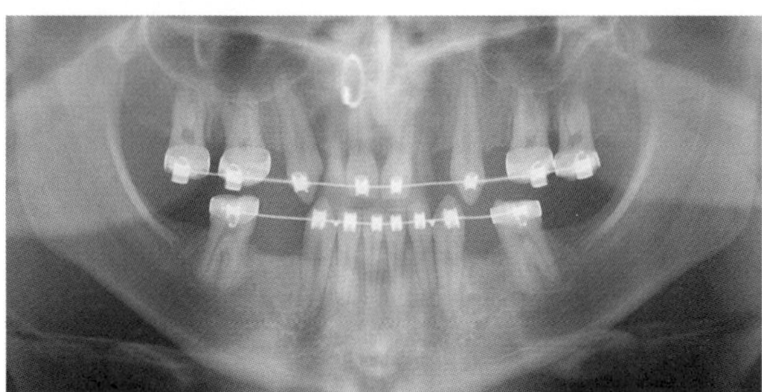

Figure 25.5 Pre-debond panoramic radiograph showing missing 16 permanent teeth and retained primary maxillary lateral incisors.

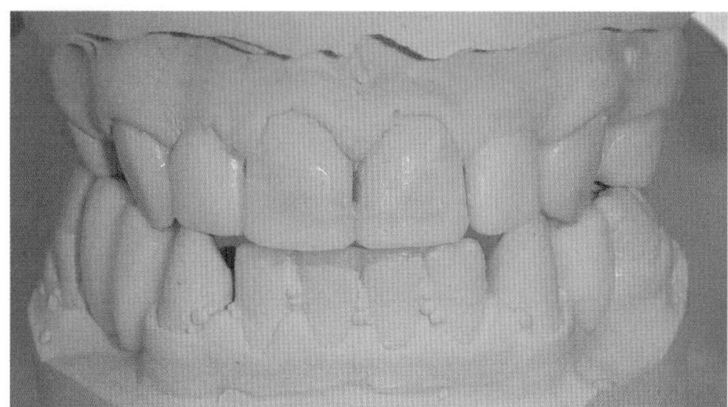

Figure 25.6 Diagnostic wax-up at an increased VD.

The following treatment procedures were carried out.

1) Preventive care, OHI, scaling and polishing.
2) Preparation of articulated study models and diagnostic wax-up at an increased vertical dimension to create restorative space (Figure 25.6).
3) Composite restorations of UR1, UR3, UL1, UL3 and UL6 at 2 mm increased VD.
4) Fabrication of surgical guide for implant placement.
5) Extraction of URB and ULB and immediate placement of implants (Figure 25.7).
6) Restoration of implants with provisional crowns.
7) Fabrication and fitting of CAD-CAM custom-made zirconia abutments and all- ceramic lithium disilicate crowns (Figure 25.8).
8) Fabrication and fitting of a cantilever RBB LL6–LL5 and a fixed-movable RBB LR6–LR3 (Figure 25.9).
9) Review and maintenance.

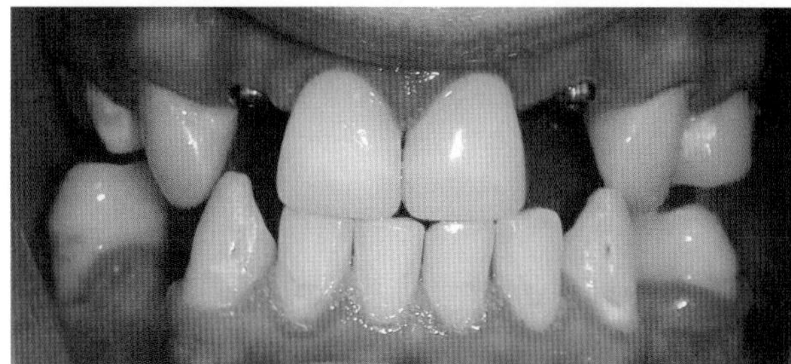

Figure 25.7 Clinical photograph of composite restorations and implants with healing abutments in the lateral incisor positions.

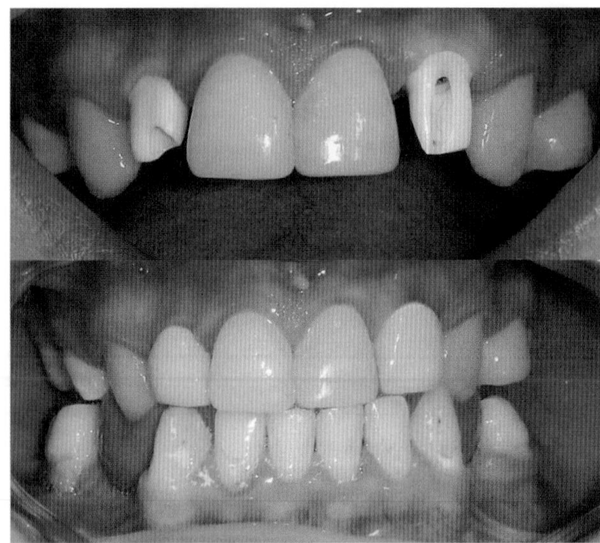

Figure 25.8 CAD-CAM zirconia abutments and all-ceramic crowns.

The patient's postoperative clinical photograph and radiographs are shown in Figures 25.10 and 25.11 respectively.

This was a challenging case and there were a number of learning points.

- Importance of plaque control and patient motivation and co-operation prior to embarking on complex restorative treatment.
- Usefulness of diagnostic wax-up to visualise the final intended treatment outcome and achieve ideal tooth size, shape and position to facilitate composite build-ups and also guide appropriate implant placement.
- Implant planning and placement (see Chapter 37).
- Aesthetic management of labially emerging implant screw access hole and thin gingival tissue using zirconia abutment (to avoid dark metal shadow) and cement-retained ceramic crown.
- Use of an RBB cantilever design was appropriate for single mandibular left premolar tooth replacement. An occlusal onlay fixed-movable adhesive bridge was chosen to

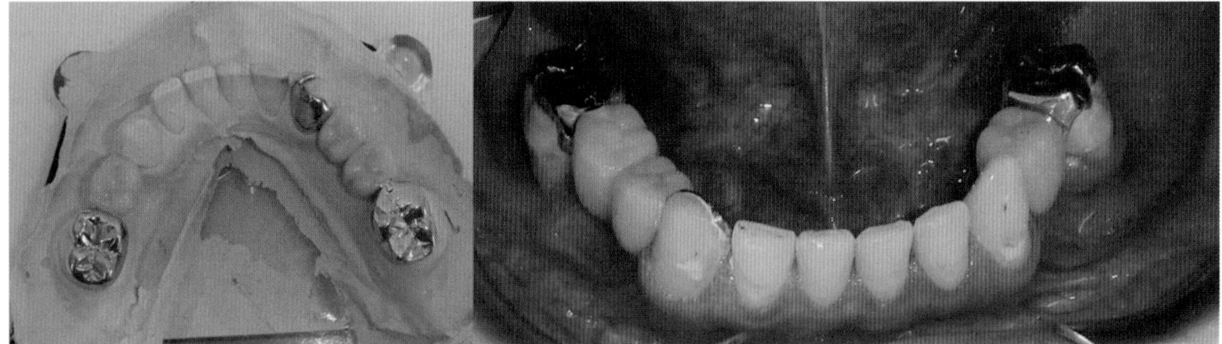

Figure 25.9 Cantilever RBB LL6–LL5 and the fixed-movable RBB LR6–LR3.

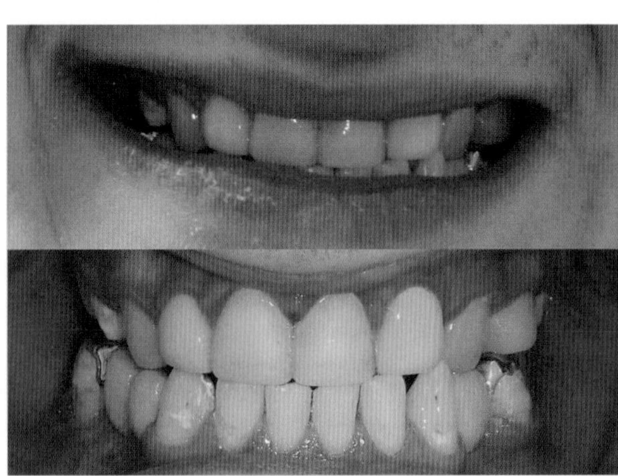

Figure 25.10 Postoperative clinical photographs.

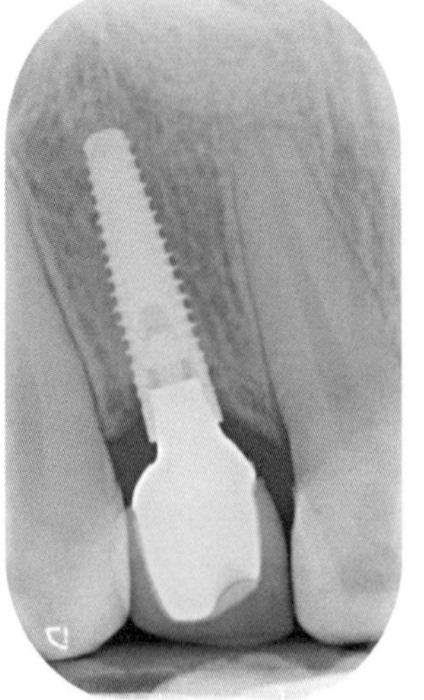

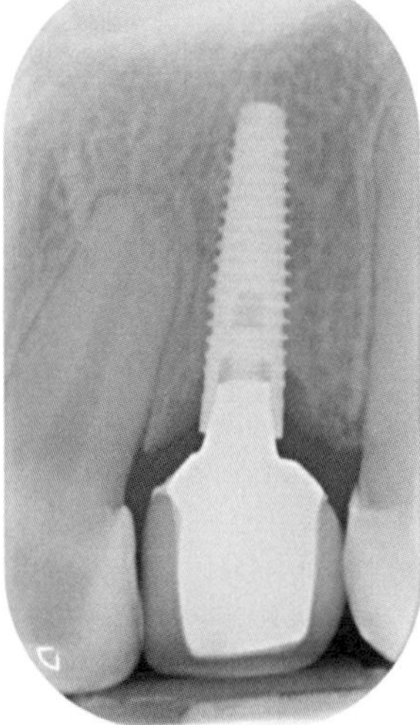

Figure 25.11 Postoperative periapical radiographs of the implant-retained crowns.

restore the longer span edentulous space in the mandibular right premolar region with severely atrophic ridge and inadequate bone for implant treatment. Limitations of bone grafting and implant treatment in atrophic mandible are discussed in Chapter 37.

The patient was very satisfied with the functional and aesthetic outcome of the treatment.

Maintenance issues in this case included the maintenance of composite restorations, resin-bonded bridges and implant-retained crowns as discussed previously in the text.

References

Addy, L., Bishop, K. and Knox, J. (2006) Modern restorative management of patients with congenitally missing teeth: 2. Orthodontic and restorative considerations. *Dent Update*, **33**, 592–595.

Aggstaller, H., Beuer, F., Edelhoff, D., Rammelsberg, P. and Gernet, W. (2008) Long-term clinical performance of resin-bonded fixed partial dentures with retentive preparation geometry in anterior and posterior areas. *J Adhes Dent*, **10**, 301–306.

Allen, P.F., Anweigi, L. and Ziada, H. (2016) A prospective study of the performance of resin bonded bridgework in patients with hypodontia. *J Dent*, **50**, 69–73.

Bishop, K., Addy, L. and Knox, J. (2006) Modern restorative management of patients with congenitally missing teeth: 1. Introduction, terminology and epidemiology. *Dent Update*, **33**, 531–534, 537.

Bishop, K., Addy, L. and Knox, J. (2007a) Modern restorative management of patients with congenitally missing teeth: 3. Conventional restorative options and considerations. *Dent Update*, **34**, 30–32, 34, 37–38.

Bishop, K., Addy, L. and Knox, J. (2007b) Modern restorative management of patients with congenitally missing teeth: 4. The role of implants. *Dent Update*, **34**, 79–80, 82–84.

Botelho, M.G. and Dyson, J.E. (2005) Long-span, fixed-movable, resin-bonded fixed partial dentures: a retrospective, preliminary clinical investigation. *Int J Prosthodont*, **18**, 371–376.

Brearley, L.J. and Mckibben, D.H. Jr (1973) Ankylosis of primary molar teeth. I. Prevalence and characteristics. *Asdc J Dent Child*, **40**, 54–63.

Breeze, J., Dover, M.S. and Williams, R.W. (2017) Contemporary Surgical Management Of Hypodontia. *Br J Oral Maxillofac Surg.*

Creugers, N. H. (1991. Resin–Bonded Bridges. A status report for the American Journal of Dentistry. *Am J Dent*, **4**, 251–255.

Dayanik, S. (2016) Resin-bonded bridges – can we cement them 'high'? *Dent Update*, **43**, 243–244, 247–250, 253.

Djemal, S., Setchell, D., King, P. and Wickens, J. (1999) Long-term survival characteristics of 832 resin-retained bridges and splints provided in a post-graduate teaching hospital between 1978 and 1993. *J Oral Rehabil*, **26**, 302–320.

Durey, K.A., Nixon, P.J., Robinson, S. and Chan, M.F. (2011) Resin bonded bridges: techniques for success. *Br Dent J*, **211**, 113–118.

Durey, K., Carter, L. and Chan, M. (2014a) The management of severe hypodontia. Part 2: Bone augmentation and the provision of implant supported prostheses. *Br Dent J*, **216**, 63–68.

Durey, K., Cook, P. and Chan, M. (2014b) The management of severe hypodontia. Part 1: Considerations and conventional restorative options. *Br Dent J*, **216**, 25–29.

Elder, A.R. and Djemal, S. (2008) Electrosurgery: a technique for achieving aesthetic and retentive resin-bonded bridges. *Dent Update*, **35**, 371–374, 376.

Garnett, M.J., Wassell, R.W., Jepson, N.J. and Nohl, F.S. (2006) Survival of resin-bonded bridgework provided for post-orthodontic hypodontia patients with missing maxillary lateral incisors. *Br Dent J*, **201**, 527–534; discussion 525.

Gill, D.S. and Barker, C.S. (2015) The multidisciplinary management of hypodontia: a team approach. *Br Dent J*, **218**, 143–149.

Harris, D., Horner, K., Grondahl, K. *et al.* (2012) E.A.O. guidelines for the use of diagnostic imaging in implant dentistry 2011. A consensus workshop organized by the European Association for Osseointegration at the Medical University of Warsaw. *Clin Oral Implants Res*, **23**, 1243–1253.

Heintze, S.D. and Rousson, V. (2010) Survival of zirconia- and metal-supported fixed dental prostheses: a systematic review. *Int J Prosthodont*, **23**, 493–502.

Hobkirk, J.A., Gill, D., Jones, S.P. *et al.* (2012) *Hypodontia: A Team Approach to Management*, Wiley-Blackwell, Oxford.

Holst, S., Geiselhoringer, H., Nkenke, E., Blatz, M.B. and Holst, A.I. (2008) Updated implant-retained restorative solutions in patients with hypodontia. *Quintessence Int*, **39**, 797–802.

Hussey, D.L. and Linden, G.J. (1996) The clinical performance of cantilevered resin-bonded bridgework. *J Dent*, **24**, 251–256.

Kellett, M., Verzijden, C.W., Smith, G.A. and Creugers, N.H. (1994) A multicentered clinical study on posterior resin-bonded bridges: the 'Manchester Trial.' *J Dent*, **22**, 208–212.

Khalaf, K., Miskelly, J., Voge, E. and Macfarlane, T.V. (2014) Prevalence of hypodontia and associated factors: a systematic review and meta-analysis. *J Orthod*, **41**, 299–316.

King, P.A., Foster, L.V., Yates, R.J., Newcombe, R.G. and Garrett, M.J. (2015) Survival characteristics of 771 resin-retained bridges provided at a UK dental teaching hospital. *Br Dent J*, **218**, 423–428; discussion 428.

Layton, D. (2011) A critical appraisal of the survival and complication rates of tooth-supported all-ceramic and metal-ceramic fixed dental prostheses: the application of evidence-based dentistry. *Int J Prosthodont*, **24**, 417–427.

Lewis, B.R., Gahan, M.J., Hodge, T.M. and Moore, D. (2010) The orthodontic-restorative interface: 2. Compensating for variations in tooth number and shape. *Dent Update*, **37**, 138–140, 142–144, 146–148 passim.

Mjor, I.A. and Odont, D. (2001) Pulp-dentin biology in restorative dentistry. Part 2: Initial reactions to preparation of teeth for restorative procedures. *Quintessence Int*, **32**, 537–551.

Morgan, C. and Howe, L. (2003) The restorative management of hypodontia with implants: I. Overview of alternative treatment options. *Dent Update*, **30**, 562–568.

Morgan, C. and Howe, L. (2004) The restorative management of hypodontia with implants: 2. Planning and treatment with implants. *Dent Update*, **31**, 22–30.

Nunn, J.H., Carter, N.E., Gillgrass, T.J. *et al.* (2003) The interdisciplinary management of hypodontia: background and role of paediatric dentistry. *Br Dent J*, **194**, 245–251.

Parkin, N., Elcock, C., Smith, R.N., Griffin, R.C. and Brook, A.H. (2009) The aetiology of hypodontia: the prevalence, severity and location of hypodontia within families. *Arch Oral Biol*, **54**(Suppl 1), S52–56.

Pjetursson, B.E. and Lang, N.P. (2008) Prosthetic treatment planning on the basis of scientific evidence. *J Oral Rehabil*, **35**(Suppl 1), 72–79.

Pjetursson, B.E., Sailer, I., Makarov, N.A., Zwahlen, M. and Thoma, D.S. (2015) All-ceramic or metal-ceramic tooth-supported fixed dental prostheses (FDPS)? A systematic review of the survival and complication rates. Part II: Multiple-unit FDPS. *Dent Mater*, **31**, 624–639.

Pjetursson, B.E., Sailer, I., Makarov, N.A., Zwahlen, M. and Thoma, D.S. (2017) Corrigendum to 'All-ceramic or metal-ceramic tooth-supported fixed dental prostheses (FDPS)? A systematic review of the survival and complication rates. Part II: Multiple-unit FDPS' [Dental Materials 31 (6) (2015) 624–639]. *Dent Mater*, **33**, E48–E51.

Raigrodski, A.J., Hillstead, M.B., Meng, G.K. and Chung, K.H. (2012) Survival and complications of zirconia-based fixed dental prostheses: a systematic review. *J Prosthet Dent*, **107**, 170–177.

Sailer, I., Pjetursson, B.E., Zwahlen, M. and Hammerle, C.H. (2007) A systematic review of the survival and complication rates of all-ceramic and metal-ceramic reconstructions after an observation period of at least 3 years. Part II: Fixed dental prostheses. *Clin Oral Implants Res*, **18**(Suppl 3), 86–96.

Sandler, J., Sira, S. and Murray, A. (2005) Photographic 'Kesling set-up'. *J Orthod*, **32**, 85–88.

Savarrio, L. and Mcintyre, G.T. (2005) To open or to close space––that is the missing lateral incisor question. *Dent Update*, **32**, 16–18, 20–22, 24–25.

Stevenson, B., Patel, D., Ricketts, D. and Cord, A. (2013) The orthodontic-restorative interface in patients with hypodontia: the patient's journey. *Dent Update*, **40**, 354–356, 358–360.

Thoma, D.S., Sailer, I., Ioannidis, A., Zwahlen, M., Makarov, N. and Pjetursson, B.E. (2017) A systematic review of the survival and complication rates of resin-bonded fixed dental prostheses after a mean observation period of at least 5 years. *Clin Oral Implants Res*, **11**, 1421–1432.

Van Heumen, C.C., Kreulen, C.M. and Creugers, N.H. (2009) Clinical studies of fiber-reinforced resin-bonded fixed partial dentures: a systematic review. *Eur J Oral Sci*, **117**, 1–6.

Yin, W. and Bian, Z. (2015) The gene network underlying hypodontia. *J Dent Res*, **94**, 878–885.

26

Internal Root Resorption

26.1 Definition

Internal root resorption is defined as the progressive destruction of intraradicular dentine of the root canal walls as a result of clastic cells activities (Patel *et al.*, 2010).

26.2 Pathogenesis

The precise mechanisms of cellular activation in internal inflammatory root resorption are not fully understood. However, the receptor activator of nuclear factor kappa beta ligand (RANKL) and osteoprotegerin (OPG) signalling pathways are believed to play a major role in the modulation of clastic activity by multinuclear odontoclast cells involved in inflammatory root resorption, a process similar to bone resorption by osteoclasts (Low *et al.*, 2005).

Exposure of the mineralised dentine to pulp cells, following damage to the organic sheath, predentine and odontoblasts can potentially initiate the internal resorption process. The progression of resorption is dependent on two factors: (1) the pulp tissue at the resorption site must be vital, and (2) the coronal pulp above the resorption site must be necrotic and infected as bacterial stimulus is essential for the continuation of the inflammatory process (Haapasalo and Endal, 2006). Internal inflammatory resorption may stop if the whole canal becomes necrotic.

26.3 Predisposing Factors

Aetiological factors for internal root resorption include trauma, dentine cracks, pulpal disease, dens invaginatus, pulpotomy, restorative treatment, autotransplantation, orthodontic treatment and viral infection such as herpes zoster (Barclay, 1993; Haapasalo and Endal, 2006).

26.4 Epidemiology

The reported prevalence of internal root resorption is between 0.01% and 1% (Haapasalo and Endal, 2006). However, microscopic examination of extracted teeth has detected the presence of small internal resorption defects in 50% of teeth with pulpitis and 77% of teeth with pulp necrosis. These lesions are unlikely to be detected during conventional radiographic examination in most cases as complete pulp necrosis stops the growth of these resorptive lesions (Gabor *et al.*, 2012).

26.5 Classification

Internal resorption can be classified into three categories (Darcey and Qualtrough, 2013a).

- Internal surface resorption, which is a self-limiting process similar to external surface resorption (see Chapter 17).
- Internal inflammatory resorption, a purely destructive form of internal resorption resulting in progressive enlargement of the resorption defect within the root canal which may lead to root perforation (Patel *et al.*, 2010).
- Internal replacement resorption, a rare condition characterised by irregular resorption of the intraradicular dentine and replacement by osteoid and cementum-like tissues which may lead to pulp canal obliteration (Ne *et al.*, 1999).

26.6 Diagnosis

Diagnosis of internal root resorption is based on accurate clinical and radiographic assessment.

Diseases and Conditions in Dentistry: An Evidence-Based Reference, First Edition. Keyvan Moharamzadeh.

Companion website: www.wiley.com/go/moharamzadeh/diseases

26.6.1 Clinical Features

Internal root resorption may present as a pink (vital) or dark grey (non-vital) coronal lesion located centrally. Initially, the pulp may be vital, resembling symptoms of pulpitis, whereas complete pulp necrosis can develop symptoms of apical periodontitis (Patel *et al.*, 2010). Therefore, assessment of the vitality of the tooth must be part of clinical examination.

Perforation of the root can occur due to progression of the lesion which may lead to development of a sinus tract or a periodontal defect if the lesion communicates with the periodontal ligament (PDL) near the crestal alveolar bone.

26.6.2 Radiographic Features

Internal inflammatory root resorption is characterised by a uniform enlarged area of the root canal with smooth, sharp, clearly defined margins of the lesion.

Internal replacement resorption shows irregular enlargement of the pulp canal with evidence of obliteration or replacement with mixed radiolucent and opaque areas on radiographic examination.

Differentiating between internal replacement resorption and external cervical resorption can be challenging because the resorptive tissue often has a similar radiographic appearance (Haapasalo and Endal, 2006). In internal replacement resorption, the radiopaque line of demarcation between the root canal and the image of resorption in dentine is absent. However, in external cervical resorption, there is often a thin dentine wall between the vital pulp and the resorption area and the original shape of the root canal is intact and visible (Patel and Ford, 2007).

Cone beam computed tomography provides additional relevant information on the location, extent and nature of resorptive lesions and can be very useful in the diagnosis and treatment planning of cases of perforating root resorption defects (Bhuva *et al.*, 2011).

26.7 Treatment Considerations

The aim of treatment is to stop the resorptive process by eliminating its causes, eradicate the intraradicular bacterial infection, seal any present perforations, obturate the root canal system and provide an effective coronal restoration. Root canal treatment is often indicated for teeth with internal resorption (Darcey and Qualtrough, 2013b; Haapasalo and Endal, 2006; Heithersay, 2007; Patel *et al.*, 2010).

Further to the general guidelines for endodontic treatment discussed in Chapter 3, below are some of the specific considerations for management of teeth with internal resorption.

- Pulpal bleeding can be controlled effectively by extirpation of the pulp and removal of the resorptive lesion using a large instrument, unless there is a perforation.
- The root canal system must be irrigated using sodium hypochlorite solution. The use of passive ultrasonic irrigation or a self-adjusting file system may further enhance the efficiency of chemomechanical debridement of the canals with resorption cavity (Topcuoglu *et al.*, 2015).
- The root canal must be dressed using non-setting calcium hydroxide-based intracanal medicament for a few days.
- The apical portion of the root canal below the resorption cavity can be obturated using different conventional obturation techniques.
- Thermo-plasticised gutta percha (GP) (e.g. Obtura system) and vertical compaction technique can be used to obturate non-perforated internal resorption cavities.
- MTA or Biodentine can be used to seal the perforated lesions.
- Flowable composite can be used in large coronal resorption areas to reinforce a tooth with thin root canal walls.
- In cases of internal replacement resorption, endodontic treatment may be complicated by the presence of calcified tissue within the resorption cavity, which it may be possible to remove using techniques such as curettage, application of trichloracetic acid and use of ultrasonic tips.

The prognosis of non-surgical endodontic treatment is usually good for non-perforated cases and is guarded for perforated teeth, depending on the size of resorption and the size and location of the perforation. The use of MTA has improved the prognosis in perforated cases (Bogen and Kuttler, 2009). Surgical treatment may be indicated in failed treatment cases (Asgary *et al.*, 2014) or in perforated teeth with associated periodontal defects (see Chapter 39).

Case Study

A 37-year-old male patient complained of persistent swelling associated with UR1 which was the abutment of a cantilever PFM bridge replacing UR2. Clinical and radiographic examination (Figure 26.1) confirmed the diagnosis of internal root resorption of UR1 and chronic apical periodontitis with a sinus tract.

The prognosis of treatment was guarded due to the presence of a large periradicular lesion, open apex and perforated internal resorption. The patient wanted to keep the tooth and consider endodontic treatment.

The root canal treatment procedure is described below.

1) Local anaesthesia and rubber dam isolation.
2) Microscope magnification.
3) Preparation of access cavity through the crown.
4) Initial debridement of the canal and removal of the necrotic pulp tissue.
5) Further exploration of the canal showed presence of a perforating resorption lesion with an open apex (apical gauge: size 100).
6) WL determination using an electronic apex locator, Root ZX II Apex Locator (J. Morita, USA).
7) Instrumentation of the canal to the WL using ProTaper files and curved hand files to engage the walls of the resorption cavity.

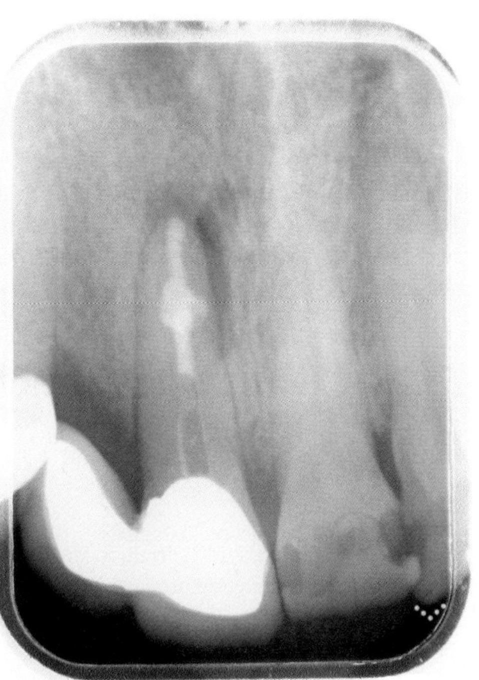

Figure 26.2 Periapical radiograph of the MTA plug at the apical half of the canal filling the perforated resorption cavity.

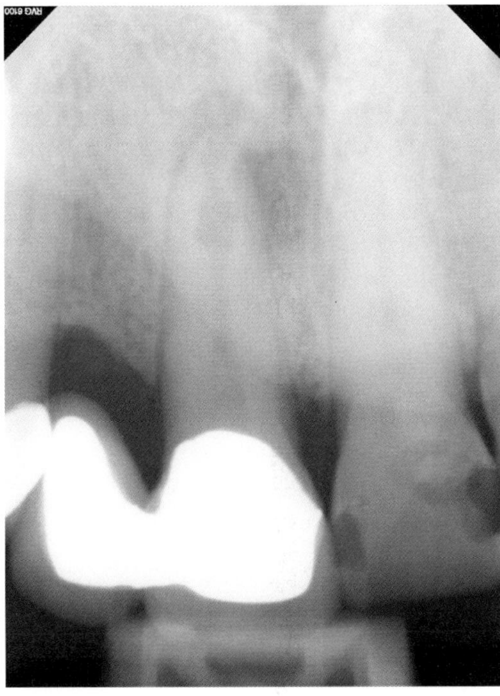

Figure 26.1 Preoperative periapical radiograph of UR1 showing the enlargement of the root canal at the apical third of the root and presence of periapical and lateral radiolucency indicating a possible laterally perforated internal root resorption lesion.

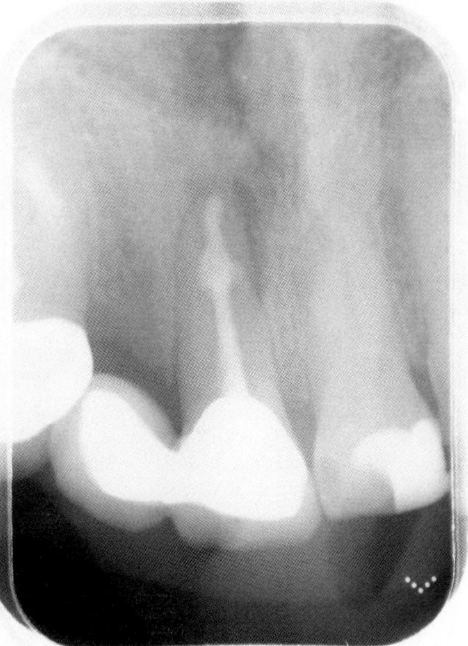

Figure 26.3 Postoperative periapical radiograph showing satisfactory root canal obturation and reduction in the size of periapical radioluceny in a short period of time compared to the preoperative radiograph.

8) Irrigation of the canal with 1% sodium hypochlorite solution. Care was taken to avoid apical extrusion of the irrigant, especially due to presence of an open apex and perforation. Normal saline solution was used at the very apical part of the canal.
9) Calcium hydroxide dressing for 2 weeks.
10) Obturation of the apical portion of the canal and the perforated resorption cavity with MTA (Figure 26.2) and backfill with thermo-plasticised GP using the Obtura system.
11) The access cavity was restored with a GIC base and composite resin.

The decision to obdurate the apical portion of the canal with MTA was made because the apical foramen was large and it appeared that the resorptive lesion had perforated the lateral wall of the root canal corresponding with the lateral radiolucency.

Chemomechanical debridement combined with dressing the canal with non-setting calcium hydroxide for 2 weeks resulted in resolution of the sinus tract and reduction of exudates in the canal, facilitating MTA plug placement.

The patient was asymptomatic at the time of obturation and there was already evidence of periapical healing on the postobturation radiograph (Figure 26.3), even within the short period of time compared to the preoperative radiograph. The patient was not available for 1-year follow-up.

References

Asgary, S., Eghbal, M.J., Mehrdad, L., Kheirieh, S. and Nosrat, A. (2014) Surgical management of a failed internal root resorption treatment: a histological and clinical report. *Restor Dent Endod*, **39**, 137–142.

Barclay, C. (1993) Root resorption. 2: Internal root resorption. *Dent Update*, **20**, 292–294.

Bhuva, B., Barnes, J.J. and Patel, S. (2011) The use of limited cone beam computed tomography in the diagnosis and management of a case of perforating internal root resorption. *Int Endod J*, **44**, 777–786.

Bogen, G. and Kuttler, S. (2009) Mineral trioxide aggregate obturation: a review and case series. *J Endod*, **35**, 777–790.

Darcey, J. and Qualtrough, A. (2013a) Resorption: Part 1. Pathology, classification and aetiology. *Br Dent J*, **214**, 439–451.

Darcey, J. and Qualtrough, A. (2013b) Resorption: Part 2. Diagnosis and management. *Br Dent J*, **214**, 493–509.

Gabor, C., Tam, E., Shen, Y. and Haapasalo, M. (2012) Prevalence of internal inflammatory root resorption. *J Endod*, **38**, 24–27.

Haapasalo, M. and Endal, U. (2006) Internal inflammatory root resorption: the unknown resorption of the tooth. *Endodontic Topics*, **14**, 60–79.

Heithersay, G.S. (2007) Management of tooth resorption. *Aust Dent J*, **52**, S105–121.

Low, E., Zoellner, H., Kharbanda, O.P. and Darendeliler, M.A. (2005) Expression of MRNA for osteoprotegerin and receptor activator of nuclear factor kappa beta ligand (RANKL) during root resorption induced by the application of heavy orthodontic forces on rat molars. *Am J Orthod Dentofacial Orthop*, **128**, 497–503.

Ne, R.F., Witherspoon, D.E. and Gutmann, J.L. (1999) Tooth resorption. *Quintessence Int*, **30**, 9–25.

Patel, S. and Ford, T.P. (2007) Is the resorption external or internal? *Dent Update*, **34**, 218–220, 222, 224–226, 229.

Patel, S., Ricucci, D., Durak, C. and Tay, F. (2010) Internal root resorption: a review. *J Endod*, **36**, 1107–1121.

Topcuoglu, H.S., Duzgun, S., Ceyhanli, K.T., Akti, A., Pala, K. and Kesim, B. (2015) Efficacy of different irrigation techniques in the removal of calcium hydroxide from a simulated internal root resorption cavity. *Int Endod J*, **48**, 309–316.

27

Irrigation Accidents

27.1 Introduction

Hulsmann *et al.* have comprehensively reviewed different types of irrigation-related accidents that may occur during endodontic treatment (Hulsmann and Hahn, 2000; Hulsmann *et al.*, 2009). This chapter contains a summary of these possible incidents and recommendations for their prevention and management.

27.2 Types of Incidents and Common Causes

Endodontic irrigation-related incidents include:

- injection of irrigants such as sodium hypochlorite into the periapical tissues (Mehdipour *et al.*, 2007; Zhu *et al.*, 2013)
- air emphysema due to hydrogen peroxide extrusion or drying root canals with compressed air or use of air-driven handpieces (Schuman *et al.*, 2001)
- allergic reactions to the irrigant's ingredients (Chia Shi Zhe *et al.*, 2016; Kaufman and Keila, 1989).

Most of these incidents happen due to wedging of the irrigating needle, inaccurate working length determination, excessive widening of the apical foramen and perforations (Guivarc'h *et al.*, 2017).

27.3 Signs and Symptoms

Common symptoms associated with most irrigation accidents include pain, swelling, ecchymosis, oedema, haemorrhage, ulceration, paraesthesia, and chlorine taste and irritation of throat in cases of injection into the maxillary sinus (Guivarc'h *et al.*, 2017; Hulsmann and Hahn, 2000).

27.4 Prevention

Appropriate precautions must be taken during endodontic treatment to minimise the risk of procedural errors that may lead to irrigant extrusion.

The irrigation needle must be safely secured and fixed to the syringe. The needle must be passive in the root canal and not be wedged into the canal. A low and constant finger pressure should be applied to the syringe during irrigation, ensuring that excess irrigant comes out of the access cavity, which should be immediately removed using the suction. A diluted but adequately effective concentration of the irrigant must be used.

Several alternative endodontic irrigation devices have been introduced to enhance the efficiency of irrigation and reduce the risk of irrigant extrusion (Pasricha *et al.*, 2015).

- The EndoVac system (Kerr Dental, Bioggio, Switzerland) uses negative vacuum pressure to deliver the irrigant into the root canal, and then pulls it up into the suction unit (Schoeffel, 2007, 2008a, b, 2009).
- The Quantec-E irrigation system (SybronEndo, Orange, CA) has a fluid delivery unit attached to an endodontic handpiece which enables continuous irrigation during rotary preparation (Walters *et al.*, 2002).
- The RinsEndo irrigation system (RinsEndo, Co. Duerr-Dental, Bittigheim-Bissingen, Germany) is based on automated irrigation using pressure and suction technology (McGill *et al.*, 2008).

EndoVac has significantly less potential for apical extrusion than photon-induced photoacoustic streaming and side-vented needle (Yost *et al.*, 2015). A systematic review has shown that apical negative pressure irrigation prevents the apical extrusion of irrigant (Romualdo *et al.*, 2017).

Diseases and Conditions in Dentistry: An Evidence-Based Reference, First Edition. Keyvan Moharamzadeh.

Companion website: www.wiley.com/go/moharamzadeh/diseases

27.5 Management

Based on the available literature evidence (Guivarc'h *et al.*, 2017; Hales *et al.*, 2001; Hulsmann *et al.*, 2009), the following recommendations can be made for the management of irrigation accidents.

- The clinician should remain calm, assist and reassure the patient, who may be anxious.
- The patient should be immediately informed about the cause and nature of the incident.
- Sodium hypochlorite solution must be removed from the tooth using an empty syringe to aspirate or using paper points and the root canal should be dressed with non-setting calcium hydroxide.
- In most mild cases no or only minimal intervention may be required.
- Local anaesthesia and prescription of appropriate analgesic medication can be helpful to reduce the acute pain.
- Cold compression can further reduce the swelling and pain.
- In severe cases where there is a high risk of infection spreading, hospital referral and antibiotic treatment are recommended.
- The patient must be reviewed daily until recovery.
- The patient should be informed that healing can take days to weeks, and that symptoms in most cases will resolve completely within 1 month (Kleier *et al.*, 2008).
- When the acute symptoms have subsided, root canal treatment can be completed. It is important to use a mild, non-irritating irrigant such as sterile normal saline solution in the apical part of the root canal or perforation area.
- In most cases, there is no indication for tooth extraction or surgical treatment. However, surgical management can be indicated in the treatment of inferior alveolar nerve injury caused by endodontic extrusion of a large amount of calcium hydroxide paste (Byun *et al.*, 2016).
- In cases where the irrigant is extruded into the maxillary sinus, radiographic examination is indicated to assess fluid levels in the sinus. Appropriate analgesia, antibiotics and referral for surgical drainage may also be indicated.
- If the patient is allergic to hypochlorite solution, it is best to avoid using chlorhexidine solution as well. A different irrigant can be used after allergy testing. Systemic corticosteroids and antihistamines may be required if a hypersensitivity reaction occurs (Hulsmann *et al.*, 2009).
- Air emphysema is self-limiting in most cases and does not require any special treatment. Pain and swelling resolve within a short period of time and only in rare cases will pain be persistent (Battrum and Gutmann, 1995). The prophylactic administration of a broad-spectrum antibiotic is recommended in these cases.

Case Study

A 57-year-old male patient was urgently referred by an undergraduate dental student for management of moderate to severe upper lip swelling and pain which had developed immediately following root canal treatment and obturation of UL3. The patient was medically fit and well.

Periapical radiograph of UL3 (Figure 27.1) showed an underextended and poorly obturated root canal filling.

Following an urgent consultation with an oral and maxillofacial consultant colleague, it was decided to admit the patient to hospital.

Immediate management included patient support, reassurance and pain control with oral paracetamol 1 g four times a day and ibuprofen 400 mg three times a day and cold compressions for the first 24 hours.

Systemic intravenous (IV) antibiotics, including amoxicillin and clavulanic acid (Augmentin) 1.2 g three times a day, were administered for 24 hours. Anti-inflammatory steroid hydrocortisone 100 mg was also given by slow IV injection.

The patient was reviewed after 24 hours and significant improvement was noticed following initial treatment. He was discharged from he hospital with prescription for oral analgesics and antibiotics – Augmentin 625 three times a day for a further 3 days.

The patient was reviewed weekly until full recovery and complete resolution of lip swelling and pain. However, the tooth remained tender to percussion and palpation.

Endodontic retreatment was carried out using retreatment rotary files to remove the old poorly obturated gutta percha and the root canal was irrigated with a low-concentration 0.5% hypochlorite solution in the coronal parts and normal saline solution in the apical part. Figure 27.2 shows the immediate postoperative radiograph following obturation of the canal.

At 9-month review, the patient was asymptomatic and radiographic examination showed complete periapical healing (Figure 27.3), indicating a successful outcome of endodontic retreatment.

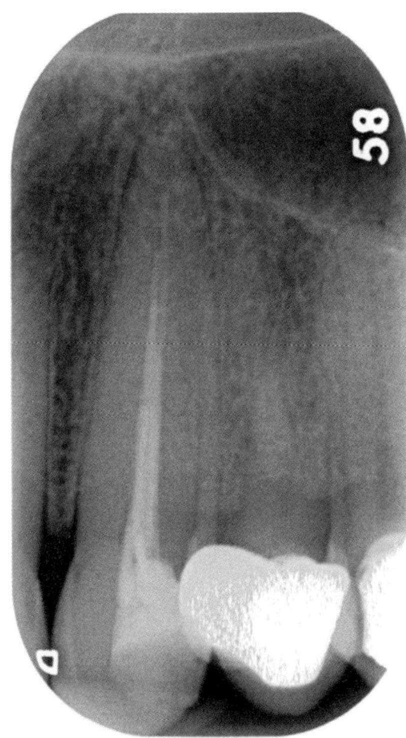

Figure 27.1 Periapical radiograph of UL3 obturated by the student showing poor-quality obturation.

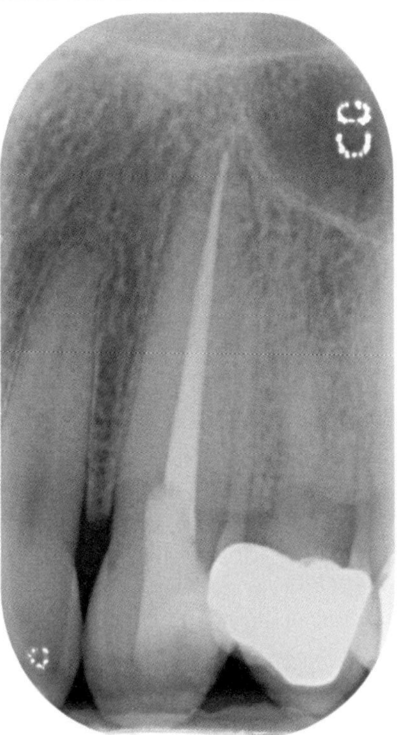

Figure 27.2 Immediate postoperative periapical radiograph showing optimal-quality obturation of the root canal.

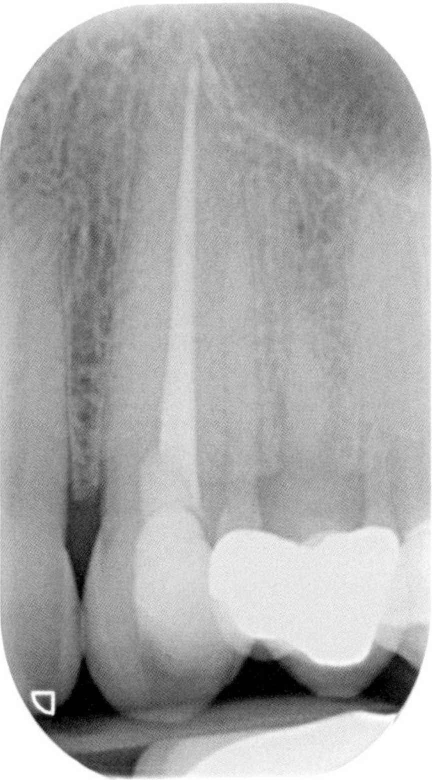

Figure 27.3 Follow-up periapical radiograph at 9 months showing complete periapical healing.

References

Battrum, D.E. and Gutmann, J.L. (1995) Implications, prevention and management of subcutaneous emphysema during endodontic treatment. *Endod Dent Traumatol*, **11**, 109–114.

Byun, S.H., Kim, S.S., Chung, H.J. *et al.* (2016) Surgical management of damaged inferior alveolar nerve caused by endodontic overfilling of calcium hydroxide paste. *Int Endod J*, **49**, 1020–1029.

Chia Shi Zhe, G., Green, A., Fong, Y.T., Lee, H.Y. and Ho, S.F. (2016) Rare case of type I hypersensitivity reaction to sodium hypochlorite solution in a healthcare setting. *BMJ Case Rep*, **2016**.

Guivarc'h, M., Ordioni, U., Ahmed, H.M., Cohen, S., Catherine, J.H. and Bukiet, F. (2017) Sodium hypochlorite accident: a systematic review. *J Endod*, **43**, 16–24.

Hales, J.J., Jackson, C.R., Everett, A.P. and Moore, S.H. (2001) Treatment protocol for the management of a sodium hypochlorite accident during endodontic therapy. *Gen Dent*, **49**, 278–281.

Hulsmann, M. and Hahn, W. (2000) Complications during root canal irrigation – literature review and case reports. *Int Endod J*, **33**, 186–193.

Hulsmann, M., Rodig, T. and Nordmeyer, S. (2009) Complications during root canal irrigation. *Endodont Top*, **16**, 27–63.

Kaufman, A.Y. and Keila, S. (1989) Hypersensitivity to sodium hypochlorite. *J Endod*, **15**, 224–226.

Kleier, D.J., Averbach, R.E. and Mehdipour, O. (2008) The sodium hypochlorite accident: experience of diplomates of the American Board of Endodontics. *J Endod*, **34**, 1346–1350.

McGill, S., Gulabivala, K., Mordan, N. and Ng, Y.L. (2008) The efficacy of dynamic irrigation using a commercially available system (Rinsendo) determined by removal of a collagen 'bio-molecular film' from an ex vivo model. *Int Endod J*, **41**, 602–608.

Mehdipour, O., Kleier, D.J. and Averbach, R.E. (2007) Anatomy of sodium hypochlorite accidents. *Compend Contin Educ Dent*, 28, 544–546, 548, 550.

Pasricha, S.K., Makkar, S. and Gupta, P. (2015) Pressure alteration techniques in endodontics – a review of literature. *J Clin Diagn Res*, 9, Ze01–06.

Romualdo, P.C., de Oliveira, K.M., Nemezio, M.A. *et al.* (2017) Does apical negative pressure prevent the apical extrusion of debris and irrigant compared with conventional irrigation? a systematic review and meta-analysis. *Aust Endod J*, **43**(3), 129–137.

Schoeffel, G.J. (2007) The Endovac method of endodontic irrigation: safety first. *Dent Today*, 26, 92, 94, 96 passim.

Schoeffel, G.J. (2008a) The Endovac method of endodontic irrigation, part 2 – efficacy. *Dent Today*, 27, 82, 84, 86–87.

Schoeffel, G.J. (2008b) The Endovac method of endodontic irrigation, part 3: system components and their interaction. *Dent Today*, **27**, 106, 108–111.

Schoeffel, G.J. (2009) The Endovac method of endodontic irrigation: part 4, clinical use. *Dent Today*, **28**, 64, 66–67.

Schuman, N.J., Owens, B.M. and Shelton, J.T. (2001) Subcutaneous emphysema after restorative dental treatment. *Compend Contin Educ Dent*, **22**, 38–40, 42.

Walters, M.J., Baumgartner, J.C. and Marshall, J.G. (2002) Efficacy of irrigation with rotary instrumentation. *J Endod*, **28**, 837–839.

Yost, R.A., Bergeron, B.E., Kirkpatrick, T.C. *et al.* (2015) Evaluation of 4 different irrigating systems for apical extrusion of sodium hypochlorite. *J Endod*, **41**, 1530–1534.

Zhu, W.C., Gyamfi, J., Niu, L.N. *et al.* (2013) Anatomy of sodium hypochlorite accidents involving facial ecchymosis – a review. *J Dent*, **41**, 935–948.

28

Low Maxillary Sinus Floor

Ian Brook - Case study

28.1 Introduction

The maxillary sinus expands inferiorly and laterally with age. Sinus pneumatisation and expansion is larger following extraction of the posterior molar teeth (Sharan and Madjar, 2008).

Sinus septa (also called Underwood septa) are present in approximately 38% of cases and are often located between the premolar and molar regions. The sinus lining is called Schneiderian membrane with a median thickness of 0.85 mm (Rancitelli *et al.*, 2015).

The presence of a low maxillary sinus floor and inadequate bone is a limiting factor for placement of dental implants in the posterior maxilla which often necessitates sinus augmentation (or sinus lift/sinus elevation/sinus graft) procedures (Pjetursson and Lang, 2015). However, options to avoid sinus augmentation in the posterior maxilla include:

- short implants (5–8 mm length) which usually require at least 6–8 mm bone height
- placement of tilted implants parallel to the mesial or distal wall of the maxillary sinus
- zygomatic implants in the lateral part of the zygomatic bone
- shortened dental arch limited to the anterior maxilla.

Different aspects of sinus augmentation procedures are described in the following sections.

28.2 Sinus Floor Elevation Techniques

There are two main techniques for elevation of the sinus floor: the lateral wall (window) approach (Wallace *et al.*, 2012) and the crestal approach (osteotome/transalveolar/Summers technique) (Pjetursson and Lang, 2014).

28.2.1 Lateral Approach

The lateral approach involves a modified Caldwell–Luc operation (Villacorta, 1967) to gain access to the sinus cavity.

28.2.1.1 Indications and Contraindications

Sinus augmentation using the lateral approach is indicated when there is severely reduced bone height (less than 6 mm remaining) for implant treatment in the posterior maxilla. This technique is also preferred over the crestal approach when there is an oblique sinus floor.

Contraindications to this approach include:

- medical reasons, including chemotherapy and radiotherapy within 6 months, severe bleeding disorders, immunocompromised patients, uncontrolled diabetes, bone metabolic diseases, drug and alcohol abuse, noncompliant patients and psychological conditions
- local factors, such as acute or chronic sinusitis, viral, bacterial, mycotic, allergic sinusitis, odontogenic sinusitis, allergic rhinitis and antral tumours
- any other conditions that contraindicate implant treatment (see Chapter 37).

28.2.1.2 Preoperative Assessment

It is important to carry out thorough preoperative assessment by obtaining a full medical and dental history, carrying out intraoral and extraoral examinations including maxillary sinus palpation as well as appropriate radiographic examination such as oral panoramic radiograph (OPT). Cone beam computed tomography (CBCT) is a useful tool which can identify interfering sinus septa, their orientation (Irinakis *et al.*, 2017) and the posterior superior alveolar artery in the lateral sinus wall (Varela-Centelles *et al.*, 2015).

Diseases and Conditions in Dentistry: An Evidence-Based Reference, First Edition. Keyvan Moharamzadeh.

Companion website: www.wiley.com/go/moharamzadeh/diseases

28.2.1.3 Surgical Approach

Sinus augmentation can be carried out as a separate surgical procedure prior to implant placement (two-stage technique) or it can be performed simultaneously at the time of implant placement (one-stage technique) (Figure 28.1) if there is at least a minimum 5 mm bone height to support the implant with good primary stability.

28.2.1.4 Bone Grafting

Although a successful outcome can still be achieved without placement of any graft material (Ellegaard *et al.*, 2006), options for graft materials that can be used include the following.

- Autologous bone grafts obtained from intraoral sites, such as mandible body, ramus and tuberosity, or extraoral sites such as iliac crest, tibial plateau, rib and calvaria; a 27–30% graft resorption rate over 10 years has been reported (Schmitt *et al.*, 2014).
- Bone substitutes which have a slower resorption rate compared to autologous bone.
- Combination of autologous bone and bone substitutes (Figure 28.2).

Systematic reviews show that the type of graft material used in sinus augmentation does not have a significant influence on implant survival (Al-Nawas and Schiegnitz, 2014; Cabezas-Mojon *et al.*, 2012; Papageorgiou *et al.*, 2016).

Barrier membranes have been used to enhance bone formation (Tarnow *et al.*, 2000) and to improve the outcome (Cabezas-Mojon *et al.*, 2012). However, there is insufficient evidence to prove that any sinus lift procedure is superior to any other in terms of implant survival (Esposito *et al.*, 2014).

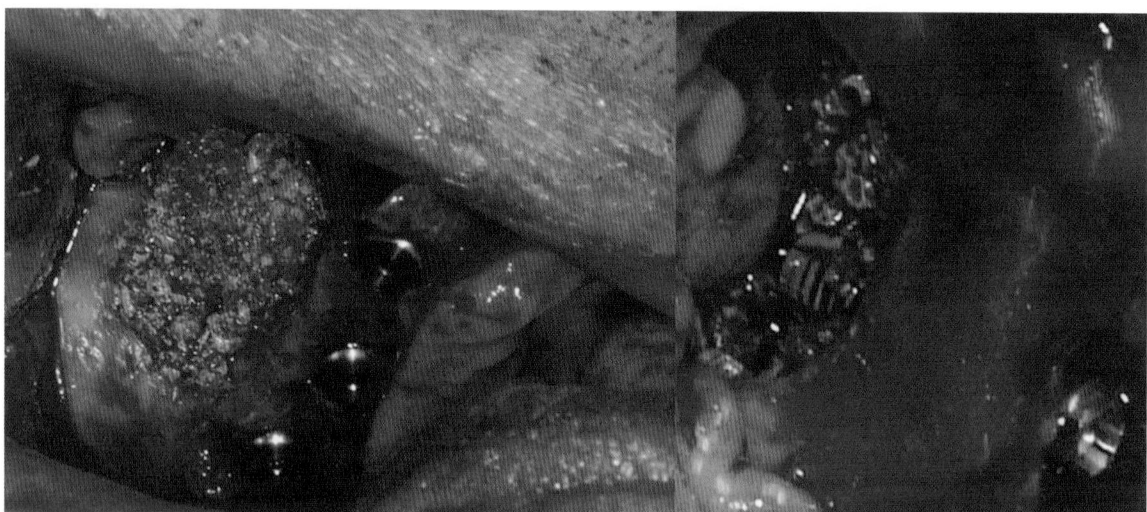

Figure 28.1 One-stage sinus augmentation procedure showing the lateral wall repaired with bone substitute following implant placement.

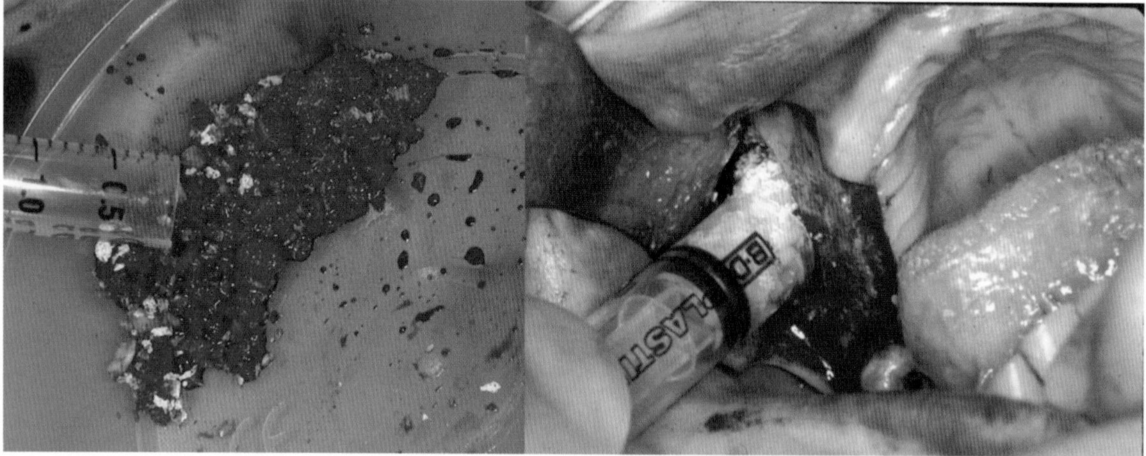

Figure 28.2 Mixture of autologous bone and bovine-derived bone graft substitute (Bio-Oss®, Geistlich, Wolhusen, Switzerland) used for sinus floor augmentation with lateral approach.

28.2.1.5 Postoperative Care and Complications

Postoperative care includes appropriate analgesia, application of a cooling pad over the sinus for the first hours to reduce swelling and advice to the patient to avoid nose blowing and sneezing. Postoperative antibiotics and chlorhexidine mouth rinse are also recommended.

Complications of the sinus augmentation procedure include the following (Pjetursson and Lang, 2015).

- Sinus membrane perforation (10–40% risk), which can be repaired using fibrin glue, suturing or membranes, depending on the size of perforation. If there is a large perforation and a stable superior border cannot be achieved, the augmentation procedure should be abandoned and re-entry attempted after 6–9 months.
- Excessive bleeding and wound dehiscence.
- Infraorbital nerve damage due to deep dissection to release the flap.
- Implant migration and hematoma.
- Damage to the adjacent teeth and sensitivity.
- Infection, graft failure, parasinusitis and the spread of infection to the orbit and brain in which case the graft must be removed and high-dose antibiotics must be administered.
- Sinusitis.
- Late failure such as chronic infection, graft exposure, graft loss, oral-antral fistula (OAF), soft tissue ingrowth and sinus cyst.

28.2.2 Crestal Approach

The crestal approach involves an intrusion osteotomy through the alveolar ridge to elevate the sinus floor and create a tent for bone graft material (Pjetursson and Lang, 2014). It is a more conservative surgical technique compared to the lateral approach and often provides good implant primary stability, although there is uncertainty about possible perforation of the sinus membrane.

This approach is indicated where there is type III and type IV bone with residual bone height of 5–7 mm, flat sinus floor and adequate crestal bone width for an implant.

Contraindications to this technique include the general contraindications for sinus augmentation as discussed above as well as inner ear complications, potential vertigo and oblique sinus floor with more than 45° inclination.

Surgical technique involves (1) depth cut and osteotomy preparation up to 2 mm from the sinus floor; (2) greenstick fracture using multiple ostetomes with increasing sizes; (3) testing sinus membrane with the Valsalva manoeuvre (nose blowing); (4) placement of bone graft material; and (5) implant placement.

Evidence shows this technique is predictable and has a high implant survival rate and a low incidence of complications (Corbella *et al.*, 2015; Tan *et al.*, 2008).

28.3 Implant Survival

Based on systematic reviews and meta-analyses, reported survival rates (over 1 year) for implants placed in augmented maxillary sinus are around 95–99.5% regardless of the augmentation technique and materials used (Esposito *et al.*, 2014; Starch-Jensen *et al.*, 2018). This is similar to implant survival in non-grafted maxillae as well as the survival of short dental implants (99%) (Atieh *et al.*, 2012; Thoma *et al.*, 2015). However, sinus augmentation procedures are associated with an increased incidence of biological complications, higher morbidity and costs and increased surgical time compared to short dental implants (Sanz *et al.*, 2015).

Case Study

A 46-year-old female patient presented with a loose upper front tooth, missing teeth, difficulty eating on the right side and inability to tolerate a removable denture on the palate.

The patient was a non-smoker and medically fit and well.

Clinical examination showed missing UR4–UR8 and LR5–LR6. The maxillary anterior teeth were heavily restored and UR1 had a failed post crown with deep secondary subgingival caries.

Radiographic examination (Figure 28.3) showed a very low maxillary sinus floor on the right side and inadequate bone in the right maxillary molar region.

The treatment strategy included the following aspects.

- Prevention and oral hygiene optimisation.
- Extraction of non-restorable UR1 and replacement of this tooth with a fixed-fixed bridge.
- New indirect restorations on the remaining maxillary anterior teeth.
- Sinus augmentation in the right side using the lateral window approach (Figure 28.4) and inlay bone grafting with autologous bone harvested from the mandible (chin).
- Placement of dental implants in UR4, UR5 and UR6 region.
- Restoration of the implants with a screw-retained fixed porcelain fused to metal (PFM) prosthesis.

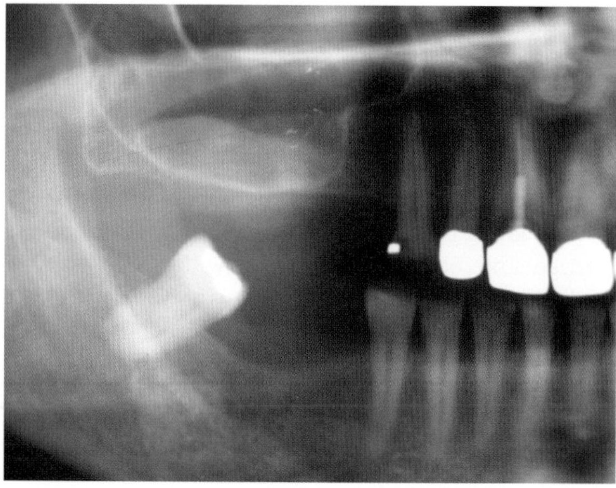

Figure 28.3 Sectional oral panoramic radiograph showing failed post crown UR1 with secondary caries and a low maxillary sinus floor with inadequate bone height in the right maxillary molar region.

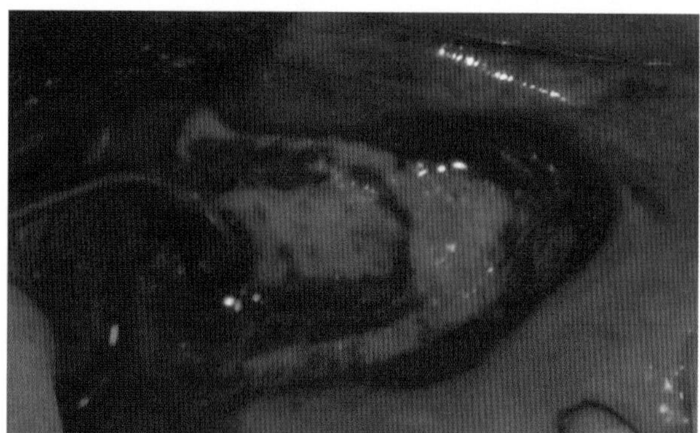

Figure 28.4 Clinical photograph of the lateral wall window access and elevation of the maxillary sinus membrane using a blunt instrument.

- Provision of a lower cobalt-chromium removable partial denture.
- Review and maintenance.

The postoperative radiograph following sinus augmentation and restoration of the implants is shown in Figure 28.5.

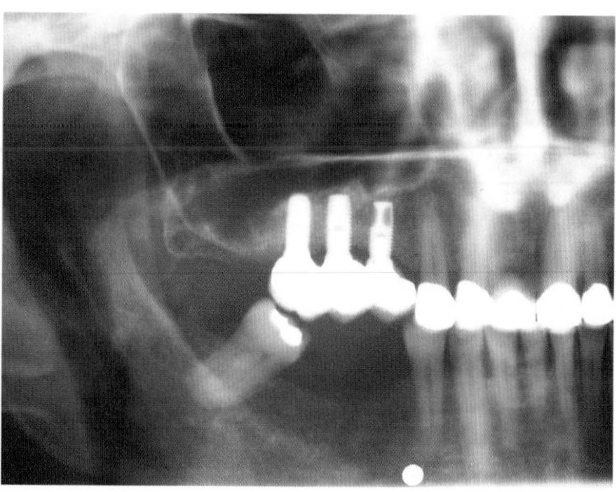

Figure 28.5 Postoperative sectional panoramic radiograph showing the implants in grafted maxillary sinus.

References

Al-Nawas, B. and Schiegnitz, E. (2014) Augmentation procedures using bone substitute materials or autogenous bone – a systematic review and meta-analysis. *Eur J Oral Implantol*, 7(Suppl 2), S219–234.

Atieh, M.A., Zadeh, H., Stanford, C.M. and Cooper, L.F. (2012) Survival of short dental implants for treatment of posterior partial edentulism: a systematic review. *Int J Oral Maxillofac Implants*, **27**, 1323–1331.

Cabezas-Mojon, J., Barona-Dorado, C., Gomez-Moreno, G., Fernandez-Caliz, F. and Martinez-Gonzalez, J.M. (2012) Meta-analytic study of implant survival following sinus augmentation. *Med Oral Patol Oral Cir Bucal*, **17**, E135–139.

Corbella, S., Taschieri, S. and del Fabbro, M. (2015) Long-term outcomes for the treatment of atrophic posterior maxilla: a systematic review of literature. *Clin Implant Dent Relat Res*, **17**, 120–132.

Ellegaard, B., Baelum, V. and Kolsen-Petersen, J. (2006) Non-grafted sinus implants in periodontally compromised patients: a time-to-event analysis. *Clin Oral Implants Res*, **17**, 156–164.

Esposito, M., Felice, P. and Worthington, H.V. (2014) Interventions for replacing missing teeth: augmentation procedures of the maxillary sinus. *Cochrane Database Syst Rev*, **5**, CD008397.

Irinakis, T., Dabuleanu, V. and Aldahlawi, S. (2017) Complications during maxillary sinus augmentation associated with interfering septa: a new classification of septa. *Open Dent J*, **11**, 140–150.

Papageorgiou, S.N., Papageorgiou, P.N., Deschner, J. and Gotz, W. (2016) Comparative effectiveness of natural and synthetic bone grafts in oral and maxillofacial surgery prior to insertion of dental implants: systematic review and network meta-analysis of parallel and cluster randomized controlled trials. *J Dent*, **48**, 1–8.

Pjetursson, B.E. and Lang, N.P. (2014) Sinus floor elevation utilizing the transalveolar approach. *Periodontology 2000*, **66**, 59–71.

Pjetursson, B.E. and Lang, N.P. (2015) Elevation of the maxillary sinus floor, in *Clinical Periodontology and Implant Dentistry*, 6th edn (eds N.P. Lang and J. Lindhe), Wiley, New York.

Rancitelli, D., Borgonovo, A.E., Cicciu, M. *et al.* (2015) Maxillary sinus septa and anatomic correlation with the Schneiderian membrane. *J Craniofac Surg*, **26**, 1394–1398.

Sanz, M., Donos, N., Alcoforado, G. *et al.* (2015) Therapeutic concepts and methods for improving dental implant outcomes. Summary and consensus statements. The 4th EAO Consensus Conference 2015. *Clin Oral Implants Res*, **26**(Suppl 11), 202–206.

Schmitt, C., Karasholi, T., Lutz, R., Wiltfang, J., Neukam, F.W. and Schlegel, K.A. (2014) Long-term changes in graft height after maxillary sinus augmentation, onlay bone grafting, and combination of both techniques: a long-term retrospective cohort study. *Clin Oral Implants Res*, **25**, E38–46.

Sharan, A. and Madjar, D. (2008) Maxillary sinus pneumatization following extractions: a radiographic study. *Int J Oral Maxillofac Implants*, **23**, 48–56.

Starch-Jensen, T., Aludden, H., Hallman, M., Dahlin, C., Christensen, A.E. and Mordenfeld, A. (2018) A systematic review and meta-analysis of long-term studies (five or more years) assessing maxillary sinus floor augmentation. *Int J Oral Maxillofac Surg*, **47**, 103–116.

Tan, W.C., Lang, N.P., Zwahlen, M. and Pjetursson, B.E. (2008) A systematic review of the success of sinus floor elevation and survival of implants inserted in combination with sinus floor elevation. *Part II: Transalveolar technique. J Clin Periodontol*, **35**, 241–254.

Tarnow, D.P., Wallace, S.S., Froum, S.J., Rohrer, M.D. and Cho, S.C. (2000) Histologic and clinical comparison of bilateral sinus floor elevations with and without barrier membrane placement in 12 patients: Part 3 of an ongoing prospective study. *Int J Periodontics Restorative Dent*, **20**, 117–125.

Thoma, D.S., Zeltner, M., Husler, J., Hammerle, C.H. and Jung, R.E. (2015) EAO Supplement Working Group 4 - EAO CC 2015 Short implants versus sinus lifting with longer implants to restore the posterior maxilla: a systematic review. *Clin Oral Implants Res*, **26**(Suppl 11), 154–169.

Varela-Centelles, P., Loira-Gago, M., Seoane-Romero, J.M., Takkouche, B., Monteiro, L. and Seoane, J. (2015) Detection of the posterior superior alveolar artery in the lateral sinus wall using computed tomography/cone beam computed tomography: a prevalence meta-analysis study and systematic review. *Int J Oral Maxillofac Surg*, **44**, 1405–1410.

Villacorta, M.G. (1967) Modified Caldwell–Luc operation. *J Philipp Dent Assoc*, **20**, 6–9.

Wallace, S.S., Tarnow, D.P., Froum, S.J. *et al.* (2012) Maxillary sinus elevation by lateral window approach: evolution of technology and technique. *J Evid Based Dent Pract*, **12**, 161–171.

29

Microdontia

29.1 Definition, Prevalence and Classification

Microdontia is defined as teeth that are smaller than normal (Poulsen and Koch, 2013). Prevalence of microdontia in the primary dentition is between 0.2% and 0.5% and in the permanent dentition between 0.5% to 3.1%, mostly affecting the maxillary lateral incisor teeth, named peg laterals (1.8%) (Hua *et al.*, 2013). Females are more commonly affected than males (Brook *et al.*, 2014).

Shafer *et al.* (1958) classified microdontia into three categories.

- True generalised microdontia, which is a rare form of microdontia where all the teeth are smaller in size but are well formed.
- Relative generalised microdontia, where the teeth appear small due to large jaws.
- Microdontia involving a single tooth, which is the most common form of microdontia.

29.2 Aetiology

Genetic and environmental factors are implicated in the aetiology of microdontia (Jeong *et al.*, 2015).

True generalised microdontia has been associated with Down's syndrome, pituitary dwarfism, Fanconi's anemia, chemotherapy and radiotherapy (Poulsen and Koch, 2013).

Other syndromes associated with microdontia include ectodermal dysplasia, Gorlin–Chaudhry–Moss syndrome, orofaciodigital syndrome, Ullrich–Turner syndrome, Hallermann–Streiff syndrome, tricho-rhino-phalangeal syndrome, Rothmund–Thomson syndrome, branchio-oculo-facial syndrome, oculo-mandibulo-facial syndrome and Williams' syndrome (Bloch-Zupan *et al.*, 2012).

Localised microdontia is often associated with hypodontia and its severity is affected by the severity of hypodontia (Brook, 1984).

29.3 Examination and Diagnosis

Past medical history (PMH) to identify any related syndromes or medical conditions, familial history (genetic disorder) and dental history (especially missing teeth) are the relevant aspects of history taking in patients with microdontia.

Useful assessment tools to aid diagnosis and treatment planning include:

- clinical photographs showing the patient's smile line
- appropriate radiographs to assess root morphology, length, size, periodontal bone levels, periapical tissues, bone volume for potential implant treatment (may also require CBCT) and any skeletal discrepancy
- articulated study models
- diagnostic wax-up to visualise the final outcome when planning restorative-only treatment and to facilitate the placement of restorations
- Kesling tooth set-up when planning orthodontic treatment
- Bolton (tooth size discrepancy) analysis to evaluate the impact of build-ups of small teeth on the functional and aesthetic outcomes of treatment of malocclusion and to establish whether the excess space will be in the mandibular or maxillary arch. Bolton's normal ratio is important for proper articulation of maxillary and mandibular teeth (Bolton, 1958). The overall ratio is the summed mesiodistal widths of 12 mandibular to maxillary teeth. The anterior ratio is the summed mesiodistal widths of six anterior mandibular to the corresponding maxillary teeth (Othman and Harradine, 2006).

29.4 Management

Treatment options depend mainly on the severity of microdontia and the patient's wishes, functional and aes-

Diseases and Conditions in Dentistry: An Evidence-Based Reference, First Edition. Keyvan Moharamzadeh.

Companion website: www.wiley.com/go/moharamzadeh/diseases

thetic requirements (Laverty and Thomas, 2016) and include:

- prevention only without any other treatment, which may not address the patient's concerns
- orthodontic treatment only to correct the position of the microdont teeth and close the spaces
- restorative treatment only to restore the microdont teeth
- combined orthodontic and restorative treatment
- extraction of the microdont tooth (especially if it has a poor prognosis and there is a need for space) and space management with either orthodontic or restorative treatment, as discussed in Chapter 25.

In some cases, it is ideal to close the spaces with orthodontic treatment to obviate the need for restorative treatment, minimising the maintenance requirements of restorations. However, this is not always practical and therefore, it is preferable to leave the residual spaces where the teeth could be built up to ideal size and shape.

Mesiodistal, apicocoronal and labiolingual position of the microdont teeth should be assessed carefully and corrected to achieve ideal aesthetics, emergence profile, gingival margin, soft tissue position and occlusion (Laverty and Thomas, 2016).

Options for the restoration of microdont teeth include direct adhesive restorations with composite resin or indirect restorations such as porcelain veneers and crowns, which are less conservative options.

Potential challenges with composite build-up of microdont teeth include (Hobkirk *et al.*, 2012):

- reduced surface area for bonding
- poor aesthetics due to a large discrepancy between the diameter of the root and the built-up crown with extensive composite addition (emergence profile issue)
- difficulty cleaning the reshaped tooth.

Very pointed and conical canine teeth may require reshaping to reduce trauma to soft tissues. However, there is a potential risk of pulp exposure during tooth preparation and therefore, composite addition to these teeth is often preferred. Crowns may lack retention form on very conical teeth. In extreme circumstances such as severe oligodontia cases, overdentures are indicated (see Chapter 16).

Regarding microdont lateral incisor teeth (peg laterals), if the amount of build-up is small, the microdont tooth should be positioned near the central incisor tooth to limit the restorative procedure to the distal surface of the lateral only and preserve the optimal mesial soft tissue papilla contour (Counihan, 2000). If the lateral incisor is very narrow, the tooth should be positioned near the centre of the space (mesiodistally) and slightly palatally to maximise the amount of labial build-up (Fortin *et al.*, 2004).

Case Study

A 19-year-old female patient was referred by her GDP for management of bilateral microdont maxillary lateral incisor teeth and spacing. She was concerned about the appearance of the teeth.

The patient was medically fit and well. Her preoperative clinical photographs and radiograph are shown in Figures 29.1 and 29.2 respectively.

Based on the clinical and radiographic examination, the following diagnoses were made.

- Localised microdontia with peg-shaped maxillary lateral incisor teeth and spacing.
- Tooth transposition of UL2 and UL3.

The treatment options below were discussed with the patient, including risks, benefits, expected outcomes and maintenance requirements.

- Prevention only with no further treatment.

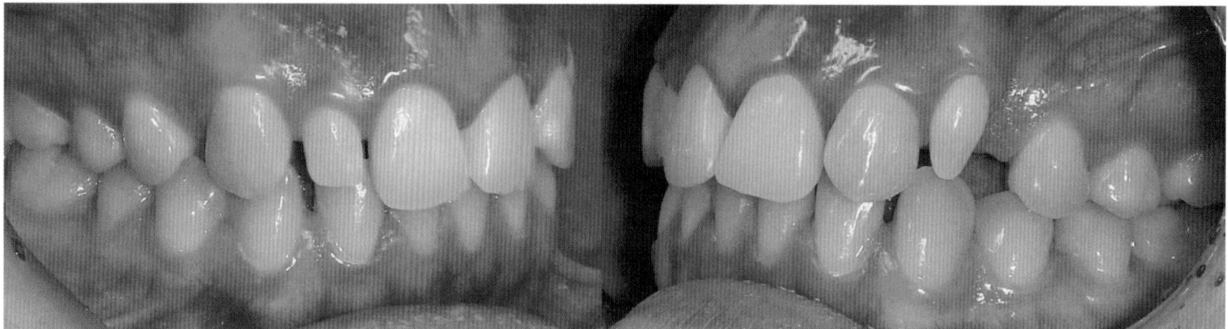

Figure 29.1 Preoperative clinical photographs showing peg-shaped UR2 and UL2. UL2 has erupted distal to UL3.

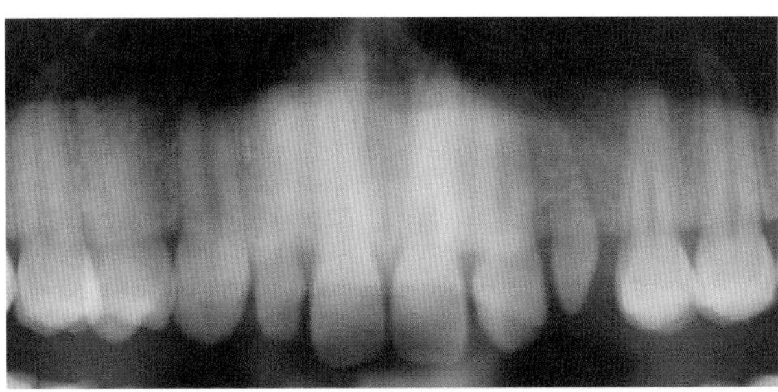

Figure 29.2 Preoperative radiograph of the anterior teeth showing the relatively small and short root of microdont UL2. UL3 has erupted in the place of UL2.

- Conservative restorative treatment only by direct composite additions to the microdont teeth and canine reshaping.
- Orthodontic treatment to idealise the spaces for subsequent restorative treatment.
- Extraction of the microdont UL2 and replacement of the tooth with a resin-bonded bridge or an implant.

The patient did not want orthodontic treatment or any extractions but preferred to build up the microdont teeth and improve the appearance. Therefore, the following treatment was provided.

1) Prevention.
2) Impressions, bite registration, face-bow record and preparation of articulated study models.
3) Diagnostic wax-up to build the maxillary lateral incisors to full shape and camouflage UL3.
4) Composite restoration of UR2, UL2 and UL3.
5) Review.

The patient's postoperative clinical photographs are shown in Figure 29.3.

This was a conservative treatment approach which obviated the need for long-term orthodontic treatment or complicated implant treatment.

This case was challenging due to the labial position of UL2. The use of a silicone putty stent made over the diagnostic wax-up on the palatal side facilitated restoration of the peg-shaped teeth. Occlusion was carefully adjusted following restoration of microdont UL2 which was in the place of UL3 to avoid any heavy occlusal contacts on lateral excursion.

Shade selection was difficult as the patient's natural teeth had different shades. Therefore, care was taken in selecting the shade for the individual teeth to match the colour of the adjacent teeth.

With careful reflection on the ideal anatomy of the teeth on composite restorations, a satisfactory aesthetic result was achieved.

The patient was satisfied with the outcome and was discharged back to her GDP for routine dental care and maintenance.

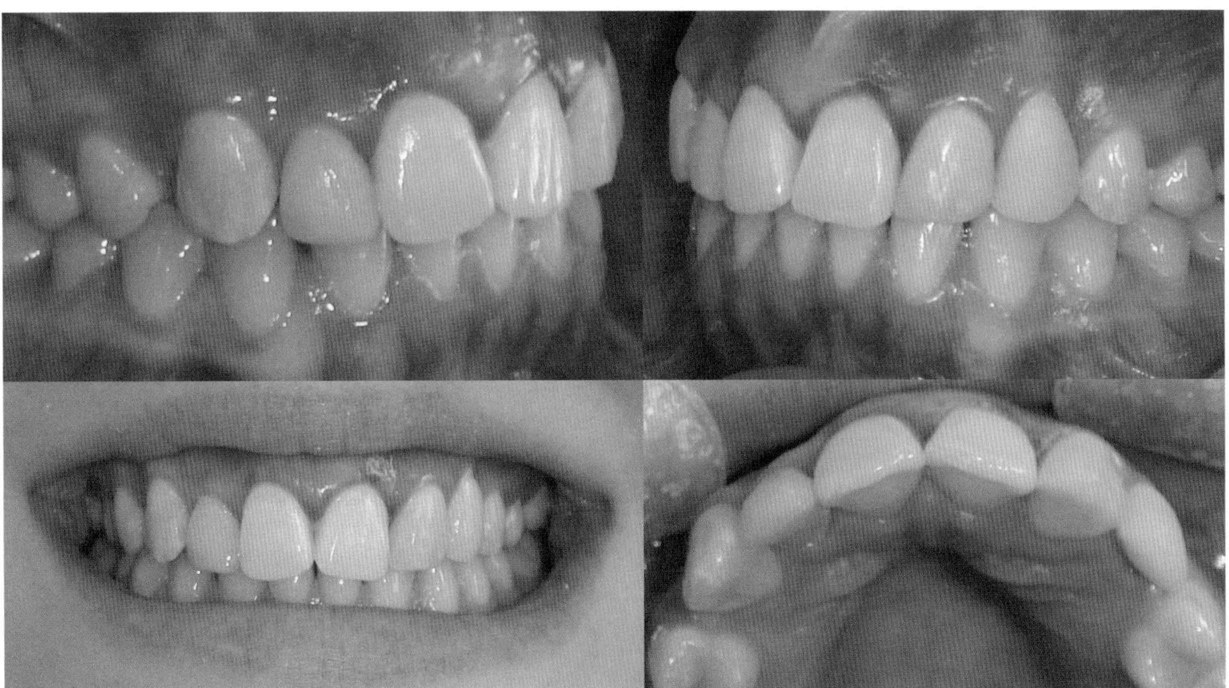

Figure 29.3 Postoperative clinical photographs following composite restorations.

References

Bloch-Zupan, A., Sedano, H. and Scully, C. (2012) *Dento/Oro/Craniofacial Anomalies and Genetics*, Elsevier, Oxford.

Bolton, W.A. (1958) Disharmony in tooth size and its relation to the analysis and treatment of malocclusion. *Angle Orthod*, **28**, 113–130.

Brook, A.H. (1984) A unifying aetiological explanation for anomalies of human tooth number and size. *Arch Oral Biol*, **29**, 373–378.

Brook, A.H., Jernvall, J., Smith, R.N., Hughes, T.E. and Townsend, G.C. (2014) The dentition: the outcomes of morphogenesis leading to variations of tooth number, size and shape. *Aust Dent J*, **59**(Suppl 1), 131–142.

Counihan, D. (2000) The orthodontic restorative management of the peg-lateral. *Dent Update*, **27**, 250–256.

Fortin, D., Guertin, G., Papadakis, A. (2004) Combining orthodontic and restorative treatment to optimize esthetics and function in space management cases. *Oral Health*, July 1.

Hobkirk, J.A., Gill, D., Jones, S.P. *et al.* (2012) *Hypodontia: A Team Approach to Management*, Wiley-Blackwell, Oxford.

Hua, F., He, H., Ngan, P. and Bouzid, W. (2013) Prevalence of peg-shaped maxillary permanent lateral incisors: a meta-analysis. *Am J Orthod Dentofacial Orthop*, **144**, 97–109.

Jeong, K.H., Kim, D., Song, Y.M., Sung, J. and Kim, Y.H. (2015) Epidemiology and genetics of hypodontia and microdontia: a study of twin families. *Angle Orthod*, **85**, 980–985.

Laverty, D.P. and Thomas, M.B. (2016) The restorative management of microdontia. *Br Dent J*, **221**, 160–166.

Othman, S.A. and Harradine, N.W. (2006) Tooth-size discrepancy and Bolton's ratios: a literature review. *J Orthod*, **33**, 45–51; discussion 29.

Poulsen, S. and Koch, G. (2013) *Pediatric Dentistry: A Clinical Approach*, 2nd edn, Wiley-Blackwell, Chichester.

Shafer, W.G., Hine, M.K. and Levy, B.M. (1958) *A Textbook of Oral Pathology*, W.B. Saunders, Philadelphia.

30

Necrotising Periodontal Diseases

30.1 Introduction

Necrotising periodontal diseases are characterised by necrosis of periodontal tissues and are classified into three groups: (1) necrotising gingivitis, which is limited to gingivae; (2) necrotising periodontitis involving the periodontal ligament and bone and causing attachment loss; and (3) necrotising stomatitis which extends beyond the mucogingival junction (Lang and Lindhe, 2015).

30.2 Epidemiology

Necrotising periodontal diseases have a low prevalence in industrialised countries, estimated to be less than 0.2% (Dufty *et al.*, 2016). However, there is a higher prevalence in developing countries, mainly affecting young adults, but they can develop at any age (Botero *et al.*, 2015).

Necrotising periodontitis is less common than necrotising gingivitis and has a reported prevalence of 0–11% in HIV-positive patients (Mataftsi *et al.*, 2011).

30.3 Predisposing Factors

Predisposing factors include systemic diseases (HIV and impaired immunity), malnutrition, poor oral hygiene, pre-existing gingivitis, history of previous necrotising periodontal disease, psychological stress, inadequate sleep, smoking and alcohol use, Caucasian ethnicity, and young age of 21–24 years (Herrera *et al.*, 2014).

30.4 Clinical Features and Diagnosis

Necrotising gingivitis presents with intense gingival pain, papillae necrosis with 'punched-out' appearance, marginal (linear) gingival erythema and spontaneous bleeding. Other possible signs and symptoms include malaise, fever, lymphadenopathy, malodour and metallic taste.

The condition can progress rapidly and develop into necrotising periodontitis characterised by attachment loss, bone necrosis, interproximal craters (negative papillae), bone exposure and sequestrum formation. If the disease is left untreated, it may subside and become chronic and reoccur later. In severe cases, the zone of destruction can extend beyond the mucogingival junction and develop into necrotising stomatitis involving the buccal and lingual mucosa and lips.

Differential diagnosis includes herpetic gingivostomatitis, gingival lesions associated with acute leukaemia and other mucous membrane diseases. Diagnosis is usually clinical, although a smear test for the presence of fusospirochaetal bacteria, and leucocytes and blood test to rule out leukaemia can be carried out (Scully, 2013).

30.5 Microbiology and Histology

Necrotic lesions in necrotising periodontal diseases contain spirochaetes and fusiform bacteria with the potential to invade the epithelium and connective tissue (Listgarten, 1965), releasing endotoxins that can activate or modify the host response and cause periodontal tissue destruction. Composition of the microbiota includes *Prevotella intermedia* and *Fusobacterium*, *Treponema* and *Selenomonas* (Loesche *et al.*, 1982). Gingival lesions in HIV-positive patients may also contain yeasts such as *Candida albicans*, herpes viruses or superinfecting bacterial species (Winkler *et al.*, 1989).

Microscopic examination of necrotising gingivitis lesions shows four distinct zones: superficial bacterial

Diseases and Conditions in Dentistry: An Evidence-Based Reference, First Edition. Keyvan Moharamzadeh.

Companion website: www.wiley.com/go/moharamzadeh/diseases

layer, neutrophil-rich zone, necrotic zone and spirochaetal infiltration zones (Listgarten, 1965).

30.6 Management

Due to the destructive nature of necrotising periodontal diseases, treatment should be initiated as soon as the diagnosis is established. Treatment stages are described below (Herrera *et al.*, 2014; Lang and Lindhe, 2015).

30.6.1 Acute Phase Treatment

The aim is to stop disease activity and reduce the patient's pain and discomfort. Therapies include the following.

- Initial daily superficial ultrasonic debridement with minimal pressure for the duration of the acute phase, which is usually 2–4 days.
- Oral hygiene instruction (OHI) to replace tooth brushing (which can be painful) with chemical plaque control until healing occurs. This includes 0.2% chlorhexidine mouthrinse (twice daily) and 3% hydrogen peroxide solution diluted 1:1 in warm water (three times daily) for up to 7 days.
- Systemic antibiotics in severe cases or systemic involvement: metronidazole 250 mg, three times daily until healing occurs.
- Review (ideally daily).

30.6.2 Treatment of Chronic Periodontal Disease

As the symptoms of the acute phase subside, it is important to treat any pre-existing conditions such as plaque-induced gingivitis or chronic periodontitis. This includes patient motivation, OHI to resume tooth brushing and interdental cleaning, professional prophylaxis and/or root surface debridement (RSD) under local anaesthesia (LA) in all sites with deep periodontal pockets equal to or greater than 4 mm as well as addressing any periodontal risk factors, as discussed in Chapter 6.

30.6.3 Corrective Phase Treatment

The aim of this phase is to correct and eliminate any gingival defects and interproximal craters caused by the destructive disease. Surgical treatment modalities involve gingivoplasty and/or gingivectomy to correct superficial soft tissue defects and periodontal flap surgery or regeneration to manage deep craters. In HIV patients, it may be best to avoid surgery but use intensive interproximal cleaning to prevent recurrence.

30.4 Maintenance

Maintenance includes supportive periodontal therapy (SPT) (see Chapter 6) and addressing any predisposing factors as described earlier in this chapter.

Case Study

A 47-year-old female patient referred by her GDP presented with recurrent gum infections, discomfort and bone exposure in the left mandibular canine region.

The patient was medically fit and well but had been smoking heavily for the past 10 years. She had a stressful job.

Clinical examination showed generalised gingival recession and the loss of interdental papillae between LL2 and LL3 with bone exposure (Figure 30.1).

Full periodontal assessment showed generalised 4–7 mm periodontal pockets and a number of teeth were grade 1 mobile. Radiographic examination showed generalised mild to moderate horizontal periodontal bone loss.

The diagnoses was necrotising periodontitis with bone sequestrum at LL2–LL3. The following treatment was provided.

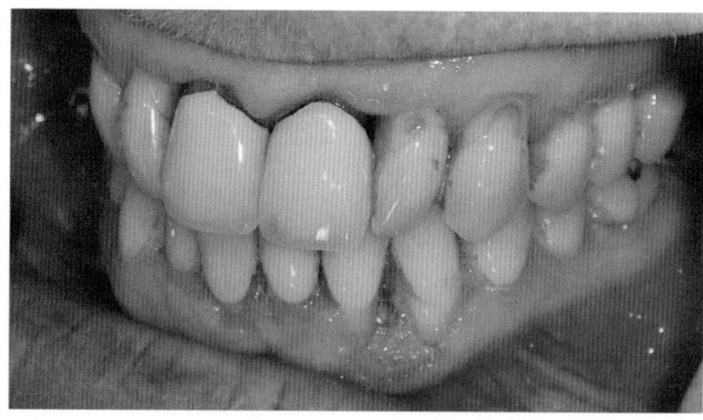

Figure 30.1 Preoperative clinical photograph showing the exposed necrotic bone between LL2 and LL3.

1) Initial local debridement and removal of loosely attached bone sequestrum at LL2–LL3.
2) OHI, including advice to use 0.2% chlorhexidine mouthrinse twice daily for 1 week.
3) Smoking cessation advice and patient referral to smoking cessation service. The patient was also advised to reduce stress and see her general medical practitioner for management of stress.

4) RSD under LA in all sites with deep pockets of 4 mm or more, and further oral hygiene reinforcement, including modified Bass and interdental brushing.
5) Postoperative oral hygiene review in 1 month and full periodontal reassessment 3 months after RSD.
6) Further RSD under LA in all sites with residual deep pockets.
7) Periodontal reassessment 3 months following the second cycle of RSD showed a very good response to non-surgical treatment, with significant improvement and reduction in pocket depth and periodontal indices.

The patient was discharged to the GDP for maintenance, SPT and routine dental care.

References

Botero, J.E., Rosing, C.K., Duque, A., Jaramillo, A. and Contreras, A. (2015) Periodontal disease in children and adolescents of Latin America. *Periodontology 2000*, **67**, 34–57.

Dufty, J., Gkranias, N., Petrie, A., McCormick, R., Elmer, T. and Donos, N. (2016) Prevalence and treatment of necrotizing ulcerative gingivitis (NUG) in the British Armed Forces: a case-control study. *Clin Oral Invest*, **21**, 1935–1944.

Herrera, D., Alonso, B., de Arriba, L., Santa Cruz, I., Serrano, C. and Sanz, M. (2014) Acute periodontal lesions. *Periodontology 2000*, **65**, 149–177.

Lang, N.P. and Lindhe, J. (2015) *Clinical Periodontology and Implant Dentistry*, Wiley-Blackwell, Oxford.

Listgarten, M.A. (1965) Electron microscopic observations on the bacterial flora of acute necrotizing ulcerative gingivitis. *J Periodontol*, **36**, 328–339.

Loesche, W.J., Syed, S.A., Laughon, B.E. and Stoll, J. (1982) The bacteriology of acute necrotizing ulcerative gingivitis. *J Periodontol*, **53**, 223–230.

Mataftsi, M., Skoura, L. and Sakellari, D. (2011) HIV Infection and periodontal diseases: an overview of the post-HAART era. *Oral Dis*, **17**, 13–25.

Scully, C. (2013) *Oral and Maxillofacial Medicine: The Basis of Diagnosis and Treatment*, 3rd edn, Churchill Livingstone, Edinburgh.

Winkler, J.R., Murray, P.A., Grassi, M. and Hammerle, C. (1989) Diagnosis and management of HIV-associated periodontal lesions. *J Am Dent Assoc*, **Suppl**, 25 s–34 s.

31

Occlusal Issues and Occlusion

31.1 Definitions

'*Static occlusion*' is the occlusal contacts between the mandibular and maxillary teeth in a static position. '*Dynamic occlusion*' is the occlusal contacts between the mandibular and maxillary teeth when the mandible is moving against the maxillae (Davies and Gray, 2001a).

'*Centric occlusion*' (CO), also called 'intercuspal position' (ICP), 'habital bite' or 'bite of convenience', is the occlusion between the teeth at maximum intercuspation.

'*Centric relation*' (CR) is defined anatomically as the position of the mandible in relation to the maxillae when the head of the condyle is at the uppermost and foremost position. Conceptually, at CR, the muscles of mastication are at their most relaxed position and geometrically, the head of the condyle is at its terminal hinge axis. CR is an important position in prosthodontics as it is a reproducible position irrespective of guidance provided by the teeth (Keshvad and Winstanley, 2000a, b, 2001).

Two types of movement normally occur in the mandible: rotational movement around its axis and translational movement, which occurs as the condyle translates within the temporomandibular joint (TMJ). Posselt (1958) described a three-dimensional '*envelope of motion*' for the border movements of the mandible in all three planes (Figure 31.1).

The mandibular movement pathways are determined by two guidance systems: posterior guidance (condylar guidance) (Aull, 1965; Lundeen and Wirth, 1973) and anterior guidance provided by the teeth (Rinchuse *et al.*, 2007).

When the mandible moves to one side (working side), the head of the condyle on the other side (non-working side) moves forwards, medially and downwards. The angle between the downwards movement and the horizontal plane is called the 'condylar angle'. The angle between medial movement and the sagittal plane is called the 'Bennet angle'. The working-side condyle also makes an initial immediate lateral movement named the 'immediate side shift' or 'Bennet movement' (Milosevic, 2003c).

Anterior guidance includes 'protrusive guidance' provided by the incisor teeth, causing separation of the posterior teeth during mandibular protrusion (Christensen phenomenon); guidance during lateral excursions such as 'canine guidance' provided by the canine teeth only on the working side during mandibular lateral excursions; and 'group function' when there are shared contacts between several teeth on the working side during mandibular lateral excursion.

Occlusal interference influencing anterior guidance can be classified into 'working-side interference', caused by a premature or heavy occlusal contact on posterior teeth on the working side, and 'non-working-side interference', caused by an occlusal contact on the posterior teeth on the non-working side during mandibular lateral excursion (Davies and Gray, 2001a).

'Freedom in centric' or 'long centric' refers to the ability of the mandible to move forward at CO for a short distance while maintaining tooth contact on the same plane (Schuyler, 1969).

31.2 Occlusal Philosophies

Several occlusal philosophies have been developed in the past. McCollum and Stuart introduced the gnathological concept in 1955 based on balanced occlusion, believing that anterior guidance was independent of the condylar path. In 1960, Stuart and Stallard adopted the concept of mutually protected (canine-guided) occlusion with cusp fossa three-point (tripod) occlusal contacts in posterior teeth (Stuart, 1973). The Pankey-Mann-Schuyler philosophy of occlusal rehabilitation was then introduced based on the spherical theory of occlusion and functionally generated wax pattern. Their principles included maximum number of teeth contacts in CR, group function occlusion, disclusion of the posterior teeth in protrusion, and disclusion of all non-working-side teeth in lateral excursions (Anderson, 1994). These ideologies

Diseases and Conditions in Dentistry: An Evidence-Based Reference, First Edition. Keyvan Moharamzadeh.

Companion website: www.wiley.com/go/moharamzadeh/diseases

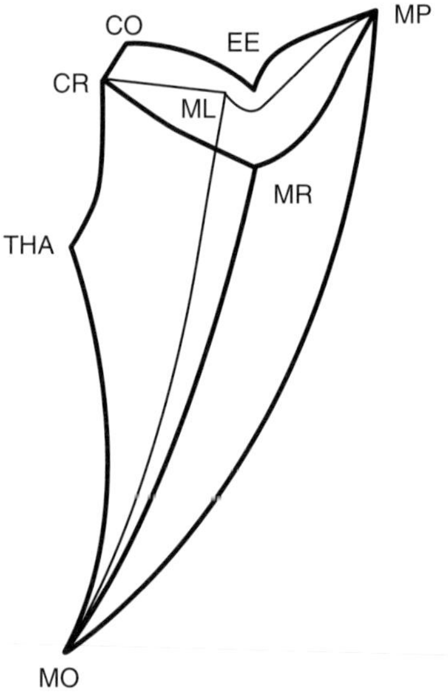

Figure 31.1 Posselt's envelope of motion showing the limits of mandibular border movements. CO, centric occlusion; CR, centric relation; EE, edge-to-edge incisor position; ML, maximum left side lateral excursion; MO, maximum mandibular opening with full translation movement; MP, maximum protrusion; MR, maximum right side lateral excursion; THA, terminal hinge axis or maximum mandibular opening without the translation of condyles (Posselt, 2001).

have undergone constant revisions over the years (Ash, 1995).

Based on the contemporary practice of prosthodontics, ideal occlusal features for dentate patients are listed below.

- CO occurring in CR with no slide.
- Anterior guidance provided by the anterior teeth (canine guidance with no posterior interferences).
- Some freedom in CO.
- Multiple simultaneous contacts.
- Occlusal forces directed down the long axis of the teeth.
- Cusp tip to flat fossa contact.
- No cuspal incline contacts.
- Smooth and shallow guidance contacts.

31.3 Assessment and Recording of Occlusion

Assessment of the patient's static and dynamic occlusion prior to any restorative treatment is important to establish whether the new restorations can be provided in a 'conformative approach' without the need to alter the patient's existing occlusion, or if a 'reorganisation approach' is required to place the restorations at a new ideal occlusion in harmony with the patient's masticatory system.

It is essential to assess CO, CR, any present slides from CR to CO, type of anterior guidance and the presence or absence of freedom in centric.

Occlusion can be recorded using different methods (Davies and Gray, 2001b).

- Two-dimensional methods such as clinical photograph, occlusal sketching diagram, articulating papers, Shimstock occlusion foil and the T-scan which uses a computer program that can also analyse the relative hardness of the contacts between the teeth.
- Three-dimensional methods such as verified articulated study models using face-bow record and bite registration materials.

31.4 Articulators

Different types of articulators have been developed for mounting study models and occlusal analysis in prosthodontics (Hobo *et al.*, 1976; Mitchell and Wilkie, 1978a, b).

- Hinge articulators which only replicate hinge movements.
- Average-value articulators permit lateral and hinge movements with an average condylar guidance angle.
- Adjustable articulators are subdivided into semi-adjustable articulators, which can replicate some of the mandibular movements, and fully adjustable articulators which can reproduce most of the mandibular movements with more accurate condylar angles, incisal angles, immediate and delayed Bennet shift (Bellanti, 1973).

Articulators can also be classified into:

- ARCON type (anatomically articulated condyle), in which the condylar elements are in the lower part and the fossae are in the upper part of the articulator, such as Denar and Whipmix articulators.
- Non-ARCON type (non-anatomically articulated condyle), in which the condylar elements are in the upper part and the fossae are in the lower part of the articulator, such as the Dentatus articulator.

The ARCON articulators reproduce mandibular movements more precisely than non-ARCON articulators (Milosevic, 2003b).

31.5 Face-bow

A face-bow is used to transfer the relationship of the maxillary arch to the temporomandibular joint which enables mounting the maxillary cast on an adjustable articulator (Squier, 2004).

There are two types of face-bow.

- Arbitrary face-bow, which positions the maxillae in relation to an arbitrary terminal hinge axis (near the external acoustic meatus).
- Kinematic face-bow, which locates the actual terminal hinge axis of the condyles.

The use of a face-bow is particularly important when significant changes to the patient's dynamic occlusion, including occlusal guidance, are being planned, for example, in occlusal rehabilitation of patients where canine guidance is altered or missing.

31.6 Conformative Approach

In the conformative approach, the bite is registered at CO without any increase in the occlusal vertical dimension (OVD) to enable the laboratory to fabricate a restoration that conforms to the patient's existing occlusion and avoid any premature contact on the new restoration that can have several adverse consequences, such as tooth hypersensitivity and mobility due to occlusal trauma, restoration fracture, tooth wear and temporomandibular problems (Davies *et al.*, 2001a).

It is important to verify the correct articulation of the study models using a second record of the bite with a different material. Minor modifications can be carried out on the models to eliminate any errors (model grooming).

'Functionally generated pathway' is a useful technique to record the movements of teeth opposing a prepared tooth (Jedynakiewicz and Martin, 2001). This is achieved by using a pattern acrylic such as Duralay built up on a prepared tooth and asking the patient to bite in CO and then go into excursions to carve out the pathway of the opposing teeth on the Duralay.

31.7 Reorganisation of Occlusion

Reorganisation of occlusion may be required in extensive occlusal rehabilitation when it is not possible (or desirable) to conform to the patient's existing occlusion (Davies *et al.*, 2001b), for example, in tooth wear cases when it is not possible to restore the worn and broken teeth to their ideal height and shape without increasing the OVD.

When reorganising occlusion, bite is often registered at the retruded contact position (RCP) which is a point in CR where the first teeth meet.

The most commonly used technique for bite registration at the RCP involves the use of a customised anterior bite plane such as a 'Lucia jig' or a stabilising splint (Milosevic, 2003a) initially to 'deprogramme' the musculature 'engram' followed by bimanual manipulation of the jaw into the RCP and registration of the bite using appropriate material.

If an arbitrary face-bow record has been taken, the study models can then be mounted on a semi-adjustable articulator with estimated condylar angles based on lateroprotrusive wax records or by adjusting the condylar angles of the articulator until the space between the non-working-side molar teeth is the same as it is in the patient's mouth.

If a kinematic face-bow has been used and pantograph tracings have been obtained, the study models can be mounted on a fully adjustable articulator. However, this technique is not used routinely in practice due to its complexity.

Following articulation of the study models, a diagnostic wax-up can be prepared as a valuable guide to provide an appropriate (ideal) occlusal scheme prior to fabrication of final restorations. A 'mock-up trial' (intraoral rehearsal) of the wax-up in the mouth can be carried out to visualise the final intended outcome of treatment. Diagnostic wax-up also provides a template for provisional restorations and enables any modifications of occlusion before proceeding to definitive restorations.

If the maxillary anterior provisional crowns have been modified to improve the patient's function and aesthetics, a customised incisal guidance table can be used by the laboratory technician to copy the guiding surfaces of the upper anterior provisional crowns to replicate the same anterior guidance in definitive restorations (Mall *et al.*, 2013).

31.8 Determinants of Posterior Occlusal Morphology

It is important to be aware that the occlusal morphology of the posterior teeth can be affected by several vertical and horizontal determinants and any restorations that are placed on the posterior teeth must be in harmony with these determinants (Aull, 1965; Jensen, 1991).

Vertical determinants of occlusion that can affect the cusp height and fossa depth of the posterior teeth include condylar guidance (steep guidance = taller cusp), anterior guidance (increased overbite and reduced overjet = taller cusps), plane of occlusion (parallel plane with condylar guidance = shorter cusps), curve of Spee (acute curve = shorter cusps) and lateral translation movement (greater movement and immediate side shift = shorter cusps).

Horizontal determinants of occlusion that can affect the ridge and groove direction (the angle between laterotrusive and mediotrusive pathways) include distance from rotating condyle (greater distance = wider angle), distance from midsagittal plane (greater distance = wider angle), lateral translating movement (greater movement = wider angle) and intercondylar distance (greater distance = smaller angle).

Case Study

A 56-year-old female patient referred by her general dental practitioner (GDP) complained of discomfort and difficulty eating due to drifted teeth and lack of adequate contacts between the upper and lower teeth.

Clinical examination showed an anterior open bite and the only occlusal contacts at CO were on the right first molars and the left first and second molar teeth (Figure 31.2). There was a significant slide from the RCP to the ICP in both horizontal and vertical directions. Non-working-side occlusal interferences were also noticed on both right and left lateral excursions.

Treatment options discussed with patient included (1) orthodontic treatment, (2) additive approach to build up the occlusal surfaces of the teeth to reduce the open bite, and (3) occlusal adjustment by selective grinding from the posterior molar teeth to improve the occlusion and reduce the open bite.

The patient preferred the third option. Therefore, study models were prepared, the bite was registered at the RCP using hard beauty wax, a face-bow record was taken using an arbitrary face-bow and the casts were mounted on a semi-adjustable articulator.

The occlusal surfaces of the molar teeth were sprayed with a golden colour (Figure 31.3) to enable visualisation of the areas of selective grinding during occlusal adjustment of the study models.

Similar occlusal adjustments were carried out inside the mouth to increase the number of occlusal contacts, eliminate the non-working-side interferences and reduce the anterior open bite. Selective grinding of the teeth on the casts was very helpful and facilitated the process of occlusal adjustment in the mouth. However, the use of articulating paper was still necessary to achieve an ideal result.

It was interesting to see how simple occlusal adjustment solved the patient's problems and resulted in immediate relief of symptoms. Following adjustment of the molar teeth, the patient's anterior open bite was improved (Figure 31.4).

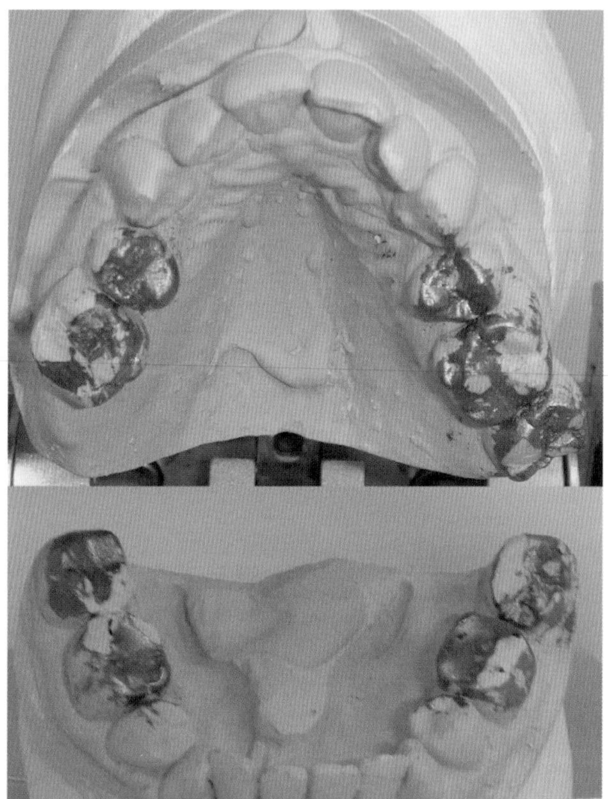

Figure 31.3 Photograph of the articulated study models following occlusal adjustment on the models showing the areas that have been selectively reduced.

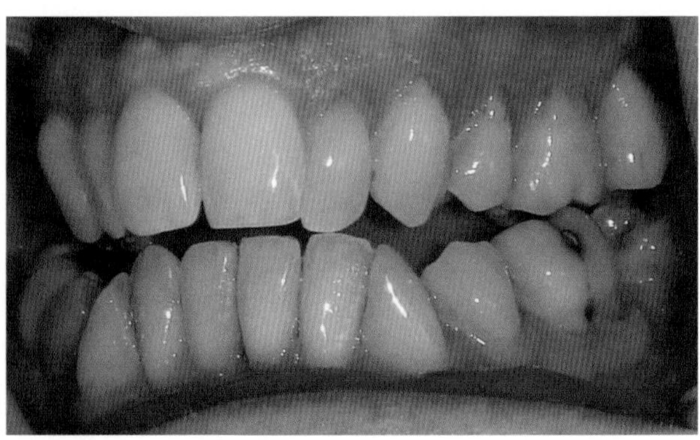

Figure 31.2 Peroperative clinic photograph of the patient's occlusion showing an anterior open bite and occlusal contacts only on the molar teeth.

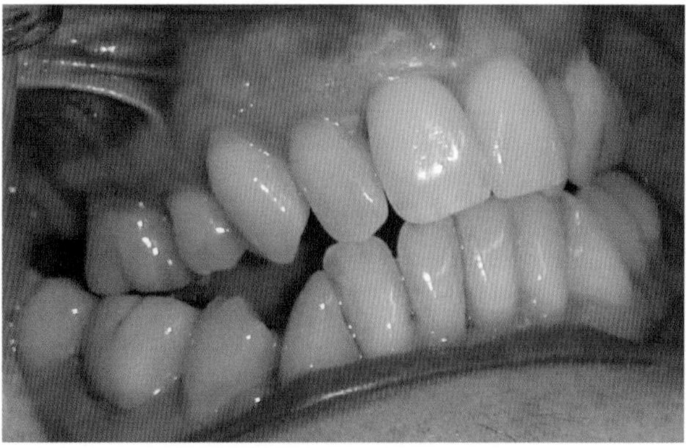

Figure 31.4 Postoperative clinical photograph showing significant reduction in open bite and increase in the number of occlusal contacts.

However, due to severe tilting and drifting of the premolar teeth, it was not possible to completely close the open bite in the right premolar area without orthodontic treatment.

The patient was very satisfied with the outcome of treatment and was discharged back to her GDP for routine dental care and maintenance.

References

Anderson, J.A. Jr (1994) The Pankey–Mann–Schuyler philosophy of restorative dentistry: an overview. *Northwest Dent*, **73**, 25–29.

Ash, M.M. Jr (1995) Philosophy of occlusion: past and present. *Dent Clin North Am*, **39**, 233–255.

Aull, A.E. (1965) Condylar determinants of occlusal patterns. *J Prosthet Dent*, **15**, 826–849.

Bellanti, N.D. (1973) The significance of articulator capabilities. I. Adjustable vs. semiadjustable articulators. *J Prosthet Dent*, **29**, 269–275.

Davies, S. and Gray, R.M. (2001a) What is occlusion? *Br Dent J*, **191**, 235–238, 241–245.

Davies, S.J. and Gray, R.M. (2001b) The examination and recording of the occlusion: why and how. *Br Dent J*, **191**, 291–296, 299–302.

Davies, S.J., Gray, R.M. and Smith, P.W. (2001a) Good occlusal practice in simple restorative dentistry. *Br Dent J*, **191**, 365–368, 371–374, 377–381.

Davies, S.J., Gray, R.M. and Whitehead, S.A. (2001b) Good occlusal practice in advanced restorative dentistry. *Br Dent J*, **191**, 421–424, 427–430, 433–434.

Hobo, S., Shillingburg, H.T. Jr and Whitsett, L.D. (1976) Articulator selection for restorative dentistry. *J Prosthet Dent*, **36**, 35–43.

Jedynakiewicz, N.M. and Martin, N. (2001) Functionally-generated pathway theory, application and development in CEREC restorations. *Int J Comput Dent*, **4**, 25–36.

Jensen, W.O. (1991) Alternate occlusal schemes. *J Prosthet Dent*, **65**, 54–55.

Keshvad, A. and Winstanley, R.B. (2000a) An appraisal of the literature on centric relation. Part I. *J Oral Rehabil*, **27**, 823–833.

Keshvad, A. and Winstanley, R.B. (2000b) An appraisal of the literature on centric relation. Part II. *J Oral Rehabil*, **27**, 1013–1023.

Keshvad, A. and Winstanley, R.B. (2001) An appraisal of the literature on centric relation. Part III. *J Oral Rehabil*, **28**, 55–63.

Lundeen, H.C. and Wirth, C.G. (1973) Condylar movement patterns engraved in plastic blocks. *J Prosthet Dent*, **30**, 866–875.

Mall, P., Singh, K., Rao, J. and Kumar, L. (2013) Rehabilitation of anterior teeth with customised incisal guide table. *BMJ Case Rep*, 2013.

Milosevic, A. (2003a) Occlusion: 2. Occlusal splints, analysis and adjustment. *Dent Update*, **30**, 416–422.

Milosevic, A. (2003b) Occlusion: 3. Articulators and related instruments. *Dent Update*, **30**, 511–515.

Milosevic, A. (2003c) Occlusion: 1. Terms, mandibular movement and the factors of occlusion. *Dent Update*, **30**, 359–361.

Mitchell, D.L. and Wilkie, N.D. (1978a) Articulators through the years. Part I. Up to 1940. *J Prosthet Dent*, **39**, 330–338.

Mitchell, D.L. and Wilkie, N.D. (1978b) Articulators through the years. Part II. From 1940. *J Prosthet Dent*, **39**, 451–458.

Posselt, U. (1958) Range of movement of the mandible. *J Am Dent Assoc*, **56**, 10–13.

Posselt, U. (2001) Terminal hinge movement of the mandible. *J Prosthet Dent*, **86**, 2–9.

Rinchuse, D.J., Kandasamy, S. and Sciote, J. (2007) A contemporary and evidence-based view of canine protected occlusion. *Am J Orthod Dentofacial Orthop*, **132**, 90–102.

Schuyler, C.H. (1969) Freedom in centric. *Dent Clin North Am*, **13**, 681–686.

Squier, R.S. (2004) Jaw relation records for fixed prosthodontics. *Dent Clin North Am*, **48**, 471–486.

Stuart, C.E. (1973) The contributions of gnathology to prosthodontics. *J Prosthet Dent*, **30**, 607–608.

32

Oncology-Related Defects in Mandible

32.1 Introduction

Cancer of the oral cavity and lips is the most common head and neck cancer and is the 15th most common cancer in Europe (Ferlay *et al.*, 2013). Worldwide, over 300 000 new cases were diagnosed in 2012, accounting for 2% of all cancer cases. Oral cancer is more common in men than in women (Kalavrezos and Scully, 2015d). Around 90% of oral cancers are squamous cell carcinomas (SCC), mostly affecting the tongue and the floor of the mouth.

Risk factors for oral cancer include age, genetics, tobacco (Kalavrezos and Scully, 2015a), smoking, alcohol, betel (Kalavrezos and Scully, 2015b), exposure to radiation (Kalavrezos and Scully, 2015c) and human papilloma virus (HPV) infection (Castellsague *et al.*, 2016).

The 5-year survival rate for early-stage, localised oral cancer is over 80%. This figure drops to above 40% if the cancer has spread to cervical lymph nodes and below 20% for advanced tumours with distant metastasis. Extracapsular spread is one of the most important prognostic factors in oral SCC (Shaw *et al.*, 2010). Other important prognostic factors include increased N stage (according to the TNM staging system), increased T stage, involved or close margins, advanced age, perineural invasion, co-morbidity and poor tumour differentiation (Rogers *et al.*, 2009). Therefore, early detection and diagnosis of oral cancer are crucial to improve its prognosis and reduce the risk of adverse treatment effects. UK referral guidelines and important diagnostic aspects of oral cancer, including the staging and grading of tumours, have been thoroughly discussed by Kalavrezos and Scully (Kalavrezos and Scully, 2016a, b).

A wide range of modalities have been used to treat oral cancer, including different types of surgery, external beam radiotherapy, intensity-modulated radiotherapy (IMRT), brachytherapy, chemotherapy, photodynamic therapy, cryotherapy, molecularly targeted therapy and immunotherapy. Common management protocols for oral SCC in most centres include primary ablative surgery with or without surgical reconstruction and postoperative radiotherapy or chemoradiotherapy in some cases (Shaw *et al.*, 2011).

32.2 Roles of the Multidisciplinary Team in Head and Neck Cancer Management

Head and neck oncology patients in the UK are managed by MDTs (Kalavrezos and Scully, 2016c) with the following members.

- Surgeons including an ear, nose and throat (ENT) surgeon, an oral and maxillofacial surgeon (OMFS) and a plastic surgeon. Their main roles are patient assessment, diagnosis, preparation, surgical management and reconstruction of the defects.
- Clinical oncologists advise on treatment modalities such as radiotherapy, chemotherapy and/or palliative care.
- Restorative dentists provide any necessary preoperative, intraoperative and postoperative dental advice and treatment as well as prosthetic rehabilitation following cancer treatment.
- Pathologists with expertise in both histopathology and cytopathology confirm the microscopic diagnosis (including depth of invasion, presence of any perineural or perivascular invasion, and extracapsular spread of the tumour), pathological staging and grading of the tumour and assess the resected specimen margins for effective clearance of the tumour.
- Radiologists advise and report on diagnostic imaging, including chest X-ray radiography, ultrasound, computed tomography (CT), magnetic resonance imaging (MRI) and positron emission tomography (PET) imaging.
- Clinical nurse specialists (CNS) play a key role in the MDT and provide both psychosocial support and co-ordination of care for patients. The CNS also works

Diseases and Conditions in Dentistry: An Evidence-Based Reference, First Edition. Keyvan Moharamzadeh.

Companion website: www.wiley.com/go/moharamzadeh/diseases

closely with other groups, including patient self-help groups, and with other members of specialist and extended teams.

- The speech and language therapist (SLT) helps patients whose cancer or treatment causes problems with communication or swallowing, and also provides psychosocial support and information for patients and carers.
- The dietitian is involved in pretreatment assessment to correct patients' pre-existing nutritional deficiencies before treatment begins, and to maintain their nutritional status during and after treatment. Dietitians provide support and advice regarding tube feeding, help to manage some of the treatment side effects and also provide education on nutritional issues for other professionals who work with cancer patients.
- The team secretary, data manager and MDT co-ordinator organise MDT meetings, provide clerical support for the MDT, record all data and decisions made by the team and communicate appropriate information promptly to all those (such as GPs) who may require it.
- Other members include anaesthetist, dental hygienist, senior nursing staff from the head and neck ward, palliative care specialist, psychiatrist and psychologist.

32.3 Consequences of Cancer Surgery in Mandible

Cancer surgery in the mandible can have several consequences (Pace-Balzan *et al.*, 2011).

- Impaired mastication due to the loss of teeth and mandibular integrity, potential damage to the temporomandibular joint, muscles of mastication, alteration of oral anatomy, reduced tongue function and patient's ability to form and manipulate a food bolus.
- Swallowing can be difficult if tongue strength and mobility are reduced. Dry mouth following radiotherapy can further exacerbate this problem.
- Speech problems if there is damage to lips and tongue. Speech can be significantly impaired if the tumour affects the maxillae or oropharynx.
- Poor saliva control due to altered oral anatomy, diminished sulci, motor and sensory impairment of lips and perioral tissues.
- Facial disfigurement caused by the tumour itself or following cancer surgery, especially with large tumours requiring neck dissection and/or free flap reconstruction. This may cause social concerns and affect the patient's self-esteem.
- Reduced ability to wear conventional dentures due to altered oral anatomy, mucositis and xerostomia following radiotherapy.

Most of the above issues can have a significant impact on head and neck cancer patients' quality of life (Rogers *et al.*, 2010, 2016).

32.4 Classification of Mandibular Defects

Defects of the mandible can be categorised based on their location and extent. Jewer (1989) classified mandibular defects into the following groups.

- Central defects that include both canines (C).
- Lateral segments excluding the condyle (L).
- Condylar resection together with the lateral mandible (hemi-mandibular resection) (H).
- Combinations of the above defects (LC, HC, LCL, HCL and HH).

This classification was further modified to describe associated soft tissue defects as well.

- 't' for tongue defect
- 'm' for mucosal defect
- 's' for an external skin defect

A similar classification based on functional and aesthetic factors has also been described (Boyd *et al.*, 1993).

Brown *et al.* (2016) proposed a new classification for mandibular defects after oncological resection based on the four corners of the mandible: class I (lateral defect), class II (hemi-mandibulectomy defect), class III (anterior defect), class IV (extensive defect). Further classes (Ic, IIc, IVc) are defined if the defect included condylectomy. The increasing defect class is related to the size of the defect, osteotomy rate, and functional and aesthetic outcome, with potential to guide the method of reconstruction.

32.5 Rehabilitation of Mandibular Defects

Rehabilitation of mandibular defects resulting from oral cancer resection may involve surgical reconstruction and prosthetic treatment, as discussed in the following sections.

32.5.1 Surgical Reconstruction of Mandibular Defects

Anterior mandibular (C) defects are often reconstructed using free vascularised bone grafts (Chim *et al.*, 2010). A free fibula bone graft is the first choice for reconstruction of anterior or large defects (Kokosis *et al.*, 2016). An iliac crest vascularised free flap was also commonly used in the past (Shenaq and Klebuc, 1994).

Lateral (L) defects can be reconstructed with free vascularised bone grafts or soft tissue flaps such as anterolateral thigh (ALT), gracilis, rectus and latissimus dorsi flaps, with or without reconstruction plates. However, reconstruction with plates is associated with lower success rates and higher risk of complications such as plate exposure (Fanzio *et al.*, 2015). Therefore, in patients with poor prognosis, soft tissue flap and plate reconstruction may be a simple adequate option but in dentate patients with favourable prognosis, free vascularised bone grafts are more durable and the preferred option (Shnayder *et al.*, 2015).

Table 32.1 summarises some of the characteristics, advantages and disadvantages of commonly used free flaps in mandibular reconstruction. Further relevant details are discussed in a previous publication by Chim *et al.* (2010).

A systematic review of 9499 mandibular defects that were reconstructed with fibular (6178), iliac crest (1380), composite radial (1127), scapular (709), serratus anterior and rib (63), metatarsal (32) and lateral arm flaps including humerus (10) showed the failure rate was higher for iliac crest (6.2%) than for fibular, radial and scapular flaps combined (3.4%). Dental implants were most commonly placed in reconstructed mandibles with iliac crest bone (Brown *et al.*, 2017).

32.5.2 Prosthetic Rehabilitation of Mandibular Defects

32.5.2.1 Pretherapy Dental Screening

Initial full dental assessment prior to cancer treatment is a crucial stage to establish and maintain the patient's oral and dental health (Butterworth *et al.*, 2016). This is particularly important if the patient is to have radiotherapy (see Chapters 36 and 44).

The aim of pretreatment screening is to identify and eliminate any dental diseases by restorative treatment or the extraction of teeth with poor prognosis, especially posterior molar teeth with compromised prognosis. Patient motivation and preventive care, including oral hygiene education (OHE), diet advice, fluoride application (for dentate patients) and denture care advice (for denture wearers), as well as smoking cessation and alcohol advice, must be initiated prior to cancer therapy and maintained during and after treatment.

32.5.2.2 Prosthetic Challenges

Prosthetic rehabilitation of mandibular defects is often challenging due to altered oral anatomy, compromised tissue support, presence of scar tissue, bulky flaps, reduced sulcus depth and the neutral zone, impaired tongue function, altered sensation, mandibular deviation and restricted mouth opening. In patients who have received radiotherapy, there is also an increased risk of development of oral mucositis, dry mouth (with low quality and

Table 32.1 Free flaps commonly used in mandibular reconstruction.

Flap name	Advantages	Disadvantages
Fibula flap	• Provides a long segment of bone. • Allows a two-team approach, where the resecting and reconstructive team can work simultaneously. Vertical distraction osteogenesis can be applied secondarily to gain adequate alveolar height	• Slight donor site morbidity, including pain on ambulation and ankle instability. Limited height which does not allow both contouring of the inferior mandibular margin and restoring sufficient alveolar height for dental implants
Iliac crest osteocutaneous flap based on the deep circumflex iliac artery	• Provides a large piece of curved corticocancellous bone with good height suitable for placement of dental implants. Donor site hidden under clothing	• Groin skin provides a poor colour match in the head and neck. Difficult to shape the curved bone in anterior mandible. Bulky soft tissue component. Donor site morbidity: pain and abdominal hernias
Scapular free osteocutaneous flap	• Large quantity of skin and soft tissue. Concealed donor site	• The bone lacks a segmental blood supply and does not tolerate osteotomies well. Limited quantity of bone. Does not permit a two-team approach as the patient needs to be turned to harvest the graft. Shoulder disability
Radial forearm osteocutaneous flap	• Provides a large quantity of soft tissue	• Only a short segment of thin monocortical bone (up to14 cm) can be harvested which does not tolerate osteotomies well. Increased risk of fracture of the radius after flap harvest. • Unsightly donor site

quantity of saliva), radiation-induced caries, trismus and osteoradionecrosis (ORN) (Siddall *et al.*, 2012).

Potential solutions to overcome some of these challenges are listed below.

- Preprosthetic surgery such as vestibuloplasty to increase the depth of sulci, debulking large soft tissue flaps and free gingival grafting to increase the amount of attached keratinised tissue (Kwasnicki and Butterworth, 2009).
- Surgical release of the tongue to improve its mobility.
- Lowering of the palatal contour of the maxillary prosthesis to enable contact with the compromised tongue and enhance its function.
- Placement of osseointegrated implants to support fixed or removable prostheses.
- Prevention and management of side effects of radiotherapy are discussed in detail in Chapters 36 and 44.

32.5.2.3 Conventional Prosthetic Management

Initially, employing conservative prosthetic treatment approaches such as base plates only without teeth, removable complete or partial dentures, simple fixed bridges and shortened dental arch enables evaluation of treatment effectiveness and the patient's acceptance of simple conventional prosthetic treatment. Functional impression techniques, artificial teeth with shallow cusp inclinations and occlusal balance and articulation are important factors to improve stability of the dentures.

Where there is loss of mandibular continuity, deviation of the residual mandible towards the affected side can occur. To reduce mandibular deviation, different methods can be used such as intermaxillary fixation, sectional or modified dentures (in edentulous patients) and mandibular guidance appliances or resection prostheses (in dentate patients) that use a mandibular guide flange or a maxillary occlusal platform (guide ramp) to guide the mandibular segment into optimal occlusal contact (Bhattacharya *et al.*, 2015; Hasanreisoglu *et al.*, 1992).

It has been shown that a significant number of oncology patients can be successfully rehabilitated with conventional mandibular prostheses (Garrett *et al.*, 2006; Tang *et al.*, 2008).

32.5.2.4 Implants in Oncology Patients

According to the UK National Multidisciplinary Guidelines on restorative dentistry and oral rehabilitation of oncology patients, dental implants should be considered for all patients having resection for head and neck cancer (Butterworth *et al.*, 2016).

32.5.2.4.1 Indications and Limitations Osseointegrated implants can be indicated in the following circumstances.

- To retain a fixed prosthesis to replace the missing teeth in patients with good prognosis for both cancer and implant treatment.
- To support a removable prosthesis and improve its retention and stability, especially when there is poor hard and soft tissue support and dry mouth.

Implants are less desirable in oncology patients with the following problems (Pace-Balzan *et al.*, 2011).

- Inadequate motivation, unrealistic expectations and lack of resources for treatment and maintenance.
- Poor oncological prognosis.
- Significantly restricted access in patients with severe trismus or very small mouth opening.
- Poor oral hygiene, existing and untreated periodontal disease, smoking, drug abuse and excessive alcohol consumption.
- Inadequate bone quantity and quality.
- Unfavourable maxillo-mandibular relationship.
- Inadequate oral function, tongue volume and mobility as well as poor motor and sensory innervation on the tissue sides that are to be in contact with the implant-retained prosthesis.
- Bisphosphonate medication, especially intravenous bisphosphonates.
- Bleeding disorders.

32.5.2.4.2 Relevant History and Preoperative Examination

Preoperative history taking must include:

- full medical history and obtaining relevant information from the MDT regarding tumour stage, grade, prognosis and the details of cancer treatment, especially radiotherapy time, dose and field
- social history, including smoking and alcohol
- dental history, including previous dental treatment, denture history for denture wearers and access to dental care and maintenance
- oral hygiene methods and use of any oral care products
- questions regarding diet, dry mouth, oral intake of solid food and liquid drinks and swallowing status.

Preoperative clinical examination must include:

- assessment of mouth opening, tongue function and the quality of the soft tissues and evaluation of any present free flaps in terms of their bulk, compressibility, hair-bearing skin and amount of keratinised tissue
- dental examination and full periodontal assessment. Sensibility testing and periapical radiographic examination of the teeth may also be required
- evaluation of any existing fixed or removable prostheses
- assessment of occlusion

- clinical and radiographic evaluation of bone volume and the position of any metal hardware. This may include cone beam computed tomography (CBCT).

32.5.2.4.3 ***Planning, Timing and Design Considerations*** Implant planning and placement as well as the management of localised and generalised ridge defects are discussed in Chapters 37, 45 and 46.

The goal must be restoration-driven implant placement which necessitates comprehensive prosthodontic planning prior to surgery.

Computer-guided implant surgery using custom-made surgical stents based on three-dimensional imaging such as CBCT is a useful approach that enables accurate, predictable and atraumatic implant placement (Dawood *et al.*, 2013). This is particularly valuable in oncology patients as it minimises surgical trauma to irradiated jaws which are at higher risk of developing ORN (Horowitz *et al.*, 2009).

When designing an implant-retained fixed prosthesis for oncology patients, it is mandatory for the suprastructure to be screw retained. This will enable easy removal of the prosthesis to allow regular inspection of the underlying tissues for potential cancer recurrence.

In irradiated jaws, it is also best to avoid mucosal contacts with the prosthesis to minimise the risk of denture trauma to irradiated sites.

Although in non-irradiated patients a mandibular overdenture supported by two implants can be sufficient, in irradiated edentulous jaws, a minimum of four implants in the anterior mandible is recommended to achieve maximum support for the prosthesis and to relieve the vulnerable underlying soft tissues, especially after radiotherapy. Atraumatic surgical technique with minimal reflection of periosteum and one-stage implant placement further minimises the risk of soft tissue trauma and development of ORN. It is also recommended to wait 4–6 months before abutment connection to allow extra time for osseointegration in irradiated sites (Schoen *et al.*, 2004).

Since most recurrences of oral malignancies manifest within 1 year after initial cancer treatment (Kissun *et al.*, 2006), it may be prudent to wait at least 1 year before secondary implant placement.

32.5.2.4.4 ***Primary Implants*** In oncology patients, dental implants can be successfully placed at the time of surgical tumour resection (primary implants) (Barber *et al.*, 2011). The advantages of placement of primary implants are as follows.

- Completion of oral rehabilitation in a shorter period of time compared to a delayed approach.
- Better access at the time of reconstruction as trismus may develop later.
- Osseointegration will take place before radiotherapy.
- Avoids the need for further surgery to place implants.

Disadvantages of primary implants include the following.

- Unknown patient prognosis as it may not always be possible to restore or use the implants in the future.
- Risk of failure due to postoperative radiotherapy.
- Less precise implant placement.
- Radiation scattering during radiotherapy.

Therefore, primary implants may be desirable for well-motivated low-risk patients with localised anterior tumours with favourable behaviour in continuous mandible and without lymph node involvement, especially if it is expected that cancer surgery will significantly hamper the prognosis of conventional prosthetic rehabilitation in the future (Siddall *et al.*, 2012).

32.5.2.4.5 ***Implants in Irradiated Bone*** A meta-analysis by Chrcanovic *et al.* (2016) showed that irradiation has a negative effect on the survival of implants, especially in patients receiving high doses of radiation (absorbed dose of higher than 55 Gy). However, there was no statistically significant difference in survival when implants were placed before or after 12 months following radiotherapy. This study and others have failed to support the effectiveness of hyperbaric oxygen therapy in irradiated patients (Esposito and Worthington, 2013).

These findings were consistent with other systematic reviews which reported mean survival rates for implants placed in irradiated jaws ranging from 46.3% to 98.0% and a significant increase in the risk of implant failure in irradiated patients with a risk ratio of 2.74. Implant failure rates were significantly higher in maxillary sites (risk ratio: 5.96) (Chambrone *et al.*, 2013).

A systematic review of 38 studies published between 1990 and 2012 showed that overall implant survival rates were 88.9% for implants placed after radiotherapy and 92.2% for implants placed before radiotherapy. The survival of implants placed after radiotherapy was significantly higher for the mandible (93.3%) than for the maxillae (78.9%) or for grafted bone (87.5%) (Nooh, 2013).

32.5.2.4.6 ***Implants in Grafted Bone Flaps*** A systematic review of 20 studies showed survival rates of implants placed in rehabilitated jaws with bone flaps were between 82.4% and 100%. The most commonly reported complications were peri-implant mucositis, soft tissue proliferation and peri-implantitis. The main reported prognostic factors were time of implant placement and radiotherapy (Zhang *et al.*, 2016).

Rohner has described a technique to prefabricate vascularised fibular flaps with implants placed and integrated into the fibula before flap harvest and tissue transfer. A provisional prosthesis that was fixed to the flap with implants *in situ* was used as a guide to accurately position the flap by placing the prosthesis into occlusion (Rohner *et al.*, 2013).

Case Study

A 49-year-old male patient was referred from the OMFS department for prosthetic rehabilitation following resection of T2 N0 M0 SCC from the floor of the mouth and reconstruction with a radial forearm flap.

The patient wanted to have some teeth to be able to chew food. He was medically fit and well and had stopped smoking 2 years before. He consumed 10 units of alcohol per week.

The patient's oral food intake was satisfactory and he was managing to swallow well although he felt some restriction of tongue movements due to the presence of the flap.

The patient was visiting a dental hygienist regularly for periodontal scaling and trimming of the hair on the floor of the mouth on the skin side of the flap.

Clinical examination showed good mouth opening, satisfactory tongue mobility and strength, an edentulous mandible with a bulky radial forearm flap on the floor of the mouth and dentate maxillae with generalised gingival recession, inflammation and cervical caries on the maxillary anterior teeth (Figure 32.1). The patient had a mild class III skeletal relationship.

The BPE scores were 3 in the upper quadrants with generalised 4–5 mm periodontal pockets and bleeding on probing.

Radiographic examination (Figure 32.2) showed the presence of a surgical plate on the anterior mandible and good bone height in both anterior and posterior mandible. Generalised moderate periodontal bone loss was noticed on the maxillary teeth.

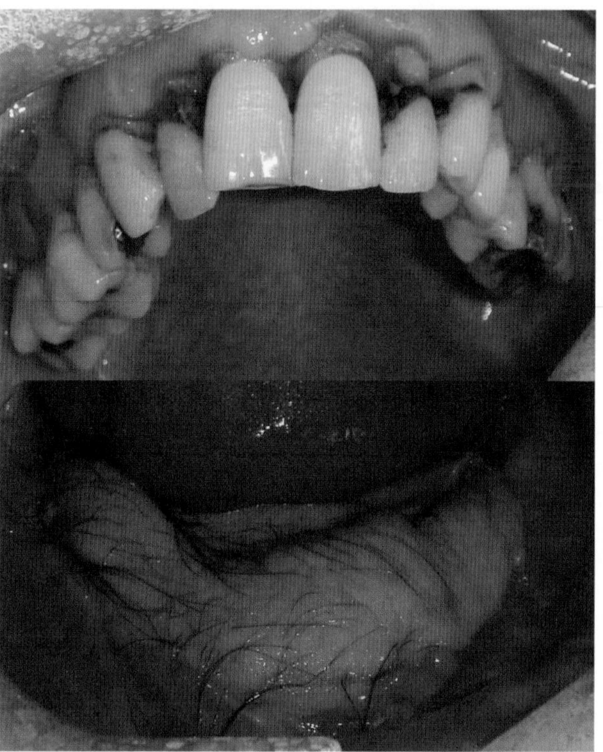

Figure 32.1 Preoperative clinical photographs.

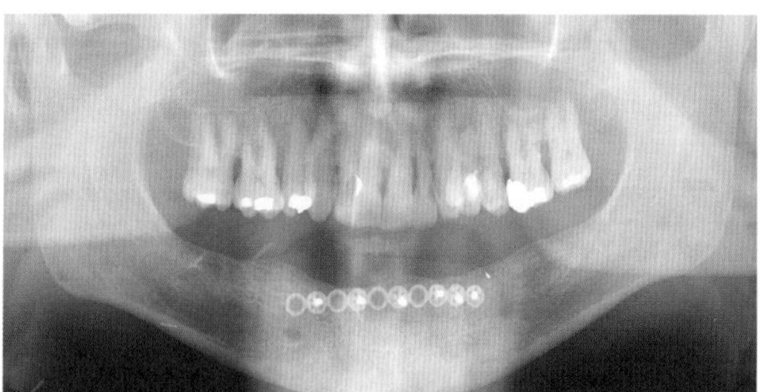

Figure 32.2 Preoperative oral panoramic radiograph.

Initial Treatment

Initial treatment included:

1) preventive care, OHE, fluoride and diet advice
2) non-surgical periodontal treatment
3) restoration of caries on the maxillary anterior teeth
4) fabrication and fitting of a temporary conventional mandibular complete denture to assess the patient's ability to wear a prosthesis and also to determine tooth position for potential future implant planning and placement
5) periodontal reassessment and maintenance.

Review of the denture showed significant lack of retention and stability due to the presence of the bulky underlying flap and diminished sulcus depth.

Following discussion of options with the patient, including risks and benefits, it was decided to rehabilitate the mandible with an implant-retained fixed prosthesis.

As part of implant planning, radiopaque markers (composite fillings) were placed within the denture teeth and a CBCT scan of the mandible was obtained with the denture *in situ* to assess the bone volume in relation to the teeth.

Adequate bone width and height were available in both the anterior and posterior mandible. Therefore, it was decided to place four regular neck (4.1 mm endosteal implant diameter) standard Straumann implants with 14 mm length in the mandible to support a fixed full-arch prosthesis (All-on-Four).

Surgical Treatment

The surgical procedure was carried out under general anaesthesia, including the following main steps.

1) Crestal incision on the attached gingivae and elevation of a full-thickness flap.
2) Careful dissection and debulking of the radial forearm flap from a safe margin to prevent damage to its main vascular pedicle (Figure 32.3).
3) Removal of the bone screws and surgical plate from the anterior mandible to allow implant placement (Figure 32.4).
4) Placement of four mandibular implants in the canine and first molar sites (Figures 32.5 and 32.6).
5) Flap repositioning and suturing to ensure presence of keratinised gingivae as much as possible around the implants.
6) Healing abutments with adequate height (5 mm) were fitted onto the implants to avoid soft tissue growing over the implants (Figure 32.7).

The option of a free gingival graft from the palate to increase the width of keratinised tissue around the implants was offered to the patient at this stage. However, he did not want further surgery and preferred to proceed with prosthetic treatment.

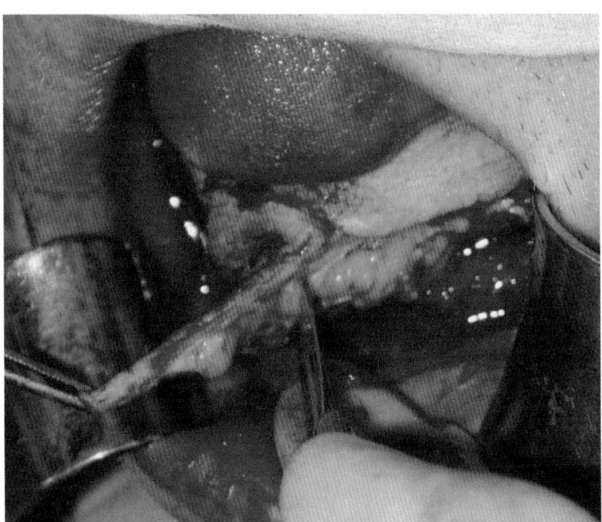

Figure 32.3 Surgical debulking of the radial forearm flap and removal of excessive hair-bearing skin.

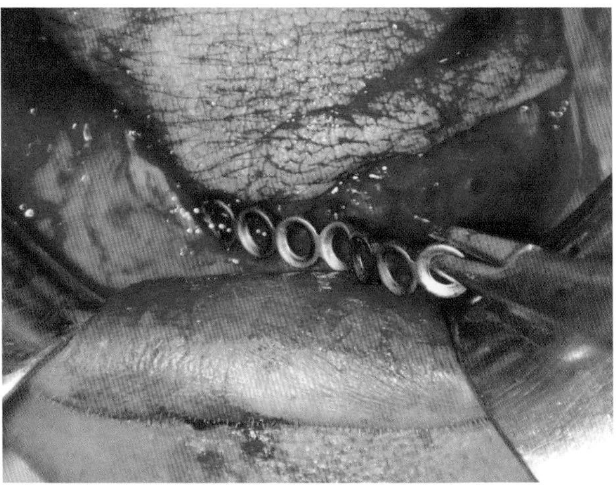

Figure 32.4 Surgical plate removal from the anterior mandible.

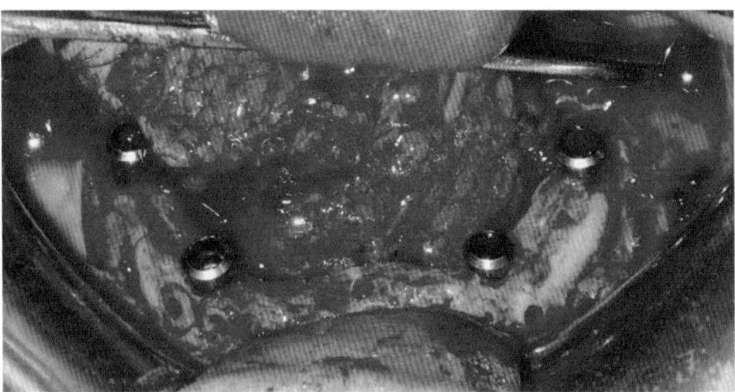

Figure 32.5 Four tissue-level implants placed in the edentulous mandible.

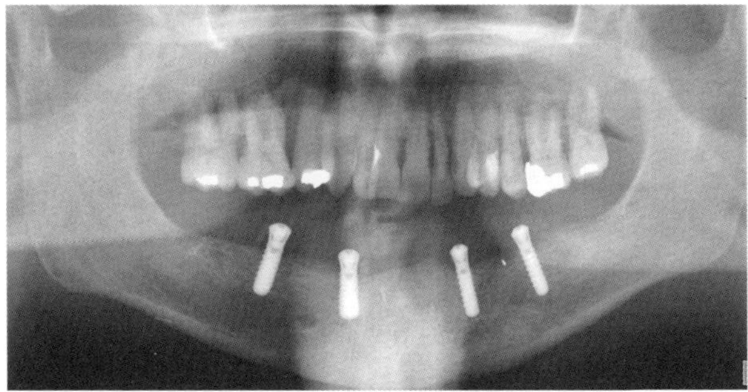

Figure 32.6 Post-implant placement panoramic radiograph.

Prosthetic Phase Treatment

The prosthetic phase of the treatment included the following stages.

1) Primary impression, fabrication of an open special tray, fitting of open-tray impression copings on the implants and fixture-head level impression of the implants with additional silicone impression material (Figure 32.8).

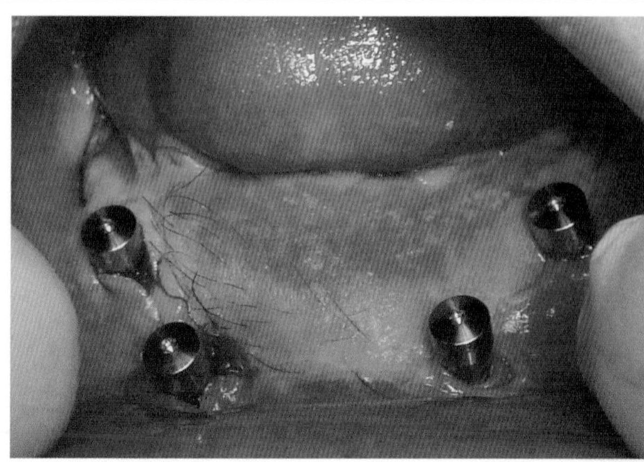

Figure 32.7 Clinical photograph showing healing abutments fitted on the implants and significant reduction in the size of the flap.

2) Preparation of the stone model with implant replicas (analogs) in place and verification of the correct position of the implants using a Duralay verification jig (Figure 32.9).
3) A screw-retained wax rim was also fabricated to enable accurate registration of the bite. Shade was also taken at the same time.
4) Preparation of articulated models to assess the available intraocclusal space and design the metal framework.
5) Trial of teeth on wax to verify final tooth position. The anterior teeth were set up at an edge-to-edge position due to skeletal class III relationship.
6) Subsequent stages included fabrication, trial of titanium metal framework, and trial insertion of the teeth on wax on the metal framework (Figure 32.10).
7) Insertion of the final processed screw-retained prosthesis, tightening the screws with a torque wrench and filling the screw access holes with composite resin.
8) Postoperative instructions, review and maintenance.

Postoperative clinical photographs of the final implant-retained prosthesis and the patient's smile are shown in Figure 32.11.

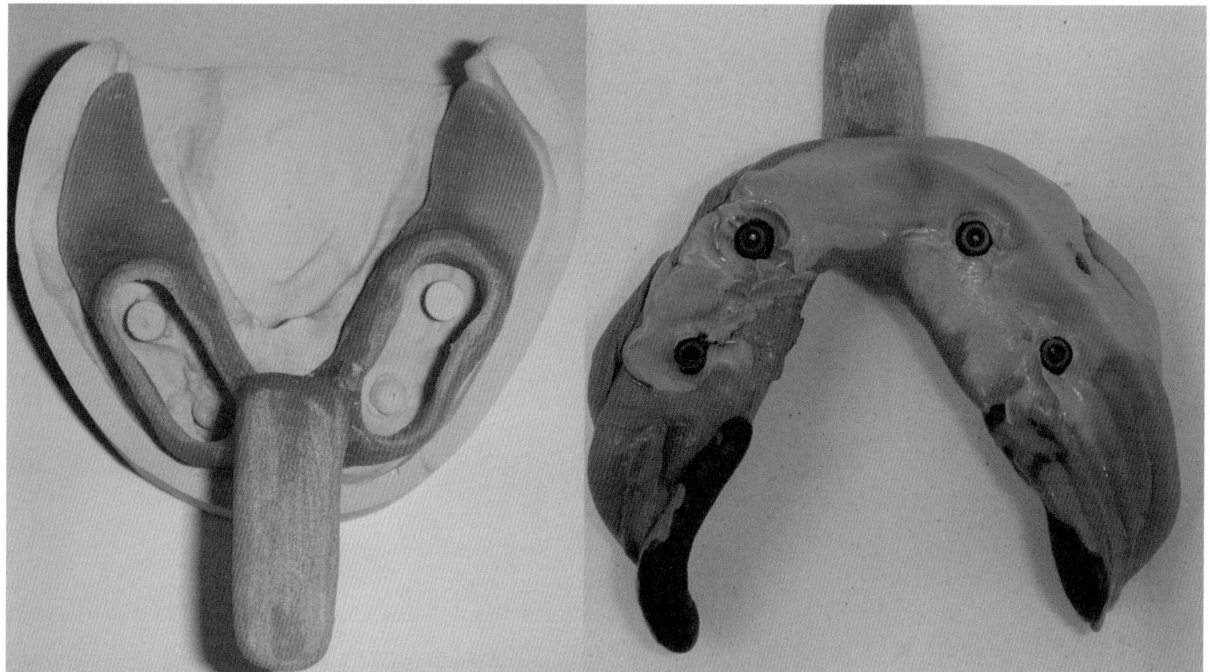

Figure 32.8 Silicone impression of the implants using an open tray impression technique.

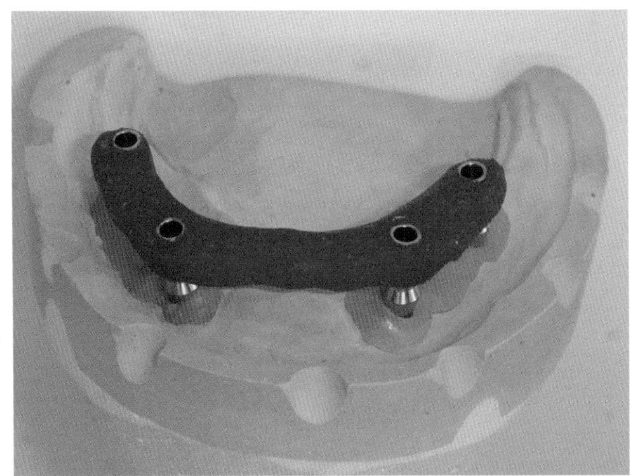

Figure 32.9 Duralay verification jig to verify the position of the implants.

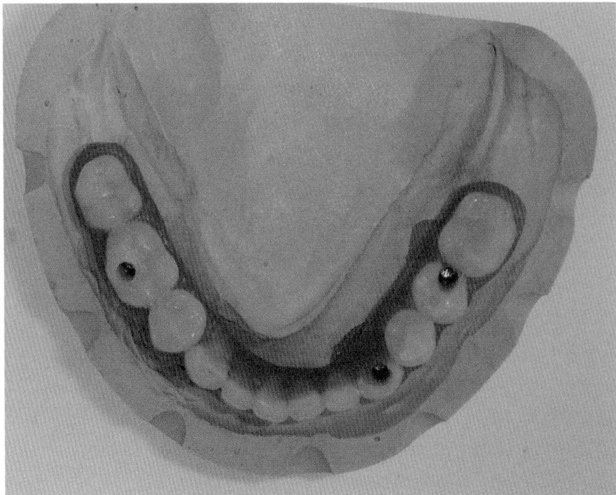

Figure 32.10 Photograph of the screw-retained acrylic teeth on wax on metal framework fitted onto the model ready for final trial insertion in the mouth.

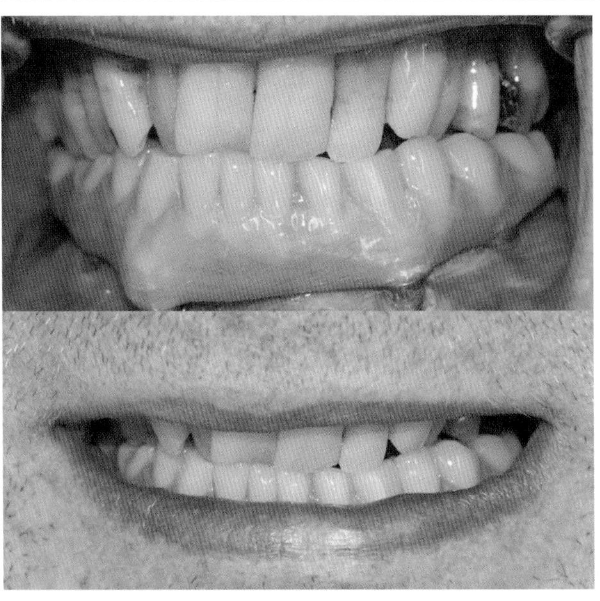

Figure 32.11 Postperative clinical photographs of the final screw-retained prosthesis and the patient's smile.

References

Barber, A.J., Butterworth, C.J. and Rogers, S.N. (2011) Systematic review of primary osseointegrated dental implants in head and neck oncology. *Br J Oral Maxillofac Surg*, **49**, 29–36.

Bhattacharya, S.R., Majumdar, D., Singh, D.K., Islam, M.D., Ray, P.K. and Saha, N. (2015) Maxillary palatal ramp prosthesis: a prosthodontic solution to manage mandibular deviation following surgery. *Contemp Clin Dent*, **6**, S111–113.

Boyd, J.B., Gullane, P.J., Rotstein, L.E., Brown, D.H. and Irish, J.C. (1993) Classification of mandibular defects. *Plast Reconstr Surg*, **92**, 1266–1275.

Brown, J.S., Barry, C., Ho, M. and Shaw, R. (2016) A new classification for mandibular defects after oncological resection. *Lancet Oncol*, **17**, E23–30.

Brown, J.S., Lowe, D., Kanatas, A. and Schache, A. (2017) Mandibular reconstruction with vascularised bone flaps: a systematic review over 25 years. *Br J Oral Maxillofac Surg*, **55**, 113–126.

Butterworth, C., Mccaul, L. and Barclay, C. (2016) Restorative dentistry and oral rehabilitation: united kingdom national multidisciplinary guidelines. *J Laryngol Otol*, **130**, S41–S44.

Castellsague, X., Alemany, L., Quer, M., Halec, G. and Quiros, B. (2016) HPV involvement in head and neck cancers: comprehensive assessment of biomarkers in 3680 patients. *J Natl Cancer Inst*, **108**, Djv403.

Chambrone, L., Mandia, J. Jr, Shibli, J.A., Romito, G.A. and Abrahao, M. (2013) Dental implants installed in irradiated jaws: a systematic review. *J Dent Res*, **92**, 119s–130s.

Chim, H., Salgado, C.J., Mardini, S. and Chen, H.C. (2010) Reconstruction of mandibular defects. *Semin Plast Surg*, **24**, 188–197.

Chrcanovic, B.R., Albrektsson, T. and Wennerberg, A. (2016) Dental implants in irradiated versus nonirradiated patients: a meta-analysis. *Head Neck*, **38**, 448–481.

Dawood, A., Tanner, S. and Hutchison, I. (2013) Computer guided surgery for implant placement and dental rehabilitation in a patient undergoing sub-total mandibulectomy and microvascular free flap reconstruction. *J Oral Implantol*, **39**, 497–502.

Esposito, M. and Worthington, H.V. (2013) Interventions for replacing missing teeth: hyperbaric oxygen therapy for irradiated patients who require dental implants. *Cochrane Database Syst Rev*, **9**, CD003603.

Fanzio, P.M., Chang, K.P., Chen, H.H. *et al.* (2015) Plate exposure after anterolateral thigh free-flap reconstruction in head and neck cancer patients with composite mandibular defects. *Ann Surg Oncol*, **22**, 3055–3060.

Ferlay, J., Steliarova-Foucher, E., Lortet-Tieulent, J. *et al.* (2013) Cancer incidence and mortality patterns in Europe: estimates for 40 countries in 2012. *Eur J Cancer*, **49**, 1374–1403.

Garrett, N., Roumanas, E.D., Blackwell, K.E. *et al.* (2006) Efficacy of conventional and implant-supported mandibular resection prostheses: study overview and treatment outcomes. *J Prosthet Dent*, **96**, 13–24.

Hasanreisoglu, U., Uctasli, S. and Gurbuz, A. (1992) Mandibular guidance prostheses following resection procedures: three case reports. *Eur J Prosthodont Restor Dent*, **1**, 69–72.

Horowitz, A., Orentlicher, G. and Goldsmith, D. (2009) Computerized implantology for the irradiated patient. *J Oral Maxillofac Surg*, **67**, 619–623.

Jewer, D.D., Boyd, J.B., Manktelow, R.T. *et al.* (1989) Orofacial and mandibular reconstruction with the iliac crest free flap: a review of 60 cases and a new method of classification. *Plast Reconstr Surg*, **84**, 391–403; discussion 404–405.

Kalavrezos, N. and Scully, C. (2015a) Mouth cancer for clinicians. Part 3: Risk factors (traditional: tobacco). *Dent Update*, **42**, 476–478, 480–483.

Kalavrezos, N. and Scully, C. (2015b) Mouth cancer for clinicians. Part 4: Risk Factors (traditional: alcohol, betel and others). *Dent Update*, **42**, 644–646, 648–650, 653–654.

Kalavrezos, N. and Scully, C. (2015c) Mouth cancer for clinicians. Part 5: Risk Factors (other). *Dent Update*, **42**, 766–768, 771–772, 775–776 passim.

Kalavrezos, N. and Scully, C. (2015d) Mouth cancer for clinicians. Part 2: Epidemiology. *Dent Update*, **42**, 354–356, 358–359.

Kalavrezos, N. and Scully, C. (2016a) Mouth cancer for clinicians. Part 7: Cancer diagnosis and pre-treatment preparation. *Dent Update*, **43**, 50–54, 57–60, 63–65.

Kalavrezos, N. and Scully, C. (2016b) Mouth cancer for clinicians. Part 8: Referral. *Dent Update*, **43**, 176–178, 181–182, 184–185.

Kalavrezos, N. and Scully, C. (2016c) Mouth cancer for clinicians. Part 9: The patient and care team. *Dent Update*, **43**, 276–278, 281–282, 285–287.

Kissun, D., Magennis, P., Lowe, D., Brown, J.S., Vaughan, E.D. and Rogers, S.N. (2006) Timing and presentation of recurrent oral and oropharyngeal squamous cell carcinoma and awareness in the outpatient clinic. *Br J Oral Maxillofac Surg*, **44**, 371–376.

Kokosis, G., Schmitz, R., Powers, D.B. and Erdmann, D. (2016) Mandibular reconstruction using the free vascularized fibula graft: an overview of different modifications. *Arch Plast Surg*, **43**, 3–9.

Kwasnicki, A. and Butterworth, C. (2009) 360 Degrees peri-implant, keratinised, soft-tissue grafting with stereolithographic-aided dressing plate. *Int J Oral Maxillofac Surg*, **38**, 87–90.

Nooh, N. (2013) Dental implant survival in irradiated oral cancer patients: a systematic review of the literature. *Int J Oral Maxillofac Implants*, **28**, 1233–1242.

Pace-Balzan, A., Shaw, R.J. and Butterworth, C. (2011) Oral rehabilitation following treatment for oral cancer. *Periodontology 2000*, **57**, 102–117.

Rogers, S.N. (2010) Quality of life perspectives in patients with oral cancer. *Oral Oncol*, **46**, 445–447.

Rogers, S.N., Brown, J.S., Woolgar, J.A. *et al.* (2009) Survival following primary surgery for oral cancer. *Oral Oncol*, **45**, 201–211.

Rogers, S.N., Semple, C., Babb, M. and Humphris, G. (2016) Quality of life considerations in head and neck cancer: United Kingdom National Multidisciplinary Guidelines. *J Laryngol Otol*, **130**, S49–S52.

Rohner, D., Bucher, P. and Hammer, B. (2013) Prefabricated fibular flaps for reconstruction of defects of the maxillofacial skeleton: planning, technique, and long-term experience. *Int J Oral Maxillofac Implants*, **28**, E221–229.

Schoen, P.J., Reintsema, H., Raghoebar, G.M., Vissink, A. and Roodenburg, J.L. (2004) The use of implant retained mandibular prostheses in the oral rehabilitation of head and neck cancer patients. a review and rationale for treatment planning. *Oral Oncol*, **40**, 862–871.

Shaw, R.J., Lowe, D., Woolgar, J.A. *et al.* (2010) Extracapsular spread in oral squamous cell carcinoma. *Head Neck*, **32**, 714–722.

Shaw, R.J., Pace-Balzan, A. and Butterworth, C. (2011) Contemporary clinical management of oral squamous cell carcinoma. *Periodontology 2000*, **57**, 89–101.

Shenaq, S.M. and Klebuc, M.J. (1994) The iliac crest microsurgical free flap in mandibular reconstruction. *Clin Plast Surg*, **21**, 37–44.

Shnayder, Y., Lin, D., Desai, S.C., Nussenbaum, B., Sand, J.P. and Wax, M.K. (2015) Reconstruction of the lateral mandibular defect: a review and treatment algorithm. *Jama Facial Plast Surg*, **17**, 367–373.

Siddall, K.Z., Rogers, S.N. and Butterworth, C.J. (2012) The prosthodontic pathway of the oral cancer patient. *Dent Update*, **39**, 98–100, 103–106.

Tang, J.A., Rieger, J.M. and Wolfaardt, J.F. (2008) A review of functional outcomes related to prosthetic treatment after maxillary and mandibular reconstruction in patients with head and neck cancer. *Int J Prosthodont*, **21**, 337–3354.

Zhang, L., Ding, Q., Liu, C., Sun, Y., Xie, Q. and Zhou, Y. (2016) Survival, function, and complications of oral implants placed in bone flaps in jaw rehabilitation: a systematic review. *Int J Prosthodont*, **29**, 115–125.

33

Oncology-Related Defects in Maxillae

33.1 Maxillary Tumours

Maxillary malignant tumours can be classified based on their tissue of origin.

- *Squamous cell carcinoma* (SCC) can arise from the paranasal sinuses or the palatal epithelium. Paranasal sinus tumours often result in larger and more disfiguring defects compared to palatal tumours.
- *Salivary gland tumours* such as adenoid cystic carcinoma and mucoepidermoid carcinomas, which can affect the hard and soft palate. High-grade tumours result in larger defects compared to low-grade tumours.
- *Mesenchymal tumours* such as fibrosarcoma, liposarcoma, chondrosarcomas and osteosarcomas.
- Other malignancies include malignant melanoma, lymphoma, basal cell carcinoma, multiple myeloma, angiosarcoma and malignant schwannoma (Chidzonga, 2006).

Resection of some benign tumours such as ameloblastoma, pleomorphic adenoma and myxoma can also result in maxillary defects.

33.2 Surgical Resection

Maxillary tumours can be accessed and removed using different surgical approaches (Truitt *et al.*, 1999).

- Alveolectomy or alveolar ostectomy is performed transorally to remove part of the alveolar bone (and teeth) associated with a tumour.
- Palatectomy is carried out transorally by initial mucosal incisions with at least 5 mm safe margins around the tumour followed by palatal bony cuts to remove the bone, mucosa and any teeth associated with the tumour.
- Maxillectomy (partial or radical) often requires an extraoral access via skin incisions (Weber–Fergusson incision) to expose the maxilla to be resected. Mucosal incisions and bony cuts are more extensive and may involve the alveolar ridges, palate, nasal bones, orbital floor, malar process, pterygoid plates and zygomatic arch.

Patients with postsurgical maxillary defects are predisposed to hypernasal speech, fluid leakage through the nose, possibility of aspiration, impaired masticatory function and poor aesthetics (Keyf, 2001). Therefore, surgical reconstruction or prosthetic treatment of maxillary defects is an essential part of rehabilitation of this group of patients.

33.3 Classification of Maxillary Defects

Aramany (1978a) classified the partially edentulous maxillectomy dental arches into six groups.

- Class I: Midline resection
- Class II: Unilateral resection (not crossing the midline)
- Class III: Central palate resection (not affecting the teeth)
- Class IV: Bilateral anteroposterior resection (crossing the midline)
- Class V: Posterior resection (not involving the anterior teeth)
- Class VI: Anterior resection (not involving the posterior teeth)

Brown *et al.* (2000) proposed a modified classification system for maxillectomy defects that described both the horizontal and vertical extent of the defect and related the likely functional and aesthetic outcomes to the method of reconstruction.

Brown and Shaw (2010) introduced a further modified version of the classification for maxillae and midface defects with recommended methods of reconstruction for each defect class.

The vertical component was classified as follows.

- Class I: Maxillectomy not causing an oronasal fistula
- Class II: Maxillectomy not involving the orbit

Diseases and Conditions in Dentistry: An Evidence-Based Reference, First Edition. Keyvan Moharamzadeh.

Companion website: www.wiley.com/go/moharamzadeh/diseases

- Class III: Maxillectomy involving the orbital adnexae with orbital retention
- Class IV: Maxillectomy with orbital enucleation or exenteration
- Class V: Orbitomaxillary defect
- Class VI: Nasomaxillary defect

The horizontal or palatal component was classified as follows.

- (a) Central palatal defect without involvement of the dental alveolus
- (b) Unilateral palatal defect less than or equal to half of the palate
- (c) Bilateral palatal defect less than or equal to half of the palate or transverse anterior defect
- (d) Palatal defect greater than half of the palate

33.4 Surgical Reconstruction

Maxillary defects can be rehabilitated with different surgical approaches, depending on the size and complexity of the defect, as described below (Brown and Shaw, 2010; Mucke *et al.*, 2009; O'Connell and Futran, 2010; Shrime and Gilbert, 2009).

33.4.1 Local and Regional Flaps

Local and regional flaps are indicated for repair of small defects.

- Palatal island flap based on the greater palatine vessels.
- Buccal fat pad can also be used in limited cases.
- Temporalis muscle flap and temporoparietal osteofascial flap can be used for orbital reconstruction.

33.4.2 Soft Tissue Free Flaps

Soft tissue free flaps used for maxillary reconstruction include:

- radial forearm free flap, frequently used for small maxillary defects. Its main disadvantage is donor site morbidity
- rectus abdominis flap
- latissimus dorsi flap
- anterolateral thigh (ALT) flap.

33.4.3 Hard Tissue or Composite Free Flaps

Hard tissue or composite free flaps are indicated for reconstruction of more extensive maxillary defects. They can support the orbit and cheek more reliably than soft-tissue free flaps or non-vascularised grafts. The most commonly used hard/composite tissue flaps for maxillary reconstruction are listed below.

- Radial forearm osteocutaneous free flap
- Fibula free flap
- Scapular free flap
- Deep circumflex iliac artery (DCIA)/internal oblique free flap
- Thoracodorsal angular artery (TDAA)/latissimus dorsi free flap

33.5 Prosthetic Treatment

In patients with maxillary defects, the aims of prosthetic treatment are to restore the partition between the oral and nasal cavities, restore palatal contours, replace the missing dentition, provide retention, stability and support for removable denture/obturator prosthesis without stressing any abutment teeth beyond their physiological tolerance, and ultimately improve speech, swallowing, masticatory function and aesthetics (Keyf, 2001).

There has been some debate on whether to aim to reconstruct and close the defects surgically, as described above, or consider prosthetic treatment using obturators to fill the defects. It is important to note that prosthetic treatment is easier and more cost-effective than surgical reconstruction. In addition, leaving the defect open allows monitoring of the tissues for tumour recurrence and prevents mucus accumulation and infection on the nasal side of the flap. An obturator prosthesis restores the palatal contours better than bulky flaps which are often overcontoured and reduce the tongue space. Bulky flaps provide poor tissue support for partial dentures and do not allow utilisation of the defect for retention, causing increased stress on the abutment teeth.

Studies have found no differences between surgical reconstruction and prosthodontic rehabilitation of maxillary defects in terms of facial attractiveness and speech outcomes (Rieger *et al.*, 2011).

Important prognostic factors for successful prosthetic rehabilitation include size of the defect, availability of supporting hard and soft tissues in the defect side, proximity of vital structures, systemic conditions, patient's attitude, motivation, expectations and ability to adapt to the prosthesis (Keyf, 2001).

33.6 Alterations at Surgery to Facilitate Prosthetic Treatment

At the time of tumour resection, the surgeon can help the prosthodontist to improve the outcome of subsequent prosthetic rehabilitation (Ali *et al.*, 2015c; El Fattah *et al.*, 2012). This can be achieved by:

- maintaining access to the defect and removal of the inferior turbinates to prevent their downgrowth
- retaining the premaxillary segment to improve support and stability of the obturator and provide an additional site for implant placement
- skin grafting the cheek side of the defect to create a keratinised lateral wall surface with undercut which can be engaged more effectively by the obturator prosthesis, improving its stability, retention and support
- retention of key teeth and bone resection through the socket next to these teeth to maintain alveolar bone around the teeth
- using the remaining palatal mucosa to cover the bony margin of the defect
- performing coronoidectomy to reduce the risk of postoperative trismus
- placement of primary osseointegrated implants as discussed in the previous chapter
- appropriate management of the remaining soft palate to help velopharyngeal closure. Functional remaining soft palate may be retained but non-functional soft palate remnants are best removed to enable proper extension of an obturator prosthesis onto the residual, functional velopharyngeal musculature. However, in edentulous patients, the remaining band of soft palate may help to improve denture retention.

33.7 Prosthetic Treatment Phases

Prosthetic rehabilitation of patients undergoing maxillectomy is usually carried out over several stages, initially with fabrication of a surgical obturator worn for the first 1–4 weeks immediately after maxillectomy, followed by an interim obturator worn for 3–6 months until the defect is stabilised and finally a definitive obturator (Pace-Balzan *et al.*, 2011).

33.7.1 Surgical Obturator

A surgical obturator separates the oral and nasal cavities in the immediate postoperative period and therefore enables relatively normal speech and deglutition and reduces the psychological impact of the surgery and the period of hospitalisation. It also provides a matrix for surgical packing and reduces the risk of contamination of the surgical wound (Huryn and Piro, 1989).

Basic design principles for an immediate obturator include the following (Carl, 1976).

- It should be extended short of the skin graft and mucosal junction and be kept simple, lightweight and low cost.
- It should reproduce normal palatal contours.
- Perforations may be placed in the interproximal areas to facilitate wire fixation.
- The defect side must be out of occlusion on posterior teeth.

It is preferable not to use the patient's existing denture as a surgical obturator because it may be underextended palatally or overcontoured buccally and may be damaged during fixation.

The procedure of fabrication of a surgical obturator includes the following steps.

1) Initial preoperative impression, preparation and duplication of the stone model.
2) Removal of the teeth in the path of the resection from the cast in the laboratory.
3) Alteration of the cast to restore normal palatal contours.
4) Trimming the cast in the canine area to minimise tension on the midline skin wound.
5) Extension of the acrylic resin to the vestibular depth on the defect side.
6) Addition of loops to engage the reline material; other retention features such as clasps and perforations for wiring; and anterior teeth for esthetics.

Following maxillectomy, the immediate obturator must be tried in and adjusted prior to fixation. It can be relined with silicone putty intraoperatively for better adaptation to the defect walls and can be fixed in place using circumdental, circumnasal or circumzygomatic wires, transalveolar screws and palatal screws (Pace-Balzan *et al.*, 2011).

33.7.2 Interim Obturator

The surgical obturator can be modified to accommodate the changes in the defect and tissues during the early postoperative phase. The interim or provisional obturator can be worn to enable speech and swallowing until wound healing is complete and the defect becomes dimensionally stable.

In most patients, the surgical obturator can be relined with appropriate denture reline material, and clasps can be added for retention. A flange can be incorporated for lip and cheek support and the anterior teeth can be added to improve aesthetics. In edentulous patients, the existing denture can also be relined and used as an interim obturator.

Alternatively, a more precise postsurgical impression can be taken to fabricate a new interim obturator.

If the patient is having radiotherapy, a light and hollow obturator is preferred as the tissues become oedematous and friable. Different fabrication techniques have been described in the literature (Rilo *et al.*, 2005; Shimizu *et al.*, 2009; Ziada and O'Donovan, 2000).

The obturator should be relined regularly to improve adaptation as the healing continues and optimal oral hygiene must be maintained.

33.7.3 Definitive Obturator

Healed and stabilised maxillectomy defects can be rehabilitated permanently with a definitive obturator. Although most maxillectomy defects heal within 3–6 months following surgery, dimensional changes may continue for over a year which may necessitate further relining of the obturator.

A definitive obturator prosthesis must be designed to have adequate support, retention and stability as generally required for any removable prosthesis to serve its intended purpose. In addition, the obturator must be able to seal the defect effectively to prevent leakage of liquid into the nasal passage (Ali *et al.*, 2015a; Aramany, 1978b).

Important factors that affect movement of the prosthesis during function include the size and shape of the defect, presence or absence of supporting palatal shelves, quality and quantity of the remaining dentition, and any implant treatment.

Adequate extension of the obturator into the defect is necessary to achieve an effective seal and improve retention and stability by engaging appropriate undercuts within the defect walls. This is particularly important in edentulous patients who are lacking retention.

In partially dentate patients, the remaining teeth can be very useful as abutments to improve the prognosis of the prosthesis. These teeth must be well maintained and care must be taken to avoid stressing the remaining dentition beyond its physiological limit. Sometimes splinting adjacent teeth can be helpful to distribute the loads.

Different obturator designs have been used, including hollow bulb, full bulb, inflatable bulb, inkwell with a removable lid, and two-piece obturators with lock-and-key or magnet systems to retain the parts together. The hollow design is often preferred to reduce the weight of the obturator prosthesis (Ali *et al.*, 2015b; Bahrami and Falahchai, 2017; Buzayan *et al.*, 2013; Kumar *et al.*, 2013; Nanda *et al.*, 2013; Vaidya *et al.*, 2016).

33.8 Soft Palate Defects

Defects involving the soft palate may result in velopharyngeal insufficiency, leading to speech problems due to nasal air escape and swallowing difficulties (Barata *et al.*, 2013).

Prosthetic rehabilitation of soft palate defects can be challenging and may involve fabrication of an obturator, a speech aid prosthesis (speech bulb) or an obturator combined with a speech aid component to re-establish velopharyngeal closure (Shetty *et al.*, 2014; Tuna *et al.*, 2010).

Alternatively, surgical reconstruction can be considered after resection of the soft palate using soft tissue flaps such as uvulopalatal flap (Gillespie and Eisele, 2000) and radial forearm free flap (Rieger *et al.*, 2009; Yoshida *et al.*, 1993).

33.9 Osseointegrated Implants

The placement of dental implants significantly improves the function of obturator prostheses. Implants can be placed at the time of tumour resection (primary implants) or at a later stage during oral rehabilitation (secondary implants) (Siddall *et al.*, 2012).

Premaxillae and maxillary tuberosity are often the most desirable locations for implant placement in patients having partial maxillectomy. However, care must be taken not to overload a few implants in extremely large defects. Zygomatic implants have also been used successfully to improve the retention and stability of large maxillary obturators (El-Sayed *et al.*, 2014).

Indications, techniques and success criteria for zygomatic implants have been discussed in detail in a review by Aparicio *et al.* (2014).

A systematic review of 68 studies, including 4556 zygomatic implants in 2161 patients, showed that the 12-year cumulative survival rate was 95.21% for zygomatic implants in general. Zygomatic implants used in rehabilitation of patients after maxillectomy had lower survival rates (ranging from 78.6% to 94.1%), with most failures occurring i the early stages (within the first 6 months) postoperatively. The main observed complications were sinusitis (2.4%), soft tissue infection (2.0%), paraesthesia (1.0%) and oroantral fistulae (0.4%) (Chrcanovic *et al.*, 2016).

Case Study

An 81-year-old male patient was referred from the OMFS department for restorative rehabilitation following resection of a T2 N0 M0 SCC on the left side of the palate.

The patient had been wearing an interim obturator for over 6 months which was leaking and had poor stability and retention. He had no other symptoms.

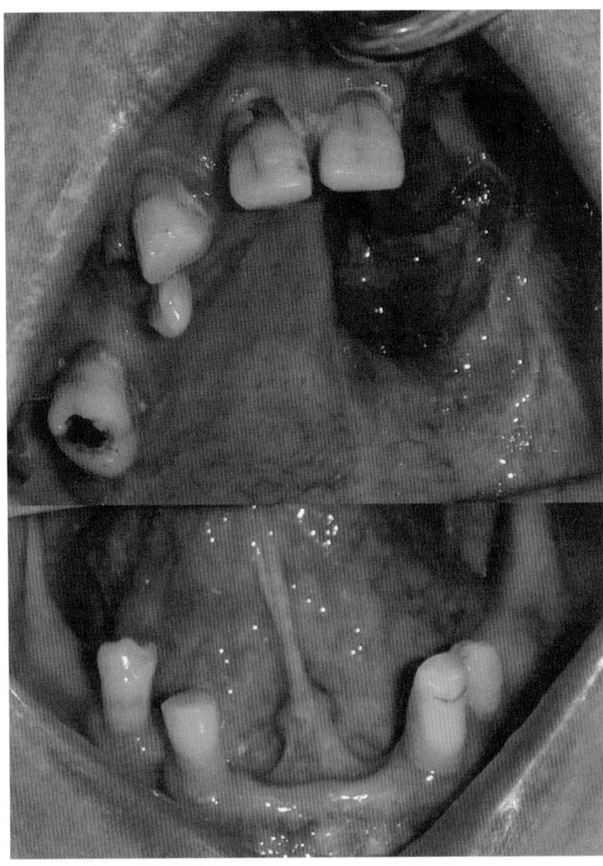

Figure 33.1 Preoperative clinical photographs showing Aramany Class II maxillary defect (unilateral resection), the remaining maxillary and mandibular teeth and fractured root-treated UR4.

The patient was partially dentate in both maxillary and mandibular arches (Figure 33.1). Periodontal examination of the remaining dentition showed the BPE scores were 2 in all dentate sextants. There was no obvious pulpal disease or any endodontic lesion associated with any of the remaining teeth.

The treatment strategy was as follows.

- Prevention, OHI and periodontal scaling.
- Smoothing and preparation of the fractured UR4 as an overdenture abutment.
- Restoration of the worn UR3 and LR3 with composite resin to ideal shape and occlusion.
- Fabrication and fitting of a definitive maxillary obturator prosthesis and a mandibular removable partial denture.
- Review and maintenance.

The basic procedural steps followed for fabrication of the definitive obturator are listed below.

1) Protection of the maxillary defect with Vaseline-impregnated gauze to prevent extrusion of impression material into the deep inaccessible parts of the defect.
2) Primary impressions with alginate impression material using a stock tray.
3) Preparation and surveying of the study models to identify an ideal path of insertion and suitable undercuts, and designing the upper and lower removable prostheses.
4) Fabrication of a two-part special tray (Figure 33.2).
5) Rest seat preparations on the abutment teeth.
6) Modification of the small obturator part of the special tray with ISO functional (compound) material (GC America) for better adaptation into the defect.
7) Border moulding of the periphery of the larger part of the special tray with thermoplastic greenstick compound material.
8) Final wash impression using additional silicone impression material with the special tray. The defect was

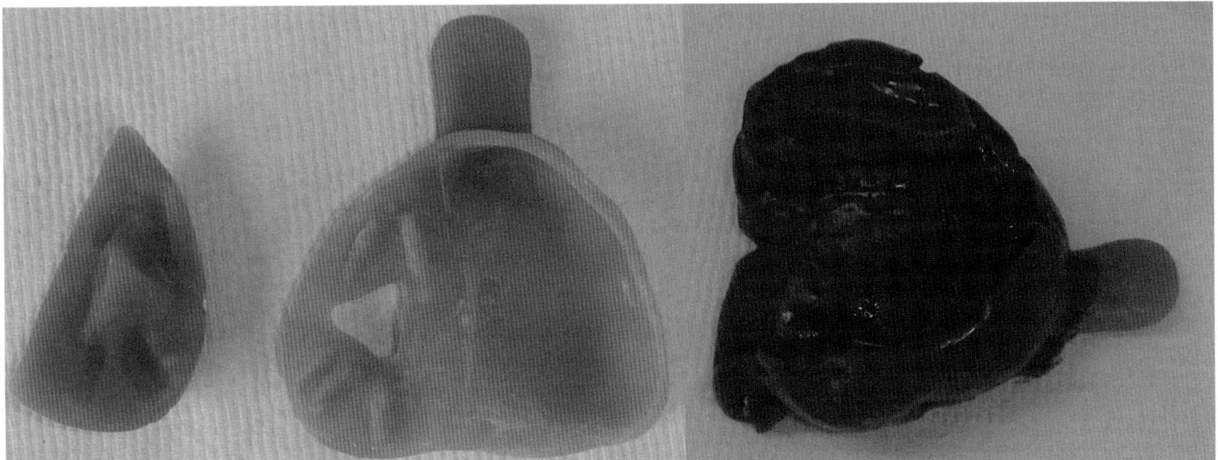

Figure 33.2 Photographs of the two-piece special tray with interlocking features and the master impression with additional silicone impression material.

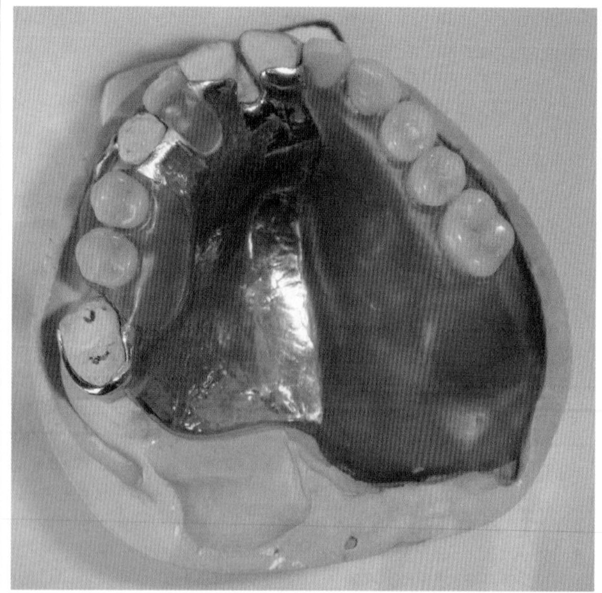

Figure 33.3 Photograph of the acrylic teeth on wax on the metal framework of the maxillary obturator prosthesis fitted on the stone model ready for trial insertion.

recorded and sealed first using the small part of the tray and then an overimpression was taken using the larger part of the tray.

9) Fabrication of a metal framework and intraoral trial.
10) Bite registration using wax blocks on the metal frameworks.
11) Trial insertion of the waxed prostheses (Figure 33.3).
12) Laboratory processing of the maxillary obturator with an open hollow bulb design and the mandibular removable partial denture.
13) Insertion of the maxillary obturator prosthesis and the mandibular removable partial denture.

The patient's postoperative clinical photograph is shown in Figure 33.4.

There were several learning points in this case. Use of the two-part special tray was very helpful in obtaining an accurate impression of the defect to achieve a good seal and minimise the risk of any leakage from around the obturator.

Using the existing undercuts within the defect contributed significantly to the retention of the obturator.

With appropriate designing of the partial denture to have good extension, support, bracing, direct and indirect retention using the remaining teeth, the retention and stability of the obturator were further enhanced.

At the final review appointment, the patient was very satisfied with both the maxillary obturator prosthesis and the mandibular removable partial denture and reported significant improvement in his quality of life.

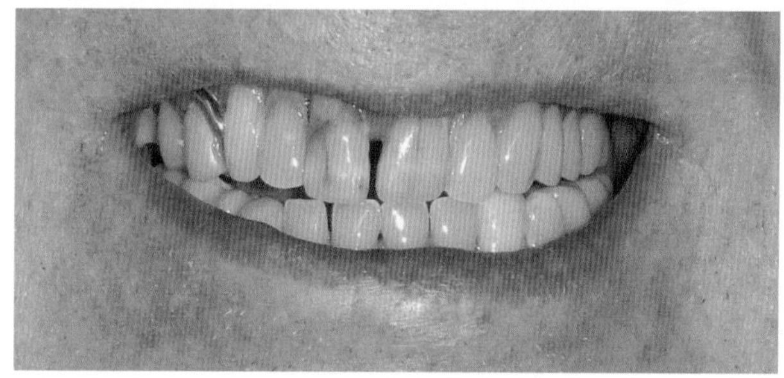

Figure 33.4 Postoperative clinical photograph of the patient's smile showing satisfactory aesthetics and free-way space.

References

Ali, R., Altaie, A. and Nattress, B. (2015a) Rehabilitation of oncology patients with hard palate defects. Part 2: Principles of obturator design. *Dent Update*, **42**, 428–430, 433–434.

Ali, R., Altaie, A. and Nattress, B. (2015b) Rehabilitation of oncology patients with hard palate defects. Part 3: Construction of an acrylic hollow box obturator. *Dent Update*, **42**, 612–614, 616, 618–620.

Ali, R., Altaie, A. and Nattress, B. (2015c) Rehabilitation of oncology patients with hard palate defects. Part 1: The surgical planning phase. *Dent Update*, **42**, 326–328, 331–332, 335.

Aparicio, C., Manresa, C., Francisco, K. *et al.* (2014) Zygomatic implants: indications, techniques and outcomes, and the zygomatic success code. *Periodontology 2000*, **66**, 41–58.

Aramany, M.A. (1978a) Basic principles of obturator design for partially edentulous patients. Part I: Classification. *J Prosthet Dent*, **40**, 554–557.

Aramany, M.A. (1978b) Basic principles of obturator design for partially edentulous patients. Part II: Design principles. *J Prosthet Dent*, **40**, 656–662.

Bahrami, M. and Falahchai, S.M. (2017) Full mouth reconstruction of a skeletal class II division 1 patient with adenoid cystic carcinoma using an interim immediate obturator and a definitive obturator. *Case Rep Dent*, **2017**, 5458617.

Barata, L.F., de Carvalho, G.B., Carrara-de Angelis, E., de Faria, J.C. and Kowalski, L.P. (2013) Swallowing, speech and quality of life in patients undergoing resection of soft palate. *Eur Arch Otorhinolaryngol*, **270**, 305–312.

Brown, J.S. and Shaw, R.J. (2010) Reconstruction of the maxilla and midface: introducing a new classification. *Lancet Oncol*, **11**, 1001–1008.

Brown, J.S., Rogers, S.N., Mcnally, D.N. and Boyle, M. (2000) A modified classification for the maxillectomy defect. *Head Neck*, **22**, 17–26.

Buzayan, M.M., Ariffin, Y.T. and Yunus, N. (2013) Closed hollow bulb obturator – one-step fabrication: a clinical report. *J Prosthodont*, **22**, 591–595.

Carl, W. (1976) Preoperative and immediate postoperative obturators. *J Prosthet Dent*, **36**, 298–305.

Chidzonga, M.M. (2006) Oral malignant neoplasia: a survey of 428 cases in two Zimbabwean hospitals. *Oral Oncol*, **42**, 177–183.

Chrcanovic, B.R., Albrektsson, T. and Wennerberg, A. (2016) Survival and complications of zygomatic implants: an updated systematic review. *J Oral Maxillofac Surg*, **74**, 1949–1964.

El Fattah, H., Zaghloul, A., Pedemonte, E. and Escuin, T. (2012) Pre-prosthetic surgical alterations in maxillectomy to enhance the prosthetic prognoses as part of rehabilitation of oral cancer patient. *Med Oral Patol Oral Cir Bucal*, **17**, E262–270.

El-Sayed, W.M., Gad, M.A. and Medra, A.M. (2014) Prosthodontic management of maxillectomy patients with dental implants in residual zygomatic bone: a preliminary report. *Int J Prosthodont*, **27**, 534–540.

Gillespie, M.B. and Eisele, D.W. (2000) The uvulopalatal flap for reconstruction of the soft palate. *Laryngoscope*, **110**, 612–615.

Huryn, J.M. and Piro, J.D. (1989) The maxillary immediate surgical obturator prosthesis. *J Prosthet Dent*, **61**, 343–347.

Keyf, F. (2001) Obturator prostheses for hemimaxillectomy patients. *J Oral Rehabil*, **28**, 821–829.

Kumar, P., Jain, V., Thakar, A. and Aggarwal, V. (2013) Effect of varying bulb height on articulation and nasalance in maxillectomy patients with hollow bulb obturator. *J Prosthodont Res*, **57**, 200–205.

Mucke, T., Loeffelbein, D.J., Hohlweg-Majert, B., Kesting, M.R., Wolff, K.D. and Holzle, F. (2009) Reconstruction of the maxilla and midface – surgical management, outcome, and prognostic factors. *Oral Oncol*, **45**, 1073–1078.

Nanda, A., Jain, V. and Nafria, A. (2013) Light is right – various techniques to fabricate hollow obturators. *Cleft Palate Craniofac J*, **50**, 237–241.

O'Connell, D.A. and Futran, N.D. (2010) Reconstruction of the midface and maxilla. *Curr Opin Otolaryngol Head Neck Surg*, **18**, 304–310.

Pace-Balzan, A., Shaw, R.J. and Butterworth, C. (2011) Oral rehabilitation following treatment for oral cancer. *Periodontology 2000*, **57**, 102–117.

Rieger, J., Bohle III, G., Huryn, J., Tang, J.L., Harris, J. and Seikaly, H. (2009) Surgical reconstruction versus prosthetic obturation of extensive soft palate defects: a comparison of speech outcomes. *Int J Prosthodont*, **22**, 566–572.

Rieger, J.M., Tang, J.A., Wolfaardt, J., Harris, J. and Seikaly, H. (2011) Comparison of speech and aesthetic outcomes in patients with maxillary reconstruction versus maxillary obturators after maxillectomy. *J Otolaryngol Head Neck Surg*, **40**, 40–47.

Rilo, B., Dasilva, J.L., Ferros, I., Mora, M.J. and Santana, U. (2005) A hollow-bulb interim obturator for maxillary resection. A case report. *J Oral Rehabil*, **32**, 234–236.

Shetty, N.B., Shetty, S., Nagraj, E, D'Souza, R. and Shetty, O. (2014) Management of velopharyngeal defects: a review. *J Clin Diagn Res*, **8**, 283–287.

Shimizu, H., Yoshida, K., Mori, N. and Takahashi, Y. (2009) An alternative procedure for fabricating a hollow interim obturator for a partial maxillectomy patient. *J Prosthodont*, **18**, 276–278.

Shrime, M.G. and Gilbert, R.W. (2009) Reconstruction of the midface and maxilla. *Facial Plast Surg Clin North Am*, **17**, 211–223.

Siddall, K.Z., Rogers, S.N. and Butterworth, C.J. (2012) The prosthodontic pathway of the oral cancer patient. *Dent Update*, **39**, 98–100, 103–106.

Truitt, T.O., Gleich, L.L., Huntress, G.P. and Gluckman, J.L. (1999) Surgical management of hard palate malignancies. *Otolaryngol Head Neck Surg*, **121**, 548–552.

Tuna, S.H., Pekkan, G., Gumus, H.O. and Aktas, A. (2010) Prosthetic rehabilitation of velopharyngeal insufficiency: pharyngeal obturator prostheses with different retention mechanisms. *Eur J Dent*, **4**, 81–87.

Vaidya, S., Parkash, H., Gupta, S., Bhargava, A. and Kapoor, C. (2016) Two-piece hollow bulb obturator for postsurgical partial maxillectomy defect in a young patient revamping lost malar prominence: a clinical report. *J Prosthodont*, **25**, 71–76.

Yoshida, H., Michi, K., Yamashita, Y. and Ohno, K. (1993) A comparison of surgical and prosthetic treatment for speech disorders attributable to surgically acquired soft palate defects. *J Oral Maxillofac Surg*, **51**, 361–365.

Ziada, H.M. and O'Donovan, S. (2000) Procedure for reducing the vertical height of a hollow box interim obturator. *J Prosthet Dent*, **83**, 589.

34

Open Apex (Immature Non-Vital Teeth)

34.1 Definition

The open apex can be defined as an unusually wide apical foramen of a root, making it challenging to prepare an apical stop during endodontic treatment. This definition varies according to different authors and is based on the minimum ISO file size used to gauge the apex of the root ranging from size 40 to 100 (Kim and Chandler, 2013).

34.2 Aetiology

Open apex can be due to (a) early cessation of root development (immature teeth) as a result of pulpal necrosis in young teeth, (b) external or internal root resorption, or (c) excessive instrumentation and apical widening or perforation of a closed root.

Caries and trauma are the most common causes of pulpal necrosis. Other developmental conditions such as dens invaginatus can also lead to early pulpal necrosis and open apex in young teeth (Flanagan, 2014).

34.3 Classification

Open apices can be classified into three types: divergent, parallel and tapering. It has been stated that the rate of root development in the labiolingual plane is slower than that in the mesiodistal direction. Therefore, a parallel-appearing apex on a radiograph may be actually more divergent in its labiolingual aspect. This makes it very difficult to thoroughly instrument the apical portion of these canals (Friend, 1966).

34.4 Management Strategies

Endodontic treatment of non-vital teeth with closed apices has been discussed in Chapter 3.

Challenges associated with management of non-vital teeth with open apices include effective and safe disinfection of the root canal, obturation of the canal with an open apex that has no barrier to prevent extrusion of the root filling material into the periapical tissues, and the susceptibility of the teeth to fracture due to fragile thin roots (Trope, 2010).

The following sections describe the relevant aspects of management of non-vital teeth with open apices.

34.4.1 Working Length Determination in Teeth with Open Apices

The European Society of Endodontology (2006) recommends the use of an electronic apex locator (EAL) followed by confirmation of the canal length with an undistorted periapical radiograph during root canal treatment. If the instrument in the canal appears to be shorter than 3 mm from the radiographic apex, the working length needs to be adjusted.

Although radiography has been the main method of determining the working length during treatment of teeth with open apices, case reports and clinical trials have reported variations in techniques, including methods such as digital tactile technique and the use of paper points (Kim and Chandler, 2013). An *in vivo* study has shown that the EAL method (Root ZX) has maximum accuracy (99.85%) followed by digital tactile (98.2%) and digital radiographic methods (97.9%) (Mandlik *et al.*, 2013). *In vitro* studies also confirm that the EAL is more reliable and accurate than the other methods in young teeth with immature apices (Diwanji *et al.*, 2014).

34.4.2 Irrigation Considerations

Care must be taken to avoid extrusion of cytotoxic irrigants beyond the apex during chemomechanical root canal debridement of teeth with open apices. The author's recommended technique is the use of 1% sodium hypochlorite solution in the coronal three-quarters of

Diseases and Conditions in Dentistry: An Evidence-Based Reference, First Edition. Keyvan Moharamzadeh.

Companion website: www.wiley.com/go/moharamzadeh/diseases

the root canal and normal saline solution for irrigation of the very apical part of the root canal with an open apex.

34.4.3 Calcium Hydroxide Apexification

Calcium hydroxide apexification has been used for many years for treatment of non-vital immature permanent teeth to induce root end closure. The technique involves removal of the coronal non-vital pulp tissue to the level of the apex and long-term placement (several months) of calcium hydroxide in the canals to induce calcified apical barrier formation before obturation of the root canal with gutta percha.

Although the success rate for this technique has been reported to be high (Chala *et al.*, 2011), it has several associated problems.

- The length of time required for formation of the apical barrier (3–24 months).
- Multiple appointments needed for repeated applications of calcium hydroxide.
- The adverse effects of long-term exposure to calcium hydroxide on the mechanical properties of dentine, based on *in vitro* studies (Rosenberg *et al.*, 2007). However, there are no clinical studies to directly support the correlation between calcium hydroxide dressing and root fracture (Yassen and Platt, 2013).

Guidelines by the European Academy of Paediatric Dentistry suggest that apexification with calcium hydroxide should be avoided and the long-term use of calcium hydroxide in the root canals of immature teeth is no longer advocated (Duggal *et al.*, 2017).

34.4.4 Placement of an Apical Plug to Create an Artificial Apical Barrier

34.4.4.1 Mineral Trioxide Aggregate

Mineral trioxide aggregate (MTA) is commonly used to repair perforated root canals and to create an artificial apical barrier in non-vital teeth with open apices (Bogen and Kuttler, 2009). It shortens treatment time significantly, requires fewer patient visits and results in more predictable barrier formation compared to calcium hydroxide apexification.

Root end closure is accomplished by placement of a minimum 4 mm long MTA plug at the apex following chemomechanical debridement of the root canal.

It has been shown that mechanically mixed MTA has better handling characteristics than manually mixed MTA. Indirect ultrasonic activation improves the adaptation of manually mixed MTA to the dentine walls (Sisli and Ozbas, 2017). In apices with divergent walls, it can be difficult to achieve good adaptation between the MTA plug and the root canal walls and there is an increased risk of extrusion of MTA beyond the open apex. The use of an absorbable collagen-based material as a barrier membrane for MTA to be condensed within the canal can improve the adaptation of the MTA plug and enhance its sealing ability (Gharechahi and Ghoddusi, 2012).

After placement of an MTA plug, thermo-plasticised gutta percha can be used to fill the remaining root canal space. If the root canal walls are thin, the remaining canal space can be filled with a hybrid composite resin instead of gutta percha to reinforce the root against fracture (Wilkinson *et al.*, 2007).

It has been shown that the use of MTA as a root end filling results in the reduction of periradicular inflammation and induces cementum-like hard tissue formation (Torabinejad *et al.*, 1995).

Systematic reviews indicate a very high success rate (as high as 95%) in terms of both clinical and radiographic outcomes with the use of MTA as an apical barrier material for endodontic treatment of immature necrotic permanent teeth. Success rates for MTA are comparable to or even higher than those of calcium hydroxide apexification (Lin *et al.*, 2016; Nicoloso *et al.*, 2017).

Current evidence and guidelines support the use of MTA followed by root canal obturation as the treatment of choice for management of non-vital traumatised young teeth with open apices (Duggal *et al.*, 2017).

34.4.4.2 Biodentine®

Biodentine is a calcium silicate-based bioceramic material that has been developed as an alternative to MTA to repair damaged dentine with reduced setting time and improved physical and biological properties (Rajasekharan *et al.*, 2014). Several case reports have shown favourable clinical and radiographic outcomes with Biodentine as an apical barrier material for the treatment of non-vital immature teeth (Bajwa *et al.*, 2015; Martens *et al.*, 2016; Vidal *et al.*, 2016). Biodentine's sealing ability is comparable to MTA (Bani *et al.*, 2015). However, further clinical studies are required to establish the long-term clinical performance of Biodentine as an apical plug material.

34.4.5 Regenerative Endodontic Treatment

Dental pulp regeneration and regenerative endodontic treatment (RET) procedures have received increasing attention recently, aiming to achieve revascularisation of the pulp tissue in immature teeth with necrotic pulp and therefore maintain the self-repair capacity of dental pulp (Hargreaves *et al.*, 2013). RET procedures allow prolonged root development in traumatised young teeth (Wigler *et al.*, 2013) and re-establish pulp vitality in mature teeth (Paryani and Kim, 2013).

Regenerative treatment of an immature tooth with necrotic pulp generally involves initial irrigation and debridement of the root canal with minimal or no instrumentation of the dentinal walls, placing an antimicrobial medicament in the canal, creating a blood clot or placement of a protein-based scaffold in the canal, placement of an intracanal barrier and maintaining effective coronal seal (Galler, 2016).

Many different RET protocols have been used in terms of type and concentration of irrigant (sodium hypochlorite, chlorhexidine, EDTA), intracanal medicament (triple/double antibiotic paste or calcium hydroxide paste), type of intracanal scaffold (blood clot, platelet-rich plasma or other biomaterials), type of barrier, restorative material and duration of treatment (Kontakiotis *et al.*, 2015; Law, 2013).

Limitations of RET include prolonged treatment time for disinfection of the root canal space, increased number of appointments, potential discolouration of teeth, unpredictable histological outcomes, unknown prognosis for further root development, failure to induce bleeding in some cases, risk of root canal calcification or obliteration and the need for subsequent root canal therapy if the treatment is not successful (Nosrat *et al.*, 2012).

A systematic review by Kahler *et al.* (2017) showed some evidence of further root development in necrotic immature permanent teeth treated with RET, although the results were variable. The level of evidence related to the use of RET is currently weak and therefore this treatment approach should only be considered in limited situations where the prognosis with other techniques is poor (Duggal *et al.*, 2017).

Case Study

A 45-year-old male patient presented with discomfort and previous frequent swellings associated with a crowned UL1. He reported a history of trauma to the anterior teeth in childhood. The patient had no relevant medical history.

Clinical examination showed that UL1 was tender to percussion, was grade I mobile and had inflamed and tender labial sulcus. There was no deep periodontal pocket.

Radiographic examination (Figure 34.1) showed UL1 had a wide root canal with an open apex and there was a large periapical radiolucency associated with this tooth.

The diagnosis was chronic apical periodontitis of UL1 with an open apex. The following treatment was provided.

1) Local anaesthesia and rubber dam isolation.
2) Access cavity preparation through the existing crown.
3) Working length determination using an apex locator.
4) Root canal debridement and irrigation with 1% hypochlorite solution in the coronal three-quarters of the root canal and normal saline solution in the apical part.
5) Drying of the canal and placement of an MTA plug at the apex using a root canal plugger and obturation of the remaining coronal part of the canal with thermoplasticised gutta percha using the Obtura system (Figure 34.2).
6) Restoration of the access cavity with resin-modified glass ionomer cement.
7) Fabrication and fitting of a definitive all-ceramic crown.
8) Review.

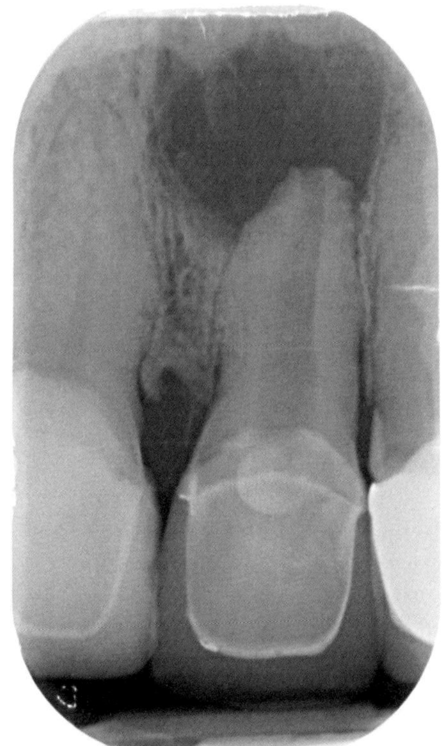

Figure 34.1 Preoperative periapical radiograph of UL1 showing an open apex and a large periapical radiolucency.

The patient remained asymptomatic following the above treatment and a 9-month follow-up radiograph showed evidence of good periapical healing (Figure 34.3), indicating a successful outcome for non-surgical endodontic treatment.

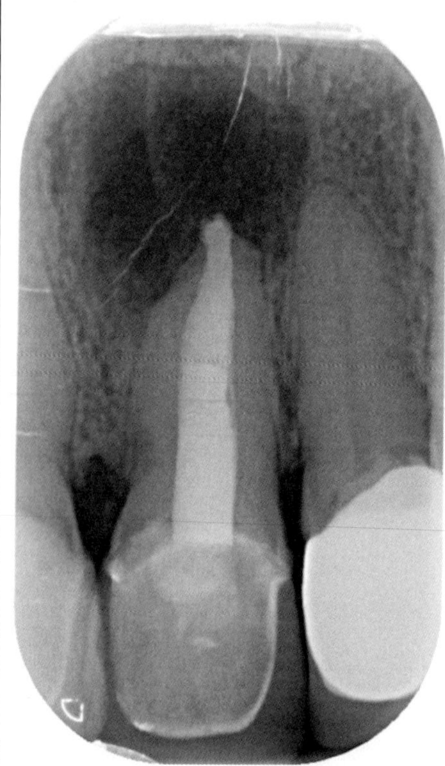

Figure 34.2 Immediate postoperative periapical radiograph after obturation of the canal with MTA plug at the apex and backfill with warm gutta percha.

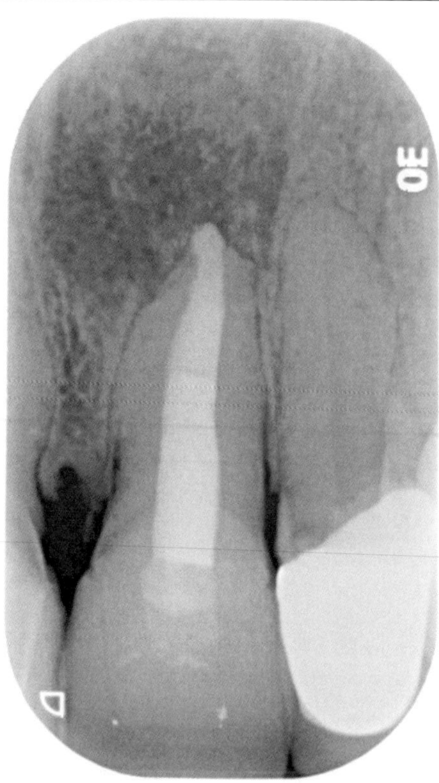

Figure 34.3 Postoperative 9-month follow-up periapical radiograph showing periapical healing.

References

Bajwa, N.K., Jingarwar, M.M. and Pathak, A. (2015) Single visit apexification procedure of a traumatically injured tooth with a novel bioinductive material (Biodentine). *Int J Clin Pediatr Dent*, **8**, 58–61.

Bani, M., Sungurtekin-Ekci, E. and Odabas, M.E. (2015) Efficacy of Biodentine as an apical plug in nonvital permanent teeth with open apices: an in vitro study. *Biomed Res Int*, **2015**, 359275.

Bogen, G. and Kuttler, S. (2009) Mineral trioxide aggregate obturation: a review and case series. *J Endod*, **35**, 777–790.

Chala, S., Abouqal, R. and Rida, S. (2011) Apexification of immature teeth with calcium hydroxide or mineral trioxide aggregate: systematic review and meta-analysis. *Oral Surg Oral Med Oral Pathol Oral Radiol Endod*, **112**, E36–42.

Diwanji, A., Rathore, A., Arora, R., Dhar, V., Madhusudan, A. and Doshi, J. (2014) Working length determination of root canal of young permanent tooth: an in vitro study. *Ann Med Health Sci Res*, **4**, 554–558.

Duggal, M., Tong, H.J., Al-Ansary, M., Twati, W., Day, P.F. and Nazzal, H. (2017) Interventions for the endodontic management of non-vital traumatised immature permanent anterior teeth in children and adolescents: a systematic review of the evidence and guidelines of the European Academy of Paediatric Dentistry. *Eur Arch Paediatr Dent*, **18**, 139–151.

ESE (2006) Quality Guidelines For Endodontic Treatment: consensus report of the European Society of Endodontology. *Int Endod J*, **39**, 921–930.

Flanagan, T.A. (2014) What can cause the pulps of immature, permanent teeth with open apices to become necrotic and what treatment options are available for these teeth? *Aust Endod J*, **40**, 95–100.

Friend, L.A. (1966) The root treatment of teeth with open apices. *Proc R Soc Med*, **59**, 1035–1036.

Galler, K.M. (2016) Clinical procedures for revitalization: current knowledge and considerations. *Int Endod J*, **49**, 926–936.

Gharechahi, M. and Ghoddusi, J. (2012) A nonsurgical endodontic treatment in open-apex and immature teeth affected by dens invaginatus: using a collagen membrane as an apical barrier. *J Am Dent Assoc*, **143**, 144–148.

Hargreaves, K.M., Diogenes, A. and Teixeira, F.B. (2013) Treatment options: biological basis of regenerative endodontic procedures. *J Endod*, **39**, S30–43.

Kahler, B., Rossi-Fedele, G., Chugal, N. and Lin, L.M. (2017) An evidence-based review of the efficacy of treatment approaches for immature permanent teeth with pulp necrosis. *J Endod*, **43**, 1052–1057.

Kim, Y.J. and Chandler, N.P. (2013) Determination of working length for teeth with wide or immature apices: a review. *Int Endod J*, **46**, 483–491.

Kontakiotis, E.G., Filippatos, C.G., Tzanetakis, G.N. and Agrafioti, A. (2015) Regenerative endodontic therapy: a data analysis of clinical protocols. *J Endod*, **41**, 146–154.

Law, A.S. (2013) Considerations for regeneration procedures. *J Endod*, **39**, S44–56.

Lin, J.C., Lu, J.X., Zeng, Q., Zhao, W., Li, W.Q. and Ling, J.Q. (2016) Comparison of mineral trioxide aggregate and calcium hydroxide for apexification of immature permanent teeth: a systematic review and meta-analysis. *J Formos Med Assoc*, **115**, 523–530.

Mandlik, J., Shah, N., Pawar, K., Gupta, P., Singh, S. and Shaik, S.A. (2013) An in vivo evaluation of different methods of working length determination. *J Contemp Dent Pract*, **14**, 644–648.

Martens, L., Rajasekharan, S. and Cauwels, R. (2016) Endodontic treatment of trauma-induced necrotic immature teeth using a tricalcium silicate-based bioactive cement. A report of 3 cases with 24-month follow-up. *Eur J Paediatr Dent*, **17**, 24–28.

Nicoloso, G.F., Potter, I.G., Rocha, R.O., Montagner, F. and Casagrande, L. (2017) A comparative evaluation of endodontic treatments for immature necrotic permanent teeth based on clinical and radiographic outcomes: a systematic review and meta-analysis. *Int J Paediatr Dent*, **27**, 217–227.

Nosrat, A., Homayounfar, N. and Oloomi, K. (2012) Drawbacks and unfavorable outcomes of regenerative endodontic treatments of necrotic immature teeth: a literature review and report of a case. *J Endod*, **38**, 1428–1434.

Paryani, K. and Kim, S.G. (2013) Regenerative endodontic treatment of permanent teeth after completion of root development: a report of 2 cases. *J Endod*, **39**, 929–934.

Rajasekharan, S., Martens, L.C., Cauwels, R.G. and Verbeeck, R.M. (2014) Biodentine material characteristics and clinical applications: a review of the literature. *Eur Arch Paediatr Dent*, **15**, 147–158.

Rosenberg, B., Murray, P.E. and Namerow, K. (2007) The effect of calcium hydroxide root filling on dentin fracture strength. *Dent Traumatol*, **23**, 26–29.

Sisli, S.N. and Ozbas, H. (2017) Comparative micro-computed tomographic evaluation of the sealing quality of proroot MTA and MTA angelus apical plugs placed with various techniques. *J Endod*, **43**, 147–151.

Torabinejad, M., Hong, C.U., Lee, S.J., Monsef, M. and Pitt Ford, T.R. (1995) Investigation of mineral trioxide aggregate for root-end filling in dogs. *J Endod*, **21**, 603–608.

Trope, M. (2010) Treatment of the immature tooth with a non-vital pulp and apical periodontitis. *Dent Clin North Am*, **54**, 313–324.

Vidal, K., Martin, G., Lozano, O., Salas, M., Trigueros, J. and Aguilar, G. (2016) Apical closure in apexification: a review and case report of apexification treatment of an immature permanent tooth with Biodentine. *J Endod*, **42**, 730–734.

Wigler, R., Kaufman, A.Y., Lin, S., Steinbock, N., Hazan-Molina, H. and Torneck, C.D. (2013) Revascularization: a treatment for permanent teeth with necrotic pulp and incomplete root development. *J Endod*, **39**, 319–326.

Wilkinson, K.L., Beeson, T.J. and Kirkpatrick, T.C. (2007) Fracture resistance of simulated immature teeth filled with resilon, gutta-percha, or composite. *J Endod*, **33**, 480–483.

Yassen, G.H. and Platt, J.A. (2013) The effect of nonsetting calcium hydroxide on root fracture and mechanical properties of radicular dentine: a systematic review. *Int Endod J*, **46**, 112–118.

35

Open Bite

35.1 Definition and Classification

Open bite is defined as no vertical overlap of the anterior teeth (anterior open bite) when the posterior teeth are in occlusion, or as no occlusion between the posterior teeth (posterior open bite) when the anterior teeth are touching as the patient bites down.

Open bite can be dental, without the influence of the vertical skeletal pattern, or it can be skeletal, where the vertical skeletal pattern is contributory (Burford and Noar, 2003).

35.2 Aetiology

Open bite has a multifactorial aetiology based on genetic and environmental factors (Rijpstra and Lisson, 2016). Some of the specific causes are:

- skeletal pattern
- influence of soft tissues such as tongue thrust
- habits such as digit sucking
- airway obstruction by enlarged tonsils and adenoids leading to prolonged mouth breathing
- neuromuscular deficiency
- iatrogenic extrusion of molars
- cleft lip and palate
- acromegaly
- rheumatoid disease
- trauma

35.3 Incidence

The incidence of anterior open bite varies among populations (Krooks *et al.*, 2016; Proffit *et al.*, 1998) and reported figures for the UK are 2–4% (Burford and Noar, 2003). After the age of 9 years, the incidence of open bite drops as the child stops the habit of digit sucking and develops normal occlusion and swallowing function. In the mid-teens, the incidence increases again due to late vertical facial growth.

35.4 Indications for Treatment

Patients with open bite may seek treatment for aesthetic reasons, functional issues such as difficulty in incising food efficiently and speech problems (Ferguson, 1995).

35.5 Treatment Options

35.5.1 Prevention

Simple cases of open bite can be treated conservatively in children with cessation of digit sucking (Huang *et al.*, 2015). Different approaches used for the cessation of non-nutritive sucking habits in children include (Borrie *et al.*, 2015):

- giving appropriate advice to parents to encourage their children to stop the habit
- behaviour modification techniques and psychological interventions such as positive and negative reinforcement
- application of an aversive taste to the digit
- fitting appliances such as palatal crib or palatal arch to make thumb sucking uncomfortable.

Stopping the sucking habit may help to close an open bite naturally, which may take several years. However, if the habit persists following growth completion, the open bite will often be permanent which may require orthodontic treatment.

35.5.2 Orthodontic Treatment

Orthodontic approaches to correct an open bite include (Sandler *et al.*, 2011):

- molar intrusion using a high pull headgear

Diseases and Conditions in Dentistry: An Evidence-Based Reference, First Edition. Keyvan Moharamzadeh.

Companion website: www.wiley.com/go/moharamzadeh/diseases

- molar intrusion using temporary anchorage devices (TAD) (mini-implants) and elastomeric chains attached to mini-screws (Alsafadi *et al.*, 2016)
- incisor extrusion using fixed appliances, which has a high relapse potential after appliance removal.

35.5.3 Orthognathic Surgery

Severe cases of open bite in adult patients with significant skeletal discrepancy may require orthognathic surgery to correct the open bite and other co-existing malocclusions. Surgical treatment often requires pre- and postsurgical orthodontics. Vertical relapse has been reported following combined orthodontic-surgical treatments (Solano-Hernandez *et al.*, 2013). With the introduction of TADs as an effective treatment modality, orthognathic surgery may be avoidable in selected anterior open bite cases (Reichert *et al.*, 2014).

35.5.4 Restorative Treatment

Restorative treatment may also be required as part of multidisciplinary patient management, especially when the open bite is associated with conditions that affect the tooth size, shape and number such as microdontia/hypodontia, amelogenesis imperfecta (Gisler *et al.*, 2010) and enamel hypoplasia (Cooke and Neesome, 1990).

Restorative options to reduce an anterior open bite include:

- selective grinding of posterior molar teeth, which is an invasive and irreversible treatment option and may cause sensitivity and pulpal exposure
- restoration of the anterior teeth with direct composite resin or indirect restorations to reduce the open bite as described in the clinical case report below.

Case Study

A 41-year-old male patient was referred by his GDP for management of anterior open bite. The patient's presenting complain was poor appearance due to open bite, spacing and a retained deciduous tooth.

The medical history was clear and the patient was a non-smoker. He reported a history of thumb sucking in childhood and pen biting in adulthood.

The patient's preoperative clinical photographs and radiograph are shown in Figures 35.1 and 35.2 respectively.

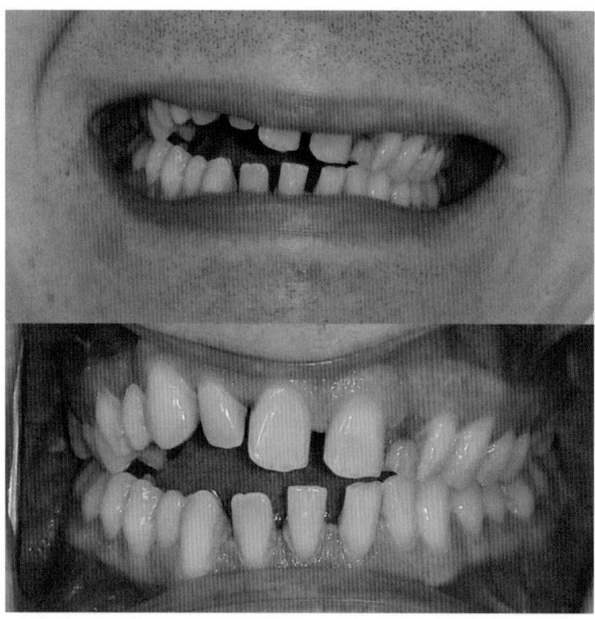

Figure 35.1 Preoperative clinical photographs showing an anterior open bite UL1–UR4, retained primary ULB, microdontia and spacing, calculus in the lower anterior region and a RBB UL4 with poor aesthetics. The patient has a low upper lip line.

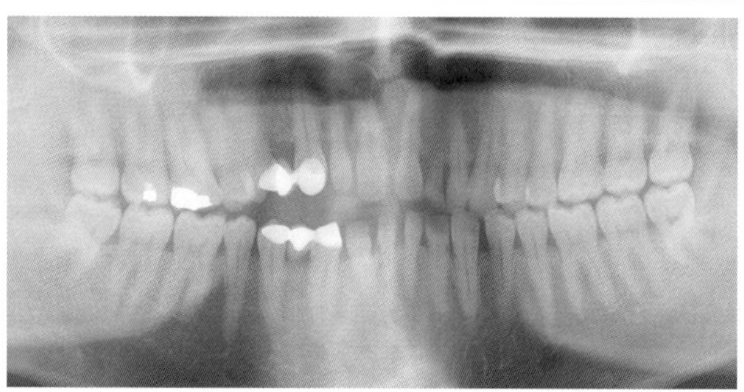

Figure 35.2 Oral panoramic radiograph showing that all the permanent teeth are present and there is a retained ULB with resorbed root.

Periodontal examination showed the BPE scores were 1 in all quadrants, except for the lower anterior region which was 2 with presence of calculus and gingival inflammation.

The following treatment options were discussed with the patient, including risks, benefits and expected outcomes.

- No treatment
- Orthodontic treatment
- Segmental osteotomy
- Restorative treatment

Important factors in decision making in this case included:

- patient's preference and co-operation as he did not want lengthy orthodontic treatment or surgery
- low lip line which was a favourable factor to hide gingival margin discrepancy and restoration margins
- reversible or irreversible nature of treatment as it was safer to consider reversible and conservative treatment

options such as adhesive composite additions to reduce the open bite in this case
- space available for restoration of the teeth.

Since the patient preferred the restorative-only option, the following treatment was provided.

1) Prevention, oral hygiene instructions (OHI), plaque control, scaling and polishing to improve periodontal condition.
2) Impressions, bite registration and preparation of articulated study models.
3) Diagnostic wax-up of UL2–UR5 to reduce the anterior open bite and intraoral rehearsal (Figure 35.3).
4) Extraction of ULB and fitting of an immediate acrylic removable partial denture (RPD) to fill the space.
5) Sectioning and removing the resin-bonded bridge (RBB) UR4 and addition of this tooth to the RPD.
6) Composite build-up of UR1, UR2, UR3, UL1 and UL2 using a silicone putty stent made over the diagnostic wax-up as a guide.
7) Fabrication and cementation of an indirect composite fused to metal onlay bridge UR4–5 to increase the height of UR5 and restore the UR4 space.
8) Composite restorations on LL1, LR1, LR2, LR3 and LR5 to close the spacing and further reduce the anterior open bite.
9) Review and maintenance.

The patient's postoperative clinical photographs are shown in Figure 35.4.

This was an example of conservative restorative management of anterior open bite which obviated the need for complicated orthodontic or surgical treatments. There were several important learning points in this case.

- Careful planning and timing of the treatment process.
- Trial and adjustment of a diagnostic wax-up to achieve ideal tooth contour, position, midline and occlusal plane.
- Technique of direct composite build-up using a stent made over the diagnostic wax-up.
- Adhesive onlay bridge with composite facing to enable better adaptation, blending of colour and hiding of the onlay margins.

The patient was very satisfied with the outcome of treatment and was discharged back to his GDP for long-term maintenance.

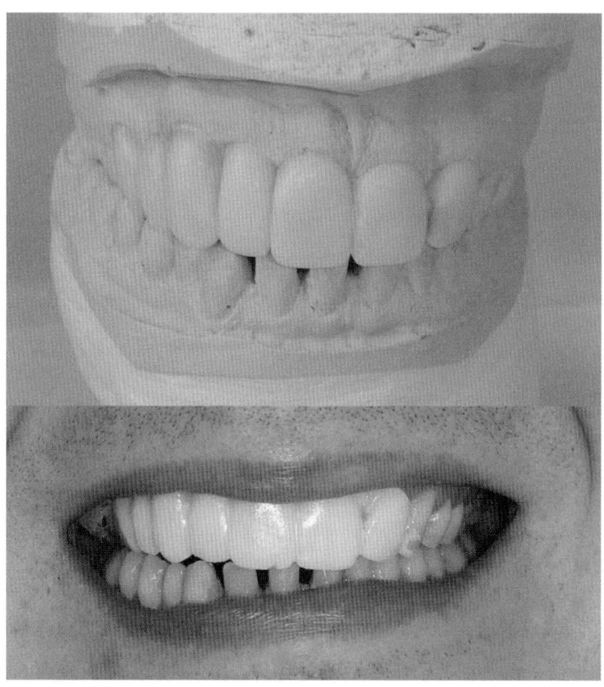

Figure 35.3 Diagnostic wax-up of UL2–UR5 to reduce the anterior open bite and intraoral trial of the wax-up using temporisation material (Protemp, 3M ESPE).

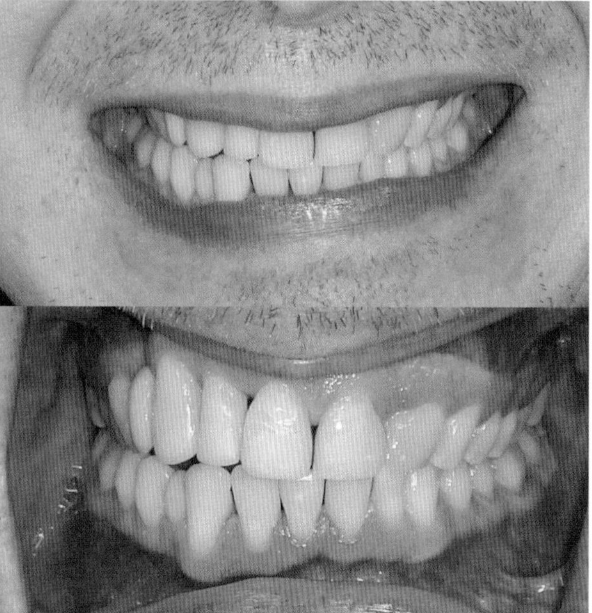

Figure 35.4 Postoperative clinical photographs showing significant improvement in aesthetics and favourable restorative treatment outcome of closing the anterior open bite.

References

Alsafadi, A.S., Alabdullah, M.M., Saltaji, H., Abdo, A. and Youssef, M. (2016) Effect of molar intrusion with temporary anchorage devices in patients with anterior open bite: a systematic review. *Prog Orthod*, **17**, 9.

Borrie, F.R., Bearn, D.R., Innes, N.P. and Iheozor-Ejiofor, Z. (2015) Interventions for the cessation of non-nutritive sucking habits in children. *Cochrane Database Syst Rev*, **3**, CD008694.

Burford, D. and Noar, J.H. (2003) The causes, diagnosis and treatment of anterior open bite. *Dent Update*, **30**, 235–241.

Cooke, M.S. and Neesome, P.R. (1990) Combined orthodontic and restorative correction of severe anterior open bite. *Quintessence Int*, **21**, 729–736.

Ferguson, J.W. (1995) The assessment and treatment of anterior open bite. *Dent Update*, **22**, 163–168.

Gisler, V., Enkling, N., Zix, J., Kim, K., Kellerhoff, N.M. and Mericske-Stern, R. (2010) A multidisciplinary approach to the functional and esthetic rehabilitation of amelogenesis imperfecta and open bite deformity: a case report. *J Esthet Restor Dent*, **22**, 282–293.

Huang, B., Lejarraga, C., Franco, C.S. *et al.* (2015) Influence of non-orthodontic intervention on digit sucking and consequent anterior open bite: a preliminary study. *Int Dent J*, **65**, 235–241.

Krooks, L., Pirttiniemi, P., Kanavakis, G. and Lahdesmaki, R. (2016) Prevalence of malocclusion traits and orthodontic treatment in a Finnish adult population. *Acta Odontol Scand*, **74**, 362–367.

Proffit, W.R., Fields, H.W. Jr and Moray, L.J. (1998) Prevalence of malocclusion and orthodontic treatment need in the United States: estimates from the NHANES III survey. *Int J Adult Orthodon Orthognath Surg*, **13**, 97–106.

Reichert, I., Figel, P. and Winchester, L. (2014) Orthodontic treatment of anterior open bite: a review article – is surgery always necessary? *Oral Maxillofac Surg*, **18**, 271–277.

Rijpstra, C. and Lisson, J.A. (2016) Etiology of anterior open bite: a review. *J Orofac Orthop*, **77**, 281–286.

Sandler, P.J., Madahar, A.K. and Murray, A. (2011) Anterior open bite: aetiology and management. *Dent Update*, **38**, 522–524, 527–528, 531–532.

Solano-Hernandez, B., Antonarakis, G.S., Scolozzi, P. and Kiliaridis, S. (2013) Combined orthodontic and orthognathic surgical treatment for the correction of skeletal anterior open-bite malocclusion: a systematic review on vertical stability. *J Oral Maxillofac Surg*, **71**, 98–109.

36

Osteoradionecrosis

36.1 Definition and Pathogenesis

Osteoradionecrosis (ORN) has been defined as a non-healing exposed irradiated bone present for over 3 months without any evidence of persisting or recurrent tumour (Dhanda *et al.*, 2016; Marx, 1983b). It is characterised by deep-seated bone pain which may have a purulent discharge and sequestrated bone (Silvestre-Rangil and Silvestre, 2011). ORN can gradually progress and result in significant bone loss and pathological jaw fractures (Nadella *et al.*, 2015).

Although the mechanism of development of ORN is still under investigation, it is widely believed that radiation damage to the endothelial cells causes microvascular inflammation (arteritis) and thrombosis which leads to hypoxia, tissue necrosis and bone destruction (Marx, 1983a). A fibroatrophic mechanism has also been proposed based on fibroblast activation and dysregulation mediated by free radicals or reactive oxygen species (ROS) and cytokines triggering an acute inflammatory response. According to this theory, disease progression involves three stages: a prefibrotic phase, an organised phase and a remodelling fibroatrophic phase (Delanian and Lefaix, 2004).

36.2 Prevalence

The prevalence of ORN reported in the literature varies from 0.4% to 56% and the most frequently reported prevalence rates for ORN are between 5% and 15% (Chronopoulos *et al.*, 2017).

According to a systematic review (Nabil and Samman, 2011), the overall incidence of ORN following tooth extraction in irradiated patients was 7%. When extractions were carried out in conjunction with systemic antibiotics, the incidence of ORN was reduced to 6%. When prophylactic hyperbaric oxygen (HBO) therapy was used with extractions, the incidence was further reduced to 4%.

36.3 Risk Factors

The risk of development of ORN is increased in the following situations (Caparrotti *et al.*, 2017; Chrcanovic *et al.*, 2010; Dhanda *et al.*, 2016; Kuhnt *et al.*, 2016; Madrid *et al.*, 2010; Owosho *et al.*, 2017).

- High dose of radiation (exceeding 60 Gy).
- Poor periodontal status of the patient and presence of infections.
- Tobacco and alcohol use.
- Large tumour in the oral cavity resected with bone surgery.
- Surgical trauma to the irradiated site, for example tooth extraction, especially in the posterior mandible.
- Prosthesis trauma, such as ill-fitting dentures.
- Xerostomia and poor oral hygiene.
- Systemic factors such as malnutrition, immunodeficiency and peripheral vascular disease.

The use of modern radiotherapy techniques such as conformal three-dimensional radiation therapy and intensity-modulated radiation therapy (IMRT) (de Felice *et al.*, 2016) is expected to result in a reduction in ORN, although there is a paucity of studies to confirm the real benefit of IMRT on ORN risk reduction (Caparrotti *et al.*, 2017; Dhanda *et al.*, 2016). Potential benefits of IMRT include improved dose distribution, salivary gland sparing and reduced xerostomia which may result in fewer instances of dental disease and post-treatment extractions (Duarte *et al.*, 2014) when coupled with meticulous prophylactic dental care.

36.4 Classification of ORN

Many different ORN classification and staging systems have been proposed based on clinical findings (Clayman, 1997), combined clinical and radiographic presentation (Coffin, 1983; Notani *et al.*, 2003; Schwartz and Kagan, 2002; Store and Boysen, 2000), disease progression

Diseases and Conditions in Dentistry: An Evidence-Based Reference, First Edition. Keyvan Moharamzadeh.

Companion website: www.wiley.com/go/moharamzadeh/diseases

(Epstein *et al.*, 1987), duration of bone exposure (Glanzmann and Gratz, 1995) and response to treatment (Morton and Simpson, 1986) such as HBO therapy (Marx, 1983b).

A systematic review (Shaw *et al.*, 2017) evaluated the consistency of 16 different mandibular ORN classification systems and recommended Notani *et al.*'s classification with the additional category of minor bone spicules for use as a suitable endpoint in clinical trials.

Notani *et al.*'s (2003) ORN classification includes the following stages.

- Stage I: ORN lesion confined to the alveolar bone.
- Stage II: ORN lesion limited to the bone above the level of the inferior alveolar (ID) canal.
- Stage III: ORN invading below the level of the ID canal and/or presence of skin fistula and/or pathological jaw fracture.

36.5 Diagnosis

Clinical diagnostic features of ORN include (Chronopoulos *et al.*, 2017):

- oral mucosal ulceration and exposure of necrotic bone for over 3 months
- pain, paraesthesia or anaesthesia
- suppuration and unpleasant odour
- trismus
- in advanced cases, pathological bone fractures, intraoral or extraoral fistulae and systemic infection can occur.

Radiographically, ORN may not be detectable in the early stages. As the disease progresses, localised osteolytic areas or extensive radiolucent lesions with bone sequestration and fracture may be visible on radiographic examination.

The most commonly used imaging technique is oral panoramic radiograph (OPT), although computed tomography (CT) scan and magnetic resonance imaging (MRI) have also been used to investigate ORN (Deshpande *et al.*, 2015). Other advanced imaging techniques that may offer some benefits in differentiating between ORN and tumour recurrence include bone scintigraphy, diffusion-weighted imaging (DWI), single photon emission computed tomography (SPECT) and positron emission tomography (PET) (Chronopoulos *et al.*, 2017).

A biopsy of the lesion is required to confirm the diagnosis and to exclude cancer recurrence or metastatic disease (Marwan *et al.*, 2016).

36.6 Prevention

36.6.1 Pre-Radiotherapy Dental Assessment and Extractions

Preoperative oral and dental assessment is an essential part of prevention that aims to plan for extraction of teeth with doubtful prognosis or those which are at risk of future dental disease and are in an area where there is an increased risk of ORN. Ideally, the extractions must be carried out as soon as possible, or at least a minimum 10 days before radiotherapy (Butterworth *et al.*, 2016).

36.6.2 Patient Education

Oral hygiene education (OHE), smoking and alcohol advice should be given and the patient must be instructed to use an appropriate daily fluoride application protocol following radiotherapy, as described in Chapter 5, to prevent radiation-induced caries. It is important to maintain regular dental care to reduce postradiotherapy complications.

36.6.3 Minimising Trauma

Soft and hard tissue trauma must be minimised after radiotherapy and ill-fitting dentures must be removed. Conservative management of teeth which develop dental diseases after radiotherapy is recommended to reduce the need for extractions. Non-vital teeth are best treated endodontically and left *in situ* to avoid extractions. In cases where extractions are unavoidable, atraumatic dental extraction is recommended.

36.6.4 Prophylactic Hyperbaric Oxygen Therapy and Antibiotics

Prophylactic hyperbaric oxygen therapy (HBOT) and antibiotics prior to dental extractions have been used to prevent ORN. Marx *et al.* (1985) conducted a randomised controlled trial indicating the benefits of HBOT over antibiotics as a preventive measure prior to extractions in irradiated jaws. Due to several limitations in this study and the lack of other clinical trials, there is a need for high-quality research to establish the value of HBOT for the prevention of ORN (Shaw and Butterworth, 2011). Although further clinical trials in HBOT are currently under way (Shaw *et al.*, 2011), HBOT has high cost and limited treatment location availability and is time-consuming, which may reduce patient compliance (Chouinard *et al.*, 2016).

36.7 Management

The Royal College of Surgeons of England and the British Society for Disability and Oral Health published a clinical guideline on the oral management of oncology patients requiring radiotherapy, chemotherapy and/or bone marrow transplantation, with useful recommendations for the management of ORN (Kumar *et al.*, 2012).

- Reducing trauma by soft diet, denture adjustment if necessary and avoiding extractions.
- Establishing and maintaining good oral hygiene.
- Relieving symptoms by topical anaesthesia or systemic analgesia.
- The use of novel therapeutic agents such as a combination of pentoxifylline-tocopherol-clodronate (PENTOCLO) may offer additional benefit (Lyons and Brennan, 2017; Robard *et al.*, 2014).
- High-dose broad-spectrum systemic antibiotics such as amoxicillin with clavulanic acid should be considered both for treatment of ORN and prior to any extractions or sequestrectomy and must be continued until healing occurs.
- Localised surgical debridement and excision of necrotic bone may help to achieve primary wound closure. They would also enable the obtaining of samples for culture and sensitivity and biopsy of the lesion for histopathology assessment to rule out malignancy.
- Ultrasound therapy has also been shown to be an effective conservative ORN management approach and may reduce the need for surgical treatment (Costa *et al.*, 2016; Harris, 1992).
- HBOT may be necessary for management of severe cases and as an adjunct to surgical intervention in the treatment of established ORN (Dhanda *et al.*, 2016). It has been shown that HBOT improves treatment outcomes for patients with late radiation tissue injury (Bennett *et al.*, 2016). However, the level of evidence for the effectiveness of HBOT in the treatment of ORN in the head and neck region is weak (Shaw and Dhanda, 2011) and there is controversy in the literature based on the limitations of a randomised clinical trial of HBOT in the treatment of ORN (Annane *et al.*, 2004). Further research is necessary to establish the optimum patient selection for HBOT and timing of treatment.
- It is important to establish the extent of bone necrosis in advanced chronic cases using appropriate imaging techniques. Fluorescent tetracycline marker can be used at the time of surgery to distinguish the healthy bone margins (Pautke *et al.*, 2010). Surgical treatment of advanced ORN which has resulted in fractures and fistulae usually involves radical resection and removal of the necrotic bone segment and reconstruction with free tissue transfer such as a fibula free flap. It has been shown that the rate of postoperative complications and failure was significantly higher in reconstructed ORN cases compared to reconstruction of defects after resection of primary tumour (Lee *et al.*, 2015).

Case Study

A 75-year-old-female edentulous patient seen in a joint restorative dentistry/oral and maxillofacial surgery (OMFS) clinic presented with pain and discomfort from a non-healing ulcer present for 4 months on the lingual aspect of the mandible on the left side (Figure 36.1).

The patient had been diagnosed with pT2 pN0 M0 moderately differentiated squamous cell carcinoma (SCC) on the left lateral border of tongue 3 years earlier and had received the following treatment.

- Elective tracheostomy, selective neck dissection, left lateral partial glossectomy and reconstruction with left radial forearm free flap.
- The patient received postsurgical adjuvant radiotherapy 60 Gy in 30 fractions over 40 days.
- The patient had surgical division of left tongue tethering 2 years after radiotherapy to improve tongue function and facilitate prosthetic rehabilitation as she was unable to wear a mandibular complete denture.

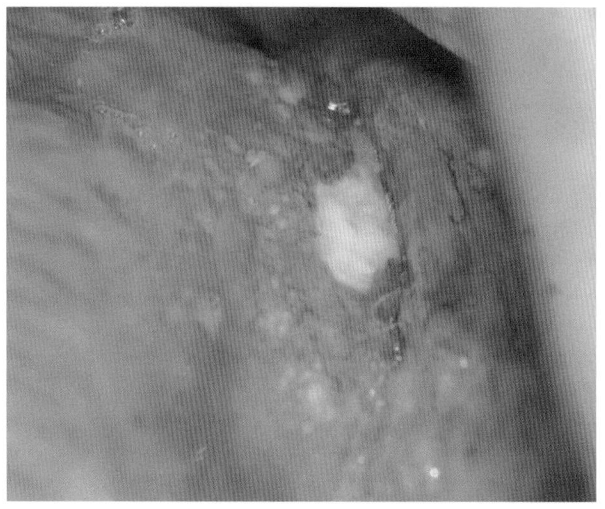

Figure 36.1 Intraoral clinical photograph of the non-healing mucosal defect.

Clinical examination showed a mucosal defect and a small area of necrotic bone exposure on the lingual surface of the mandible on the left side consistent with features seen in osteoradionecrosis. The following treatment was provided.

1) Pain relief with oral paracetamol 1 g four times per day and ibuprofen 400 mg three times per day when required.
2) Patient advice including soft diet, avoiding trauma on the left side and oral hygiene education including daily use of 0.2% chlorhexidine mouthrinse.
3) Localised debridement, removal of necrotic bone and primary wound closure.
4) Samples were sent for culture and sensitivity and histopathology assessment.
5) Oral systemic antibiotics – amoxicillin 500 mg with clavulanic acid 125 mg three times per day for the duration of healing.
6) Follow-up assessment showed complete healing of the wound and resolution of the symptoms (Figure 36.2).
7) Prosthetic rehabilitation with a set of well-fitting conventional complete dentures (Figure 36.3) to be worn comfortably without causing any further irritation or trauma.
8) Regular reviews and maintenance.

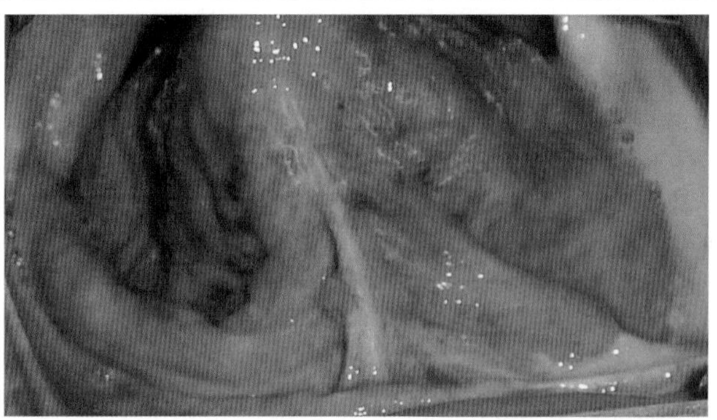

Figure 36.2 Intraoral clinical photograph of the mandible following treatment showing well-healed oral mucosa.

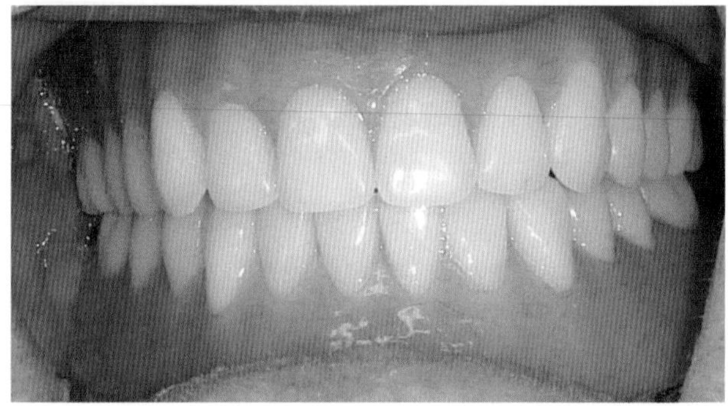

Figure 36.3 Postoperative clinical photograph of the complete dentures.

References

Annane, D., Depondt, J., Aubert, P. *et al.* (2004) Hyperbaric oxygen therapy for radionecrosis of the jaw: a randomized, placebo-controlled, doubleblind trial from the ORN96 study group. *J Clin Oncol*, **22**, 4893–4900.

Bennett, M.H., Feldmeier, J., Hampson, N.B., Smee, R. and Milross, C. (2016) Hyperbaric oxygen therapy for late radiation tissue injury. *Cochrane Database Syst Rev*, **4**, CD005005.

Butterworth, C., Mccaul, L. and Barclay, C. (2016) Restorative dentistry and oral rehabilitation: United Kingdom national multidisciplinary guidelines. *J Laryngol Otol*, **130**, S41–S44.

Caparrotti, F., Huang, S.H., Lu, L. et al. (2017) Osteoradionecrosis of the mandible in patients with oropharyngeal carcinoma treated with intensity-modulated radiotherapy. *Cancer*, **123**, 3691–3700.

Chouinard, A.F., Giasson, L. and Fortin, M. (2016) Hyperbaric oxygen therapy for head and neck irradiated patients with special attention to oral and maxillofacial treatments. *J Can Dent Assoc*, **82**, G24.

Chrcanovic, B.R., Reher, P., Sousa, A.A. and Harris, M. (2010) Osteoradionecrosis of the jaws – a current overview – Part 1: Physiopathology and risk and predisposing factors. *Oral Maxillofac Surg*, **14**, 3–16.

Chronopoulos, A., Zarra, T., Ehrenfeld, M. and Otto, S. (2017) Osteoradionecrosis of the jaws: definition, epidemiology, staging and clinical and radiological findings. A concise review. *Int Dent J*, June 25 (epub ahead of print).

Clayman, L. (1997) Clinical controversies in oral and maxillofacial surgery: Part Two. Management of dental extractions in irradiated jaws: a protocol without hyperbaric oxygen therapy. *J Oral Maxillofac Surg*, **55**, 275–281.

Coffin, F. (1983) The incidence and management of osteoradionecrosis of the jaws following head and neck radiotherapy. *Br J Radiol*, **56**, 851–857.

Costa, D.A., Costa, T.P., Netto, E.C. et al. (2016) New perspectives on the conservative management of osteoradionecrosis of the mandible: a literature review. *Head Neck*, **38**, 1708–1716.

de Felice, F., Musio, D. and Tombolini, V. (2016) Osteoradionecrosis and intensity modulated radiation therapy: an overview. *Crit Rev Oncol Hematol*, **107**, 39–43.

Delanian, S. and Lefaix, J.L. (2004) The radiation-induced fibroatrophic process: therapeutic perspective via the antioxidant pathway. *Radiother Oncol*, **73**, 119–131.

Deshpande, S.S., Thakur, M.H., Dholam, K., Mahajan, A., Arya, S. and Juvekar, S. (2015) Osteoradionecrosis of the mandible: through a radiologist's eyes. *Clin Radiol*, **70**, 197–205.

Dhanda, J., Pasquier, D., Newman, L. and Shaw, R. (2016) Current concepts in osteoradionecrosis after head and neck radiotherapy. *Clin Oncol (R Coll Radiol)*, **28**, 459–466.

Duarte, V.M., Liu, Y.F., Rafizadeh, S., Tajima, T., Nabili, V. and Wang, M.B. (2014) Comparison of dental health of patients with head and neck cancer receiving IMRT vs conventional radiation. *Otolaryngol Head Neck Surg*, **150**, 81–86.

Epstein, J.B., Wong, F.L. and Stevenson-Moore, P. (1987) Osteoradionecrosis: clinical experience and a proposal for classification. *J Oral Maxillofac Surg*, **45**, 104–110.

Glanzmann, C. and Gratz, K.W. (1995) Radionecrosis of the mandibula: a retrospective analysis of the incidence and risk factors. *Radiother Oncol*, **36**, 94–100.

Harris, M. (1992) The conservative management of osteoradionecrosis of the mandible with ultrasound therapy. *Br J Oral Maxillofac Surg*, **30**, 313–318.

Kuhnt, T., Stang, A., Wienke, A., Vordermark, D., Schweyen, R. and Hey, J. (2016) Potential risk factors for jaw osteoradionecrosis after radiotherapy for head and neck cancer. *Radiat Oncol*, **11**, 101.

Kumar, N., Brooke, A., Burke, M., John, R., O'Donnell, A. and Soldani, F. (2012) *The Oral Management Of Oncology Patients Requiring Radiotherapy, Chemotherapy And/Or Bone Marrow Transplantation. Clinical Guidelines*. Royal College of Surgeons of England and British Society for Disability and Oral Health. Available at: www.bsdh.org/documents/pBSDH_RCS_Oncol_Radio_BMT_update_2012.pdf (accessed 28 December 2017).

Lee, M., Chin, R.Y., Eslick, G.D., Sritharan, N. and Paramaesvaran, S. (2015) Outcomes of microvascular free flap reconstruction for mandibular osteoradionecrosis: a systematic review. *J Craniomaxillofac Surg*, **43**, 2026–2033.

Lyons, A.J. and Brennan, P.A. (2017) Pentoxifylline – a review of its use in osteoradionecrosis. *Br J Oral Maxillofac Surg*, **55**, 230–234.

Madrid, C., Abarca, M. and Bouferrache, K. (2010) Osteoradionecrosis: an update. *Oral Oncol*, **46**, 471–474.

Marwan, H., Green, J.M. 3rd, Tursun, R. and Marx, R.E. (2016) Recurrent malignancy in osteoradionecrosis specimen. *J Oral Maxillofac Surg*, **74**, 2312–2316.

Marx, R.E. (1983a) A new concept in the treatment of osteoradionecrosis. *J Oral Maxillofac Surg*, **41**, 351–357.

Marx, R.E. (1983b) Osteoradionecrosis: a new concept of its pathophysiology. *J Oral Maxillofac Surg*, **41**, 283–288.

Marx, R.E., Johnson, R.P. and Kline, S.N. (1985) Prevention of osteoradionecrosis: a randomized prospective clinical trial of hyperbaric oxygen versus penicillin. *J Am Dent Assoc*, **111**, 49–54.

Morton, M.E. and Simpson, W. (1986) The management of osteoradionecrosis of the jaws. *Br J Oral Maxillofac Surg*, **24**, 332–341.

Nabil, S. and Samman, N. (2011) Incidence and prevention of osteoradionecrosis after dental extraction in irradiated patients: a systematic review. *Int J Oral Maxillofac Surg*, **40**, 229–243.

Nadella, K.R., Kodali, R.M., Guttikonda, L.K. and Jonnalagadda, A. (2015) Osteoradionecrosis of the jaws: clinico-therapeutic management: a literature review and update. *J Maxillofac Oral Surg*, **14**, 891–901.

Notani, K., Yamazaki, Y., Kitada, H. et al. (2003) Management of mandibular osteoradionecrosis corresponding to the severity of osteoradionecrosis and the method of radiotherapy. *Head Neck*, **25**, 181–186.

Owosho, A.A., Tsai, C.J., Lee, R.S. et al. (2017) The prevalence and risk factors associated with osteoradionecrosis of the jaw in oral and oropharyngeal cancer patients treated with intensity-modulated radiation therapy (IMRT): the Memorial Sloan Kettering Cancer Center experience. *Oral Oncol*, **64**, 44–51.

Pautke, C., Bauer, F., Bissinger, O. et al. (2010) Tetracycline bone fluorescence: a valuable marker for osteonecrosis characterization and therapy. *J Oral Maxillofac Surg*, **68**, 125–129.

Robard, L., Louis, M.Y., Blanchard, D., Babin, E. and Delanian, S. (2014) Medical treatment of osteoradionecrosis of the mandible by PENTOCLO: preliminary results. *Eur Ann Otorhinolaryngol Head Neck Dis*, **131**, 333–338.

Schwartz, H.C. and Kagan, A.R. (2002) Osteoradionecrosis of the mandible: scientific basis for clinical staging. *Am J Clin Oncol*, **25**, 168–171.

Shaw, R.J. and Butterworth, C. (2011) Hyperbaric oxygen in the management of late radiation injury to the head and neck. Part II: Prevention. *Br J Oral Maxillofac Surg*, **49**, 9–13.

Shaw, R.J. and Dhanda, J. (2011) Hyperbaric oxygen in the management of late radiation injury to the head and neck. Part I: Treatment. *Br J Oral Maxillofac Surg*, **49**, 2–8.

Shaw, R., Forner, L., Butterworth, C. et al. (2011) Randomised controlled trials in HBO: "A call to arms" for HOPON and DAHANCA-21. *Br J Oral Maxillofac Surg*, **49**, 76–77.

Shaw, R., Tesfaye, B., Bickerstaff, M., Silcocks, P. and Butterworth, C. (2017) Refining the definition of mandibular osteoradionecrosis in clinical trials: the Cancer Research UK HOPON Trial (Hyperbaric Oxygen for the Prevention of Osteoradionecrosis). *Oral Oncol*, **64**, 73–77.

Silvestre-Rangil, J. and Silvestre, F.J. (2011) Clinico-therapeutic management of osteoradionecrosis: a literature review and update. *Med Oral Patol Oral Cir Bucal*, **16**, E900–904.

Store, G. and Boysen, M. (2000) Mandibular osteoradionecrosis: clinical behaviour and diagnostic aspects. *Clin Otolaryngol Allied Sci*, **25**, 378–384.

37

Partial Edentulism – Implant Treatment

37.1 Introduction

This chapter focuses on the replacement of missing teeth in partially dentate patients with osseointegrated dental implants. Management of partially dentate patients with conventional removable partial dentures will be discussed in Chapter 38.

Osseointegration is defined as a direct structural and functional connection between vital bone and the surface of a loaded implant (Albrektsson *et al.*, 1981).

Albrektsson *et al.* (1986) outlined the following minimum criteria for successful dental implant treatment.

- Immobile unattached dental implant.
- Absence of peri-implant radiolucency.
- Less than 0.2 mm annual vertical bone loss after the first year.
- Absence of signs and symptoms (pain, infection, neuropathies, paraesthesia or violation of the mandibular canal).
- A success rate of 85% at 5 years and 80% at 10 years.

Additional success criteria, including aesthetics and patient satisfaction, have also been suggested (Papaspyridakos *et al.*, 2012).

37.2 Preoperative Patient Assessment

Preoperative assessment of patients for dental implant treatment includes history taking, clinical examination and special investigations (Barker, 2012).

37.2.1 History

Relevant aspects of patient history for implant treatment are listed below.

- Chief complaint and its history.
- Dental history including previous treatment, parafunctional habits, bruxism and clenching.
- Family history of relevant genetic disorders and aggressive periodontal disease.
- Patient's expectations, motivation and compliance.
- Social history including smoking and alcohol intake.
- Medical history including bone diseases, diabetes, bleeding disorders, cardiovascular diseases, mucosal diseases, immune system disorders, history of cancer and any relevant treatment, drug addiction and psychiatric conditions (Donos and Calciolari, 2014).
- Medications, history of chemotherapy, radiotherapy, bisphosphonates and antimetabolics.

37.2.2 Clinical Examination

It is important to perform extraoral examination of mouth opening, temporomandibular joints (TMJ), lymph nodes, facial asymmetry and evaluation of smile line and lip support, especially when planning implants in the aesthetic zone.

Intraoral examination must include oral soft tissues, edentulous spaces in terms of available mesiodistal and occlusogingival space, bone height, width, volume and quality, gingival phenotype and the level of gingivae in relation to the cementoenamel junction (CEJ) of adjacent teeth, periodontal examination, aesthetic assessment of shape, position and height-to-width ratio of clinical crowns in the anterior region, assessment of occlusion, overjet, overbite, interocclusal space, anterior guidance, occlusal plane, malpositioned teeth, asymmetry, restorative assessment and endodontic status of the remaining teeth.

37.2.3 Special Investigations

Relevant special investigations may include the following.

- Sensibility testing of the teeth adjacent to the planned implant site.
- Radiographic examination such as oral panoramic radiograph for an overall view of the teeth, bone levels and anatomical structures and periapical radiographs

Diseases and Conditions in Dentistry: An Evidence-Based Reference, First Edition. Keyvan Moharamzadeh.

Companion website: www.wiley.com/go/moharamzadeh/diseases

of the teeth adjacent to the edentulous areas for detailed relevant information.
- Cone beam computed tomography may be indicated when clinical examination and conventional radiography have failed to provide adequate information for safe and successful implant treatment. Examples of these situations include ridge defects requiring significant bone grafting, sinus augmentation, distraction osteogenesis, zygomatic implants and computer-guided implant surgery (Harris *et al.*, 2012).

37.3 Risk Factors

Risk factors for implant failure can be grouped into local, systemic and behavioural aspects (Lang and Lindhe, 2015).

37.3.1 Local Risk Factors

Local risk factors include the following.

- Poor oral hygiene is a significant risk indicator for secondary implant failure due to peri-implantitis (Tecco *et al.*, 2017).
- History of periodontal disease decreases the survival rate of implants (Sousa *et al.*, 2016) and the factors that increase the risk of periodontitis also increase the risk of implant failure (Chrcanovic *et al.*, 2014b). Elimination of periodontitis lesions before implant placement and the establishment of a high standard of infection control are decisive factors for the success of implant therapy in periodontally compromised patients.
- Endodontic infections in the adjacent teeth can lead to retrograde peri-implantitis (Ramanauskaite *et al.*, 2016).
- Parafunction and excessive loading can increase the risk of failure, especially technical and mechanical complications (Salvi and Bragger, 2009).

37.3.2 Systemic Risk Factors

Systemic risk factors include the following.

- *Smoking* is a significant risk factor for implant failure and postoperative biological complications (Chrcanovic *et al.*, 2015d) as it impairs the immune response and interferes with wound healing. Therefore, smoking cessation is strongly recommended as part of treatment planning for dental implants.
- *Diabetes*: evidence suggests that implant survival in well-controlled diabetes patients is similar to that in non-diabetic patients. However, patients with diabetes in general show higher marginal bone loss around implants compared to non-diabetic patients (Chrcanovic *et al.*, 2014a). Patients with poorly controlled diabetes have an elevated risk of wound healing problems, infections and biological complications of implants, especially during the period of osseointegration and the first year of loading (Annibali *et al.*, 2016).
- *Bisphosphonates* increase the risk of medication-related osteonecrosis of jaw (MRONJ), especially in patients receiving intravenous (IV) bisphosphonates (see Chapter). There is a rare but real risk of implant failure with oral bisphosphonates and the risk depends on the dose and length of the drug treatment although the level of evidence is low (Chrcanovic *et al.*, 2016a). Dental implant treatment is not recommended for patients receiving IV bisphosphonates and those on long-term oral bisphosphonates (Scully *et al.*, 2006). Also, bone grafting and sinus lift procedures are not recommended in this group of patients.
- *Radiotherapy*: implants in irradiated bone have been discussed in Chapter 32.
- *Chemotherapy*: although it has been shown that certain chemotherapeutic agents do not have negative effects on the survival of dental implants (Chrcanovic *et al.*, 2016b; Kovacs, 2001), chemotherapy can cause delayed wound healing and immunosuppression and thorough periodontal care and implant maintenance are very important in these patients.
- *Anticoagulants*: patients on oral anticoagulants with an international normalised ratio (INR) of 2–4 are not at significantly higher risk of postoperative bleeding than normal patients or those who discontinue the medication. Topical haemostatic agents would be effective in preventing postoperative bleeding in these patients and discontinuation of oral anticoagulant is not recommended for single tooth extraction or simple dental implant placement which does not require autogenous bone grafts or extensive flaps (Madrid and Sanz, 2009). Patients with severe liver disease, thrombocytopenia, congenital bleeding disorders (such as haemophilia and von Willebrand's disease) and clotting factor deficiencies are at significantly increased risk of bleeding and any oral surgery procedure should be managed in the hospital setting after liaison with the patient's haematologist (Renton *et al.*, 2013).
- *Immunosuppression*: dental implants can be placed successfully in HIV-positive patients, especially if the condition is controlled by highly active antiretroviral therapy (HAART) medication (Gay-Escoda *et al.*, 2016). However, the failure rate is increased in smoker HIV-positive patients (Gherlone *et al.*, 2016). Strict

maintenance protocol must be implemented to reduce the risk of peri-implant diseases.

- *Metabolic bone disease*: it has been shown that there is no significant difference in implant survival rate between patients with and without osteoporosis. However, a meta-analysis showed an increase in peri-implant bone loss in patients with osteoporosis (de Medeiros *et al.*, 2017).
- *Mucosal and autoimmune disorders*: patients with scleroderma may have stiff lips and restricted mouth opening, which can cause access problems and difficulty maintaining good oral hygiene and so rigorous maintenance is required. Patients with systemic lupus erythematosus (SLE) can be susceptible to bacteraemia and therefore, antibiotic cover is recommended for these patients. It has been shown that implant survival rates in patients with mucosal diseases such as oral lichen planus, Sjögren's syndrome, epidermolysis bullosa and systemic sclerosis are comparable to those of patients without oral mucosal diseases (Reichart *et al.*, 2016).
- Certain haematological and lymphoreticular disorders, such as agranulocytosis, acquired and cyclic neutropenias, leucocyte adhesion deficiency (LAD) and aplastic anaemia, can all increase susceptibility to periodontitis. There are no well-controlled studies on implant success in this area. As these patients lose their teeth early in life, dental implants can be placed under control or in the remission phase of the disease and a strict postoperative maintenance protocol is required in these patients (see Chapter 43).
- Genetic disorders such as Down's syndrome (Limeres Posse *et al.*, 2016) and Papillon–Lefevre syndrome (Nickles *et al.*, 2013) can cause early tooth loss due to susceptibility to infections. Dental implants may have a lower survival rate in these patients and effective postoperative care and long-term maintenance are essential.

37.3.3 Behavioural Risk Factors

Behavioural risk factors include the following.

- Poor compliance with oral hygiene and attendance.
- Unrealistic expectations, lack of understanding and poor communication.
- Alcohol and/or drug abuse may reduce the patient's co-operation and make them poor candidates for implant treatment.
- Psychiatric or psychological issues can also affect the patient's co-operation and complicate the treatment. However, patients with medically controlled depression can be treated with dental implants.

37.4 Risk Assessment and Patient Consent

It is important to carry out patient-specific risk assessment to establish whether the patients belong to the low-, medium- or high-risk category, depending on the factors described above.

Patients must be fully informed about treatment benefits, risks, complications, costs, future maintenance requirements and alternative approaches and written consent must be obtained prior to treatment.

37.5 Treatment Considerations

The aim of treatment is functional and aesthetic restoration of missing teeth. Careful presurgical planning is required to enable restoration-driven implant placement to achieve this goal.

37.5.1 Planning Stage

In addition to full preoperative patient assessment as described above, preparation of articulated study models and diagnostic wax-up is important for implant planning to analyse the available prosthetic space and enable fabrication of a surgical stent that can be used to facilitate implant placement with correct position and angulation. Diagnostic wax-up will also help to modify the existing teeth to ideal shape, height and occlusion if necessary prior to placement and restoration of implants.

Fabrication of a radiographic stent using radiopaque denture teeth worn by the patient during imaging can help to establish the position of planned implant-retained crowns in relation to the available bone. This technique is often used in computer-assisted implant planning and placement.

A minimum of 7 mm mesiodistal space is required for a regular implant with approximately 4 mm diameter. A minimum of 4 mm vertical distance from the top of ridge mucosa to the opposing teeth is also required.

Important anatomical structures that should be avoided to reduce the risk of damage during implant placement include the following.

- *Inferior alveolar nerve*: it is important to have at least a 2 mm safety zone above the upper border of the mandibular canal when planning for implant placement in the posterior mandible.
- *Mental nerve*: implant placement immediately anterior to the mental foramen must be avoided due to the possible presence of an anterior loop and a 4 mm safety zone must be considered.

- *Blood vessels* including the sublingual artery (branch of the lingual artery) and submental artery (branch of the facial artery), both close to lingual cortical plates.
- *Floor of the mouth* can be protected by reflecting the lingual flap to the level of the implant depth to prevent perforation of the lingual plate and damage to the vessels.
- *Nasal cavity and maxillary sinuses.*
- *Adjacent teeth.*

37.5.2 Surgical Stage

Surgical implant placement protocols include one-stage or two-stage implant placement.

In the one-stage approach, implant and abutment penetrate the mucosa from placement and no further surgery is required to expose the implant. It requires good primary stability of the implant and prosthodontic care can start immediately (immediate function). This procedure can be undertaken using either open or flapless surgery.

Flapless guided surgery techniques have been developed to enable precise and predictable implant placement utilising a surgical stent made with the help of computer software following analysis of the CT data obtained from the patient with a radiographic stent. The advantages of computer-guided implant placement are minimal invasive keyhole surgery, less postoperative swelling and pain, immediate recovery and cost savings (Hultin *et al.*, 2012). Although guided implant placement can be accurate, the potential risk of significant deviations should be taken into account (van Assche *et al.*, 2012).

The two-stage technique involves placement of cover screws on the implant once inserted into the bone and submerging the implant under soft tissues, which will require a second surgery to expose the implant and place the healing abutment. This technique is indicated when there is poor primary stability and/or need for simultaneous bone grafting procedure. It allows modification of soft tissues at second stage surgery but delays prosthetic care and increases treatment time.

Aseptic surgical technique is extremely important to minimise the risk of postsurgical infection.

It has been shown that prophylactic antibiotics (2 g of amoxicillin given orally 1 hour preoperatively) significantly reduce the failure rate of dental implants placed in normal conditions (Esposito *et al.*, 2010; Keenan and Veitz-Keenan, 2015).

Atraumatic implant surgery must be performed and the osteotomy drill speed must be kept below 800 rpm, with adequate cooling with normal saline solution to minimise tissue damage.

To achieve adequate primary stability of the implant, it is important to use implants with optimal height and width. In weak bone, the use of parallel-walled implants or implants with actively engaging threads (especially in extraction sockets) can enhance primary stability. However, care must be taken to avoid overambitious fixation of the implant as this can increase the risk of implant fracture during insertion.

37.5.3 Prosthetic Treatment

Osseointegrated implants can be restored with a fixed implant-retained prosthesis or removable implant-supported overdentures. Fixed implant-retained prostheses include single crowns, fixed bridges and full-arch fixed prostheses. Full-arch fixed implant-retained prostheses and removable implant-supported overdentures are discussed in Chapter 45.

Implant-retained single crowns and bridges can be screw retained or cement retained, with comparable clinical performance (Lemos *et al.*, 2016; Sherif *et al.*, 2014). Screw-retained restorations are usually preferred as they are easy to restore and retrieve and are free from residual cement. However, the presence of the screw access hole may weaken the crown and the access hole filling material can be lost. These restorations are also more sensitive to passive fit and susceptible to screw-related biomechanical complications, as discussed later in this chapter. In addition, if the access hole emerges from the labial aspect of the crown due to the angulation of the implant, it may cause significant aesthetic concern.

Cement-retained crowns can hide the access hole and improve the aesthetics in situations where the screw access hole cannot be placed palatally. Limitations of cement retention include biological risks associated with remaining excess cement and difficult retrievability of the crown.

The development of angled screw systems enables shifting the screw access hole palatally to some extent and may offer a reliable and retrievable alternative to cement-retained restorations (Greer *et al.*, 2017).

The European Association for Osseointegration (EAO) made the following clinical recommendations regarding the method of retention for reconstructions on implants (Gotfredsen *et al.*, 2012).

- For single crowns, both types of fixation methods (screw retained and cement retained) can be recommended.
- In case of cementation of the reconstruction, proper removal of cement excess is crucial to prevent biological complications.
- Extensive implant reconstructions as partial or full-arch fixed prosthesis should be screw retained.

Different materials have been used for fabrication of fixed implant superstructures, including porcelain fused to metal, gold framework and acrylic teeth, and all-ceramic restorations using zirconia abutment framework. Abutments can be prefabricated or custom made with different angulations.

In order to design an appropriate prosthesis and restore the implants, it is important to take an accurate impression of the implants and verify the position of the fixtures. Bhakta *et al.* (2011) have provided detailed step-by-step instructions for taking impressions of dental implants using closed- and open-tray impression techniques as well as recommendations for appropriate use of verification jigs.

Periapical radiographs can be taken to verify correct seating of impression copings and abutments.

The ideal occlusion for implant-retained single crowns or fixed bridges would have the following features (Davies, 2010; Kim *et al.*, 2005; Sheridan *et al.*, 2016).

- Cusp to fossa relationship.
- Narrow occlusal table.
- Only axial loading.
- Light contacts on posterior implant teeth. It is advised that the occlusal contact on an implant-supported crown should be about 30 μm 'lighter' than on the adjacent teeth (as a guide, shimstock is 10 μm thick).
- No or minimal contact in mandibular excursions.
- No guidance on implants. Ideally, canine guidance on natural teeth or group function.

37.5.4 Replacement of the Anterior Teeth with Implants

To achieve an optimal outcome for the implant crown and soft tissue aesthetics, the implant shoulder should be placed 1–2 mm more apically to the labial CEJ of the adjacent teeth (where the bone level should ideally be), and at least a 1 mm bone plate on the buccal aspect of the implant must be maintained. If there is a ridge defect, augmentation procedures would be recommended (see Chapter 46).

The emergence profile from the implant shoulder to the gingival margin should be flat and similar to the contralateral tooth.

A slightly palatal incision would help to preserve maximum keratinised tissue on the labial aspect of the implant and further improve the aesthetics. The papillae of the neighbouring teeth should not be included in the flap in the aesthetic zone unless the space is very tight for a single tooth implant.

Abutment selection depends on:

- implant shoulder depth in relation to the labial mucosal margin
- buccolingual implant shoulder position with respect to the future line of emergence of the superstructure
- the long axis of the implant.

If the peri-implant labial mucosa is thin, zirconia abutment may be considered to avoid dark metal show through the mucosa in the aesthetic zone.

It is often best to avoid two single implants next to each other in the aesthetic zone as bone saucerisation happens in adjacent implant sites as a result of establishment of the biological widths. It may be better to use a single implant with a cantilever pontic for better aesthetics.

Peri-implant soft tissue conditioning with temporary restorations can be helpful to achieve the ideal gingival contour.

Slightly long contact points with slightly palatal contact lines and mini-wings with more saturated shade are recommended to avoid black triangles.

37.5.5 Replacement of the Posterior Teeth with Implants

For replacing up to four teeth distal to the canine teeth, a three- or four-unit fixed-fixed implant-retained bridge on two implants can be safely used. For replacing more than four posterior teeth on one side, three implants are preferred to two to avoid overloading the abutments (Jemt and Lekholm, 1993).

Wide dental implants are desirable in the posterior region and show promising survival rates (Lee *et al.*, 2016).

A minimum interimplant distance of 3 mm is required for premolar and 4 mm for molar teeth. The minimum mesiodistal space required for a premolar implant is 7 mm and for a molar implant is 8 mm. Minimum distance of an implant from a tooth surface is 1.5 mm.

It is best to avoid splinting the adjacent implants to each other to enable better access for plaque control. It is also best to avoid splinting implants to the natural teeth to avoid long-term biomechanical and biological complications (Pjetursson and Lang, 2008).

37.5.6 Considerations in Bruxist Patients

Functional loading of implants may enhance osseointegration (Duyck and Vandamme, 2014). However, occlusal loads have to exceed the physiological range substantially before they can jeopardise the tissue integrity of an implant (Lang and Lindhe, 2015).

The consequences of overload on dental implants may include the following.

- Early biological failure of the implant due to insufficient osseointegration as a result of micromovement of the implant under excessive lateral loads.

- Late biological failure after osseointegration due to pathological bone loss in the presence of inflammation.
- Mechanical and technical failure of the implant and its superstructure.

It has been documented that occlusal parafunction, such as bruxism, affects the outcome of implant prostheses, but there is little data available for a causal relation between failure and overload of dental implants (Manfredini *et al.*, 2011) and the real effect of bruxism on the osseointegration and survival of dental implants is still not well established (Chrcanovic *et al.*, 2015a).

Bragger *et al.* (2001) recognised a causal relation between bruxism and the fracture of implant superstructure. Retrospective studies by Chrcanovic *et al.* (2016c) showed that implant failure rates were 13% for patients with bruxism and 4.6% for patients without parafunctional habits and it was concluded that bruxism may significantly increase both the risk of implant failure and the rate of mechanical and technical complications of implant-supported restorations (Chrcanovic *et al.*, 2017).

Suggestions to minimise the risk of implant complications in patients with bruxism include monitoring parafunctional habits, occlusal splints, reducing cantilevers, narrowing the occlusal table, decreasing cuspal inclines, increasing the number of implants and contact points, progressive loading in patients with poor bone quality, use of metal restorations instead of porcelain for molar teeth, and the use of acrylic teeth in extensive restorations (Manfredini *et al.*, 2011; Sheridan *et al.*, 2016).

37.5.7 Maintenance

To improve the long-term success of dental implant treatment, it is important to establish and maintain an effective maintenance programme to reduce the risk of potential biological complications and also manage any biomechanical complications that may arise.

A minimum recall interval of 5–6 months for peri-implant maintenance therapy has been suggested (Monje *et al.*, 2016), although this must be tailored to the individual patient risk profile, especially in patients with history of periodontal disease.

A reference postoperative periapical radiograph must be taken when definitive restorations are placed. Subsequent radiographs can be taken to monitor the bone levels. Some marginal bone loss takes place around implants during the first few years after placement due to adaptive bone response to surgical trauma and implant loading, which is usually around 0.9–1.5 mm during the first year and 0.1 mm per year thereafter in the absence of disease (normal bone remodelling). Further significant crestal bone resorption after the first year (aseptic loosening) can be due to biological reaction to non-optimal implant or prosthetic components, compromised surgical/prosthetic treatment or patient factors (Albrektsson *et al.*, 2017). This initial self-limiting marginal bone loss must be distinguished from peri-implantitis which is a late complication and a rapidly progressive infectious disease (see Chapter 40).

37.5.8 Implant Complications

Implant-related complications can be divided into biological, mechanical (technical) and aesthetic aspects.

37.5.8.1 Biological Complications

- Surgical complications such as haemorrhage, nerve damage and mandible fracture.
- Early implant loss due to lack of osseointegration, infection, contamination, trauma and overload (see above).
- Peri-implant complications including peri-implant mucosal inflammation, soft tissue proliferation, dehiscence, fistula and peri-implantitis.
- Malpositioned implants, which can be avoided by careful preoperative planning.

37.5.8.1 Mechanical Complications

- Fracture of the restoration due to increased occlusal force (greater than 200 N) on implants due to lack of periodontal ligament shock absorption.
- Wear of restoration or opposing teeth.
- Screw-related complications such as screw loosening or fracture. The absence of passivity between implant components can increase the internal stress accumulation in the screw (preload) and cause loosening or fracture. Anti-rotation features are essential for screw success and an internal connection design with minimal taper (2–15°) results in significantly better mechanical and clinical behaviour than external abutment connections (Gracis *et al.*, 2012).
- Abutment-related complications such as incomplete seating and abutment fracture.

According to a systematic review by Salvi and Bragger (2009), risk factors for mechanical and technical complications include:

- the absence of a metal framework in overdentures
- the presence of cantilever extension(s) greater than 15 mm
- bruxism
- the length of the reconstruction
- history of repeated complications.

None of the above risk factors had an impact on implant survival and success rates.

37.5.8.1 Aesthetic Complications

Aesthetic complications can be grouped into (1) white tissue aesthetic problems, such as failures in crown position, alignment, shape, size, proportions, symmetry, colour, contour and emergence profile, and (2) pink tissue failures, such as recession, black triangle, gingival asymmetry and metal shadow showing through the gingivae (Fuentealba and Jofre, 2015).

The risk of aesthetic complications is increased in patients with high aesthetic expectations, high smile line, compromised periodontal tissues and inadequate hard and soft tissues in the aesthetic zone.

37.5.8.1 Evidence

Reported figures for implant-related complications are as high as 33.6%. The most frequently reported complications are veneer fractures (13.5%), peri-implantitis and soft tissue problems (8.5%), loss of access hole restoration (5.4%), screw or abutment loosening (5.3%) and loss of retention of cemented restorations (4.7%) (Jung *et al.*, 2012; Pjetursson *et al.*, 2012; Romeo and Storelli, 2012; Scheuber *et al.*, 2012). The incidence of aesthetic complications has decreased in more recent studies, but the incidence of biological complications has remained similar compared with older studies. There has been a significant reduction in screw or abutment loosening in implant-supported prostheses. However, the overall incidence of mechanical complications and fracture of the veneering material has significantly increased in the newer studies (Pjetursson *et al.*, 2014).

37.6 Implant Survival

Due to improvements in implant dentistry, the 5-year overall survival rate of implant-supported prostheses has significantly increased in newer studies (97.1%) compared with older studies (93.5%) (Pjetursson *et al.*, 2014).

37.6.1 Implant-Retained Single Crowns

Based on a meta-analysis by Jung *et al.* (2012), survival of implants supporting single crowns was 97.2% at 5 years and 95.2% at 10 years. The survival of implant-supported single crowns was 96.3% at 5 years and 89.4% at 10 years.

A further review showed a 10-year implant survival rate of 93.8% (at patient level) and 95.0% (at implant level data) (Hjalmarsson *et al.*, 2016). The corresponding survival rate for the crown restorations was 89.5%.

37.6.2 Implant-Retained Bridge

According to a meta-analysis by Pjetursson *et al.* (2012), the estimated survival of implants supporting fixed dental prostheses was 95.6% after 5 years and 93.1% after 10 years. When only rough surface implants were included in the analysis (excluding machined surface implants), the survival rate increased to 97.2% after 5 years. The survival rate of implant-supported fixed prostheses was 95.4% after 5 years and 80.1% after 10 years of function. When only metal-ceramic restorations were included in the analysis (excluding the old gold-acrylic fixed prostheses), the survival rate increased significantly to 96.4% after 5 years and 93.9% after 10 years.

37.7 Timing of Implant Placement after Tooth Extraction

Timing of implant placement after tooth extraction has been classified to four protocols: type I to type IV (Hammerle *et al.*, 2004).

Type I (immediate placement) involves placement of the implant immediately after tooth extraction at the same surgical session. This protocol reduces the number of surgical treatment sessions and the overall treatment time. However, it is technique sensitive as the placement and anchorage can be affected by the site morphology, and flap adaptation can be difficult due to lack of soft tissues. Furthermore, immediate implant placement does not seem to counteract alveolar ridge modelling after tooth extraction and evidence for the efficacy of a concomitant regenerative technique is inconclusive (Clementini *et al.*, 2015). Therefore, immediate placement is desirable when there is intact labial bone with thick walls and thick gingival biotype (Kinaia *et al.*, 2017) to minimise the risk of recession and aesthetic complications.

Type II (early placement with soft tissue healing) refers to placement of the implant after soft tissue coverage of the socket (4–8 weeks). Its advantages include increased volume of soft tissues and it allows assessment of the resolution of any infection in the socket. However, this protocol increases treatment time and is also technique sensitive. Type II placement is desirable when there is sufficient bone volume available apically to stabilise the implant.

Type III (substantial bone healing) involves implant placement after substantial bone fill in the socket (12–16 weeks). This protocol facilitates implant placement and improves its primary stability. However, treatment time is increased and the socket walls may resorb variably during the healing period. This technique may be desirable when there is a large periapical bone lesion which does not allow type I or type II placement.

Type IV (delayed placement) is placement of implants in completely healed sites (over 4–6 months). It has the advantages of implant placement in the clinically healed ridge with mature soft tissue. However, it significantly delays treatment and various amounts of ridge resorption may have occurred. This protocol is preferred when the patient is not suitable for type I–III placement, requires extra time to consider different treatment options and will allow assessment of the healed ridge for the need for any bone augmentation procedure. Socket preservation techniques can be used to reduce the rate of bone resorption in extracted sockets. This topic is discussed in Chapter 46.

It has been shown that insertion of implants in fresh extraction sockets may affect failure rates. The reported failure rate for implants in fresh extraction sockets is 4% compared to a 3.09% failure rate for implants in healed sites (Chrcanovic *et al.*, 2015b). The immediate placement of an implant into an infected site may slightly increase the risk of implant failure when compared to immediate implant placement into a non-infected site (Zhao *et al.*, 2016). The risk can be minimised by meticulous cleaning, socket curettage and debridement, and the use of chlorhexidine 0.12% rinse prior to implant placement in infected sockets (Chrcanovic *et al.*, 2015e).

37.8 Timing of Implant Loading

Implant loading protocols can be classified into immediate loading (earlier than 1 week following implant placement), early loading (between 1 week and 2 months) and conventional loading (after 2 months) (Morton and Pollini, 2017).

The advantages of immediate loading are:

- immediate restoration of function, phonetics and aesthetics
- reduced treatment time and clinical visits
- reduced postoperative discomfort
- significant improvement in patient satisfaction and quality of life
- successful osseointegration under normal functional occlusal loads.

Good bone quality and quantity and implant primary stability are important prerequisites for early or immediate implant loading. A minimum implant stability quotient (ISQ) value of 60 is recommended for immediate loading. Immediately loaded implants in multiunit situations should be rigidly splinted by the use of superstructures.

Conventional (delayed) implant loading is recommended in the following situations.

- Poor implant primary stability.
- Substantial bone augmentation.
- Implants with reduced dimensions.
- Compromised host conditions such as bruxism and parafunctional habits.

A number of systematic reviews have shown that clinical outcomes and survival rates of immediately and early loaded implants are comparable to those of conventionally loaded implants (Esposito *et al.*, 2013; Zhang *et al.*, 2017). However, other systematic reviews have shown slightly increased failure rates for immediately loaded implants compared to conventionally loaded implants although the survival rates were still high for both groups (Chrcanovic *et al.*, 2015c; Sanz-Sanchez *et al.*, 2015). These reports should be interpreted with caution due to the potentially high risk of bias in some studies included in the systematic reviews.

Case Study

A 25-year-old male patient was referred to the restorative dentistry department for the management of traumatic loss of maxillary anterior teeth.

The patient's presenting complaint was lost upper front teeth and poor aesthetics. He had fallen from his bicycle 4 months earlier and had sustained bilateral condylar fractures, damage and loss of maxillary anterior teeth. He had been initially treated by intermaxillary fixation using screws and stainless steel wires.

The patient attended his GDP regularly and had good oral hygiene. Medical history was clear with no medications. He was a non-smoker and drank 12 units of alcohol per week.

Clinical examination showed lost UR1, UR2, UR3, UR4, UL1 and enamel/dentine fracture of UL2 which was slightly discoloured (Figure 37.1). The patient had a low smile line. Examination of occlusion showed class II skeletal relationship and an anterior open bite with crowded mandibular anterior teeth.

Periodontal examination showed healthy periodontal tissues with BPE scores of 0 in all quadrants. Sensibility testing with an electric pulp tester showed UL2 was non-vital.

Radiographic examination showed bilateral condylar fractures, unerupted third molars and periapical radiolucency associated with UL2 (Figures 37.2 and 37.3).

Based on the clinical and radiographic examinations, the following diagnoses were made.

- Enamel and dentine fracture of UL2 and chronic apical periodontitis.

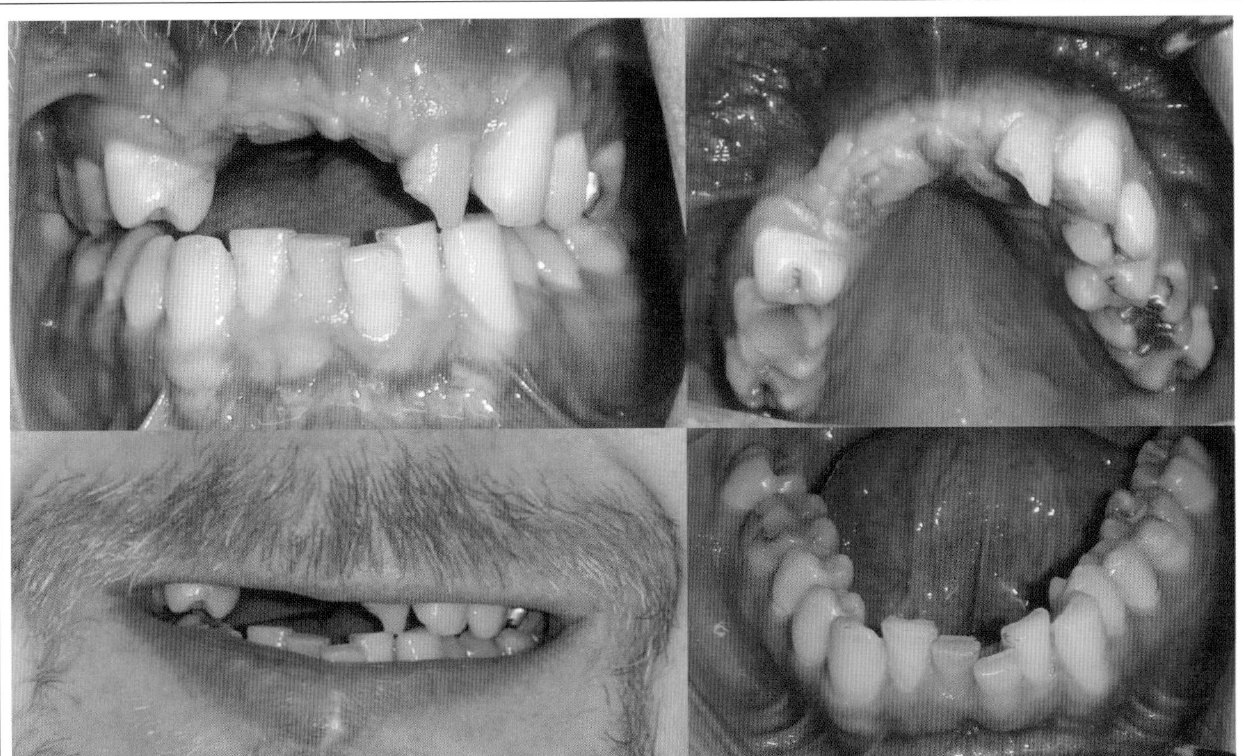

Figure 37.1 Preoperative clinical photographs showing lost UR4–UL1, fractured UL2 and mild-moderate edentulous ridge defect in the anterior maxilla in both horizontal and vertical directions.

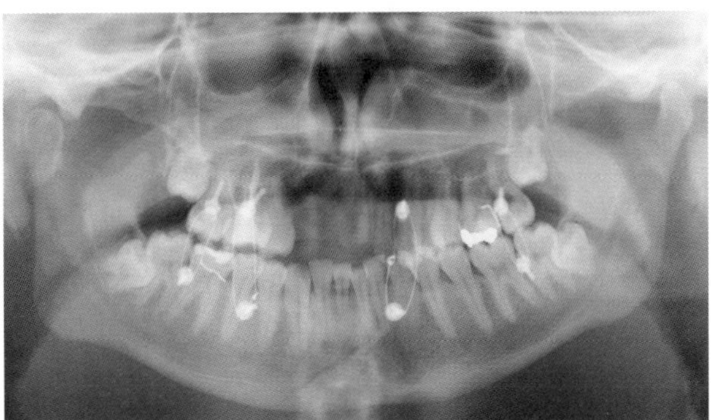

Figure 37.2 Oral panoramic radiograph following intermaxillary fixation (IMF) showing bilateral condylar fractures and IMF screws and wires.

- Bilateral condylar fractures treated by intermaxillary fixation (IMF).
- Traumatic loss of UR1, UR2, UR3, UR4 and UL1.
- Anterior open bite and crowding.
- Impacted third molar teeth.

The following treatment options were discussed with the patient, including risks and benefits.

- Endodontic treatment or extraction and replacement of UL2.

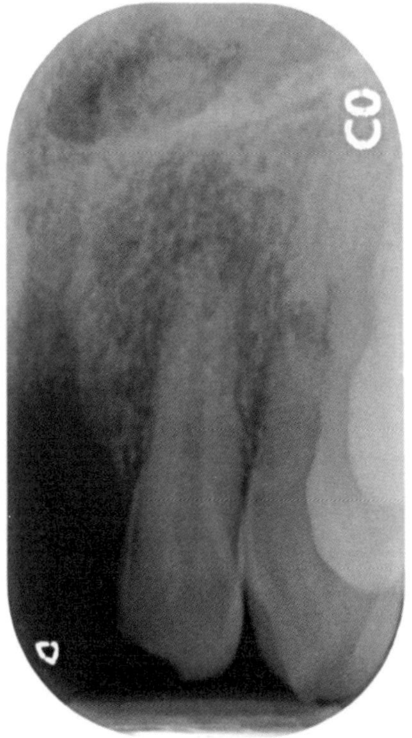

Figure 37.3 Periapical radiograph of UL2 showing a large periapical radiolucency.

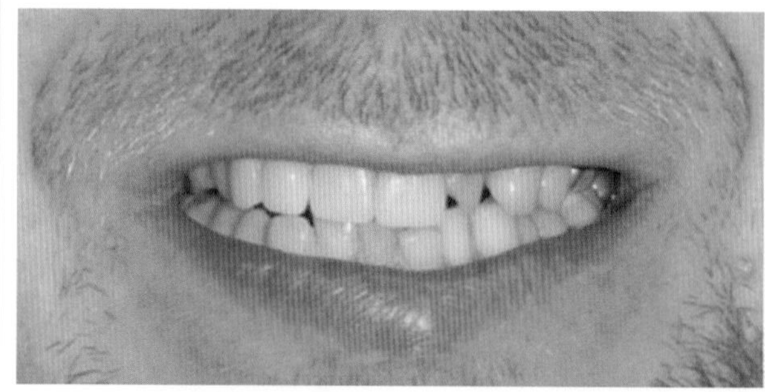

Figure 37.4 Intraoral trial of the diagnostic wax-up using denture teeth showing midline shift and malpositioned UL2.

- Removable partial denture (RPD).
- Fixed bridge including resin-bonded bridge (RBB), which would be a very long-span bridge and not recommended.
- Dental implants which may require bone grafting.
- Orthodontic treatment to correct the position of the teeth prior to replacement of the missing teeth.

The patient preferred extraction of UL2 and replacement of the missing teeth with an implant-retained fixed prosthesis without prior orthodontic treatment.

Implant planning involved the following steps.

1) Clinical photographs.
2) Preparation of articulated study models.
3) Diagnostic wax-up and intraoral trial (Figure 37.4).
4) Cone beam computed tomography (CBCT) and assessment of bone width and height using implant planning software (iCAT Vision Software) (Figure 37.5).
5) Fabrication of a surgical stent using the diagnostic wax-up.

A two-stage surgical technique was used in this case to enable simultaneous bone augmentation and submerging of the implants. The first stage included the following procedures.

1) Preoperative antibiotics: 2 g amoxicillin orally.
2) Extraction of UL2 under local anaesthesia and thorough debridement, curettage and irrigation of the socket with normal saline solution.

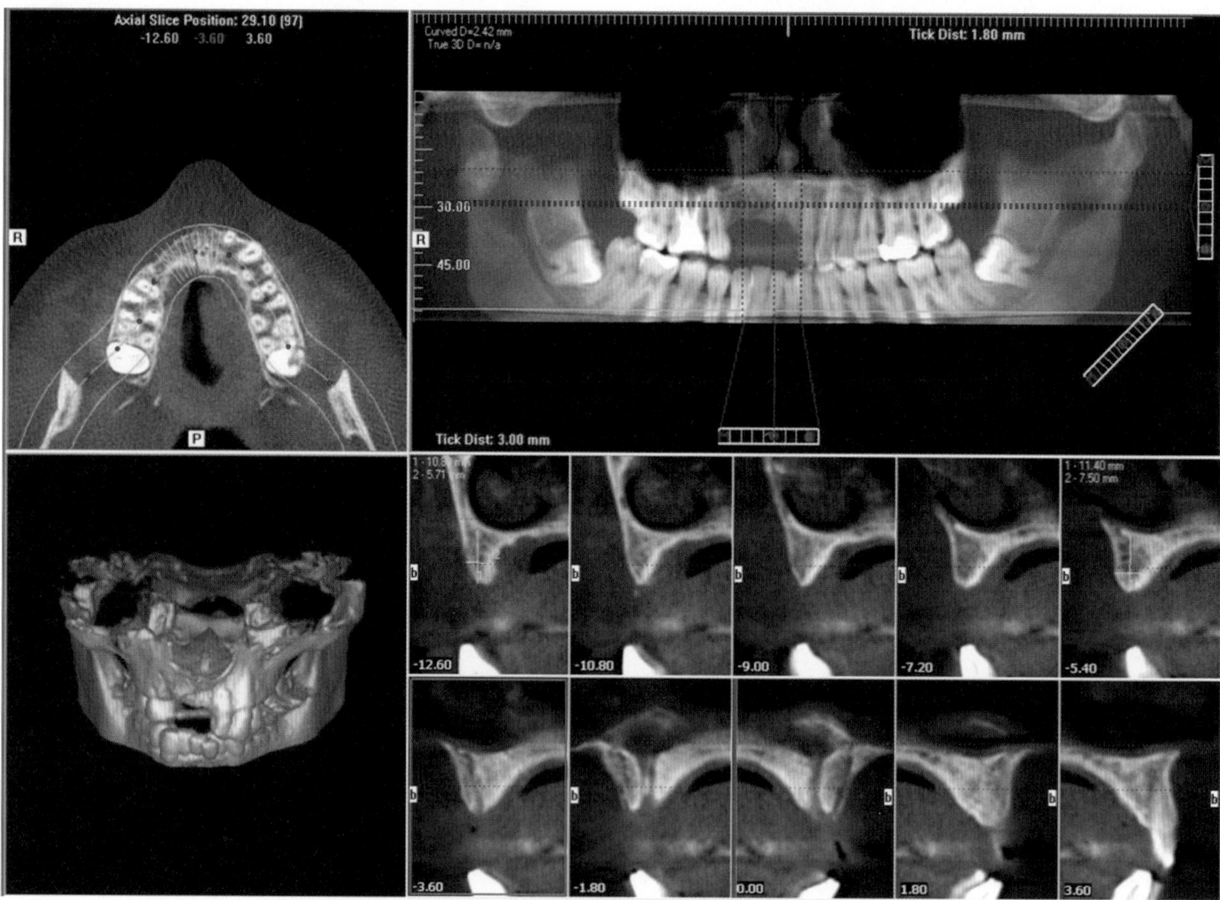

Figure 37.5 Three-dimensional CBCT image analysis using iCAT implant-planning software. Multiple cross-sectional images of the edentulous ridge in the anterior maxilla showing the measurements of bone width and height in different areas. Incisive canal is visible on the images next to the maxillary midline marked by a red vertical line.

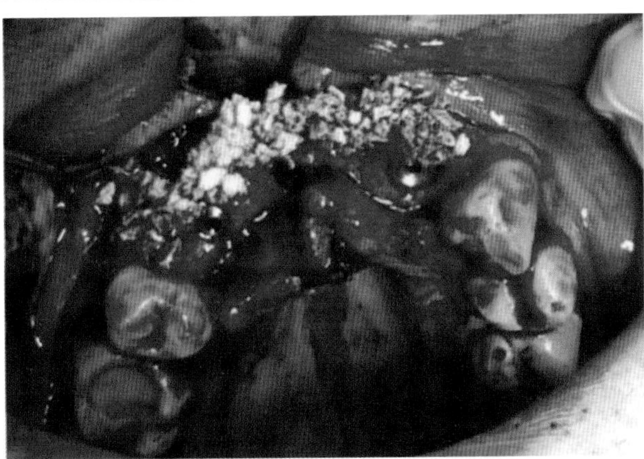

Figure 37.6 Photograph of the surgical site showing three implants placed in the bone and the graft material on the labial aspect of the alveolar ridge and the implants.

3) Incision from UR5 to UL3 and elevation of full-thickness buccal and palatal mucoperiosteal flaps.
4) Placement of three implants (NobelReplace Tapered Groovy, Nobel Biocare) in UL2 (regular platform, RP, 4.3 × 13 mm), UR1 (narrow platform, NP, 3.5 × 10 mm) and UR3 (NP).
5) Fitting cover screws on the implants.
6) Simultaneous bone defect augmentation with bovine-derived bone graft substitute (Bio-Oss®, Geistlich, Wolhusen, Switzerland) (Figure 37.6) and porcine-derived sterile resorbable bilayer collagen membrane (Bio-Gide®, Geistlich).
7) Periosteal releasing incisions to enable advancement of the labial flap and tension-free soft tissue coverage of the augmented ridge and submerging of the implants.
8) Suturing of the wound.
9) Postoperative instructions.

Edentulous ridge height was significantly improved following implant placement and guided bone augmentation (GBR) (Figure 37.7).

The second stage surgery after 4 months involved crestal incision under local anaesthesia and exposure of the implants, fitting healing abutments, suturing soft tissues around the abutments and adjustment of the patient's denture to fit over the healing abutments.

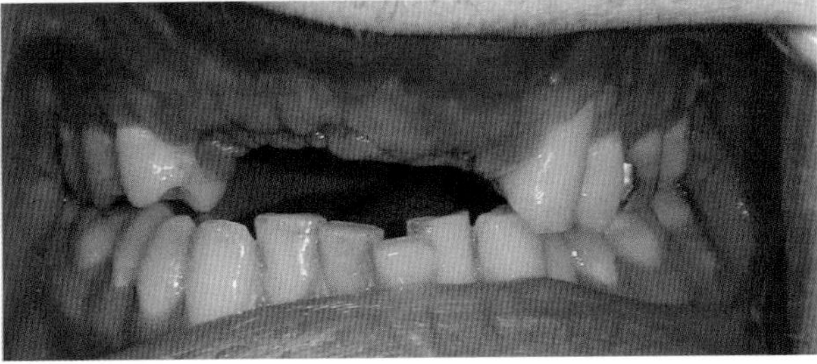

Figure 37.7 Clinical photograph of the ridge following implant placement and GBR showing satisfactory increase in ridge height and width and improvement in the ridge profile.

Prosthetic treatment procedures included the following.

1) Primary impressions and fabrication of a special tray with an open window.
2) Removal of healing abutments, fitting open-tray impression copings on the implants and fixture head level impression using additional silicone impression material in the open special tray.
3) Bite registration and shade selection.
4) Fabrication and fitting of a provisional implant-retained fixed prosthesis to shape gingival soft tissues and verify the position and aesthetics of the teeth (Figure 37.8).
5) New impression of the implants and modified soft tissues after 1 month.
6) Verification of the correct position of the implants using a Duralay verification jig (Figure 37.9).
7) Fabrication and trial of titanium metal framework.
8) Addition of the teeth onto the metal framework and final trial insertion.

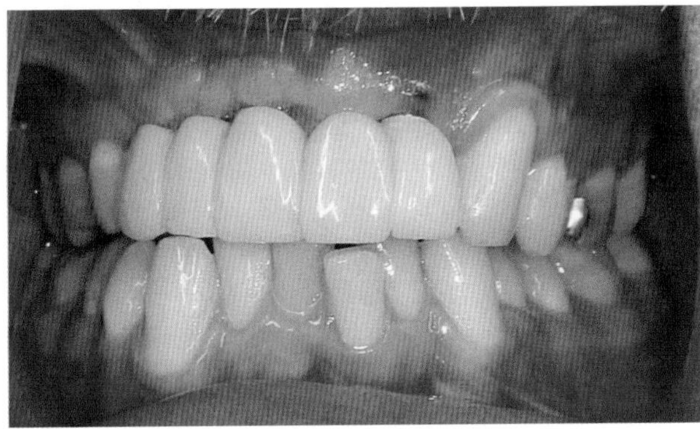

Figure 37.8 Provisional implant-retained prosthesis.

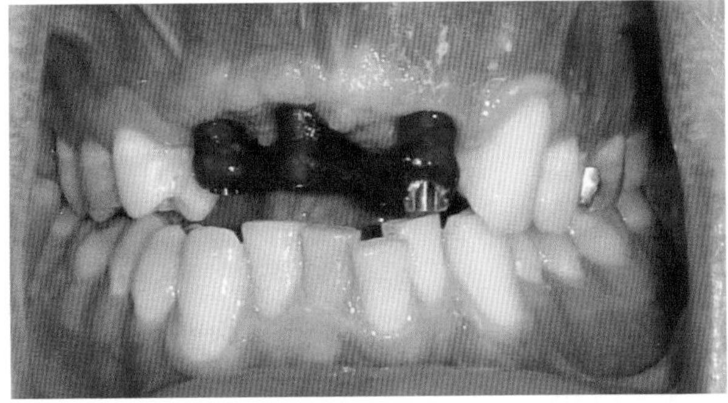

Figure 37.9 Duralay verification jig fitted onto the implants in the mouth to verify correct position of the implants in the stone model and help to achieve accurate and passive fit of the prosthesis.

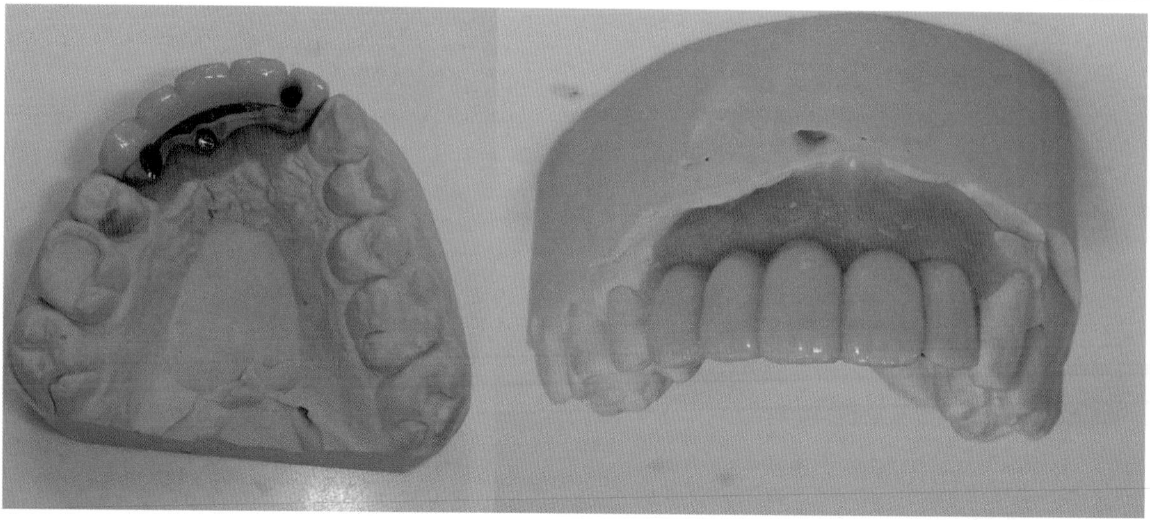

Figure 37.10 Photograph of the definitive PFM screw-retained fixed prosthesis.

9) Fitting of the final PFM screw-retained fixed prosthesis (Figure 37.10).
10) Postoperative instructions, review and maintenance.

The patient's postoperative clinical photographs and radiographs are shown in Figures 37.11 and 37.12 respectively.

The patient was satisfied with the outcome of the treatment. Long-term 6-monthly follow-ups showed satisfactory performance of the prosthesis without any biological or biomechanical complications and the patient maintained an excellent oral hygiene.

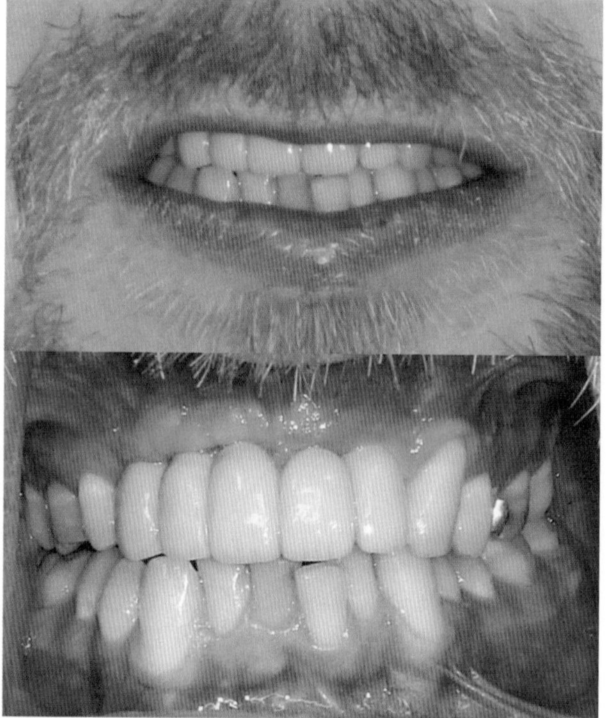

Figure 37.11 Postoperative clinical photographs of the definitive implant-retained fixed prosthesis.

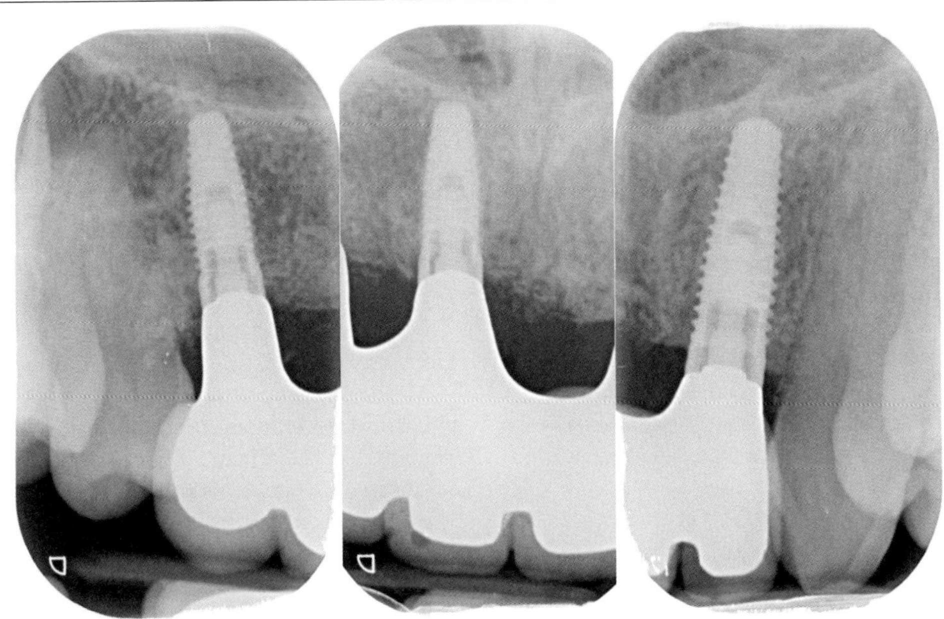

Figure 37.12 Postoperative periapical radiographs of the implants after fitting the definitive fixed screw-retained prosthesis.

References

Albrektsson, T., Branemark, P.I., Hansson, H.A. and Lindstrom, J. (1981) Osseointegrated titanium implants. Requirements for ensuring a long-lasting, direct bone-to-implant anchorage in man. *Acta Orthop Scand*, **52**, 155–170.

Albrektsson, T., Zarb, G., Worthington, P. and Eriksson, A.R. (1986) The long-term efficacy of currently used dental implants: a review and proposed criteria of success. *Int J Oral Maxillofac Implants*, **1**, 11–25.

Albrektsson, T., Chrcanovic, B., Ostman, P.O. and Sennerby, L. (2017) Initial and long–term crestal bone responses to modern dental implants. *Periodontology 2000*, **73**, 41–50.

Annibali, S., Pranno, N., Cristalli, M.P., La Monaca, G. and Polimeni, A. (2016) Survival analysis of implant in patients with diabetes mellitus: a systematic review. *Implant Dent*, **25**, 663–674.

Barker, D. (2012) Implant assessment. *Dent Update*, **39**, 128–132, 134.

Bhakta, S., Vere, J., Calder, I. and Patel, R. (2011) Impressions in implant dentistry. *Br Dent J*, **211**, 361–367.

Bragger, U., Aeschlimann, S., Burgin, W., Hammerle, C.H. and Lang, N.P. (2001) Biological and technical complications and failures with fixed partial dentures (FPD) on implants and teeth after four to five years of function. *Clin Oral Implants Res*, **12**, 26–34.

Chrcanovic, B.R., Albrektsson, T. and Wennerberg, A. (2014a) Diabetes and oral implant failure: a systematic review. *J Dent Res*, **93**, 859–867.

Chrcanovic, B.R., Albrektsson, T. and Wennerberg, A. (2014b) Periodontally compromised vs. periodontally healthy patients and dental implants: a systematic review and meta-analysis. *J Dent*, **42**, 1509–1527.

Chrcanovic, B.R., Albrektsson, T. and Wennerberg, A. (2015a) Bruxism and dental implants: a meta-analysis. *Implant Dent*, **24**, 505–516.

Chrcanovic, B.R., Albrektsson, T. and Wennerberg, A. (2015b) Dental implants inserted in fresh extraction sockets versus healed sites: a systematic review and meta-analysis. *J Dent*, **43**, 16–41.

Chrcanovic, B.R., Albrektsson, T. and Wennerberg, A. (2015c) Immediately loaded non-submerged versus delayed loaded submerged dental implants: a meta-analysis. *Int J Oral Maxillofac Surg*, **44**, 493–506.

Chrcanovic, B.R., Albrektsson, T. and Wennerberg, A. (2015d) Smoking and dental implants: a systematic review and meta-analysis. *J Dent*, **43**, 487–498.

Chrcanovic, B.R., Martins, M.D. and Wennerberg, A. (2015e) Immediate placement of implants into infected sites: a systematic review. *Clin Implant Dent Relat Res*, **17** Suppl 1, E1–E16.

Chrcanovic, B.R., Albrektsson, T. and Wennerberg, A. (2016a) Bisphosphonates and dental implants: a meta-analysis. *Quintessence Int*, **47**, 329–342.

Chrcanovic, B.R., Albrektsson, T. and Wennerberg, A. (2016b) Dental implants in patients receiving chemotherapy: a meta-analysis. *Implant Dent*, **25**, 261–271.

Chrcanovic, B.R., Kisch, J., Albrektsson, T. and Wennerberg, A. (2016c) Bruxism and dental implant failures: a multilevel mixed effects parametric survival analysis approach. *J Oral Rehabil*, **43**, 813–823.

Chrcanovic, B.R., Kisch, J., Albrektsson, T. and Wennerberg, A. (2017) Bruxism and dental implant treatment complications: a retrospective comparative study of 98 bruxer patients and a matched group. *Clin Oral Implants Res*, **28**, E1–E9.

Clementini, M., Tiravia, L., de Risi, V., Vittorini Orgeas, G., Mannocci, A. and de Sanctis, M. (2015) Dimensional changes after immediate implant placement with or without simultaneous regenerative procedures: a systematic review and meta-analysis. *J Clin Periodontol*, **42**, 666–677.

Davies, S.J. (2010) Occlusal considerations in implantology: good occlusal practice in implantology. *Dent Update*, **37**, 610–612, 615–616, 619–620.

de Medeiros, F., Kudo, G.A.H., Leme, B.G. et al. (2017) Dental implants in patients with osteoporosis: a systematic review with metaanalysis. *Int J Oral Maxillofac Surg*, June 23 (epub ahead of print).

Donos, N. and Calciolari, E. (2014) Dental implants in patients affected by systemic diseases. *Br Dent J*, **217**, 425–430.

Duyck, J. and Vandamme, K. (2014) The effect of loading on peri-implant bone: a critical review of the literature. *J Oral Rehabil*, **41**, 783–794.

Esposito, M., Worthington, H.V., Loli, V., Coulthard, P. and Grusovin, M.G. (2010) Interventions for replacing missing teeth: antibiotics at dental implant placement to prevent complications. *Cochrane Database Syst Rev*, **7**, CD004152.

Esposito, M., Grusovin, M.G., Maghaireh, H. and Worthington, H.V. (2013) Interventions for replacing missing teeth: different times for loading dental implants. *Cochrane Database Syst Rev*, **3**, CD003878.

Fuentealba, R. and Jofre, J. (2015) Esthetic failure in implant dentistry. *Dent Clin North Am*, **59**, 227–246.

Gay-Escoda, C., Perez-Alvarez, D., Camps-Font, O. and Figueiredo, R. (2016) Long-term outcomes of oral rehabilitation with dental implants in HIV-positive patients: a retrospective case series. *Med Oral Patol Oral Cir Bucal*, **21**, E385–391.

Gherlone, E.F., Cappare, P., Tecco, S. et al. (2016) A prospective longitudinal study on implant prosthetic rehabilitation in controlled HIV-positive patients with 1-year follow-up: the role of CD4+ level, smoking habits, and oral hygiene. *Clin Implant Dent Relat Res*, **18**, 955–964.

Gotfredsen, K., Wiskott, A. and Working, G. (2012) Consensus Report – Reconstructions on Implants. The Third EAO Consensus Conference 2012. *Clin Oral Implants Res*, **23** Suppl 6, 238–241.

Gracis, S., Michalakis, K., Vigolo, P., Vult von Steyern, P., Zwahlen, M. and Sailer, I. (2012) Internal vs. external connections for abutments/reconstructions: a systematic review. *Clin Oral Implants Res*, **23** Suppl 6, 202–216.

Greer, A.C., Hoyle, P.J., Vere, J.W. and Wragg, P.F. (2017) Mechanical complications associated with angled screw channel restorations. *Int J Prosthodont*, **30**, 258–259.

Hammerle, C.H., Chen, S.T. and Wilson, T.G. Jr. (2004) Consensus statements and recommended clinical procedures regarding the placement of implants in extraction sockets. *Int J Oral Maxillofac Implants*, **19** Suppl, 26–28.

Harris, D., Horner, K., Grondahl, K. et al. (2012) E.A.O. Guidelines for the Use of Diagnostic Imaging in Implant Dentistry 2011. A Consensus Workshop Organized by the European Association for Osseointegration at the Medical University of Warsaw. *Clin Oral Implants Res*, **23**, 1243–1253.

Hjalmarsson, L., Gheisarifar, M. and Jemt, T. (2016) A systematic review of survival of single implants as presented in longitudinal studies with a follow-up of at least 10 years. *Eur J Oral Implantol*, **9** Suppl 1, S155–162.

Hultin, M., Svensson, K.G. and Trulsson, M. (2012) Clinical advantages of computer-guided implant placement: a systematic review. *Clin Oral Implants Res*, **23** Suppl 6, 124–135.

Jemt, T. and Lekholm, U. (1993) Oral implant treatment in posterior partially edentulous jaws: a 5-year follow-up report. *Int J Oral Maxillofac Implants*, **8**, 635–640.

Jung, R.E., Zembic, A., Pjetursson, B.E., Zwahlen, M. and Thoma, D.S. (2012) Systematic review of the survival rate and the incidence of biological, technical, and aesthetic complications of single crowns on implants reported in longitudinal studies with a mean follow-up of 5 years. *Clin Oral Implants Res*, **23** Suppl 6, 2–21.

Keenan, J.R. and Veitz-Keenan, A. (2015) Antibiotic prophylaxis for dental implant placement? *Evid Based Dent*, **16**, 52–53.

Kim, Y., Oh, T.J., Misch, C.E. and Wang, H.L. (2005) Occlusal considerations in implant therapy: clinical guidelines with biomechanical rationale. *Clin Oral Implants Res*, **16**, 26–35.

Kinaia, B.M., Ambrosio, F., Resident, P. et al. (2017) Soft tissue changes around immediately placed implants: a systematic review and meta-analyses with at least

12 months follow up after functional loading. *J Periodontol*, **9**, 876–886.

Kovacs, A.F. (2001) Influence of chemotherapy on endosteal implant survival and success in oral cancer patients. *Int J Oral Maxillofac Surg*, **30**, 144–147.

Lang, N.P. and Lindhe, J. (2015) *Clinical Periodontology and Implant Dentistry*, Wiley-Blackwell, Oxford.

Lee, C.T., Chen, Y.W., Starr, J.R. and Chuang, S.K. (2016) Survival analysis of wide dental implant: systematic review and meta-analysis. *Clin Oral Implants Res*, **27**, 1251–1264.

Lemos, C.A., de Souza Batista, V.E., Almeida, D.A., Santiago Junior, J.F., Verri, F.R. and Pellizzer, E.P. (2016) Evaluation of cement-retained versus screw-retained implant-supported restorations for marginal bone loss: a systematic review and meta-analysis. *J Prosthet Dent*, **115**, 419–427.

Limeres Posse, J., Lopez Jimenez, J., Ruiz Villandiego, J.C. et al. (2016) Survival of dental implants in patients with down syndrome: a case series. *J Prosthet Dent*, **116**, 880–884.

Madrid, C. and Sanz, M. (2009) What influence do anticoagulants have on oral implant therapy? A systematic review. *Clin Oral Implants Res*, **20** Suppl 4, 96–106.

Manfredini, D., Bucci, M.B., Sabattini, V.B. and Lobbezoo, F. (2011) Bruxism: overview of current knowledge and suggestions for dental implants planning. *Cranio*, **29**, 304–312.

Monje, A., Aranda, L., Diaz, K.T. et al. (2016) Impact of maintenance therapy for the prevention of peri-implant diseases: a systematic review and meta-analysis. *J Dent Res*, **95**, 372–379.

Morton, D. and Pollini, A. (2017) Evolution of loading protocols in implant dentistry for partially dentate arches. *Periodontology 2000*, **73**, 152–177.

Nickles, K., Schacher, B., Ratka-Kruger, P., Krebs, M. and Eickholz, P. (2013) Long-term results after treatment of periodontitis in patients with Papillon–Lefevre syndrome: success and failure. *J Clin Periodontol*, **40**, 789–798.

Papaspyridakos, P., Chen, C.J., Singh, M., Weber, H.P. and Gallucci, G.O. (2012) Success criteria in implant dentistry: a systematic review. *J Dent Res*, **91**, 242–248.

Pjetursson, B.E. and Lang, N.P. (2008) Prosthetic treatment planning on the basis of scientific evidence. *J Oral Rehabil*, **35** Suppl 1, 72–79.

Pjetursson, B.E., Thoma, D., Jung, R., Zwahlen, M. and Zembic, A. (2012) A systematic review of the survival and complication rates of implant-supported fixed dental prostheses (FDPS) after a mean observation period of at least 5 years. *Clin Oral Implants Res*, **23** Suppl 6, 22–38.

Pjetursson, B.E., Asgeirsson, A.G., Zwahlen, M. and Sailer, I. (2014) Improvements in implant dentistry over the last decade: comparison of survival and complication rates in older and newer publications. *Int J Oral Maxillofac Implants*, **29** Suppl, 308–324.

Ramanauskaite, A., Juodzbalys, G. and Tozum, T.F. (2016) Apical/retrograde periimplantitis/implant periapical lesion: etiology, risk factors, and treatment options: a systematic review. *Implant Dent*, **25**, 684–697.

Reichart, P.A., Schmidt-Westhausen, A.M., Khongkhunthian, P. and Strietzel, F.P. (2016) Dental implants in patients with oral mucosal diseases – a systematic review. *J Oral Rehabil*, **43**, 388–399.

Renton, T., Woolcombe, S., Taylor, T. and Hill, C.M. (2013) Oral Surgery: Part 1. introduction and the management of the medically compromised patient. *Br Dent J*, **215**, 213–223.

Romeo, E. and Storelli, S. (2012) Systematic review of the survival rate and the biological, technical, and aesthetic complications of fixed dental prostheses with cantilevers on implants reported in longitudinal studies with a mean of 5 years follow-up. *Clin Oral Implants Res*, **23** Suppl 6, 39–49.

Salvi, G.E. and Bragger, U. (2009) Mechanical and technical risks in implant therapy. *Int J Oral Maxillofac Implants*, **24** Suppl, 69–85.

Sanz-Sanchez, I., Sanz-Martin, I., Figuero, E. and Sanz, M. (2015) Clinical efficacy of immediate implant loading protocols compared to conventional loading depending on the type of the restoration: a systematic review. *Clin Oral Implants Res*, **26**, 964–982.

Scheuber, S., Hicklin, S. and Bragger, U. (2012) Implants versus short-span fixed bridges: survival, complications, patients' benefits. a systematic review on economic aspects. *Clin Oral Implants Res*, **23** Suppl 6, 50–62.

Scully, C., Madrid, C. and Bagan, J. (2006) Dental endosseous implants in patients on bisphosphonate therapy. *Implant Dent*, **15**, 212–218.

Sheridan, R.A., Decker, A.M., Plonka, A.B. and Wang, H.L. (2016) The role of occlusion in implant therapy: a comprehensive updated review. *Implant Dent*, **25**, 829–838.

Sherif, S., Susarla, H.K., Kapos, T., Munoz, D., Chang, B.M. and Wright, R.F. (2014) A systematic review of screw- versus cement-retained implant-supported fixed restorations. *J Prosthodont*, **23**, 1–9.

Sousa, V., Mardas, N., Farias, B. et al. (2016) A systematic review of implant outcomes in treated periodontitis patients. *Clin Oral Implants Res*, **27**, 787–844.

Tecco, S., Grusovin, M.G., Sciara, S., Bova, F., Pantaleo, G. and Cappare, P. (2017) The association between three attitude-related indexes of oral hygiene and secondary implant failures: a retrospective longitudinal study. *Int J Dent Hyg*, July 11 (epub ahead of print).

van Assche, N., Vercruyssen, M., Coucke, W., Teughels, W., Jacobs, R. and Quirynen, M. (2012) Accuracy of computer-aided implant placement. *Clin Oral Implants Res*, **23** Suppl 6, 112–123.

Zhang, S., Wang, S. and Song, Y. (2017) Immediate loading for implant restoration compared with early or conventional loading: a meta-analysis. *J Craniomaxillofac Surg*, **45**, 793–803.

Zhao, D., Wu, Y., Xu, C. and Zhang, F. (2016) Immediate dental implant placement into infected vs. non-infected sockets: a meta-analysis. *Clin Oral Implants Res*, **27**, 1290–1296.

38

Partial Edentulism – Partial Denture Treatment

38.1 Introduction

Removable partial dentures (RPDs) are indicated for the replacement of missing teeth in partially dentate patients as temporary or definitive treatments (Davenport *et al.*, 2000a).

Removable partial dentures are simpler, quicker and cheaper than other fixed tooth replacement options such as bridges and implants and they can replace multiple anterior and/or posterior missing teeth at the same time. However, they are removable and may not be initially desirable for some patients, although there is some evidence showing they can possibly improve the patient's quality of life (Ali *et al.*, 2017; Ozhayat and Gotfredsen, 2012). Important factors influencing the patient's satisfaction with RPDs include age, number of replaced occluding teeth, replacement of anterior teeth and the nature of the opposing arch (de Kok *et al.*, 2017).

Removable partial dentures increase the level of plaque and incidence of gingivitis as well as the risk of development of caries, especially root caries (Preshaw *et al.*, 2011). Therefore RPDs require regular recalls and a strict periodontal maintenance programme and the patient must maintain a high standard of oral hygiene to achieve long-term success (Lynch, 2012).

38.2 Removable Partial Denture Types

Based on the type of material used for fabrication, RPDs can be classified as follows.

- Conventional acrylic dentures made of polymethylmethacrylate (PMMA) resin and high-impact acrylic dentures containing rubber-modified PMMA, glass and ultra-high molecular weight polyethylene (UHMWP) fibres (Rickman *et al.*, 2012a).
- Cobalt-chromium (Co-Cr) dentures which include a metal framework with acrylic saddles.
- Flexible dentures made of nylon such as Valplast, Sunflex, Lucitone dentures (Hill *et al.*, 2014).
- Hypoallergenic denture base resins such as MMA-free modified methacrylates (Pfeiffer and Rosenbauer, 2004).
- New composite dentures incorporating a composite polymer framework such as polyether-ether-ketone (PEEK) (Najeeb *et al.*, 2016).

Based on type of support, RPDs can be classified into tooth-borne, tissue (mucosa)-borne and tooth-tissue-borne groups.

38.2.1 Acrylic Dentures

Acrylic RPDs are cheaper, easier to construct and repair, and have better aesthetics compared to Co-Cr RPDs. However, they have lower strength, poorer thermal conductivity and are less retentive and less hygienic (cover more mucosa). If poorly designed, acrylic mucosa-borne RPDs can have detrimental effects on the soft tissues ('gum-stripping' dentures). To minimise the potential damage to periodontium, an acrylic RPD should be kept free of the marginal gingivae as much as possible, and where it contacts teeth, some tooth support can be obtained by bringing the acrylic resin on the tooth above the survey line (Walmsley, 2003).

Acrylic RPDs may be desirable as temporary or immediate dentures to allow healing of soft tissues, alterations to the remaining dentition prior to definitive treatment, and assessment of the patient's ability to wear removable dentures. They can also be useful where the remaining dentition has questionable prognosis and can be designed to accommodate the loss of any teeth with poor prognosis in the future.

38.2.2 Cobalt-Chromium RPDs

Cobalt-chromium RPDs are stronger, thinner, better heat conductors, more hygienic (less mucosal coverage) and more retentive than acrylic RPDs. However, they are more expensive, technique sensitive and time consuming and less aesthetic than acrylic dentures

Diseases and Conditions in Dentistry: An Evidence-Based Reference, First Edition. Keyvan Moharamzadeh.

Companion website: www.wiley.com/go/moharamzadeh/diseases

due to the presence of visible metal framework components.

Cobalt-chromium RPDs are considered to be the ideal definitive removable tooth replacement option. With careful planning, obtaining appropriate tooth and mucosa support, keeping gingival margins free when possible and a good maintenance programme, Co-Cr RPDs can be successful in the long term (Bergman *et al.*, 1995).

38.2.3 Flexible Dentures

Flexible RPDs have the advantages of light weight, improved aesthetics of clasps and patient acceptance. Flexible RPDs can be useful for patients with limited mouth opening as they can be easily placed and removed (Rickman *et al.*, 2012b). However, they have the following disadvantages.

- Mucosa borne and increased risk of gingival recession.
- Increased area of gingival coverage, plaque retention and risk of periodontal disease.
- Decreased balancing force due to increased flexibility.
- Increased risk of ridge resorption due to masticatory forces being directed on a limited area of the ridge due to elasticity of the denture base.
- Potential risk of abutment tooth movement due to clasp torqueing.

38.2.4 Hypoallergenic Dentures

Hypoallergenic denture base materials are indicated for patients with proven allergic reaction to components of conventional MMA-based RPDs. Patch testing can be used to identify the materials to which the patient is allergic. Hypoallergenic alternatives include Sinomer (modified methacrylate), Polyan (modified methacrylate), Promysan (enterephthalate-based) and Microbase (polyurethane-based) materials (Pfeiffer and Rosenbauer, 2004).

38.2.5 PEEK-based RPDs

Polyether-ether-ketone-based material is a strong, lightweight and metal-free material that can be converted to a RPD framework which is designed digitally and produced using CAD-CAM technology.

The main advantages include (Zoidis *et al.*, 2016):

- biocompatibility and suitable for patients with metal allergy
- improved aesthetics of the framework
- high strength to weight ratio
- elastic properties similar to human bone
- resistant to corrosion and low water absorption.

However, this is a new material with little evidence on its clinical performance as RPD framework material and there is a need for clinical studies to assess its long-term survival and complications in partially dentate patients.

38.3 Classification of Partially Dentate Arches

The most commonly used classification system for partially dentate arches is Kennedy's (1928) classification.

- Class I: bilateral posterior edentulous areas
- Class II: unilateral posterior edentulous area
- Class III: unilateral or bilateral edentulous area(s) bounded by remaining teeth
- Class IV: single edentulous area anterior to remaining teeth and crossing the midline

38.4 General Guidelines

Readers are strongly recommended to refer to the British Society for Prosthodontics guidelines (Ogden, 1996) on the standards for partial dentures in relation to the clinical practice and procedure of partial denture construction. Additional aspects of removable partial denture treatment are discussed in the following sections.

38.5 RPD Design

38.5.1 Surveying

It is important to survey the study models to identify a unique path of insertion for the denture, locate and measure the areas of undercut that can be used for retention and identify the need for any necessary modifications of oral and dental tissues (Davenport *et al.*, 2000c).

38.5.2 Occlusal Analysis

Preparation of articulated study models is useful to identify and correct any occlusal issues such as uneven occlusal plane and occlusal interferences prior to denture fabrication. Analysis of occlusion would also help to design the denture and place the rest seats and minor connectors in areas that would not interfere with occlusion.

38.5.3 Replacing Anterior Teeth

When replacing the anterior teeth with the RPD, it is essential to prepare an initial try-in of denture teeth on wax to establish the anterior extension of the metal framework prior to its fabrication to minimise the need for adjusting the extension of the metal framework at a later stage.

38.5.4 Milled Crowns

Abutment teeth with large restorations, tooth wear or undesirable crown angulation may be modified using indirect restorations such as milled crowns or onlays incorporating the features of the RPD, including appropriate guide planes, rest seats and bulbosity for creating undercuts suitable for engaging retentive clasps.

38.5.5 Components of RPD Design

The main features of RPD design include the following (Davenport *et al.*, 2000d, 2001a).

- Saddle areas to accommodate prosthetic teeth to replace the missing teeth.
- Support provided by rests on the abutment teeth and denture-bearing mucosa coverage.
- Direct retention provided by retentive clasps.
- Indirect retention to prevent occlusal displacement of the distal extension bases.
- Bracing to resist against horizontal displacing forces on the saddles.
- Reciprocation to provide resistance against retentive forces.
- Connectors, including major and minor connectors.

38.5.6 Saddle Areas

Saddle areas are often relieved with wax to provide space for an acrylic base under the metal framework.

Some important considerations in free end saddle areas include the following.

- Using an RPI system (mesial rest, distal proximal plate and an I-bar) to reduce torque forces on distal abutment teeth (Davenport *et al.*, 2001b).
- Using an altered cast impression technique to improve tissue support and reduce sinking of the saddles into the soft tissues (Sajjan, 2010).
- Reducing the size of the occlusal table to reduce the pressure to the underlying ridge.

38.5.7 Rests

Different types of rests can be used, such as conventional occlusal rest, cingulum ball, cingulum ledge and incisal ledge (Davenport *et al.*, 2001e). The cingulum can be raised with adhesive composite restoration if necessary or the rest seat can be incorporated into an indirect restoration. Rest seat with ring design has been used as an alternative approach for a severely tilted distal molar abutment allowing the use of existing occlusal contact and avoiding an overcontoured clasp design (Al-Helal *et al.*, 2017).

38.5.8 Retentive Clasps

Retentive clasps can be in the form of occlusally approaching or gingivally approaching clasps made of cast alloy or wrought wire which is soldered or laser welded to the framework (Davenport *et al.*, 2000b, 2001b).

If there are no natural undercuts on the potential abutment teeth, artificial undercuts can be created by adhesive composite additions.

38.5.9 Indirect Retainer

In Kennedy class I and class II arches without anterior modifications, indirect retention can be provided by a rest placed on a tooth anterior to the fulcrum line on the side opposite the extension base.

In Kennedy class IV arches, indirect retention can be provided by posterior extension of the framework and rests on the posterior teeth (Davenport *et al.*, 2001d).

38.5.10 Mandibular Major Connectors

Different types of mandibular major connectors include the following (Davenport *et al.*, 2001c).

- A lingual bar should be approximately 4 mm in height with the superior border at least 3 mm from free gingival margins. The bar is half pear shaped in cross-section with the thickest part along the inferior border.
- A sublingual bar can be used when the lingual sulcus is shallow and the bar can be kept away from the gingival margins as it is oriented more horizontally compared to a lingual bar.
- A dental bar can be used when there is inadequate sulcus depth for a lingual or sublingual bar and the clinical crowns of the anterior teeth are long enough to accommodate a bar on the lingual surface above the cingulum.
- A lingual plate can be used when the distance from the free gingival margin to the floor of the mouth is less than 7 mm or when the anterior teeth have questionable prognosis so if they are extracted, prosthetic teeth can be added onto the denture in the future. The superior border of the plate is placed at the junction of the incisal and middle third of the teeth. As this type of connector covers the gingival margins, it is very important to maintain a high standard of plaque control.
- A labial bar can be used when there is severe lingual inclination of the teeth that would not allow the use of other types of connectors.

38.5.11 Maxillary Major Connectors

Different types of maxillary major connectors are listed below (Davenport *et al.*, 2001c).

- A palatal strap is used mainly in Kennedy class III arches and the width of strap varies depending on the clinical situation.
- A modified palatal plate can be used to connect multiple saddle areas. The anterior border can be extended short of the rugae region with a minimum distance of 6 mm from the gingival margins. The posterior part of the plate can be combined with an acrylic resin extension to enable adjustment of the post dam.
- A palatal ring connector can be used when the maxillary torus restricts the use of a palatal plate, provided there is a minimum of 5 mm distance between the posterior aspect of the torus and the vibrating line.
- A horse-shoe connector can be used in patients with a strong gag reflex. If coverage of the gingival margin is unavoidable, there should be a close contact without any relief between the connector and gingival margin to avoid gingival proliferation.

38.5.12 Minor Connectors

The junction between a minor connector and rest must be at least 1.5 mm thick and placed interproximally if possible. The minor connector should join the major connector at a right angle. The minor connector should be located at least 5 mm from the other vertical components of the metal framework.

38.6 Swing-Lock RPD

The swing-lock design RPD includes a labial bar with retentive struts, hinged at one end and locked with a latch at the other end, together with a reciprocating lingual plate to gain maximum retention and stability (Lynch and Allen, 2004).

It can be used in the following situations.

- Maxillofacial defects and reduced bone support (McKenna *et al.*, 2013; Razaq *et al.*, 2012).
- Missing posterior teeth and remaining anterior teeth, especially if the teeth have marked recession; the aesthetics can be improved by adding an acrylic labial facing to the RPD to cover the recession areas.
- Unfavourable undercuts on terminal abutments and unilateral abutments.

The swing-lock design is contraindicated in patients with poor plaque control, poor manual dexterity, soft tissue limitations (such as shallow sulcus), aesthetic issues, high smile line, severe class II division II with deep bite, and alveolar ridge limitations (such as prominent buccal ridge) (Chan *et al.*, 1998).

It is important to perform an initial trial with labial wax rim to check the sulcus depth and patient compliance.

Clinical studies have shown good patient acceptance and minimal periodontal complications but the remaining teeth may develop caries (Schulte and Smith, 1980). Therefore, prevention, oral hygiene, diet and fluoride are important aspects of swing-lock design RPD maintenance.

Case Study

A 56-year-old male patient referred by his GDP presented with lost multiple posterior teeth and worn remaining anterior teeth. The patient had a strong gag reflex and could not tolerate a previous plastic denture with a palatal coverage.

The patient reported a positive history of parafunctional habits, such as bruxism.

There were no relevant dietary factors or any history of gastrointestinal disease or vomiting.

The patient used a normal toothbrush and toothpaste to brush his teeth. He was a non-smoker and medically fit and well.

Clinical examination showed that the temporomandibular joints (TMJ) and soft tissues were normal. Periodontal examination showed healthy periodontal tissues. Examination of occlusion showed reduced occlusal vertical dimension and corresponding wear facets on the remaining anterior teeth in protrusion and lateral excursive movements.

The patient's preoperative clinical photographs are shown in Figure 38.1.

Sensibility testing with an electric pulp tester showed positive response from all the remaining teeth.

Based on the above findings, the following diagnosis was made: moderate tooth wear mainly due to attrition in a partially dentate patient.

The prognosis for restoration of the worn teeth with direct adhesive composite restorative material was good as there was plenty of enamel present for bonding. The prognosis for the RPD was favourable due to the presence of both distal molar abutment teeth in the maxillary arch and one bounded saddle area in the mandibular arch.

The treatment procedures are listed below.

1) Impressions, initial bite registration (using wax blocks) and preparation of articulated study models.
2) Diagnostic wax-up of worn maxillary and mandibular remaining teeth to an ideal shape at an increased vertical dimension (by 2 mm).
3) Intraoral trial of the wax-up.

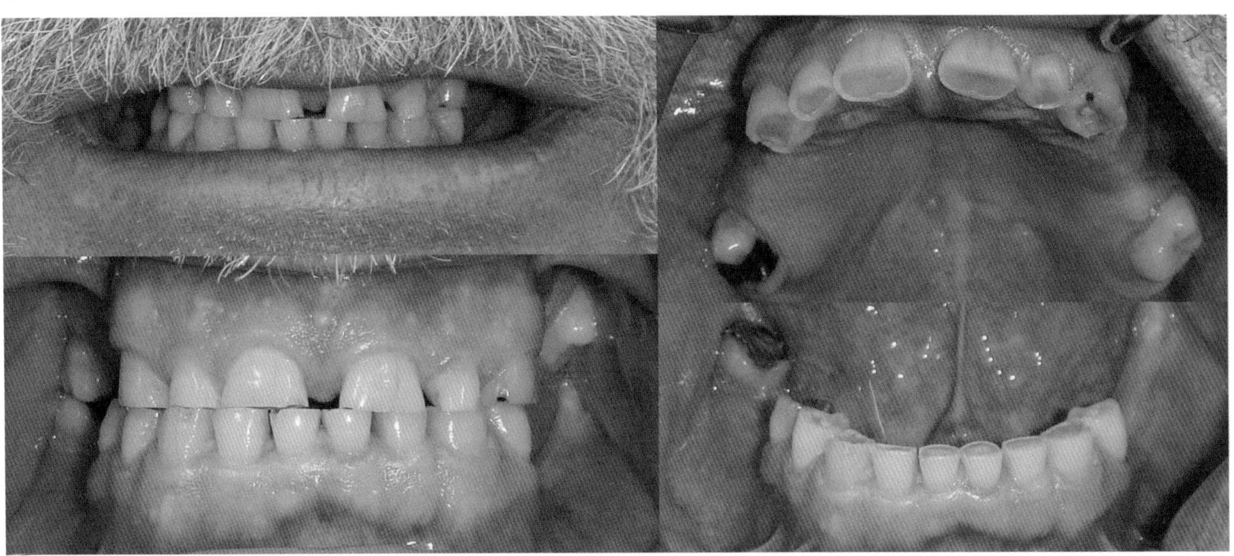

Figure 38.1 Preoperative clinical photographs showing partially dentate maxillary arch (Kennedy class III, modification I) and mandibular arch (Kennedy class II, modification I) as well as moderate tooth surface loss on the remaining anterior teeth.

4) Composite build-up (Figure 38.2) of worn teeth using a guide stent made over the diagnostic wax-up.
5) Primary impressions of the restored teeth and preparation of new study models.
6) Surveying of the study models using a surveyor.
7) New bite registration and preparation of articulated study models to enable RPD design.
8) Preparation of rest seats, adjusting and border moulding of special trays and secondary impression using regular-viscosity additional silicone impression material.
9) Fabrication and try-in of Co-Cr metal framework (Figure 38.3).

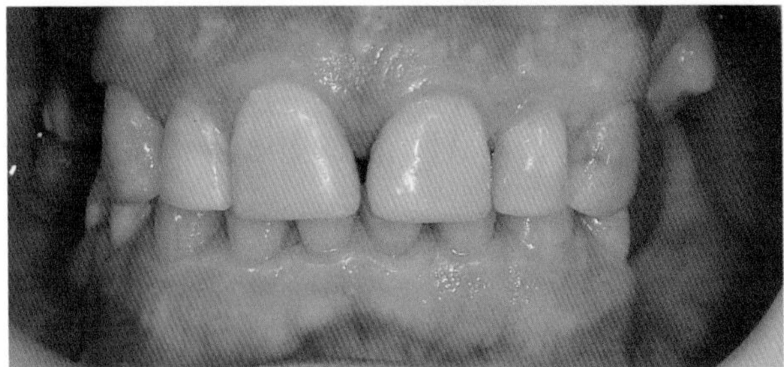

Figure 38.2 Clinical photographs of the restored worn teeth with direct adhesive composite resin.

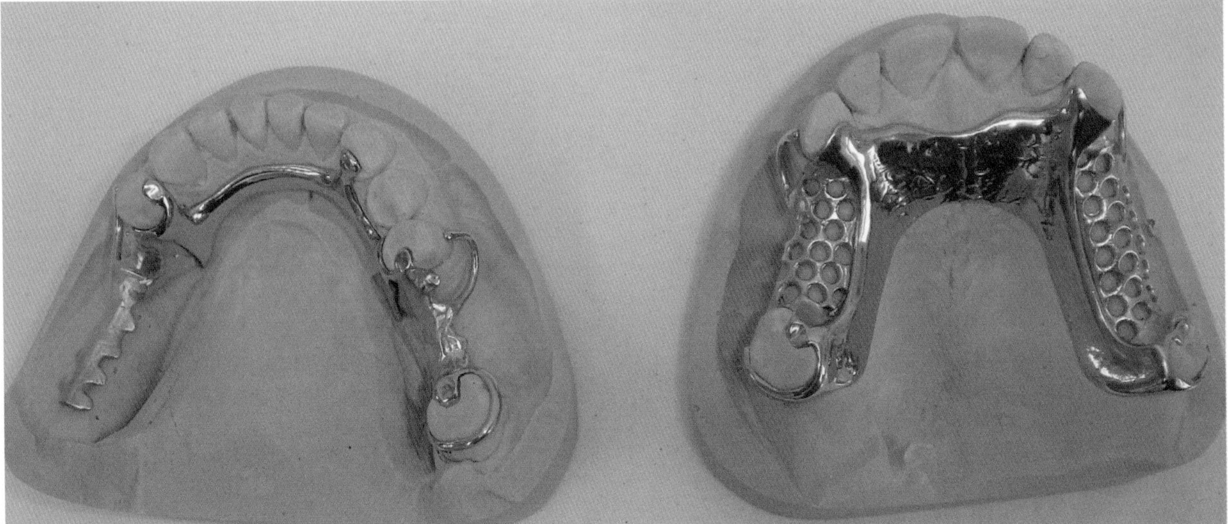

Figure 38.3 Co-Cr metal frameworks on the stone models showing a maxillary horse-shoe palatal connector without covering the gingival margins of the incisor teeth, ring clasps on the molar teeth, gingivally approaching clasps on the anterior abutment teeth, mandibular lingual bar connector, an RPI system in the left mandibular free-end saddle area and an indirect retainer cingulum rest on LR3.

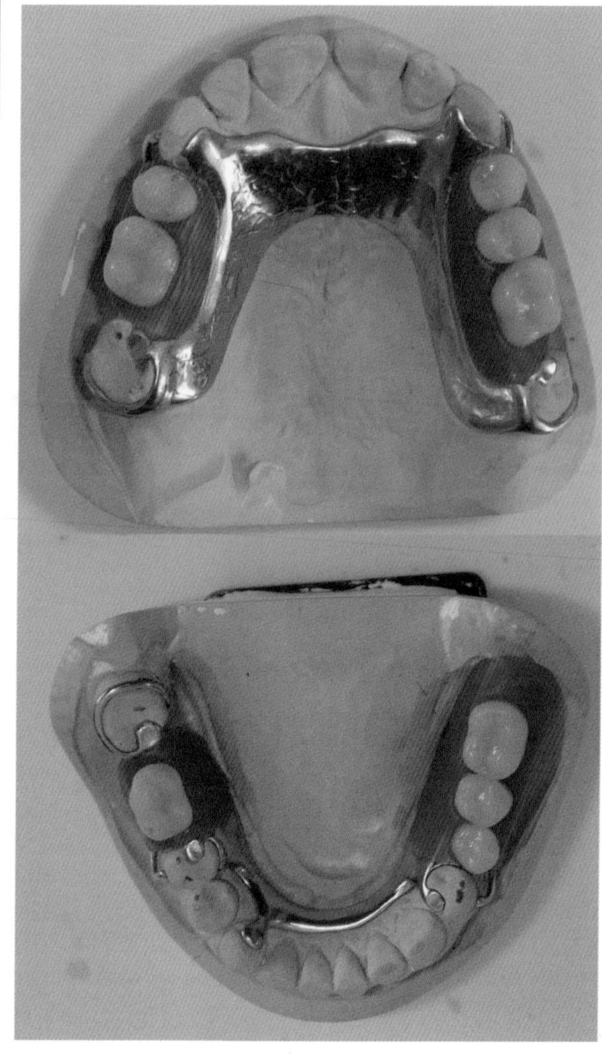

Figure 38.4 Photograph of the teeth on wax on metal framework fitted into the stone models.

10) Confirmation of bite registration with wax blocks on metal framework and shade selection.
11) Trial insertion of teeth on wax on framework (Figure 38.4).
12) Final insertion of RPDs as shown in the postoperative clinical photographs (Figure 38.5).
13) Review.

The patient was able to tolerate the horse-shoe palatal connector and was very satisfied with the outcome of treatment. He was discharged back to his GDP for long-term maintenance.

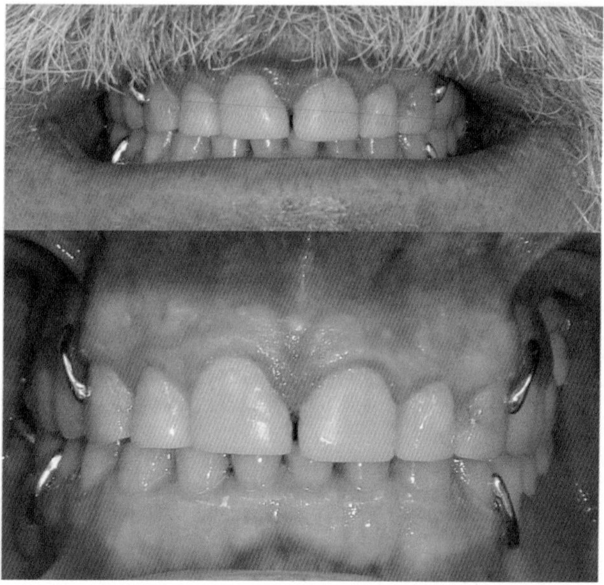

Figure 38.5 Postoperative clinical photographs.

References

Al-Helal, A., Kattadiyil, M.T. and Jekki, B. (2017) Ring rest seat design for severely tilted molar abutment tooth: an alternative option. *J Prosthodont*, **26**, 327–330.

Ali, Z., Baker, S., Barabari, P. and Martin, N. (2017) Efficacy of removable partial denture treatment: a retrospective oral health-related quality of life evaluation. *Eur J Prosthodont Restor Dent*, **25**, 101–107.

Bergman, B., Hugoson, A. and Olsson, C.O. (1995) A 25 year longitudinal study of patients treated with removable partial dentures. *J Oral Rehabil*, **22**, 595–599.

Chan, M.F., Adams, D. and Brudvik, J.S. (1998) The swing-lock removable partial denture in clinical practice. *Dent Update*, **25**, 80–84.

Davenport, J.C., Basker, R.M., Heath, J.R., Ralph, J.P. and Glantz, P.O. (2000a) Removable partial dentures. 1. Need and demand for treatment. *Br Dent J*, **189**, 364–368.

Davenport, J.C., Basker, R.M., Heath, J.R., Ralph, J.P. and Glantz, P.O. (2000b) Retention. *Br Dent J*, **189**, 646–657.

Davenport, J.C., Basker, R.M., Heath, J.R., Ralph, J.P. and Glantz, P.O. (2000c) Surveying. *Br Dent J*, **189**, 532–542.

Davenport, J.C., Basker, R.M., Heath, J.R., Ralph, J.P. and Glantz, P.O. (2000d) A system of design. *Br Dent J*, **189**, 586–590.

Davenport, J.C., Basker, R.M., Heath, J.R., Ralph, J.P., Glantz, P.O. and Hammond, P. (2001a) Bracing And reciprocation. *Br Dent J*, **190**, 10–14.

Davenport, J.C., Basker, R.M., Heath, J.R., Ralph, J.P., Glantz, P.O. and Hammond, P. (2001b) Clasp design. *Br Dent J*, **190**, 71–81.

Davenport, J.C., Basker, R.M., Heath, J.R., Ralph, J.P., Glantz, P.O. and Hammond, P. (2001c) Connectors. *Br Dent J*, **190**, 184–191.

Davenport, J.C., Basker, R.M., Heath, J.R., Ralph, J.P., Glantz, P.O. and Hammond, P. (2001d) Indirect retention. *Br Dent J*, **190**, 128–q32.

Davenport, J.C., Basker, R.M., Heath, J.R., Ralph, J.P., Glantz, P.O. and Hammond, P. (2001e) Tooth preparation. *Br Dent J*, **190**, 288–294.

De Kok, I.J., Cooper, L.F., Guckes, A.D. *et al.* (2017) Factors influencing removable partial denture patient-reported outcomes of quality of life and satisfaction: a systematic review. *J Prosthodont*, **26**, 5–18.

Hill, E.E., Rubel, B. and Smith, J.B. (2014) Flexible removable partial dentures: a basic overview. *Gen Dent*, **62**, 32–36.

Kennedy, E. (1928) Partial denture construction. *Dent Items Interest*, **1**, 3–8.

Lynch, C.D. (2012) Successful removable partial dentures. *Dent Update*, **39**, 118–120, 122–126.

Lynch, C.D. and Allen, P.F. (2004) The swing-lock denture: its use in conventional removable partial denture prosthodontics. *Dent Update*, **31**, 506–508.

Mckenna, G., Ziada, H. and Allen, P.F. (2013) Prosthodontic rehabilitation of a patient using a swing-lock lower denture after segmental mandibulectomy. *Eur J Prosthodont Restor Dent*, **21**, 141–144.

Najeeb, S., Zafar, M.S., Khurshid, Z. and Siddiqui, F. (2016) Applications of polyetheretherketone (PEEK) in oral implantology and prosthodontics. *J Prosthodont Res*, **60**, 12–19.

Ogden, A. (1996) *Guidelines in Prosthetic and Implant Dentistry*, British Society for the Study of Prosthetic Dentistry, Liverpool.

Ozhayat, E.B. and Gotfredsen, K. (2012) Effect of treatment with fixed and removable dental prostheses. an oral health-related quality of life study. *J Oral Rehabil*, **39**, 28–36.

Pfeiffer, P. and Rosenbauer, E.U. (2004) Residual methyl methacrylate monomer, water sorption, and water solubility of hypoallergenic denture base materials. *J Prosthet Dent*, **92**, 72–78.

Preshaw, P.M., Walls, A.W., Jakubovics, N.S., Moynihan, P.J., Jepson, N.J. and Loewy, Z. (2011) Association of removable partial denture use with oral and systemic health. *J Dent*, **39**, 711–719.

Razaq, I., Durey, K. and Nattress, B. (2012) Provision of a swing lock denture for a patient with Gorlin Goltz syndrome. *Eur J Prosthodont Restor Dent*, **20**, 141–144.

Rickman, L.J., Padipatvuthikul, P. and Satterthwaite, J.D. (2012a) Contemporary denture base resins: part 1. *Dent Update*, **39**, 25–28, 30.

Rickman, L.J., Padipatvuthikul, P. and Satterthwaite, J.D. (2012b) Contemporary denture base resins: part 2. *Dent Update*, **39**, 176–178, 180–182, 184 passim.

Sajjan, C. (2010) An altered cast procedure to improve tissue support for removable partial denture. *Contemp Clin Dent*, **1**, 103–106.

Schulte, J.K. and Smith, D.E. (1980) Clinical evaluation of swinglock removable partial dentures. *J Prosthet Dent*, **44**, 595–603.

Walmsley, A.D. (2003) Acrylic partial dentures. *Dent Update*, **30**, 424–429.

Zoidis, P., Papathanasiou, I. and Polyzois, G. (2016) The use of a modified poly-ether-ether-ketone (PEEK) as an alternative framework material for removable dental prostheses. A clinical report. *J Prosthodont*, **25**, 580–584.

39

Perforation

39.1 Definition

Perforation is defined as abnormal communication between the pulp space and the periradicular tissues.

39.2 Causes

Perforations can be iatrogenic or pathological (Saed *et al.*, 2016). Iatrogenic perforations are caused by:

- excessive removal of coronal dentine during access cavity preparation and searching for canals
- incorrect endodontic instrumentation and aggressive canal enlargement
- zipping and transportation in curved canals (Schafer and Dammaschke, 2009)
- careless preparation of post space.

Pathological perforations can be due to:

- external root resorption (see Chapter 17)
- internal root resorption (see Chapter 26)
- extensive caries (see Chapter 5).

39.3 Pathogenesis

Perforation causes damage to periodontal tissues which results in inflammation, loss of periodontal fibre attachment, resorption of bone and replacement with granulation tissue. In coronal perforations near the crestal bone, epithelial proliferation may ultimately result in the development of a periodontal pocket (Seltzer *et al.*, 1970).

39.4 Epidemiology

The reported incidence of perforations is between 3% and 10% (Fuss and Trope, 1996). Post space preparation accounts for 53% of iatrogenic perforations and 47% are caused during endodontic treatment.

Perforations in maxillary anterior teeth are more likely to occur at the labial aspect of the root due to the palatal inclination of the root. Perforations in multirooted teeth can occur in furcation area during access cavity preparation (Kvinnsland *et al.*, 1989).

39.5 Classification

Perforations have been classified based on their site into gingival sulcus, supracrestal, equicrestal, subcrestal, furcation, coronal third of the root, midroot and apical perforations (Tsesis and Fuss, 2006).

39.6 Diagnosis

Clinical features of perforations are listed below.

- Profuse bleeding from iatrogenic perforations.
- Fresh blood on paper points inserted into the canal.
- Apex locator showing zero reading at the site of perforation.
- Visible perforated area when assessed using microscope magnification.
- Deep periodontal pockets may be present in some cases of pre-existing perforations.

Radiographs with different angulations may confirm the presence of perforations and reveal any associated periradicular radiolucency in cases of pre-existing and pathological perforations.

Cone beam computed tomography (CBCT) produces a three-dimensional image of perforation and can be extremely useful in determining the extent of pathological perforations which are often not clinically visible (Khojastepour *et al.*, 2015).

Diseases and Conditions in Dentistry: An Evidence-Based Reference, First Edition. Keyvan Moharamzadeh.

Companion website: www.wiley.com/go/moharamzadeh/diseases

39.7 Prognosis

The prognosis of teeth with perforation depends on a number of factors (Alhadainy, 1994).

- *Location of perforation*: the prognosis of perforations in the cervical part of the root and in furcation areas is poorer compared to other sites due to their proximity to the gingival junctional epithelium and increased risk of epithelial attachment loss, formation of periodontal defects and contamination of perforation (Sinai, 1977).
- *Size of perforation*: small perforations have better prognosis as they are often associated with less severe damage to periodontal tissues and are easier to seal compared to large perforations (Tsesis and Fuss, 2006).
- *Time lapse between perforation and repair*: immediately repaired sterile and sealed perforations have better prognosis than old and infected perforations (Tsesis and Fuss, 2006).
- *Biocompatibility and sealing ability of material used to repair the perforation*: the use of mineral trioxide aggregate (MTA) and Biodentine has been shown to result in favourable histopathological outcome for repair of perforations (Silva *et al.*, 2017). MTA is composed of tricalcium silicate, tricalcium aluminate, tricalcium oxide, silicate oxide, mineral oxide and bismuth oxide. It has shown a higher percentage of complete sealing and greater amount of newly formed mineralised tissue compared to other materials (Ford *et al.*, 1995; Silva *et al.*, 2017; Torabinejad and Parirokh, 2010). Its main disadvantages include long setting time, washout and potential coronal discolouration (Felman and Parashos, 2013).

39.8 Management

Management options for perforated teeth include extraction, non-surgical treatment and surgical treatment (Roda, 2001).

39.8.1 Extraction

Extractions are indicated for non-restorable teeth, and in situations where it is impossible to access and repair the perforation or complete the root canal treatment, such as large pathological perforations and sclerotic canals. Successful intentional reimplantation of extracted perforated teeth following extraoral repair of perforation has been reported (Poi *et al.*, 1999).

39.8.2 Non-Surgical Treatment

The aim of non-surgical treatment is to repair and seal the perforation defect, complete chemomechanical debridement and obturation of the root canal(s) and re-establish healthy periodontal tissues.

Fresh perforations are best repaired immediately to prevent contamination of the perforated area. Gingival sulcus and supracrestal perforations can be restored with glass ionomer cement with good prognosis. Subcrestal, furcation, midroot and apical perforations are best sealed using MTA or Biodentine.

Immediate repair of perforation enables completion of root canal treatment without the risk of agitating the perforated area with endodontic instruments, controls haemostasis and minimises the risk of extrusion of toxic irrigants through the perforation.

Subsequent root canal treatment can be initiated after MTA has set or immediately after the repair of perforation if MTA is protected with a layer of restorative material or if Biodentine has been used. It is important to maintain the patency of the root canal during the repair procedure. In cases of sterile perforations, normal saline solution can be used to irrigate the perforated area. Haemostasis can be achieved using collagen- or cellulose-based membranes, calcium sulfate or calcium hydroxide.

Pre-existing and infected perforations may require removal of any restorative materials or hyperplastic/granulation tissue from within the perforation, further enlargement using burs and ultrasonic tips under microscope magnification (Arens and Torabinejad, 1996), and careful debridement of the perforated area prior to repair. The author recommends gentle application of a small micro-brush or paper points soaked in 2.5% sodium hypochlorite solution with dabbing action on the margins of the perforation followed by thorough irrigation of the perforated area using normal saline solution.

In cases where there is a large bone cavity around the perforation, barrier membranes and matrices can be used to facilitate placement and condensation of MTA, although it has been shown that MTA can be successfully used alone in these situations without barrier membrane (Al-Daafas and Al-Nazhan, 2007).

39.8.3 Surgical Treatment

Root perforations can be repaired externally using a surgical approach by elevating a full-thickness mucoperiosteal flap, preparing and cleaning the defect and placement of appropriate repair material (Figure 39.1).

Surgical management is indicated when non-surgical treatment is not possible due to the nature, location or

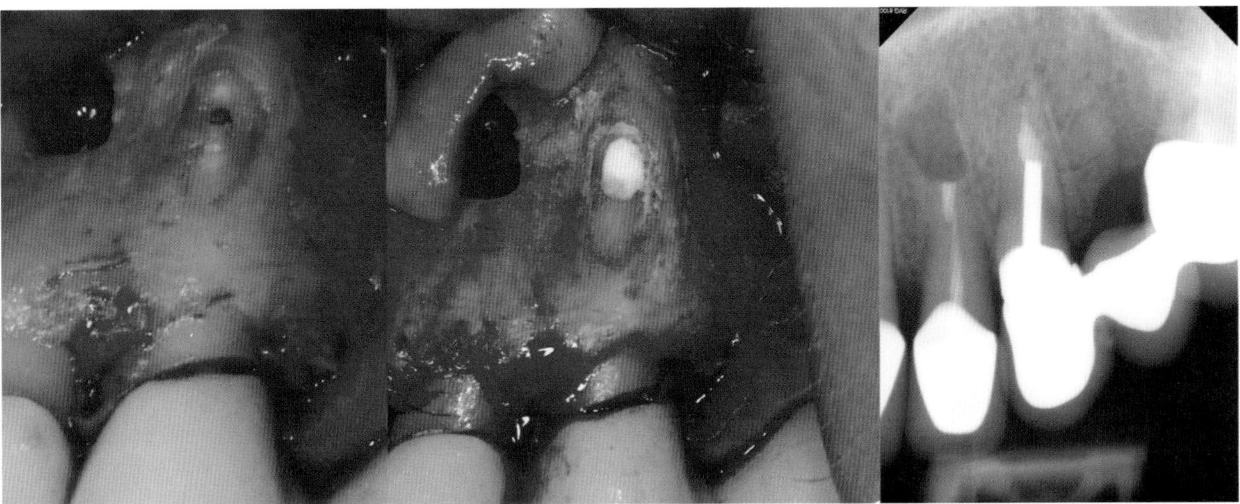

Figure 39.1 Surgical management of a dual pathology: root perforation of UL3 (bridge abutment), which had been caused by post space preparation, and chronic apical periodontitis of UL2 which had not responded to non-surgical endodontic retreatment. A full-thickness mucoperiosteal flap was raised in the UL1–UL4 region. Perforation on the labial aspect of the UL3 root was identified and repaired externally with MTA. A periapical lesion of UL2 was removed, root end resected and prepared with ultrasonic tips, and MTA retrograde filling was placed under microscopic magnification.

size of the perforation or problems with gaining internal access. Surgery can also be attempted if the tooth does not respond to non-surgical treatment or when surgical periodontal treatment is required to manage an associated periodontal defect (Regan *et al.*, 2005; Saed *et al.*, 2016).

Orthodontic extrusion or crown-lengthening surgery may be helpful in moving a subcrestal perforation above the alveolar crest.

Apical root perforations are often difficult to repair non-surgically. Periapical surgery offers an alternative solution in these situations.

In cases of furcation perforation where non-surgical treatment has failed, surgical tooth hemi-section, root resection or root separation (bicuspidisation) can be considered.

It is important to remember that freshly mixed MTA can washed out if there is a large bone defect around the repair site or when there is significant communication between the oral cavity and MTA through a periodontal defect. To solve this problem, MTA can be used to repair a perforation in conjunction with regenerative surgical periodontal approaches using bone graft materials to fill the associated osseous defects (Azim *et al.*, 2014; White and Bryant, 2002). Alternatively, a fast-setting equivalent material such as Biodentine can be used in combination with resective periodontal surgery.

39.9 Treatment Outcomes

A systematic review of 17 studies and meta-analysis of 12 studies showed an overall estimated success rate of 72.5% for non-surgical repair of root perforations. The use of MTA increased the success rate to 80.9%, although the difference was not statistically significant. The presence of pre-existing radiolucency around the perforation site was associated with a lower chance of success after treatment. Maxillary teeth demonstrated a significantly higher success rate than mandibular teeth (Siew *et al.*, 2015).

Case Study

A 46-year-old female patient was referred by an undergraduate dental student for endodontic retreatment of UL2 and UL3. The patient complained of persistent pain and swelling following the initial root canal treatment.

The patient was a non-smoker and had a clear medical history.

Clinical examination showed presence of a sinus tract on the labial aspect of the attached gingivae between UL2 and UL3. Both teeth were tender to percussion. There were no deep periodontal pockets and the teeth were not mobile.

Radiographic examination of the teeth with an inserted gutta percha (GP) cone in the sinus tract (Figure 39.2)

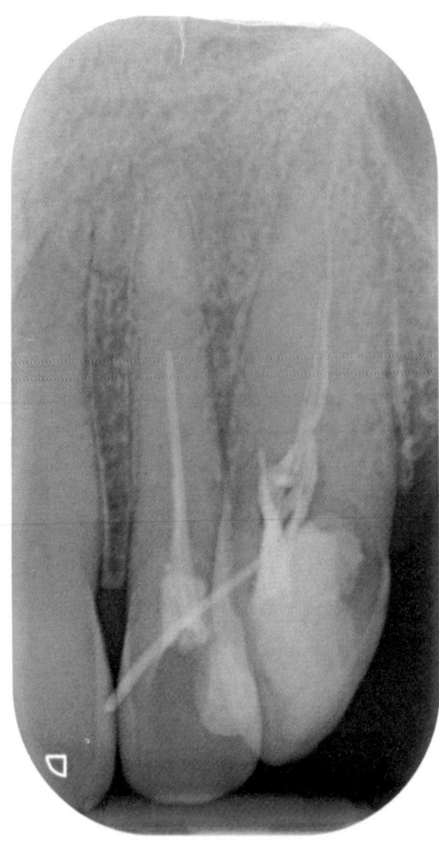

Figure 39.2 Preoperative periapical radiograph showing poor obturation of the root-filling material on UL2 and UL3 and the GP cone tracing to a potential cervical root perforation on UL3.

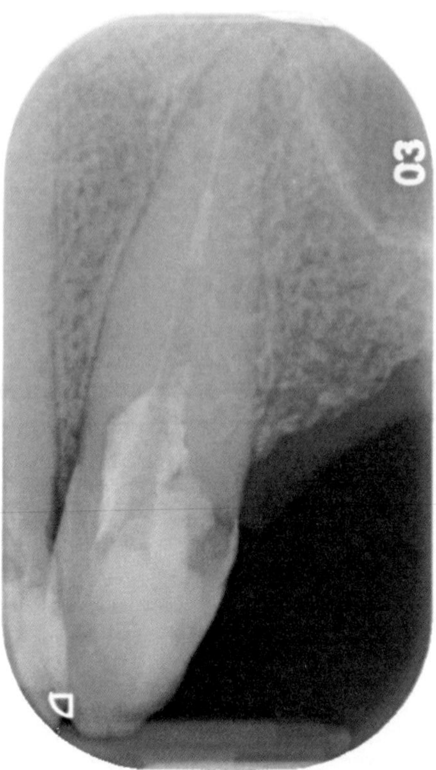

Figure 39.3 Periapical radiograph of UL3 following repair of the perforation with MTA.

showed poorly obturated and underextended root fillings of UL2 and UL3 and the GP traced to the cervical part of the UL3 root at crestal level, indicating a potential perforation.

The diagnoses were:

- poor-quality root filling of UL3 with suspected perforation, sinus tract and apical periodontitis
- chronic apical periodontitis of UL2 with underextended root filling.

Factors affecting the prognosis of treatment were:

- location and size of perforation
- presence of infection at the site of perforation
- absence of periodontal defect or pocketing
- root length was good in case of any potential future bone loss
- quality of the existing root canal filling that can be improved
- possible canal blockage at the apical part of the UL2.

The chosen treatment strategy was non-surgical exploration of UL3, attempting to repair any pre-existing perforation, and endodontic retreatment of UL3 and UL2.

The following treatment was provided.

1) Local anesthesia.
2) Rubber dam isolation.
3) Access cavity preparation on both UL2 and UL3 and exploration under operating microscope magnification.
4) Removal of the loose and poorly condensed GP from the pulp chamber and root canals using rotary retreatment files.
5) Identification of a large perforation defect on the mesiobuccal aspect of UL3 at the cervical region extending from the cementoenamel junction to the root below at subcrestal level.
6) Initial debridement and irrigation of the perforated area with normal saline solution.
7) Refining the edges of the perforation with an ultrasonic tip and removing a small amount of infected dentine.
8) Gentle application of a small micro-brush soaked with 2.5% sodium hypochlorite to the edges of the perforation.

9) Further irrigation with normal saline solution until haemostasis was achieved.
10) Repair of the perforation with MTA. A GP cone was placed in the root canal to maintain its patency and MTA was mixed and packed into the defect.
11) Non-setting calcium hydroxide was placed in the apical part of the canal and a paper point soaked in saline solution was placed in the coronal part of the canal near the MTA. The access cavity was then sealed with GIC (Figure 39.3).
12) At a subsequent visit, complete setting of MTA was confirmed, working length (WL) was determined using an apex locator, and the root canal was cleaned and shaped to the WL using ProTaper files and obturated with Thermafil (Figure 39.4).
13) Endodontic retreatment of UL2 was also completed, the root canal was successfully negotiated to its full length, cleaned, shaped and obturated.
14) Coronal seal was provided.

At the 9-month follow-up visit, the patient remained asymptomatic and the sinus tract had resolved. The teeth were not tender to percussion and there were no deep periodontal pockets. Periapical radiograph (Figure 39.5) showed absence of any obvious periapical or periodontal pathology which indicated a successful outcome of non-surgical treatment.

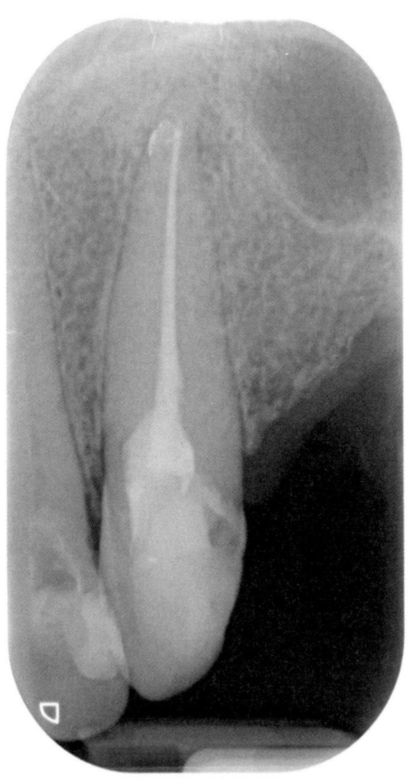

Figure 39.4 Immediate postoperative periapical radiograph of UL3 following obturation.

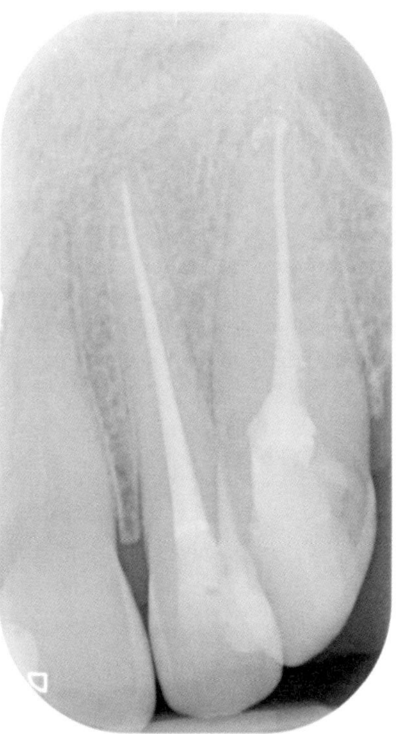

Figure 39.5 Follow-up periapical radiograph at 9 months showing improved quality of obturation on both UL2 and UL3 and evidence of periapical and periodontal healing.

References

Al-Daafas, A. and Al-Nazhan, S. (2007) Histological evaluation of contaminated furcal perforation in dogs' teeth repaired by MTA with or without internal matrix. *Oral Surg Oral Med Oral Pathol Oral Radiol Endod*, **103**, E92–99.

Alhadainy, H.A. (1994) Root perforations. A review of literature. *Oral Surg Oral Med Oral Pathol*, **78**, 368–374.

Arens, D.E. and Torabinejad, M. (1996) Repair of furcal perforations with mineral trioxide aggregate: two case reports. *Oral Surg Oral Med Oral Pathol Oral Radiol Endod*, **82**, 84–88.

Azim, A.A., Lloyd, A. and Huang, G.T. (2014) Management of longstanding furcation perforation using a novel approach. *J Endod*, **40**, 1255–1259.

Felman, D. and Parashos, P. (2013) Coronal tooth discoloration and white mineral trioxide aggregate. *J Endod*, **39**, 484–487.

Ford, T.R., Torabinejad, M., McKendry, D.J., Hong, C.U. and Kariyawasam, S.P. (1995) Use of mineral trioxide aggregate for repair of furcal perforations. *Oral Surg Oral Med Oral Pathol Oral Radiol Endod*, **79**, 756–763.

Fuss, Z. and Trope, M. (1996) Root perforations: classification and treatment choices based on prognostic factors. *Endod Dent Traumatol*, **12**, 255–264.

Khojastepour, L., Moazami, F., Babaei, M. and Forghani, M. (2015) Assessment of root perforation within simulated internal resorption cavities using cone-beam computed tomography. *J Endod*, **41**, 1520–1523.

Kvinnsland, I., Oswald, R.J., Halse, A. and Gronningsaeter, A.G. (1989) A clinical and roentgenological study of 55 cases of root perforation. *Int Endod J*, **22**, 75–84.

Poi, W.R., Sonoda, C.K., Salineiro, S.L. and Martin, S.C. (1999) Treatment of root perforation by intentional reimplantation: a case report. *Endod Dent Traumatol*, **15**, 132–134.

Regan, J.D., Witherspoon, D.E. and Foyle, D.M. (2005) Surgical repair of root and tooth perforations. *Endod Topics*, **11**, 152–178.

Roda, R.S. (2001) Root perforation repair: surgical and nonsurgical management. *Pract Proced Aesthet Dent*, **13**, 467–472; quiz 474.

Saed, S.M., Ashley, M.P. and Darcey, J. (2016) Root perforations: aetiology, management strategies and outcomes. The hole truth. *Br Dent J*, **220**, 171–180.

Schafer, E. and Dammaschke, T. (2009) Development and sequelae of canal transportation. *Endod Topics*, **15**, 75–90.

Seltzer, S., Sinai, I. and August, D. (1970) Periodontal effects of root perforations before and during endodontic procedures. *J Dent Res*, **49**, 332–339.

Siew, K., Lee, A.H. and Cheung, G.S. (2015) Treatment outcome of repaired root perforation: a systematic review and meta-analysis. *J Endod*, **41**, 1795–1804.

Silva, L.A.B., Pieroni, K., Nelson-Filho, P. et al. (2017) Furcation perforation: periradicular tissue response to Biodentine as a repair material by histopathologic and indirect immunofluorescence analyses. *J Endod*, **43**, 1137–1142.

Sinai, I.H. (1977) Endodontic perforations: their prognosis and treatment. *J Am Dent Assoc*, **95**, 90–95.

Torabinejad, M. and Parirokh, M. (2010) Mineral trioxide aggregate: a comprehensive literature review – Part Ii: leakage and biocompatibility investigations. *J Endod*, **36**, 190–202.

Tsesis, I. and Fuss, Z. (2006) Diagnosis and treatment of accidental root perforations. *Endod Topics*, **13**, 95–107.

White, C. Jr and Bryant, N. (2002) Combined therapy of mineral trioxide aggregate and guided tissue regeneration in the treatment of external root resorption and an associated osseous defect. *J Periodontol*, **73**, 1517–1521.

40

Peri-Implant Diseases

40.1 Definitions

Peri-implant diseases involve inflammatory reactions in the tissues surrounding an implant (Zitzmann and Berglundh, 2008) and can be divided into peri-implant mucositis and peri-implantitis. as described below (Albrektsson and Isidor, 1994):

Peri-implant mucositis is an reversible inflammatory process in the soft tissues surrounding a functioning implant. Peri-implantitis is the inflammatory process additionally characterised by loss of peri-implant bone.

40.2 Aetiology

Peri-implant plaque composition and biofilm development are similar to those in natural teeth (Berglundh *et al.*, 1992). Adherent plaque biofilm on the implant surface appears to be the major aetiological factor in the initiation and progression of peri-implant diseases in a process very similar to the development of periodontitis in natural teeth (Lang *et al.*, 2011; Quirynen *et al.*, 2006). However, biofilm accumulation leads to a higher incidence of bleeding around implants in comparison with natural teeth and experimental models of peri-implantitis have shown that tissue destruction is faster and more extensive around implants than in experimental periodontitis sites (Salvi *et al.*, 2017).

Microbiota of peri-implantitis sites often have high levels of motile rods, spirochaetes and fusiform bacteria similar to those found in periodontal infections. In addition, other bacteria such as staphylococci, peptostreptococci and entric rods may also be present (Mombelli and Decaillet, 2011). A systematic review of microbiological studies has associated *Porphyromonas gingivalis*, *Treponema denticola*, *Tannerella forsythia*, *Prevotella intermedia* and *Campylobacter rectus* with the aetiology of peri-implantitis (Perez-Chaparro *et al.*, 2016).

40.3 Risk Factors

Risk factors for the development of peri-implant diseases include poor oral hygiene, history of periodontitis, smoking, poorly controlled diabetes, excess cement, lack of supportive therapy and genetic traits such as IL-1 gene polymorphism (Heitz-Mayfield, 2008; Howe, 2017; Laine *et al.*, 2006; Naujokat *et al.*, 2016; Renvert and Quirynen, 2015).

40.4 Prevalence

A recent systematic review of 47 studies and meta-analyses showed that the prevalence of peri-implant diseases has increased over time (Lee *et al.*, 2017). The weighted mean prevalence of peri-implant mucositis was 29.48% (based on implants) or 46.83% (based on patient subjects). The weighted mean prevalence of peri-implantitis was 9.25% (based on implants) or 19.83% (based on patient subjects).

A higher incidence of peri-implant diseases has been reported for smokers, with a summary estimate of 36.3% (Atieh *et al.*, 2013).

40.5 Diagnostic Criteria

The main diagnostic feature of peri-implant mucositis is bleeding on probing with no bone loss. The most commonly used diagnostic criteria for peri-implantitis are probing depth of equal to or greater than 4 mm, bleeding on probing/suppuration and radiographic bone loss

Diseases and Conditions in Dentistry: An Evidence-Based Reference, First Edition. Keyvan Moharamzadeh.

Companion website: www.wiley.com/go/moharamzadeh/diseases

ranging from 1.8 to 3 mm according to different studies (Figuero *et al.*, 2014).

40.6 Patient Assessment

40.6.1 Implant Identification

It is important to first identify the type of implants and the nature of the suprastructure used when assessing implants. Implant pass (certificate) and implant recognition softwares may help to identify the implant system (Michelinakis *et al.*, 2006).

40.6.2 Relevant History

Further relevant information includes details of previous surgery/bone graft, history of complications, any changes to the implant-supported restorations, bleeding gums around implants/suppuration, and method of cleaning.

The patient should be asked about the risk factors of peri-implant diseases discussed above as well as general risk factors associated with implant failure as described in Chapter 37.

40.6.3 Assessment of Suprastructure

The suprastructures should be examined for any defects, abnormalities, available access for cleaning and occlusal problems. Stable restorations do not need to be dismantled. However, loose restorations can be dismantled to enable better assessment of the individual implants.

40.6.4 Assessment of Individual Fixtures

Individual implants can be examined for the following.

- Mobility, using clinical mobility testing (of unattached implant) and electrical tools to assess the quality of osseointegration such as Periotest reading, resonance frequency analysis and measurement of implant stability quotient (ISQ) (Choi *et al.*, 2014; Park *et al.*, 2010).
- Bacterial deposits, by assessment of presence or absence of plaque at the emergence portion of the implant restoration.

40.6.5 Assessment of Peri-Implant Soft Tissue

- Mucosal assessment for visual signs of inflammation and infection.
- Palpation to identify suppuration, swelling and tenderness.
- Bleeding on probing.
- Pocketing and attachment loss.
- Recession.
- Soft tissue aesthetic assessment including papillae, interdental space, type of mucosa and width of keratinised tissue around implant.

40.6.6 Radiographic Assessment

Intraoral periapical radiographs have been used to assess the amount of peri-implant bone loss and are still recommended as the preferred method of evaluating bone loss around dental implants (Kuhl *et al.*, 2016). It is important to identify an appropriate reference point against which to measure the amount of peri-implant bone loss. Comparison of previous radiographs can be very helpful in determining the rate of disease progression.

40.7 Management of Peri-Implant Mucositis

Peri-implant mucositis is similar to gingivitis and can be reversed with effective treatment (Lang *et al.*, 2011; Salvi and Ramseier, 2015). Review of the existing evidence indicates that non-surgical mechanical therapy alone is effective in the treatment of peri-implant mucositis, regardless of the use of adjunctive measures such as antiseptic mouthrinses or antimicrobials (Schwarz *et al.*, 2015b). Mechanical treatment includes supra- and subgingival debridement of the implant surface and transmucosal components using different curettes and ultrasonic devices with modified tips (Figuero *et al.*, 2014). Furthermore, effective plaque control by the patient using manual or powered toothbrushes as well as interproximal aids is an important factor for treatment success (Figuero *et al.*, 2014; Renvert and Polyzois, 2015).

40.8 Management of Peri-Implantitis

Evidence suggests that non-surgical treatment with mechanical debridement alone offers only modest and unpredictable clinical outcomes for the treatment of peri-implantitis lesions (Suarez-Lopez del Amo *et al.*, 2016). Various protocols have been used for non-surgical management, including self-performed cleaning techniques and professional mechanical debridement with or without adjunctive measures such as locally delivered or systemic antibiotics (Renvert and Polyzois, 2015), photodynamic therapy and lasers (Mizutani *et al.*, 2016) and air-abrasive devices (Schwarz *et al.*, 2015a). These alternative/adjunctive measures may improve the efficacy of conventional non-surgical treatments at peri-implantitis sites (Schwarz *et al.*, 2015c).

However, surgical treatment is often indicated in many patients with advanced lesions when the initial non-surgical treatment is unable to achieve significant improvements in clinical parameters (Figuero *et al.*, 2014).

Prior to surgery, it is essential to establish and maintain optimal oral hygiene and address any underlying systemic risk factors (e.g. smoking and diabetes) or local plaque-retentive factors such as poorly designed prostheses which may require modification to improve access for oral hygiene.

The aim of surgical treatment is to provide adequate access for effective implant surface decontamination to minimise the risk of disease progression and promote peri-implant hard tissue healing (reosseointegration) and soft tissue reattachment (Renvert and Polyzois, 2015).

Surface modification and removal of the implant threads have been suggested as an adjunctive measure to reduce plaque retention on the implant surface. However, a rough implant surface allows better reosseointegration by stabilising the blood clot in the bone crater (Persson *et al.*, 2001). Therefore, it may be best to limit implantoplasty to non-aesthetic sites and only to the suprabony part of peri-implant defects (Schwarz *et al.*, 2011).

Different mechanical and chemical techniques have been used for implant surface decontamination, including mechanical brushing, lasers, photodynamic therapy, air-abrasion, citric acid, hydrogen peroxide, chlorhexidine and delmopinol (Mellado-Valero *et al.*, 2013). However, the literature does not clearly indicate the superiority of a specific decontamination protocol (Froum *et al.*, 2016).

Depending on the morphology of the osseous defect and aesthetic considerations, resective surgery (ideally for suprabony defects in posterior implants) or regenerative surgical treatment (for intrabony defects in the aesthetic zone) can be employed. Regenerative approaches include the use of autogenous bone or bone substitutes and porous titanium granules, with or without the use of barrier membranes. Systematic literature reviews show improvement of clinical parameters after surgical treatment of peri-implantitis. However, further research is required to establish the adjunctive benefits of regenerative approaches over non-regenerative surgical treatment (Daugela *et al.*, 2016; Schwarz *et al.*, 2015c).

Case Study

A 39-year-old male patient referred by his GDP complained of bleeding gums around an implant-retained upper front tooth. The implant had been in function for 9 years.

The patient was an irregular dental attender and had been smoking 10–15 cigarettes per day for 8 years. He brushed his teeth twice a day using a manual toothbrush and occasionally used dental floss for interdental cleaning. He had a clear medical history.

Clinical examination showed that the UR1 implant had a cement-retained crown with no mobility and normal occlusal function. Periodontal examination revealed isolated 9 mm and 11 mm deep pockets on the midlabial and distopalatal aspects of UR1 respectively, with bleeding on probing and suppuration upon palpation of the buccal aspect of the gingival mucosa over the implant. There was no recession of the soft tissues around the implant.

The patient had a low smile line (toothy smile).

Radiographic examination showed extensive peri-implant bone loss exposing the threads of the implant mesially and distally (Figure 40.1).

Based on the clinical and radiographic findings, the diagnosis of peri-implantitis (UR1) was made. The prognosis was guarded due to the extent of bone loss and depended on the patient's compliance with oral hygiene and smoking cessation. Prognosis for the aesthetics was fair as the patient had a low lip line and the interdental crestal bone height was satisfactory on both sides of the implant, indicating a low risk of gingival recession following surgical treatment. The

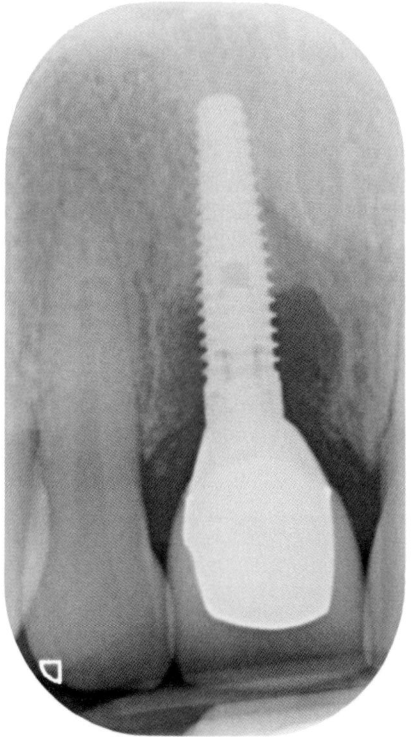

Figure 40.1 Preoperative periapical radiograph of the UR1 implant showing extensive peri-implant bone loss exposing eight threads on the distal aspect and 12 threads on the mesial aspect of the tapered implant.

presence of a deep, narrow, vertical intrabony defect would also increase the chance of potential bone regeneration and reosseointegration following surgical treatment.

The treatment strategy included the following steps.

1) Oral hygiene education, tooth brushing with modified Bass technique and interproximal cleaning using interdental brushes.
2) Smoking cessation advice.
3) Initial non-surgical debridement under local anaesthesia using an ultrasonic scaler to help to reduce inflammation.
4) Postoperative review in 1 month to assess oral hygiene and compliance with smoking cessation and preparation of the patient for surgical treatment as well as obtaining informed written consent to be reconfirmed on the day of surgery.
5) Surgical debridement of the UR1 implant as described below.
   - Local anaesthesia.
   - Crevicular incisions UL1 to UR2 labially and palatally, preserving the interdental papillae and full-thickness mucoperiosteal flap elevation.
   - Curettage and complete removal of chronically inflamed granulation tissue around the implant and within the bone defect (Figure 40.2).
   - Implant surface decontamination using ultrasonic scaler and irrigation with normal saline solution.
   - Flap repositioning, adaptation and suturing (Figure 40.3).
   - Postoperative instructions including appropriate analgesia, advice not to drink or eat anything too hot for the rest of the day, avoiding mouth rinsing for 24 hours, advice to use chlorhexidine mouthwash afterwards for 2 weeks, not to disturb the wound, avoid brushing the surgery area for 1 week and then start gentle tooth brushing of the area with a soft toothbrush after suture removal in 1 week.
6) Prescription of adjunctive systemic antibiotics, azithromycin 500mg, once a day for 3 days starting on the day of surgery.

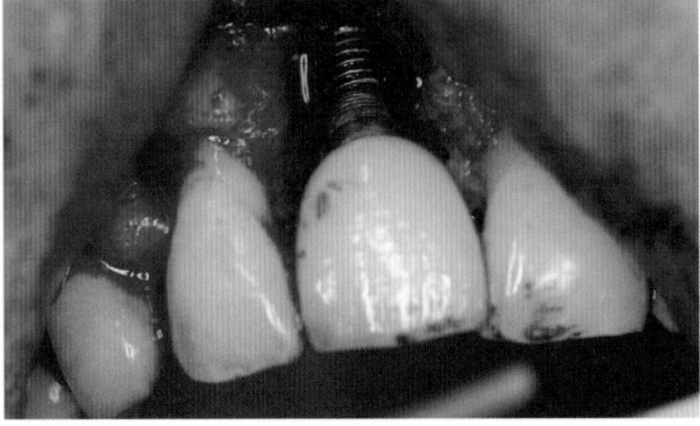

Figure 40.2 Clinical photograph of the bone defect and exposed implant threads following removal of the granulation tissue.

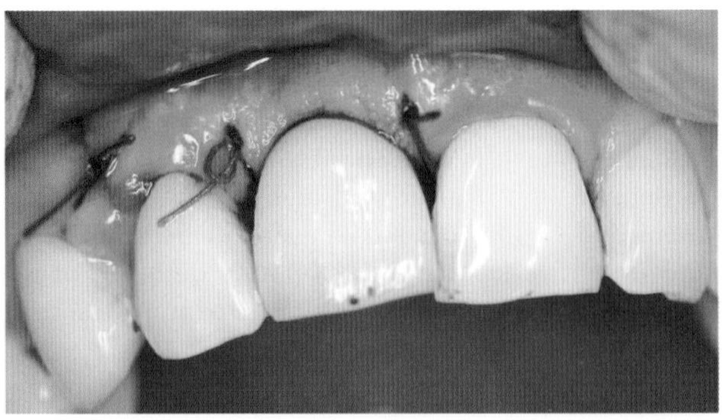

Figure 40.3 Clinical photograph of the sutured surgical wound.

7) Strict postoperative maintenance programme including monitoring and optimising the patient's plaque control and monthly professional supragingival scaling.

Periodontal reassessment in 6 months showed good patient compliance, resolution of symptoms and significant improvement of the clinical parameters. Soft tissues were normal and probing pocket depths had reduced to 4mm on both labial and palatal aspects of the implant. There was no bleeding on probing or suppuration.

Radiographic examination showed significant bone infill on both mesial and distal aspects of the implant and evidence of peri-implant hard tissue regeneration and reosseointegration indicating a successful outcome of treatment (Figure 40.4).

The patient was very satisfied with the outcome of treatment and therefore he was discharged back to his GDP for further monitoring of healing and long-term maintenance.

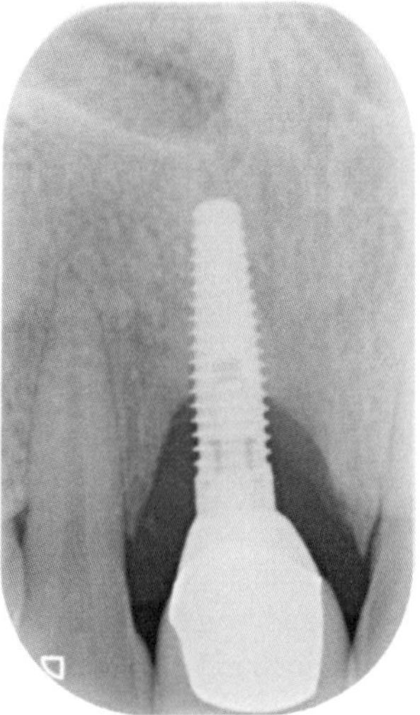

Figure 40.4 Postoperative periapical radiograph 6 months following surgical debridement of the implant showing excellent healing and regeneration of the peri-implant intrabony defect (compared to the preoperative radiograph), evidence of reosseointegration of the newly formed bone onto the implant surface as well as re-establishment of the biological width around the abutment.

References

Albrektsson, T. and Isidor, F. (1994) Consensus report of session IV, in *Proceedings of the First European Workshop on Periodontology* (eds N.P. Lang and T. Karring), Quintessence, London, pp. 365–369.

Atieh, M.A., Alsabeeha, N. ., Faggion, C.M. Jr.and Duncan, W.J. (2013) The frequency of peri-implant diseases: a systematic review and meta-analysis. *J Periodontol*, **84**, 1586–1598.

Berglundh, T., Lindhe, J., Marinello, C., Ericsson, I. and Liljenberg, B. (1992) Soft tissue reaction to de novo plaque formation on implants and teeth. An experimental study in the dog. *Clin Oral Implants Res*, **3**, 1–8.

Choi, H.H., Chung, C.H., Kim, S.G. and Son, M.K. (2014) Reliability of 2 implant stability measuring methods in assessment of various periimplant bone loss: an in vitro study with the Periotest and Osstell Mentor. *Implant Dent*, **23**, 51–56.

Daugela, P., Cicciu, M. and Saulacic, N. (2016) Surgical regenerative treatments for peri-implantitis: meta-analysis of recent findings in a systematic literature review. *J Oral Maxillofac Res*, **7**, E15.

Figuero, E., Graziani, F., Sanz, I., Herrera, D. and Sanz, M. (2014) Management of peri-implant mucositis and peri-implantitis. *Periodontology 2000*, **66**, 255–273.

Froum, S.J., Dagba, A.S., Shi, Y., Perez-Asenjo, A., Rosen, P.S. and Wang, W.C. (2016) Successful surgical protocols in the treatment of peri-implantitis: a narrative review of the literature. *Implant Dent*, **25**, 416–426.

Heitz-Mayfield, L.J. (2008) Peri-implant diseases: diagnosis and risk indicators. *J Clin Periodontol*, **35**, 292–304.

Howe, M.S. (2017) Implant maintenance treatment and peri-implant health. *Evid Based Dent*, **18**, 8–10.

Kuhl, S., Zurcher, S., Zitzmann, N.U., Filippi, A., Payer, M. and Dagassan-Berndt, D. (2016) Detection of peri-implant bone defects with different radiographic techniques – a human cadaver study. *Clin Oral Implants Res*, **27**, 529–534.

Laine, M.L., Leonhardt, A., Roos-Jansaker, A.M. et al. (2006) IL-1rn gene polymorphism is associated with peri-implantitis. *Clin Oral Implants Res*, **17**, 380–385.

Lang, N.P., Berglundh, T. and Working Group 4 of Seventh European Workshop on Periodontology (2011) Periimplant diseases: where are we now? Consensus of the Seventh European Workshop on Periodontology. *J Clin Periodontol*, **38** Suppl 11, 178–181.

Lee, C.T., Huang, Y.W., Zhu, L. and Weltman, R. (2017) Prevalences of peri-implantitis and peri-implant mucositis: systematic review and meta-analysis. *J Dent*, **62**, 1–12.

Mellado-Valero, A., Buitrago-Vera, P., Sola-Ruiz, M.F. and Ferrer-Garcia, J.C. (2013) Decontamination of dental implant surface in peri-implantitis treatment: a literature review. *Med Oral Patol Oral Cir Bucal*, **18**, E869–876.

Michelinakis, G., Sharrock, A. and Barclay, C.W. (2006) Identification of dental implants through the use of implant recognition software (IRS). *Int Dent J*, **56**, 203–208.

Mizutani, K., Aoki, A., Coluzzi, D. et al. (2016) Lasers in minimally invasive periodontal and peri-implant therapy. *Periodontology 2000*, **71**, 185–212.

Mombelli, A. and Decaillet, F. (2011) The characteristics of biofilms in peri-implant disease. *J Clin Periodontol*, **38** Suppl 11, 203–213.

Naujokat, H., Kunzendorf, B. and Wiltfang, J. (2016) Dental implants and diabetes mellitus – a systematic review. *Int J Implant Dent*, **2**, 5.

Park, J.C., Kim, H.D., Kim, S.M., Kim, M.J. and Lee, J.H. (2010) A comparison of implant stability quotients measured using magnetic resonance frequency analysis from two directions: a prospective clinical study during the initial healing period. *Clin Oral Implants Res*, **21**, 591–597.

Perez-Chaparro, P.J., Duarte, P.M., Shibli, J.A. et al. (2016) The current weight of evidence of the microbiologic profile associated with peri-implantitis: a systematic review. *J Periodontol*, **87**, 1295–1304.

Persson, L.G., Berglundh, T., Lindhe, J. and Sennerby, L. (2001) Re-osseointegration after treatment of peri-implantitis at different implant surfaces. An experimental study in the dog. *Clin Oral Implants Res*, **12**, 595–603.

Quirynen, M., Vogels, R., Peeters, W., van Steenberghe, D., Naert, I. and Haffajee, A. (2006) Dynamics of initial subgingival colonization of 'pristine' peri-implant pockets. *Clin Oral Implants Res*, **17**, 25–37.

Renvert, S. and Polyzois, I.N. (2015) Clinical approaches to treat peri-implant mucositis and peri-implantitis. *Periodontology 2000*, **68**, 369–404.

Renvert, S. and Quirynen, M. (2015) Risk indicators for peri-implantitis. A narrative review. *Clin Oral Implants Res*, **26** Suppl 11, 15–44.

Salvi, G.E. and Ramseier, C.A. (2015) Efficacy of patient-administered mechanical and/or chemical plaque control protocols in the management of peri-implant mucositis. A systematic review. *J Clin Periodontol*, **42** Suppl 16, S187–201.

Salvi, G.E., Cosgarea, R. and Sculean, A. (2017) Prevalence and mechanisms of peri-implant diseases. *J Dent Res*, **96**, 31–37.

Schwarz, F., Sahm, N., Iglhaut, G. and Becker, J. (2011) Impact of the method of surface debridement and decontamination on the clinical outcome following combined surgical therapy of peri-implantitis: a randomized controlled clinical study. *J Clin Periodontol*, **38**, 276–284.

Schwarz, F., Becker, K. and Renvert, S. (2015a) Efficacy of air polishing for the non-surgical treatment of peri-implant diseases: a systematic review. *J Clin Periodontol*, **42**, 951–959.

Schwarz, F., Becker, K. and Sager, M. (2015b) Efficacy of professionally administered plaque removal with or without adjunctive measures for the treatment of peri-implant mucositis. a systematic review and meta-analysis. *J Clin Periodontol*, **42** Suppl 16, S202–213.

Schwarz, F., Schmucker, A. and Becker, J. (2015c) Efficacy of alternative or adjunctive measures to conventional treatment of peri-implant mucositis and peri-implantitis: a systematic review and meta-analysis. *Int J Implant Dent*, **1**, 22.

Suarez-Lopez del Amo, F., Yu, S.H. and Wang, H.L. (2016) Non-surgical therapy for peri-implant diseases: a systematic review. *J Oral Maxillofac Res*, **7**, E13.

Zitzmann, N.U. and Berglundh, T. (2008) Definition and prevalence of peri-implant diseases. *J Clin Periodontol*, **35**, 286–291.

41

Periodontal Abscess

41.1 Definition and Classification

The International Workshop for Classification of Periodontal Diseases and Conditions in 1999 classified and defined abscesses of the periodontium into the following categories (Meng, 1999).

- Gingival abscess is a painful localised swelling involving the marginal and interdental gingivae which is usually caused by subgingival impaction of foreign bodies and may occur in healthy gingivae.
- Periodontal abscess is a painful localised swelling in sites affected by periodontitis, often associated with deep pockets, vertical bone loss and furcation defects, and is usually located on the gingivae coronal to the mucogingival line.
- Pericoronal abscess is usually associated with a partially erupted tooth.
- Periapical abscess is associated with necrotic pulp (see Chapter 3).

41.2 Pathogenesis

Periodontal abscess can develop as a result of:

- exacerbation of a chronic periodontal lesion with deep pocket due to marginal closure, poor drainage, subgingival microbial changes and/or compromised host response (DeWitt *et al.*, 1985)
- post-treatment periodontal abscess such as:
  - after non-surgical periodontal scaling due to entrapment of calculus fragments (Dello Russo, 1985)
  - after surgical periodontal treatment due to incomplete calculus removal or residual foreign bodies (Newman, 1993)
  - after antibiotic treatment due to superinfection from resistant subgingival biofilm (Helovuo *et al.*, 1993).

41.3 Prevalence

Periodontal abscess accounts for 6–14% of all dental emergencies and molar teeth are the most commonly affected sites (50%) due to the presence of furcation and complex anatomy (Herrera *et al.*, 2014). Although periodontal abscess is most commonly seen in patients with untreated periodontitis, it can also occur in patients under supportive periodontal therapy (SPT) and is the main cause of tooth extraction during SPT (Silva *et al.*, 2008).

41.4 Microbiology

Periodontal abscesses are usually polymicrobial, dominated mainly by gram-negative anaerobic rods such as *Porphyromonas gingivalis* (Herrera *et al.*, 2000a), similar to the microbiota found in chronic periodontitis lesions (see Chapter 6).

41.5 Diagnosis

Periodontal abscess can be acute or chronic (Corbet, 2004).

Acute periodontal abscess is characterised by pain, tenderness to palpation, swelling and suppuration from a deep periodontal pocket upon gentle pressure.

Some cases of periodontal abscess may have systemic manifestations such as fever, malaise and regional lymphadenopathy (Herrera *et al.*, 2000a). Dissemination of infection due to bacteraemia before or during treatment can also occur.

Chronic periodontal abscess is usually asymptomatic and is associated with a sinus tract which needs to be differentiated from a periapical abscess associated with necrotic pulp. Sensibility testing can be helpful in some cases if there is no simultaneous endodontic lesion. Radiographic examination of the affected site may show

Diseases and Conditions in Dentistry: An Evidence-Based Reference, First Edition. Keyvan Moharamzadeh.

Companion website: www.wiley.com/go/moharamzadeh/diseases

evidence of periodontal bone loss. A gutta percha point placed in the sinus tract may also trace to an intrabony pocket or the furcation defect of the affected tooth.

41.6 Differential Diagnosis

Differential diagnosis of periodontal abscess includes the following (Herrera *et al.*, 2000c, 2014).

- Periapical abscess (see Chapter 3) which is often associated with a non-vital tooth, caries, large restorations, sinus tract tracing to the apex of the involved root, and periapical radiolucency. There may be previous root canal treatment or endodontic errors such as perforation.
- Vertical root fracture where a fracture line can be visualised under microscope magnification and there is a mobile part of the tooth.
- Periodontic-endodontic lesion (see Chapter 42).
- Lateral periodontal cyst where the affected teeth are usually vital and not infected.
- Tumours and malignancies which would not respond to periodontal treatment and require a biopsy for definitive diagnosis.

41.7 Treatment

Management strategies to control the acute phase of periodontal abscess include the following.

- Drainage of the abscess through the pocket or an external incision.
- Mechanical root surface debridement (RSD) under local anaesthesia to remove bacterial and calculus deposits from the root surface and any foreign bodies occluding the pocket.
- Systemic antibiotic therapy can be indicated when there is diffuse progressive swelling or systemic involvement (Blair and Chapple, 2014). Various antibiotics such as metronidazole, amoxicillin/clavulanic acid and azithromycin have been used (Herrera *et al.*, 2000b; Smith and Davies, 1986).
- For teeth with hopeless prognosis and non-restorable teeth, extraction may be the best course.

The patient should be reviewed 1–2 days after the initial treatment.

Once the acute phase has resolved, the underlying periodontal condition and any residual disease must be reassessed and treated as described in Chapter 6.

Case Study

A 31-year-old male patient referred by his GDP complained of loose teeth, pus discharge from gums and bad taste in the mouth.

The patient was an irregular dental attender and had only had one cycle of periodontal scaling without local anaesthesia in the past. He reported a positive familial history of periodontitis. He was medically fit and well but had been smoking 20 cigarettes per day for the past 8 years.

Clinical examination showed poor oral hygiene, presence of plaque, calculus, generalised gingival inflammation, bleeding on probing and suppuration from multiple teeth with increased mobility. Four teeth had already been lost. Gingival swelling and a discharging sinus tract was noticed on the labial aspect of LL3 (Figure 41.1) which was vital as tested by an electric pulp tester.

Periodontal charting (Figure 41.2) showed the presence of deep periodontal pockets, mainly on the remaining first molars, maxillary incisors and mandibular canine teeth.

Radiographic examination (Figure 41.3) showed advanced periodontal bone loss with vertical pattern affecting the remaining first molar teeth, maxillary left central incisor and mandibular canine teeth.

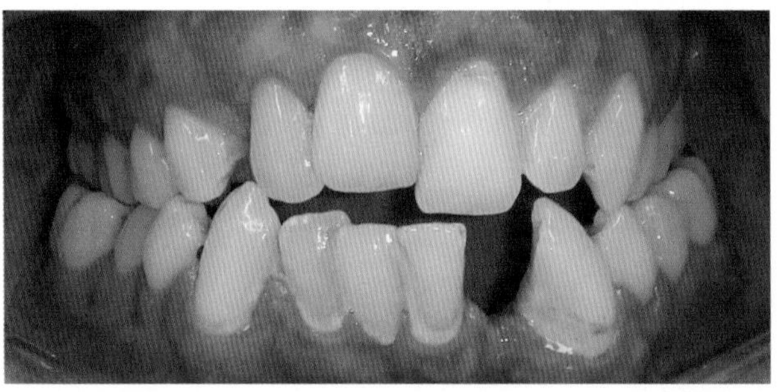

Figure 41.1 Preoperative clinical photograph showing missing teeth, plaque, gingival swelling and a sinus tract on the labial aspect of LL3.

Based on the history, clinical and radiographic findings, the following diagnoses were made.

- Localised aggressive periodontitis
- Periodontal abscess LL3 with a sinus tract
- Missing UR3, UL6, LL2, LR1
- Impacted mandibular third molar teeth

The following treatment was provided.

1) Oral hygiene education.

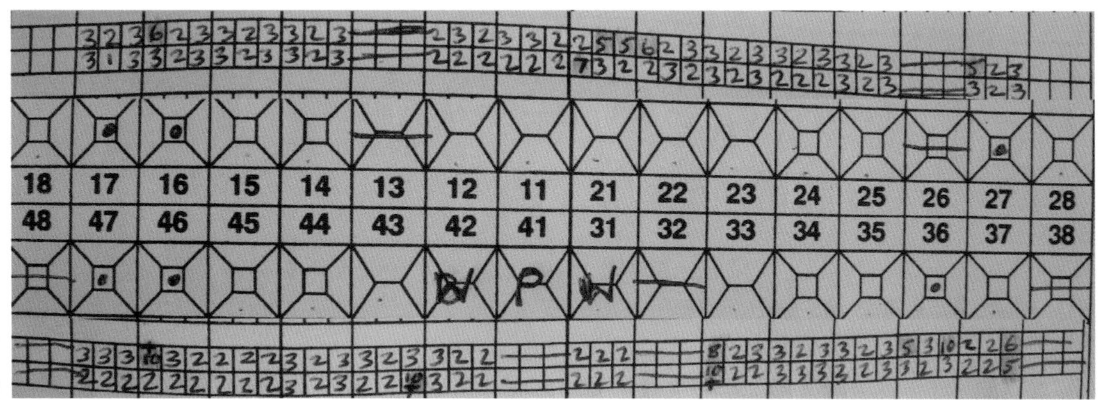

Figure 41.2 Baseline periodontal 6-point probing pocket depth chart.

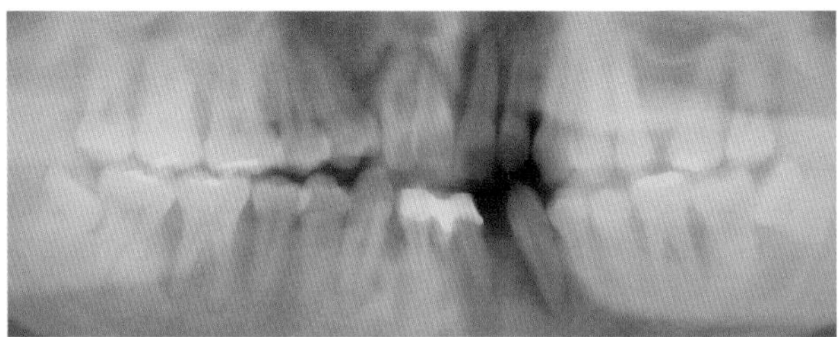

Figure 41.3 Preoperative oral panoramic radiograph showing missing UR3, UL6, LL2, LR1, impacted mandibular third molars, and advanced vertical bone loss on UR6, UL1, LL6, LL3, LR3 and LR6.

2) Smoking cessation advice.
3) Full-mouth scaling and RSD under local anaesthesia.
4) Systemic antibiotic prescription, including azithromycin 500 mg to be taken orally once a day for 3 days starting on the day of RSD.
5) Review of oral hygiene in 1 month.
6) Full periodontal reassessment in 3 months.

Some improvement was noticed following the first cycle of non-surgical periodontal treatment with adjunctive systemic azithromycin. The sinus tract and suppuration were completely resolved and the pocket depths and bleeding on probing were reduced in most sites at 3-month reassessment (Figure 41.4). There were still residual deep periodontal pockets present which required further treatment.

However, the patient had very poor plaque control despite serious attempts to educate and motivate him. The patient also refused to stop smoking and failed to attend subsequent specialist treatment sessions. Therefore, due to very poor compliance, he was discharged back to his GDP for the extraction of teeth with hopeless prognosis, continuation of non-surgical periodontal treatment of the remaining teeth and maintenance.

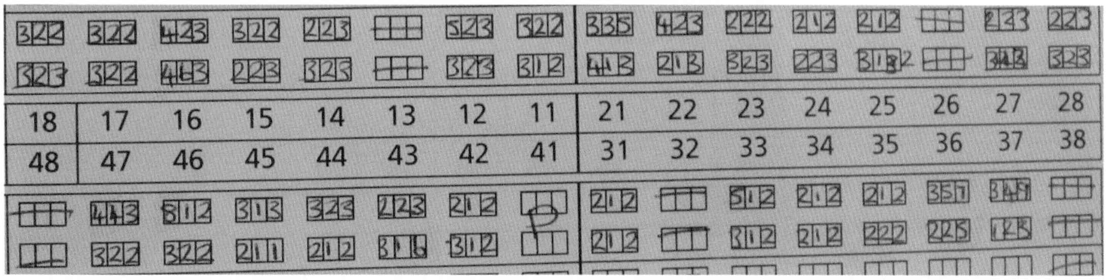

322	322	423	322	223		523	322	335	423	222	212	212		233	223
323	322	463	223	323		323	312	413	213	323	223	312		343	323
18	17	16	15	14	13	12	11	21	22	23	24	25	26	27	28
48	47	46	45	44	43	42	41	31	32	33	34	35	36	37	38
	443	812	313	323	223	212	P	212		512	212	212	357	345	
	322	322	211	212	316	312		212		312	212	222	225	123	

Figure 41.4 Periodontal probing pocket depth chart at 3-month reassessment.

References

Blair, F.M. and Chapple, I.L. (2014) Prescribing for periodontal disease. *Prim Dent J*, **3**, 38–43.

Corbet, E.F. (2004) Diagnosis of acute periodontal lesions. *Periodontology 2000*, **34**, 204–216.

Dello Russo, N.M. (1985) The post-prophylaxis periodontal abscess: etiology and treatment. *Int J Periodontics Restorat Dent*, **5**, 28–37.

Dewitt, G.V., Cobb, C.M. and Killoy, W.J. (1985) The acute periodontal abscess: microbial penetration of the soft tissue wall. *Int J Periodontics Restorat Dent*, **5**, 38–51.

Helovuo, H., Hakkarainen, K. and Paunio, K. (1993) Changes in the prevalence of subgingival enteric rods, staphylococci and yeasts after treatment with penicillin and erythromycin. *Oral Microbiol Immunol*, **8**, 75–79.

Herrera, D., Roldan, S., Gonzalez, I. and Sanz, M. (2000a) The periodontal abscess (I). Clinical and microbiological findings. *J Clin Periodontol*, **27**, 387–394.

Herrera, D., Roldan, S., O'Connor, A. and Sanz, M. (2000b) The periodontal abscess (II). Short-term clinical and microbiological efficacy of 2 systemic antibiotic regimes. *J Clin Periodontol*, **27**, 395–404.

Herrera, D., Roldan, S. and Sanz, M. (2000c) The periodontal abscess: a review. *J Clin Periodontol*, **27**, 377–386.

Herrera, D., Alonso, B., de Arriba, L., Santa Cruz, I., Serrano, C. and Sanz, M. (2014) Acute periodontal lesions. *Periodontology 2000*, **65**, 149–177.

Meng, H.X. (1999) Periodontal abscess. *Ann Periodontol*, **4**, 79–83.

Newman, M.G. (1993) The role of infection and anti-infection treatment in regenerative therapy. *J Periodontol*, **64**, 1166–1170.

Silva, G.L., Soares, R.V. and Zenobio, E.G. (2008) Periodontal abscess during supportive periodontal therapy: a review of the literature. *J Contemp Dent Pract*, **9**, 82–91.

Smith, R.G. and Davies, R.M. (1986) Acute lateral periodontal abscesses. *Br Dent J*, **161**, 176–178.

42

Periodontic-Endodontic Lesion

42.1 Definition and Classification

Periodontic-endodontic lesion is defined as simultaneous pulpal and periodontal disease simulating a single periodontal lesion (Meng, 1999).

Combined periodontic and endodontic lesions can be classified as follows (Rotstein and Simon, 2006).

- Primary endodontic disease with secondary periodontal involvement. This can occur in untreated suppurating primary endodontic lesions, perforations and root fractures where the initial endodontic lesion leads to development of a secondary periodontal defect in the presence of plaque.
- Primary periodontal disease with secondary endodontic involvement. This can arise due to the apical migration of a periodontal pocket progressing towards periapical tissues leading to pulpal necrosis caused by bacteria entering via lateral canals or the apical foramen.
- True combined periodontal and endodontic diseases can occur when an independent endodontic lesion progresses coronally and joins with a pre-existing infected periodontal pocket which is spreading apically.

42.2 Diagnosis

Below is the list of helpful history and assessment tools to establish the nature of suspected periodontic-endodontic lesions.

- History of previous periodontal disease, risk factors and any previous treatment.
- History of trauma, endodontic infections and any previous treatment.
- Assessment of clinical status of teeth, including caries and restorations.
- Sensibility testing to confirm the vitality status of the pulp.
- Periodontal probing to identify any present deep pockets around the suspected tooth.
- Full periodontal assessment to identify periodontal lesions in any other sites which would indicate the presence of pre-existing generalised periodontal disease.
- Radiographic examination to determine the presence of any periodontal bone defects, periapical radiolucency, root fracture, resorption defects and perforations. Placement of an opaque gutta percha point in the defect can help to demonstrate the extent and direction of the defect.
- The presence or absence of oral spirochaetes can be used to differentiate between endodontic and periodontal lesions (Dahle *et al.*, 1996). A dark-field microscopy spirochaete count of over 30% can indicate a pocket with periodontal disease origin and a spirochaete count of less than 10% may indicate a sinus tract associated with a purely endodontic lesion (Trope *et al.*, 1992).

42.3 Prognosis

The main prognostic factors are the pulp vitality, type and extent of the periodontal defect, and restorability of the tooth.

The prognosis of a primary endodontic lesion with secondary periodontal disease depends on the nature of the endodontic lesion and the extent of periodontal breakdown.

The prognosis of a primary periodontal lesion with secondary endodontic disease depends primarily on the extent and severity of the periodontal disease and the response of periodontium to treatment.

The prognosis of true combined disease can be guarded. If the initial endodontic treatment is efficient, the pulpal component of the disease will heal. Therefore, the long-term prognosis of combined diseases depends on the efficacy of periodontal treatment (Rotstein, 2017).

Diseases and Conditions in Dentistry: An Evidence-Based Reference, First Edition. Keyvan Moharamzadeh.

Companion website: www.wiley.com/go/moharamzadeh/diseases

42.4 Management

The treatment of choice for non-restorable teeth with hopeless prognosis is extraction and replacement of the tooth.

Periodontally compromised teeth with vital pulps will require appropriate periodontal management.

Restorable teeth with adequate remaining bone support but non-vital pulps will require appropriate endodontic treatment in the first instance. Root-treated teeth with periapical disease may also require endodontic retreatment to ensure elimination of the endodontic element of periodontic-endodontic disease. The tooth will need to be reassessed 2–3 months after the initial endodontic treatment to establish the need for periodontal treatment.

True combined periodontic-endodontic lesions may require early endodontic and periodontal interventions to stop the progression of both diseases.

In situations where it is difficult to establish the primary cause of a periodontic-endodontic lesion in non-vital teeth, treatment of periodontal disease should be delayed until healing is assessed after endodontic treatment to avoid damaging the cementum layer of the root, which may be intact and will help healing of the periodontium following appropriate endodontic treatment.

If signs of periodontal healing fail to appear within 2 months of endodontic treatment, a residual bony defect is probably associated with marginal periodontitis and would require appropriate periodontal management which may include non-surgical treatment or surgical periodontal treatment such as resective or regenerative treatment (Lang and Lindhe, 2015).

Case Study

A 56-year-old male patient was referred by his GDP for periodontal treatment. The patient's presenting complaint was frequent infections, swellings and discomfort in the lower left molar region.

The patient attended the GDP once a year and had an implant placed in the left mandibular second molar site 6 years ago.

The patient was medically fit and well and was a non-smoker. He had suboptimal oral hygiene and there was some calculus present on clinical examination.

The BPE scores were:

1	0	1
4	2	4*

There were isolated deep periodontal pockets measuring 10 mm on the distal aspect of LR6 and 12 mm on the distal aspect of LL6 and mesial aspect of LL7. There was a class III (through-and-through) furcation involvement on LL6.

Radiographic examination (Figure 42.1) showed a periodontic-endodontic lesion associated with the distal root of

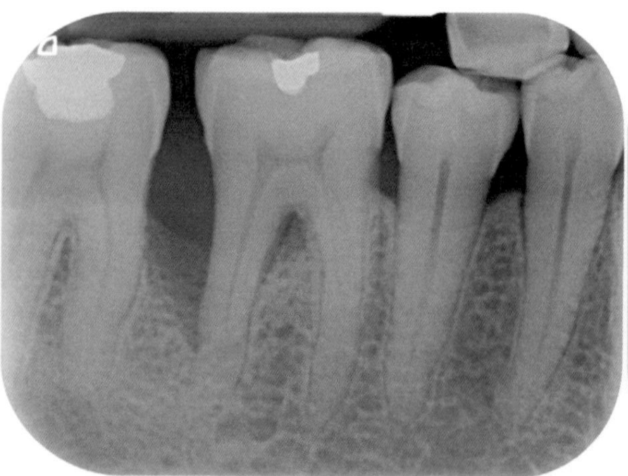

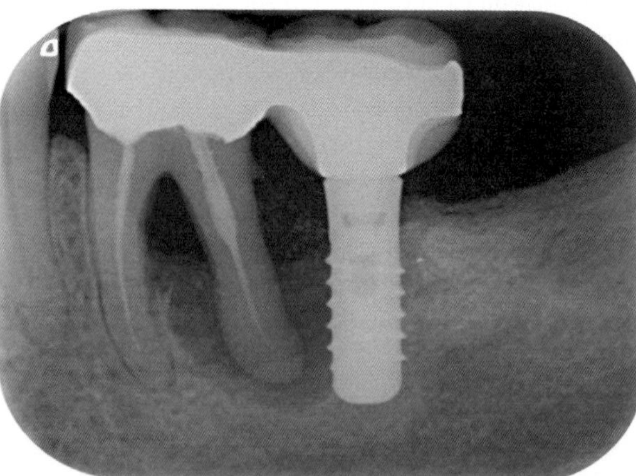

Figure 42.1 Preoperative periapical radiograph of LR6 (*right image*) showing moderate-advanced periodontal bone loss with vertical pattern. Periapical radiograph of LL6 and LL7 (*left image*) showing visible calculus deposit and advanced periodontal bone loss around the distal root of LL6 with grade III furcation involvement, severe bone loss on the mesial aspect of the LL7 implant affecting all the implant threads and periapical radiolucency associated with the distal root of LL6 which had an underextended root filling and a post crown linked to the implant-retained crown on LL7.

LL6 and peri-implant bone loss of the mesial aspect of the LL7 implant. Localised moderate-advanced vertical periodontal bone loss was also noticed on the distal aspect of LR6.

Based on the clinical and radiographic findings, the following diagnoses were made.

- Localised moderate-advanced chronic periodontitis LR6
- Chronic apical periodontitis and true combined periodontic-endodontic lesion LL6
- Peri-implantitis LL7

The following treatment options were discussed with the patient, including risks and benefits.

- No treatment.
- Extraction of LL6.
- Dismantling post crown on LL6 and non-surgical endodontic retreatment followed by periodontal treatment.
- Surgical periodontal treatment including open flap debridement of LR6, root resection (amputation) of the distal root of the LL6 and debridement of the LL7 implant surface.

The patient wanted to save the tooth but not dismantle the linked crowns on LL6 and LL7. Therefore, his preferred treatment option was surgical periodontal treatment and root resection of the distal root of LL6.

The following treatment was provided.

1) Oral hygiene instructions including modified Bass technique, interdental brushing and the use of water jet irrigator in sites with deep periodontal pockets to enhance subgingival plaque removal.
2) Initial non-surgical periodontal scaling to further reduce inflammation.
3) Periodontal flap surgery in LL6–LL7 site under local anaesthesia, resection of the distal root of LL6, removal of the chronically infected granulation tissue, root surface debridement (mesial root of LL6) and implant surface decontamination (LL7) using ultrasonic scaler and irrigation with normal saline solution.
4) Postoperative adjunctive systemic antibiotics, azithromycin 500 mg, once a day for 3 days.
5) Surgical periodontal treatment on LR6, including open flap debridement using minimally invasive surgical technique (MIST).
6) Review and reassessment.

The patient maintained excellent plaque control following the above treatment and 3-monthly periodontal reassessments showed significant improvement in periodontal condition, resolution of symptoms and bleeding, reduction in probing pocket depth and significant gain in clinical attachment level (CAL).

Radiographic examination at 6 months (Figure 42.2) showed evidence of periodontal regeneration and bone infill in both defects on LR6 and LL6–LL7.

Radiographic follow-up at 18 months (Figure 42.3) showed further bone regeneration and reosseointegration in previously diseased sites.

The patient was very satisfied with the outcome of treatment and was discharged back to his GDP for routine dental care, supportive periodontal therapy and maintenance.

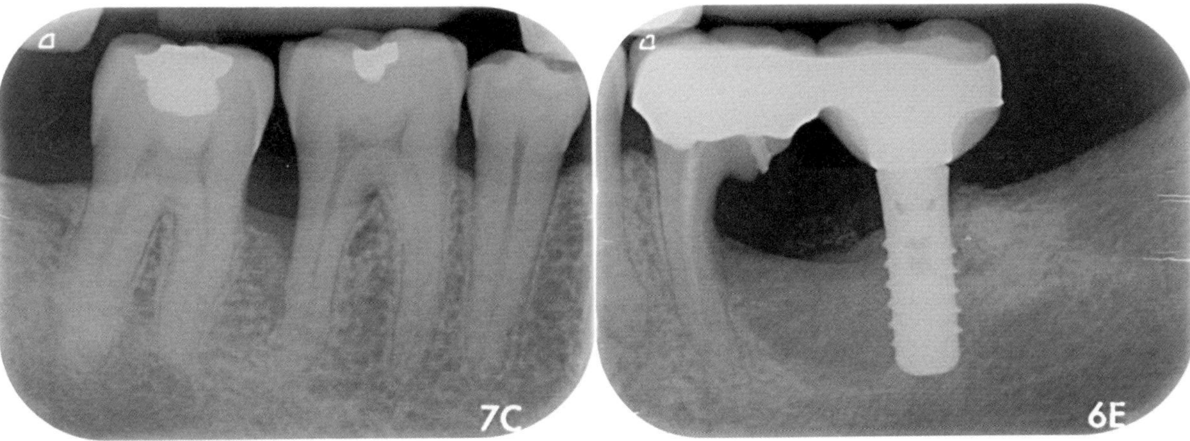

Figure 42.2 Postoperative periapical radiograph 6 months following surgical periodontal treatment showing bone infill and regeneration on the distal aspect of LR6, distal aspect of LL6 and mesial aspect of the LL7 implant.

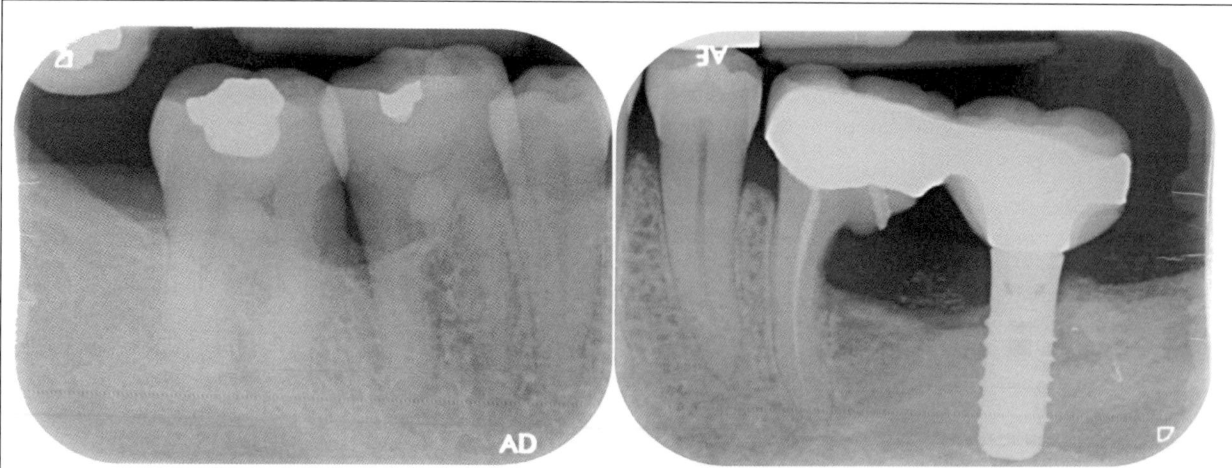

Figure 42.3 Follow-up periapical radiographs of LR6, LL6 and LL7 showing excellent bone regeneration, reosseointegration of the newly formed bone covering all the implant threads and absence of any obvious periodontal, peri-implant or periapical pathology.

References

Dahle, U.R., Tronstad, L. and Olsen, I. (1996) Characterization of new periodontal and endodontic isolates of spirochetes. *Eur J Oral Sci*, **104**, 41–47.

Lang, N.P. and Lindhe, J. (2015) *Clinical Periodontology and Implant Dentistry*, Wiley-Blackwell, Oxford.

Meng, H.X. (1999) Periodontic-endodontic lesions. *Ann Periodontol*, **4**, 84–90.

Rotstein, I. (2017) Interaction between endodontics and periodontics. *Periodontology 2000*, **74**, 11–39.

Rotstein, I. and Simon, J.H.S. (2006) The endo-perio lesion: a critical appraisal of the disease condition. *Endod Topics*, **13**, 34–56.

Trope, M., Rosenberg, E. and Tronstad, L. (1992) Darkfield microscopic spirochete count in the differentiation of endodontic and periodontal abscesses. *J Endod*, **18**, 82–86.

43

Periodontitis as a Manifestation of Systemic Disease

43.1 Introduction

Periodontitis as a manifestation of systemic diseases was defined as one of the categories of periodontitis by the 1999 International Workshop for Classification of Periodontal Disease and Conditions (Armitage, 1999). It was also further classified into three different subgroups, including periodontitis associated with haematological disorders, periodontitis associated with genetic disorders, and not otherwise specified group. These systemic diseases can have a serious impact on the onset and progression of periodontitis and its response to treatment in children and adults, and may lead to premature loss of teeth at a young age (Meyle and Gonzales, 2001).

43.2 Periodontitis Associated with Haematological Disorders

The main haematological conditions that can have periodontal manifestations are listed below.

- *Acquired neutropenia*, which can be autoimmune (caused by antineutrophil antibodies) or caused by infections and drugs that alter neutrophil function (Newburger, 2016).
- *Leukaemia* is the most common neoplastic disorder of the white blood cells and has frequent oral manifestations affecting the periodontium which are caused by either direct infiltration of leukaemic cells or underlying neutropenia, thrombocytopenia and impaired granulocyte function (Cousin, 1997; Francisconi *et al.*, 2016). Readers are strongly encouraged to refer to the Royal College of Surgeons of England's clinical guidelines on the oral management of oncology patients requiring radiotherapy, chemotherapy and/or bone marrow transplantation which includes comprehensive oral and dental considerations for before, during and after cancer treatment in this group of patients (Kumar *et al.*, 2013).

43.3 Periodontitis Associated with Genetic Disorders

Below is a list of genetic systemic diseases with significant periodontal manifestations.

- *Benign familial neutropenia* is a rare condition characterised by chronic decline in blood neutrophils and has oral manifestations such as persistent periodontitis, recurrent neutropenic ulceration and oral *Candida* infections (Casey *et al.*, 2011).
- *Cyclic neutropenia* is a rare benign, congenital haematological disorder which is characterised by recurrent episodes of severe neutropenia with 21-day intervals. It can present with recurrent oral ulcers and severe periodontitis in young children and adults (Rylander and Ericsson, 1981; Scully *et al.*, 1982). It is important to establish and maintain a high standard of oral hygiene as well as regular dental visits and strict periodontal maintenance in this group of patients (Pernu *et al.*, 1996).
- *Chediak–Higashi syndrome* (CHS) is a rare genetic immunodeficiency disorder characterised by large lysosomal vesicles in granulocytes, causing defects in neutrophil and monocyte function in terms of chemotaxis, degranulation and bactericidal action. CHS leads to susceptibility to infections and intermittent febrile episodes and has been associated with oculocutaneous albinism (Introne *et al.*, 1993). It has also been linked to severe periodontitis and early loss of teeth in children and adolescents (Delcourt-Debruyne *et al.*, 2000). However, it has been shown that it is possible to successfully manage periodontitis in a patient with a mild type of CHS which required regular dental visits, long-term systemic antimicrobial treatments and high levels of patient compliance (Bailleul-Forestier *et al.*, 2008).
- *Leucocyte adhesion deficiency (LAD) syndromes* are rare inherited primary immunodeficiency disorders resulting in recurrent infections. There are three

Diseases and Conditions in Dentistry: An Evidence-Based Reference, First Edition. Keyvan Moharamzadeh.

Companion website: www.wiley.com/go/moharamzadeh/diseases

subtypes (LAD-I, -II and -III). LAD-I is the most common type and is characterised by defects in phagocytic function due to the lack of expression of leucocyte cell surface beta-2 integrin molecules that play an important role in leucocyte adhesion to endothelial cells and chemotaxis (Cox and Weathers, 2008). If patients survive beyond infancy, they manifest a progressive and severe form of periodontitis, leading to premature loss of the primary and permanent dentitions (Nagendran *et al.*, 2012). It has been shown that the underlying aetiology of periodontal infection in LAD-I may involve a dysregulated host response that results in overexpression of the proinflammatory cytokine IL-17 and subsequent inflammation and bone resorption (Hajishengallis and Moutsopoulos, 2014).

- *Papillon–Lefèvre syndrome* (PLS) is a rare genetic disease with autosomal recessive inheritance and is caused by a mutation of the cathepsin C gene. PLS is characterised by diffuse palmoplantar hyperkeratosis and a severe form of periodontitis leading to premature loss of both deciduous and permanent dentitions (Dhanrajani, 2009). The teeth are involved in almost the same order as they erupt. Periodontal treatment may reduce the rate of disease progression in some patients with PLS and involves strict plaque control, combined mechanical and antibiotic treatment and an intensive maintenance programme as well as microbiological monitoring and treatment of the infection with *Aggregatibacter actinomycetemcomitans* (Nickles *et al.*, 2011). Implant treatment in PLS patients may have a high risk of peri-implantitis and implant loss, especially if the patient does not follow a maintenance programme (Nickles *et al.*, 2013). Some successful cases of rehabilitation of PLS patients with dental implants have been reported (Senel *et al.*, 2012).
- *Histiocytosis syndromes* are a group of clinical syndromes characterised by abnormal proliferation of histiocytes. Childhood histiocytoses are now named Langerhans cell histiocytosis (LCH), which is a rare disease caused by monoclonal proliferation of specific dendritic cells and primarily affects bones, but can also affect other organs. Different types of LCH were previously called histiocytosis X, including eosinophilic granuloma (unifocal), Hand–Schuller–Christian disease (multifocal unisystem) and Letterer–Siwe disease (multifocal multisystem) (Merglova *et al.*, 2014). Oral manifestations include periodontal lesions similar to aggressive periodontitis, loss of alveolar bone, premature loss of teeth, oral mucosal ulceration, delayed wound healing, suppuration and halitosis, which often require multidisciplinary management (Cisternino *et al.*, 2015; Klein *et al.*, 2006; Meyle and Gonzales, 2001; Panis *et al.*, 2016; Ryan *et al.*, 2012).
- *Down's syndrome*, caused by autosomal trisomy of chromosome 21, has been related to a high prevalence and severity of periodontal disease in children (Reuland-Bosma and van Dijk, 1986). Studies have suggested that the factors involved in rapid periodontal destruction in patients with Down's syndrome include dysregulation of enzymes and T-lymphocyte immunodeficiency, malfunction of polymorphonuclear leucocytes and monocytes, potential differences in collagen synthesis, abnormal capillary morphology and hyperinnervation of the gingiva together with poor plaque control (Frydman and Nowzari, 2012; Meyle and Gonzales, 2001). A systematic review has shown that early periodontal intervention, parent/carer participation in supervising oral hygiene, regular and frequent dentist attendance, plaque disclosure and use of chemical adjuvants such as chlorhexidine mouthrinse seem to improve the outcomes of periodontal disease prevention and different treatment modalities in patients with Down's syndrome (Ferreira *et al.*, 2016). Dental implants have been used for prosthetic rehabilitation of patients with Down's syndrome (Saponaro *et al.*, 2016). However, survival of dental implants is lower in this group of patients compared to the general population (Limeres Posse *et al.*, 2016).
- *Glycogen storage disease* is caused by defects in glycogen synthesis or breakdown which lead to accumulation of glycogen in the liver, kidneys and muscles. Oral ulceration and periodontitis have been reported in affected patients due to severe neutropenia and impaired neutrophil migration which characterises the onset of this rare disorder (Salapata *et al.*, 1995).
- *Infantile genetic agranulocytosis* or Kostmann's syndrome is a rare inherited autosomal recessive condition characterised by severe neutropenia. Periodontitis is a common oral manifestation in affected patients which requires intensive prevention and management (Gonzalez and Frydman, 2014; Saglam *et al.*, 1995).
- *Cohen's syndrome* is a hereditary disorder caused by a gene mutation in chromosome 8 which can cause mental retardation, obesity, craniofacial dysmorphism and neutropenia. These patients have an increased susceptibility to early periodontal disease due to neutropenia (Alaluusua *et al.*, 1997).
- *Ehlers–Danlos syndrome* (EDS) is a genetic connective tissue disorder characterised by abnormality of type I or III collagen and has 10 types based on clinical symptoms and inheritance pattern. Clinical features include joint hypermobility, skin fragility, easy bruising, cardiovascular disorders and variable musculoskeletal symptoms. Type IV (Badauy *et al.*, 2007) and type VIII (Karrer *et al.*, 2000) EDS have been associated with early-onset periodontitis which may lead to premature

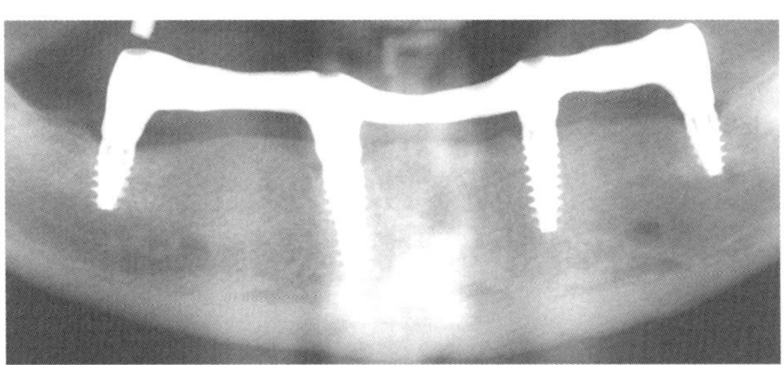

Figure 43.5 Radiographic evaluation 3 years following the placement of implants in the mandible.

References

Alaluusua, S., Kivitie-Kallio, S., Wolf, J., Haavio, M.L., Asikainen, S. and Pirinen, S. (1997) Periodontal findings in Cohen syndrome with chronic neutropenia. *J Periodontol*, **68**, 473–478.

Armitage, G.C. (1999) Development of a classification system for periodontal diseases and conditions. *Ann Periodontol*, **4**, 1–6.

Badauy, C.M., Gomes, S.S., Sant'ana Filho, M. and Chies, J.A. (2007) Ehlers-Danlos syndrome (EDS) type IV: review of the literature. *Clin Oral Invest*, **11**, 183–187.

Bailleul-Forestier, I., Monod-Broca, J., Benkerrou, M., Mora, F. and Picard, B. (2008) Generalized periodontitis associated with Chediak–Higashi syndrome. *J Periodontol*, **79**, 1263–1270.

Beumer, J. 3rd, Trowbridge, H.O., Silverman, S. Jr and Eisenberg, E. (1973) Childhood hypophosphatasia and the premature loss of teeth. A clinical and laboratory study of seven cases. *Oral Surg Oral Med Oral Pathol*, **35**, 631–640.

Casey, C., Brooke, T., Davies, R. and Franklin, D. (2011) Case report of a family with benign familial neutropenia and the implications for the general dental practitioner. *Dent Update*, **38**, 106–108, 110.

Cisternino, A., Asa'ad, F., Fusco, N., Ferrero, S. and Rasperini, G. (2015) Role of multidisciplinary approach in a case of Langerhans cell histiocytosis with initial periodontal manifestations. *Int J Clin Exp Pathol*, **8**, 13539–13545.

Cousin, G.C. (1997) Oral manifestations of leukaemia. *Dent Update*, **24**, 67–70.

Cox, D.P. and Weathers, D.R. (2008) Leukocyte adhesion deficiency type 1: an important consideration in the clinical differential diagnosis of prepubertal periodontitis. a case report and review of the literature. *Oral Surg Oral Med Oral Pathol Oral Radiol Endod*, **105**, 86–90.

Delcourt-Debruyne, E.M., Boutigny, H.R. and Hildebrand, H.F. (2000) Features of severe periodontal disease in a teenager with Chediak–Higashi syndrome. *J Periodontol*, **71**, 816–824.

Dhanrajani, P.J. (2009) Papillon–Lefevre syndrome: clinical presentation and a brief review. *Oral Surg Oral Med Oral Pathol Oral Radiol Endod*, **108**, E1–7.

Ferreira, R., Michel, R.C., Greghi, S.L. *et al.* (2016) Prevention and periodontal treatment in Down syndrome patients: a systematic review. *Plos One*, **11**, E0158339.

Francisconi, C.F., Caldas, R.J., Oliveira Martins, L.J., Fischer Rubira, C.M. and da Silva Santos, P.S. (2016) Leukemic oral manifestations and their management. *Asian Pac J Cancer Prev*, **17**, 911–915.

Frydman, A. and Nowzari, H. (2012) Down syndrome-associated periodontitis: a critical review of the literature. *Compend Contin Educ Dent*, **33**, 356–361.

Gonzalez, S. and Frydman, A. (2014) The non-surgical management of a patient with Kostmann syndrome-associated periodontitis: a case report. *J Oral Sci*, **56**, 315–318.

Hajishengallis, G. and Moutsopoulos, N.M. (2014) Etiology of leukocyte adhesion deficiency-associated periodontitis revisited: not a raging infection but a raging inflammatory response. *Expert Rev Clin Immunol*, **10**, 973–975.

Introne, W.J., Westbroek, W., Golas, G.A. and Adams, D. (1993) Chediak–Higashi syndrome, in *Genereviews* (eds R.A. Pagon, M.P. Adam, H.H. Ardinger, *et al.*), University of Washington, Seattle.

Jensen, J.L. and Storhaug, K. (2012) Dental implants in patients with Ehlers–Danlos syndrome: a case series study. *Int J Prosthodont*, **25**, 60–62.

Kapferer-Seebacher, I., Pepin, M., Werner, R. *et al.* (2016) Periodontal Ehlers–Danlos syndrome is caused by mutations in C1r and C1s, which encode subcomponents C1r and C1s of complement. *Am J Hum Genet*, **99**, 1005–1014.

Karrer, S., Landthaler, M. and Schmalz, G. (2000) Ehlers–Danlos type VIII. Review of the literature. *Clin Oral Invest*, **4**, 66–69.

Klein, F., Krigar, D., Petzoldt, D. and Eickholz, P. (2006) Periodontal manifestation of Langerhans' cell histiocytosis in a young man: case report with a 24-month follow-up. *Quintessence Int*, **37**, 175–182.

Kumar, N., Brooke, A., Burke, M., John, R., O'Donnell, A. and Soldani, F. (2013) The Oral Management of Oncology Patients Requiring Radiotherapy, Chemotherapy and/or Bone Marrow Transplantation. Clinical Guidelines. Available online at: www.bsdh.org/documents/pBSDH_RCS_Oncol_Radio_BMT_update_2012.pdf (accessed 3 January 2018).

Limeres Posse, J., Lopez Jimenez, J., Ruiz Villandiego, J.C. *et al.* (2016) Survival of dental implants in patients with Down syndrome: a case series. *J Prosthet Dent*, **116**, 880–884.

Merglova, V., Hrusak, D., Boudova, L., Mukensnabl, P., Valentova, E. and Hosticka, L. (2014) Langerhans cell histiocytosis in childhood – review, symptoms in the oral cavity, differential diagnosis and report of two cases. *J Craniomaxillofac Surg*, **42**, 93–100.

Meyle, J. and Gonzales, J.R. (2001) Influences of systemic diseases on periodontitis in children and adolescents. *Periodontology 2000*, **26**, 92–112.

Nagendran, J., Prakash, C., Anandakrishna, L., Gaviappa, D. and Ganesh, D. (2012) Leukocyte adhesion deficiency: a case report and review. *J Dent Child*, **79**, 105–110.

Newburger, P.E. (2016) Autoimmune and other acquired neutropenias. *Hematology Am Soc Hematol Educ Program*, **2016**, 38–42.

Nickles, K., Schacher, B., Schuster, G., Valesky, E. and Eickholz, P. (2011) Evaluation of two siblings with Papillon–Lefevre syndrome 5 years after treatment of periodontitis in primary and mixed dentition. *J Periodontol*, **82**, 1536–1547.

Nickles, K., Schacher, B., Ratka-Kruger, P., Krebs, M. and Eickholz, P. (2013) Long-term results after treatment of periodontitis in patients with Papillon-Lefevre syndrome: success and failure. *J Clin Periodontol*, **40**, 789–798.

Panis, V., Nikitakis, N., Daskalopoulos, A., Maragkou, T., Tsiklakis, K. and Sklavounou, A. (2016) Langerhans cell histiocytosis mimicking aggressive periodontitis: challenges in diagnosis and management. *Quintessence Int*, **47**, 731–738.

Perez, L.A., Al-Shammari, K.F., Giannobile, W.V. and Wang, H.L. (2002) Treatment of periodontal disease in a patient with Ehlers–Danlos syndrome. A case report and literature review. *J Periodontol*, **73**, 564–570.

Pernu, H.E., Pajari, U.H. and Lanning, M. (1996) The importance of regular dental treatment in patients with cyclic neutropenia. Follow-up of 2 cases. *J Periodontol*, **67**, 454–459.

Reibel, A., Manière, M., Clauss, F. *et al.* (2009) Orodental phenotype and genotype findings in all subtypes of hypophosphatasia. *Orphanet J Rare Dis*, **4**, 6.

Reuland-Bosma, W. and van Dijk, J. (1986) Periodontal disease in Down's syndrome: a review. *J Clin Periodontol*, **13**, 64–73.

Ryan, P.L., Piper, K.M. and Hughes, F.J. (2012) Langerhans cell histiocytosis: a diagnostic dilemma. *Dent Update*, **39**, 716–718, 720.

Rylander, H. and Ericsson, I. (1981) Manifestations and treatment of periodontal disease in a patient suffering from cyclic neutropenia. *J Clin Periodontol*, **8**, 77–87.

Saglam, F., Atamer, T., Onan, U., Soydinc, M. and Kirac, K. (1995) Infantile genetic agranulocytosis (Kostmann type). A case report. *J Periodontol*, **66**, 808–810.

Salapata, Y., Laskaris, G., Drogari, E., Harokopos, E. and Messaritakis, J. (1995) Oral manifestations in glycogen storage disease type 1b. *J Oral Pathol Med*, **24**, 136–139.

Saponaro, P.C., Deguchi, T. and Lee, D.J. (2016) Implant therapy for a patient with Down syndrome and oral habits: a clinical report. *J Prosthet Dent*, **116**, 320–324.

Scully, C., Macfadyen, E. and Campbell, A. (1982) Oral manifestations in cyclic neutropenia. *Br J Oral Surg*, **20**, 96–101.

Senel, F.C., Altintas, N.Y., Bagis, B. *et al.* (2012) A 3-year follow-up of the rehabilitation of Papillon–Lefevre syndrome by dental implants. *J Oral Maxillofac Surg*, **70**, 163–167.

Watanabe, H., Umeda, M., Seki, T. and Ishikawa, I. (1993) Clinical and laboratory studies of severe periodontal disease in an adolescent associated with hypophosphatasia. A case report. *J Periodontol*, **64**, 174–180.

44

Radiotherapy Side Effects

44.1 Introduction

Radiotherapy of the head and neck region can have several adverse side effects (Eliyas *et al.*, 2013). Short-term side effects include oral mucositis (Maria *et al.*, 2017), xerostomia (Mercadante *et al.*, 2017) and oral infections such as candidiasis (Worthington *et al.*, 2010). Long-term side effects include trismus (Rapidis *et al.*, 2015), radiation-induced caries (Aguiar *et al.*, 2009) and osteoradionecrosis (Caparrotti *et al.*, 2017).

Radiation-induced caries has been discussed in Chapter 5 and osteoradionecrosis was reviewed in Chapter 36.

General guidelines for prevention and management of oral and dental side effects of radiotherapy, chemotherapy and/or bone marrow transplantation have been published by the Royal College of Surgeons of England and the British Society for Disability and Oral Health (Kumar *et al.*, 2013). Further recommendations for restorative dentistry and oral rehabilitation were published as the United Kingdom National Multidisciplinary Guidelines (Butterworth *et al.*, 2016).

The following sections will focus on specific aspects of the management of radiation-induced oral mucositis, xerostomia, oral infections and trismus.

44.2 Radiation-Induced Oral Mucositis

Radiation-induced oral mucositis is an acute inflammation of the oral mucosa, tongue, and pharynx due to tissue injury after exposure to radiation, which usually lasts between 1 and 14 weeks (Maria *et al.*, 2017). It affects up to 80% of irradiated head and neck cancer patients (Elting *et al.*, 2007) and can cause oral pain, odynophagia, reduced oral intake and secondary infections.

Different grading systems have been introduced to describe the severity of radiation-induced mucositis, including the World Health Organization (WHO), Radiation Therapy Oncology Group (RTOG), Hickey, van der Schueren and Makkonen scoring systems (Etiz *et al.*, 2002).

The RTOG grading criteria, which are widely used (Mallick *et al.*, 2016), are as follows.

- Grade I: erythema (usually starts in the second week of radiotherapy)
- Grade II: focal areas of desquamation (usually develop in the third week)
- Grade III: confluent mucositis (occurs by weeks 4–5)
- Grade IV: ulceration and necrosis (happen in weeks 5–6)

Risk factors affecting the development, severity and duration of radiation-induced mucositis include age, sex, genetic susceptibility, co-morbidity, xerostomia, tobacco smoking, alcohol, dose, field and fractionation of radiotherapy, and concurrent chemotherapy (Rosenthal and Trotti, 2009).

Preventive strategies to reduce the severity of radiation-induced oral mucositis and some recommended management options are listed below (Kumar *et al.*, 2013).

- Using mucosal shields, tongue depressor and bite blocks during radiotherapy to protect the soft tissues.
- Using intensity-modulated radiotherapy (IMRT).
- Benzydamine hydrochloride mouthwash (15%) 4–8 times daily, starting before radiotherapy and continuing during and for 2–3 weeks after radiotherapy.
- Oral cooling and the use of ice chips for 30 minutes prior to chemotherapy.
- Using 2% lidocaine mouthwash prior to eating.
- Avoiding alcohol, smoking, irritant food, drinks and mouthrinses and irritating dentures.
- Atraumatic tooth brushing with a soft toothbrush or oral sponges.
- Intravenous administration of keratinocyte growth factor-1 (palifermin) in patients receiving high-dose chemotherapy or total body irradiation for stem cell transplantation.
- Pain management and treatment of any co-existing infections.

Diseases and Conditions in Dentistry: An Evidence-Based Reference, First Edition. Keyvan Moharamzadeh.

Companion website: www.wiley.com/go/moharamzadeh/diseases

- Prophylactic low-level laser therapy and photobiomodulation may also offer some benefits (Zecha *et al.*, 2016a, b).

44.3 Xerostomia

Head and neck radiotherapy can cause xerostomia due to injury to the parenchymal cells of the salivary glands and damage to blood vessels, nerves or connective tissue (Grundmann *et al.*, 2009). Damage can be caused directly by the radiation or indirectly by infiltration of inflammatory cells in response to radiation (Schaue and McBride, 2012). Radiation doses above 20 Gy can lead to the loss of up to 90% of salivary acinar cells (Henriksson *et al.*, 1994).

Xerostomia can have debilitating consequences, including development of fungal infections, altered taste or burning sensation, halitosis, difficulty swallowing and chewing and wearing dentures, which can significantly affect quality of life (Tanasiewicz *et al.*, 2016). It is also a major risk factor for the development of dental caries (Moore *et al.*, 2012).

Strategies to reduce the risk of xerostomia and treatment options for patients who have developed xerostomia following radiotherapy are discussed below (Borkent and Moharamzadeh, 2017).

44.3.1 Organ-Sparing Radiotherapy

Intensity-modulated radiotherapy is an advanced organ-sparing radiotherapy technique that delivers highly accurate radiation doses to specific areas within the tumour (Lee and Terezakis, 2008). Studies suggest that the use of salivary gland-sparing IMRT resulted in a significant reduction in xerostomia in head and neck oncology patients (Jensen *et al.*, 2010; Mendenhall *et al.*, 2014; Nutting *et al.*, 2011). However, 40% of patients still experience xerostomia following IMRT (Beetz *et al.*, 2014).

Proton beam therapy is another advanced radiotherapy technique that can spare salivary glands and reduce the risk of xerostomia by approximately up to 70% (van de Water *et al.*, 2012).

44.3.2 Salivary Gland Tissue Transfer

This technique was introduced by Jha *et al.* (2000), transferring submandibular gland tissue into the submental space before radiotherapy and shielding the gland to protect its function. Surgical salivary gland tissue transfer has become an accepted preventive option (Seikaly *et al.*, 2001). Submandibular gland tissue transfer has reduced the risk of acute and late postradiation xerostomia by 69% and 81% respectively without causing any major adverse events (Wu *et al.*, 2015).

44.3.3 Preventive Medication

Various drugs have been used to increase resistance of the salivary glands and reduce their sensitivity to radiation (Vissink *et al.*, 2015). These medications include amifostine, pilocarpine, insulin-like growth factor, keratinocyte growth factor (Jensen *et al.*, 2010), roscovitine (Martin *et al.*, 2012) and fibroblast growth factor (Kojima *et al.*, 2011). However, there is some controversy regarding the efficacy and even safety of some of these agents (Ma *et al.*, 2009).

44.3.4 Salivary Stimulation

Saliva production can be stimulated by (Kumar *et al.*, 2013):

- sugar-free chewing gums
- pilocarpine, 5–10 mg orally three times a day after radiotherapy, which can only be effective if there is some residual salivary gland function
- acupuncture.

44.3.5 Saliva Substitution

Strategies for saliva substitution include the use of frequent sips of water or a spray bottle of water, carboxymethyl cellulose saliva substitute or oral balance gel. Acidic salivary stimulants should not be used by dentate patients (Butterworth *et al.*, 2016).

44.4 Oral Infections

Cancer patients undergoing chemotherapy and radiotherapy often become immunocompromised and develop increased susceptibility to bacterial, viral and fungal infections. The most common oral infection following chemotherapy or radiotherapy is candidiasis (Lalla *et al.*, 2010).

It is extremely important to maintain a high standard of oral hygiene and denture hygiene in denture wearers to minimise the risk of development of oral infections (Noone and Barclay, 2017). The use of an alcohol-free chlorhexidine mouthwash can help to further improve short-term plaque control, considering its potential adverse effects.

Antifungal medication can be effective in treatment of oral candidiasis. Recommended regimens are as follows (Kumar *et al.*, 2013).

- Miconazole oral gel 24 mg/mL, 10 mL applied four times daily and continued for 48 hours after resolution of the lesions (Zhang *et al.*, 2016). Miconazole gel can be applied to the fitting surface of the denture in edentulous patients.
- Nystatin sugar-free oral suspension 100 000 units per mL four times daily for at least 7 days and 48 hours after resolution of lesions. However, compliance may be poor due to the unpleasant taste.
- Systemic agents such as fluconazole (50 mg daily for 7–14 days) have more consistent treatment efficacy and are recommended for oropharyngeal candidiasis or unresponsive oral *Candida* infection.

It is important to be aware that miconazole and fluconazole are contraindicated in patients taking warfarin or statins.

44.5 Trismus (Restricted Mouth Opening)

Head and neck oncology patients may develop trismus following cancer treatment due to surgical scarring or radiation-induced tissue fibrosis and contraction of muscles of mastication. The frequency and severity of trismus can be unpredictable and depend on the type and dose of radiotherapy, tumour site and stage, type of surgery and reconstruction, patient factors and co-morbidity (Moore *et al.*, 2012; Scott *et al.*, 2008). Trismus usually develops 3–6 month after radiotherapy and may become a permanent problem (Ichimura and Tanaka, 1993).

Reported prevalence of trismus is 25.4% in patients following conventional radiotherapy and 5% in patients after IMRT (Bensadoun *et al.*, 2010).

Trismus can interfere with eating, swallowing and speaking and may limit access for oral hygiene as well as dental treatment, which can be particularly uncomfortable for patients and may have an impact on their quality of life (Loh *et al.*, 2017; Scott *et al.*, 2008).

Strategies for the management of trismus in head and neck oncology patients include the following (Moore *et al.*, 2012; Scherpenhuizen *et al.*, 2015; Vissink *et al.*, 2003).

- Jaw exercises.
- Using stacked tongue spatulas to make a wedge to improve mouth opening at least 3–4 times daily.
- The use of dynamic bite openers such as TheraBite® Jaw Motion Rehabilitation System™ or OraStretch™ Press system.
- The use of Open Wide® Disposable Mouth Rest can be effective at maintaining oral access for oral hygiene or dental treatment.
- Trigger point injections, analgesics and muscle relaxants.
- Maintaining a shortened dental arch to minimise the need for dental treatment in the posterior region.

Case Study

A 63-year-old male patient was referred from the oral and maxillofacial department for prosthetic rehabilitation following treatment of T4 N1 M0 squamous cell carcinoma (SCC) of left lateral tongue by left partial glossectomy, neck dissection, reconstruction with a radial forearm free flap and postoperative adjuvant radiotherapy.

The patient complained of missing teeth, dry mouth and difficulty eating. He was medically fit and well, a former smoker and had good oral hygiene. BPE scores were 1 in all quadrants.

Preoperative clinical photographs are shown in Figure 44.1.

Based on the history, clinical and radiographic examination, the following diagnoses were made.

- T4 N1 M0 SCC left lateral tongue treated by left partial glossectomy, neck dissection and reconstruction with radial forearm free flap and radiotherapy
- Loss of multiple teeth
- Buccal abrasion lesions UR7 and tooth wear LL8
- Mild generalised gingival recession
- Staining of teeth caused by chlorhexidine mouthrinse
- Chronic apical periodontitis LR4
- Xerostomia

The treatment strategy was as follows.

1) Preventive measures, oral hygiene instructions, fluoride application, diet advice, instruction to take frequent sips of water, and prescription of Biotene® oral balance saliva replacement gel for the management of xerostomia.
2) Scaling and polishing of the teeth to remove staining and improve appearance.
3) Endodontic treatment of LR4 using ProTaper® files and obturation with Thermafil®.
4) Restoration of UR7 and LL8 with direct composite resin.
5) Fabrication and fitting of upper and lower Co-Cr removable partial dentures (Figure 44.2).
6) Review and maintenance.

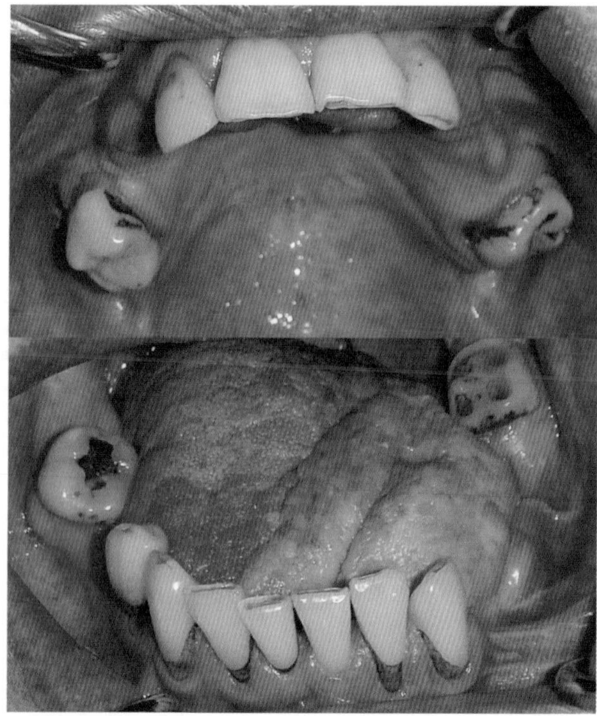

Figure 44.1 Preoperative intraoral clinical photographs showing partially dentate maxillary and mandibular arches and radial forearm flap on the left side of the floor of the mouth.

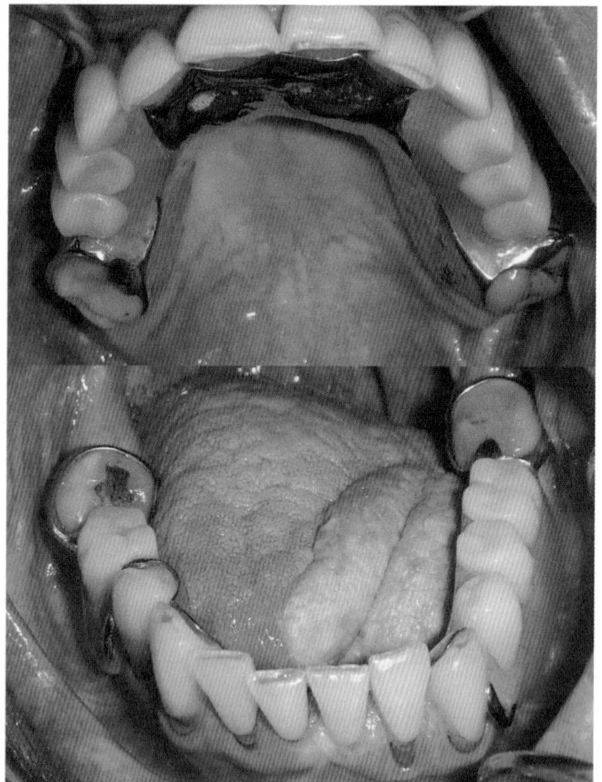

Figure 44.2 Clinical photographs of the RPDs *in situ*.

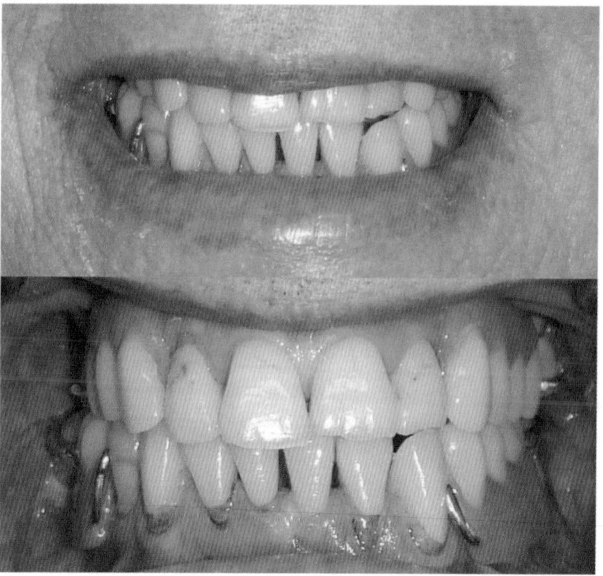

Figure 44.3 Postoperative photographs of the patient's occlusion and smile.

The patient's postoperative photographs are shown in Figure 44.3.

This was a challenging case because of the presence of the bulky flap on the left side of the mouth and the xerostomia. Taking the following steps resulted in satisfactory management of xerostomia and rehabilitation with Co-Cr partial dentures.

- Effective preventive measures and the use of Biotene oral balance saliva replacement gel to reduce the symptoms of xerostomia.
- Appropriate impression technique using a customised special tray and border moulding with green stick to enable an accurate impression around the flap with silicone impression material.
- Careful analysis of the articulated study models prior to designing the partial denture and appropriate design of the RPDs, taking into account the anatomical limitations.
- Accurate registration of the bite conforming to the existing occlusion without introducing occlusal interferences.
- Appropriate shade selection.

The patient was happy with his new dentures and reported significant improvement in the symptoms of xerostomia. Long-term maintenance with the help of the patient's general dental practitioner and a dental hygienist was very important to maintain periodontal health and prevent the development of caries.

References

Aguiar, G.P., Jham, B.C., Magalhaes, C.S., Sensi, L.G. and Freire, A.R. (2009) A review of the biological and clinical aspects of radiation caries. *J Contemp Dent Pract*, **10**, 83–89.

Beetz, I., Steenbakkers, R.J., Chouvalova, O. *et al.* (2014) The Quantec criteria for parotid gland dose and their efficacy to prevent moderate to severe patient-rated xerostomia. *Acta Oncol*, **53**, 597–604.

Bensadoun, R.J., Riesenbeck, D., Lockhart, P.B., Elting, L.S., Spijkervet, F.K. and Brennan, M.T. (2010) A systematic review of trismus induced by cancer therapies in head and neck cancer patients. *Support Care Cancer*, **18**, 1033–1038.

Borkent, D. and Moharamzadeh, K. (2017) Tissue engineering of salivary glands, in *Biomaterials for Oral and Dental Tissue Engineering* (eds L. Tayebi and K. Moharamzadeh), Woodhead Publishing, Duxford, pp. 337–351.

Butterworth, C., McCaul, L. and Barclay, C. (2016) Restorative dentistry and oral rehabilitation: United Kingdom National Multidisciplinary Guidelines. *J Laryngol Otol*, **130**, S41–S44.

Caparrotti, F., Huang, S.H., Lu, L. *et al.* (2017) Osteoradionecrosis of the mandible in patients with oropharyngeal carcinoma treated with intensity-modulated radiotherapy. *Cancer*, **123**, 3691–3700.

Eliyas, S., Porter, R., Briggs, P. and Patel, R.R. (2013) Effects of radiotherapy to the jaws. I: The scale of the problem. *Eur J Prosthodont Restor Dent*, **21**, 161–169.

Elting, L.S., Cooksley, C.D., Chambers, M.S. and Garden, A.S. (2007) Risk, outcomes, and costs of radiation-induced oral mucositis among patients with head-and-neck malignancies. *Int J Radiat Oncol Biol Phys*, **68**, 1110–1120.

Etiz, D., Orhan, B., Demirustu, C., Ozdamar, K. and Cakmak, A. (2002) Comparison of radiation-induced oral mucositis scoring systems. *Tumori*, **88**, 379–384.

Grundmann, O., Mitchell, G.C. and Limesand, K.H. (2009) Sensitivity of salivary glands to radiation: from animal models to therapies. *J Dent Res*, **88**, 894–903.

Henriksson, R., Frojd, O., Gustafsson, H. *et al.* (1994) Increase in mast cells and hyaluronic acid correlates to radiation-induced damage and loss of serous acinar cells in salivary glands: the parotid and submandibular glands differ in radiation sensitivity. *Br J Cancer*, **69**, 320–326.

Ichimura, K. and Tanaka, T. (1993) Trismus in patients with malignant tumours in the head and neck. *J Laryngol Otol*, **107**, 1017–1020.

Jensen, S.B., Pedersen, A.M., Vissink, A. *et al.* (2010) A systematic review of salivary gland hypofunction and xerostomia induced by cancer therapies: management strategies and economic impact. *Support Care Cancer*, **18**, 1061–1079.

Jha, N., Seikaly, H., McGaw, T. and Coulter, L. (2000) Submandibular salivary gland transfer prevents radiation-induced xerostomia. *Int J Radiat Oncol Biol Phys*, **46**, 7–11.

Kojima, T., Kanemaru, S., Hirano, S. *et al.* (2011) The protective efficacy of basic fibroblast growth factor in radiation-induced salivary gland dysfunction in mice. *Laryngoscope*, **121**, 1870–1875.

Kumar, N., Brooke, A., Burke, M., John, R., O'Donnell, A. and Soldani, F. (2013) *The Oral Management of Oncology Patients Requiring Radiotherapy, Chemotherapy and/or Bone Marrow Transplantation. Clinical Guidelines*. Available online at: www.bsdh.org/documents/pBSDH_RCS_Oncol_Radio_BMT_update_2012.pdf (accessed 3 January 2018).

Lalla, R.V., Latortue, M.C., Hong, C.H. *et al.* (2010) A systematic review of oral fungal infections in patients receiving cancer therapy. *Support Care Cancer*, **18**, 985–992.

Lee, N.Y. and Terezakis, S.A. (2008) Intensity-modulated radiation therapy. *J Surg Oncol*, **97**, 691–696.

Loh, S.Y., McLeod, R.W.J. and Elhassan, H.A. (2017) Trismus following different treatment modalities for head and neck cancer: a systematic review of subjective measures. *Eur Arch Otorhinolaryngol*, **274**, 2695–2707.

Ma, C., Xie, J., Chen, Q., Wang, G. and Zuo, S. (2009) Amifostine for salivary glands in high-dose radioactive iodine treated differentiated thyroid cancer. *Cochrane Database Syst Rev*, **4**, CD007956.

Mallick, S., Benson, R. and Rath, G.K. (2016) Radiation induced oral mucositis: a review of current literature on prevention and management. *Eur Arch Otorhinolaryngol*, **273**, 2285–2293.

Maria, O.M., Eliopoulos, N. and Muanza, T. (2017) Radiation-induced oral mucositis. *Front Oncol*, **7**, 89.

Martin, K.L., Hill, G.A., Klein, R.R., Arnett, D.G., Burd, R. and Limesand, K.H. (2012) Prevention of radiation-induced salivary gland dysfunction utilizing a CDK inhibitor in a mouse model. *Plos One*, **7**, E51363.

Mendenhall, W.M., Mendenhall, C.M. and Mendenhall, N.P. (2014) Submandibular gland-sparing intensity-modulated radiotherapy. *Am J Clin Oncol*, **37**, 514–516.

Mercadante, V., Al Hamad, A., Lodi, G., Porter, S. and Fedele, S. (2017) Interventions for the management of radiotherapy-induced xerostomia and hyposalivation: a systematic review and meta-analysis. *Oral Oncol*, **66**, 64–74.

Moore, S., Burke, M.C., Fenlon, M.R. and Banerjee, A. (2012) The role of the general dental practitioner in managing the oral care of head and neck oncology patients. *Dent Update*, **39**, 694–696, 698–700, 702.

Noone, J. and Barclay, C. (2017) Head and neck cancer patients – information for the general dental practitioner. *Dent Update*, **44**, 209–215.

Nutting, C.M., Morden, J.P., Harrington, K.J. *et al.* (2011) Parotid-sparing intensity modulated versus conventional radiotherapy in head and neck cancer (PARSPORT): a phase 3 multicentre randomised controlled trial. *Lancet Oncol*, **12**, 127–136.

Rapidis, A.D., Dijkstra, P.U., Roodenburg, J.L. *et al.* (2015) Trismus in patients with head and neck cancer: etiopathogenesis, diagnosis and management. *Clin Otolaryngol*, **40**, 516–526.

Rosenthal, D.I. and Trotti, A. (2009) Strategies for managing radiation-induced mucositis in head and neck cancer. *Semin Radiat Oncol*, **19**, 29–34.

Schaue, D. and McBride, W.H. (2012) T lymphocytes and normal tissue responses to radiation. *Front Oncol*, **2**, 119.

Scherpenhuizen, A., van Waes, A.M., Janssen, L.M., van Cann, E.M. and Stegeman, I. (2015) The effect of exercise therapy in head and neck cancer patients in the treatment of radiotherapy-induced trismus: a systematic review. *Oral Oncol*, **51**, 745–750.

Scott, B., Butterworth, C., Lowe, D. and Rogers, S.N. (2008) Factors associated with restricted mouth opening and its relationship to health-related quality of life in patients attending a maxillofacial oncology clinic. *Oral Oncol*, **44**, 430–438.

Seikaly, H., Jha, N., McGaw, T., Coulter, L., Liu, R. and Oldring, D. (2001) Submandibular gland transfer: a new method of preventing radiation-induced xerostomia. *Laryngoscope*, **111**, 347–352.

Tanasiewicz, M., Hildebrandt, T. and Obersztyn, I. (2016) Xerostomia of various etiologies: a review of the literature. *Adv Clin Exp Med*, **25**, 199–206.

van de Water, T.A., Lomax, A.J., Bijl, H.P., Schilstra, C., Hug, E.B. and Langendijk, J.A. (2012) Using a reduced spot size for intensity-modulated proton therapy potentially improves salivary gland-sparing in oropharyngeal cancer. *Int J Radiat Oncol Biol Phys*, **82**, E313–319.

Vissink, A., Burlage, F.R., Spijkervet, F.K., Jansma, J. and Coppes, R.P. (2003) Prevention and treatment of the consequences of head and neck radiotherapy. *Crit Rev Oral Biol Med*, **14**, 213–225.

Vissink, A., van Luijk, P., Langendijk, J.A. and Coppes, R.P. (2015) Current ideas to reduce or salvage radiation damage to salivary glands. *Oral Dis*, **21**, E1–10.

Worthington, H.V., Clarkson, J.E., Khalid, T., Meyer, S. and McCabe, M. (2010) Interventions for treating oral candidiasis for patients with cancer receiving treatment. *Cochrane Database Syst Rev*, **7**, CD001972.

Wu, F., Weng, S., Li, C., Sun, J., Li, L. and Gao, Q. (2015) Submandibular gland transfer for the prevention of postradiation xerostomia in patients with head and neck cancer: a systematic review and meta-analysis. *Orl J Otorhinolaryngol Relat Spec*, **77**, 70–86.

Zecha, J.A., Raber-Durlacher, J.E., Nair, R.G. *et al.* (2016a) Low-level laser therapy/photobiomodulation in the management of side effects of chemoradiation therapy in head and neck cancer: Part 2: Proposed applications and treatment protocols. *Support Care Cancer*, **24**, 2793–2805.

Zecha, J.A., Raber-Durlacher, J.E., Nair, R.G. *et al.* (2016b) Low level laser therapy/photobiomodulation in the management of side effects of chemoradiation therapy in head and neck cancer: Part 1: Mechanisms of action, dosimetric, and safety considerations. *Support Care Cancer*, **24**, 2781–2792.

Zhang, L.W., Fu, J.Y., Hua, H. and Yan, Z.M. (2016) Efficacy and safety of miconazole for oral candidiasis: a systematic review and meta-analysis. *Oral Dis*, **22**, 185–195.

45

Ridge Defects (Generalised)

45.1 Introduction

The alveolar ridge continues to resorb following extraction of teeth in both mandible and maxillae. The pattern of ridge resorption in the maxillae is mainly labial or buccal bone resorption. In the anterior mandible, resorption occurs more on the labial side of the ridge, and in the posterior mandible, it occurs more on the lingual aspect (Tallgren, 2003).

The rate of ridge resorption is influenced by factors such as history of extractions, wearing prosthesis and its quality, parafunctional habits and systemic diseases including diabetes and osteoporosis. Socket preservation techniques may reduce postextraction alveolar ridge dimensional changes, but they are unable to stop ridge resorption completely (Morjaria *et al.*, 2014; Willenbacher *et al.*, 2016).

This chapter focuses on different strategies for the management of generalised alveolar ridge resorption in edentulous patients.

45.2 Classifications

Cawood and Howell (1988) proposed the following classification of edentulous jaws based on a randomised cross-sectional study of 300 dried skulls.

- Class I: dentate ridge
- Class II: ridge directly after extraction
- Class III: broad and rounded ridge with adequate height and width
- Class IV: knife-edge ridge with sufficient height but insufficient width
- Class V: flat ridge with insufficient height and width
- Class VI: depressed ridge with a cup-shaped surface

Lekholm and Zarb (1985) classified the quality of residual alveolar bone into four types.

- Type I: full-thickness cortical bone
- Type II: thick cortical bone layer surrounding a dense trabecular bone
- Type III: thin cortical bone layer surrounding a dense trabecular bone
- Type IV: thin cortical bone layer surrounding a sparse trabecular bone

45.3 Neutral Zone Impression Technique for Resorbed Ridges

The neutral zone impression technique is recommended for highly atrophic mandibular ridges in patients with history of non-retentive and unstable complete denture (Gahan and Walmsley, 2005; Lynch and Allen, 2006). The procedure is described below.

- Impressions and preparation of master casts.
- Construction of a maxillary wax rim and a mandibular acrylic special tray which is adapted to the ridge, without a handle but with wire loops projecting upwards.
- The maxillary wax rim is adjusted the same way as routine registration for a complete denture.
- The mandibular special tray is placed in the mouth and two occlusal pillars are then built up with green stick compound or acrylic material to the correct height (to provide adequate free-way space) on both sides of the mandibular arch.
- A soft denture liner material is placed on the mandibular special tray around the pillars and the patient is instructed to close the mouth and move the cheeks and lips until the material is set.
- The impression is sent to the laboratory and indexed with plaster which indicates the borders of the neutral zone.
- The teeth are then placed into the neutral zone.

Diseases and Conditions in Dentistry: An Evidence-Based Reference, First Edition. Keyvan Moharamzadeh.

Companion website: www.wiley.com/go/moharamzadeh/diseases

45.4 Magnet-Retained Conventional Overdenture

Root-treated teeth can be used as overdenture abutments with incorporated magnet-based precision attachments to further improve the retention and stability of conventional overdentures (Walmsley, 2002).

The procedure involves fitting preformed or cast magnetisable alloy root elements (keepers) onto decoronated root-treated teeth. Magnets can then be fitted into the denture base directly chairside using cold-cure acrylic resin or indirectly in the laboratory.

The main advantages of magnet attachments are self-adjustment, stress breaking and automatic repositioning after denture displacement (Gillings, 1984). A 5-year multicentre study of 131 patients with magnetic attachments on natural overdenture abutments showed high (97%) patient satisfaction (Gonda *et al.*, 2013). Magnet complications include periodontal disease, pain and mobility of the abutment teeth, detachment and loss of magnetic power.

45.5 Implant-Supported Overdentures

Osseointegrated implants with different precision attachment systems have been used to improve the retention and stability of complete overdentures as well as patient satisfaction and quality of life (Kutkut *et al.*, 2018; Thomason *et al.*, 2012).

The McGill consensus statement, based on the opinion of a panel of relevant experts in the field, stated that '*The available evidence suggests that the restoration of the edentulous mandible with a conventional denture is no longer the most appropriate first choice prosthodontic treatment and there is overwhelming evidence that a two-implant overdenture should become the first choice of treatment for the edentulous mandible*' (Feine *et al.*, 2002).

Later, in 2009, the York consensus statement was released by the British Society for the Study of Prosthetic Dentistry (BSSPD) which concluded that '*A substantial body of evidence is available to demonstrate that patients' satisfaction and quality of life with implant-supported mandibular overdentures is significantly greater than for conventional dentures. Whilst it is accepted that the two-implant overdenture is not the gold standard of implant treatment, it is the minimum standard that should be sufficient for most people, taking into account performance, patient satisfaction, cost and clinical time*' (Thomason *et al.*, 2009).

The recommended number of implants for mandibular overdentures are two mandibular implants in the canine regions (Roccuzzo *et al.*, 2012). Regarding maxillary implant-supported overdentures, the use of 4–6 implants has been recommended. A higher implant failure rate has been reported in the maxillae compared to the mandible, especially with machined and short implants (length <10 mm) (Sadowsky and Zitzmann, 2016) and when less than four implants with a non-splinted anchorage are used (Raghoebar *et al.*, 2014). Although both splinted and solitary implant attachment systems are advocated, the maintenance requirement is higher for solitary attachments. Soft tissue inflammation is increased under the bar attachments and long-term maintenance care is essential for all designs (Sadowsky and Zitzmann, 2016).

Different precision attachment systems that can be used in implant-supported overdentures are listed in Table 45.1.

Table 45.1 Implant-supported precision attachments for removable overdentures.

Attachment type	Advantages	Disadvantages
Ball attachment	• Improved retention and stability • Straightforward procedure	• Need for adequate space (15 mm) • Need for parallelism • Loss of retention over time
Locator attachment	• Improved retention and stability • Straightforward procedure • Minimal space requirement • Can correct angulated implants	• Loss of retention over time • Locator maintenance
Magnets	• Improved retention and stability • Self-adjusting • Easy to wear	• Need for adequate space • Magnet complications • Need for maintenance

Table 45.1 (Continued)

Attachment type	Advantages	Disadvantages
Bar and clip	• Improved retention and stability • Splinting effect on implants	• Need for adequate space • Difficulty cleaning under the bar • Potential for peri-implant inflammatory disease
Milled bar combined with other types of attachments	• Highly improved retention and stability • Splinting effect on implants • CAD-CAM technology	• Need for adequate space • Difficulty cleaning under the bar • Potential for peri-implant inflammatory disease • High cost

The implant survival rates of mandibular overdentures are high (93–100%) regardless of the attachment system used (Kim *et al.*, 2012). The most commonly encountered prosthetic maintenance issues are replacement of an assay for magnet attachments and activation of a matrix or clip for ball or bar attachments. Other complications include fracture of attachment system or denture components and prosthesis-related adjustments (Andreiotelli *et al.*, 2010; Goodacre *et al.*, 2003; Kim *et al.*, 2012).

45.6 Full-Arch Implant-Retained Fixed Prosthesis

General preoperative assessment and planning considerations for implant treatment have been discussed in Chapter 37. Regarding full-arch fixed restorations, initial diagnostic tooth set-up is an important step in planning for implant treatment. A duplicate of the patient's existing denture with radiopaque markers (if the denture is satisfactory) can also be used and converted to a radiographic and/or surgical stent.

For implant-retained full-arch fixed prostheses, using 4–6 implants is a well-documented treatment option with high survival rates for both implants and prostheses (Heydecke *et al.*, 2012).

In the non-resorbed mandible, implants can be placed above the ID nerve and the distal implants should be placed with slight mesial angulation to facilitate restoration. In the resorbed mandible, implants can be placed in the anterior region mesial to the mental nerve, preferably with the distal implants having distal angulation to enable distal extension of the prosthesis (all-on-four concept) (Malo *et al.*, 2005). Alternatively, short implants can be used in resorbed mandibular ridges or vertical ridge augmentation procedures can be considered.

In the resorbed maxillae, the most distal implants can be placed with a distal angulation parallel with the mesial wall of the maxillary sinus (all-on-four concept). Alternatively, short implants or long implants with sinus augmentation procedures (Thoma *et al.*, 2015) or zygomatic implants (Aparicio *et al.*, 2014) can be used.

Based on systematic reviews (Patzelt *et al.*, 2014), the all-on-four treatment concept offers a predictable approach to treat atrophic jaws in patients who do not prefer ridge augmentation procedures, with reported survival rates of 99.8% for over 24 months (Soto-Penaloza *et al.*, 2017).

The framework for full-arch prostheses can be made using different materials such as gold, base metal alloys, titanium, zirconia and polyether-ether-ketone (PEEK). Various techniques have been used for processing the metal framework (Abduo *et al.*, 2011).

- One-piece casting.
- Sectioning and reconnection.
- Spark erosion with an electric discharge machine.
- Framework bonding to prefabricated abutment cylinders.
- Computer-aided design/computer-assisted manufacturing (CAD/CAM) which provides an excellent fit of frameworks.

The facing of the prosthesis can be made of acrylic teeth or porcelain. Pink acrylic or porcelain can be useful when hard or soft tissue deficiency cannot be fully repaired with ridge/soft tissue augmentation procedures.

Ideally, a minimum of 15 mm vertical space is required from the ridge crest to the planned incisal edge to accommodate the prosthetic components. If there is insufficient vertical space for a fixed full-arch prosthesis, an edentulous arch can be restored with a series of short-span fixed implant-retained bridges without the need for precision fit of a full-arch prosthesis.

Cantilever extensions were first advocated in the Toronto study (Zarb and Schmitt, 1990) and complications arise when the cantilever extension is beyond 15 mm. Distal cantilevers must be avoided in bruxist patients.

Recommended occlusal schemes for full-arch implant-retained fixed prosthesis are as follows (Kim *et al.*, 2005; Sheridan *et al.*, 2016).

- Bilaterally balanced occlusion if the opposing arch is a complete denture.
- Group function occlusion or canine-guided occlusion with shallow anterior guidance if the opposing arch is natural dentition.
- Group function if both arches are implant-retained fixed prostheses.
- No working or balancing occlusal contacts on cantilever extensions.
- Lighter occlusion on cantilever segments.

Case Study

A 55-year-old female patient presented with an old maxillary complete denture and a loose mandibular implant-supported overdenture. The patient had two Branemark implants placed in the mandibular canine areas with ball attachments which had lost their retention.

Clinical examination showed that the mandible was severely atrophic and the peri-implant mucosa was slightly inflamed (Figure 45.1), with no deep pockets. The mandibular overdenture had poor stability and retention and the attachment components were missing from inside the denture. Free-way space was also inadequate due to the space required for ball attachments.

The diagnosis was edentulous and atrophic mandible, unstable old denture, peri-implant mucositis and failed ball attachment.

The treatment strategy was fabrication of a new maxillary complete denture and a mandibular implant-supported overdenture with conversion of ball attachments to locator attachments.

The following clinical procedures were carried out.

1) Oral hygiene instructions and non-surgical debridement of mandibular implants.
2) Primary impressions and fabrication of special trays.
3) Secondary impressions with silicone impression material.
4) Bite registration and shade selection.
5) Trial insertion of dentures.
6) Replacement of ball abutments with locator abutments (Figure 45.2).
7) Insertion of dentures with spaces and vents in mandibular implant areas and fitting locator attachments chairside using cold-cured acrylic resin inside the denture (Figure 45.3).
8) Review and maintenance.

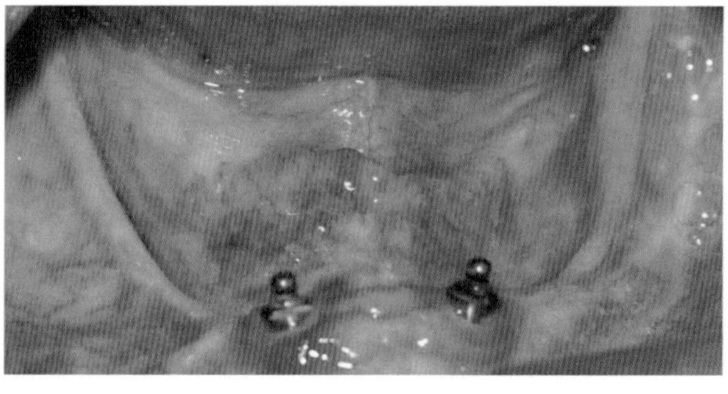

Figure 45.1 Preoperative intraoral clinical photograph of atrophic mandible and ball abutments.

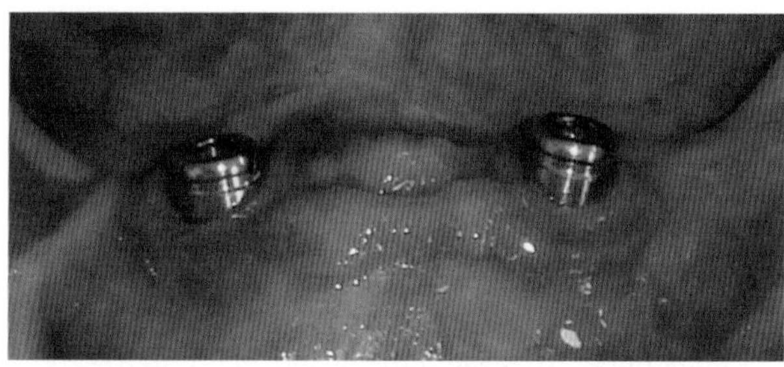

Figure 45.2 Clinical photograph of mandibular locator abutments.

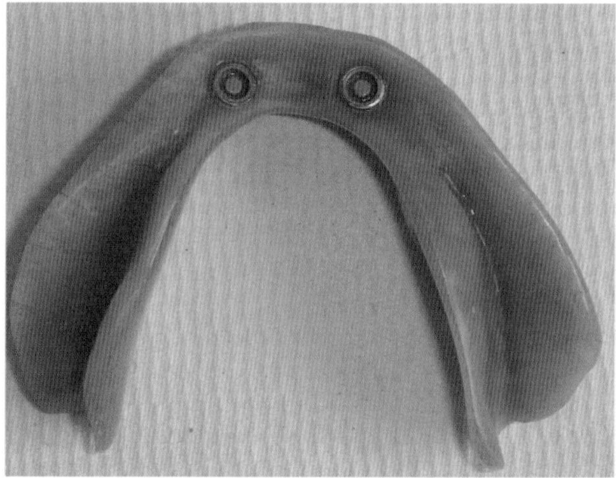

Figure 45.3 Photograph of the fitting surface of the mandibular overdenture with incorporated locator housings and pink retention inserts.

One of the challenges in this case was the class III skeletal jaw relationship. By carefully broadening the maxillary arch and placing the mandibular teeth on the ridge, a satisfactory class I relationship was achieved (Figure 45.4).

Retention of the mandibular overdenture was significantly improved after fitting locator attachments. Short locator abutments also enabled provision of adequate free-way space.

The patient was satisfied with the outcome of treatment and the new implant-supported overdenture was well maintained in the long term.

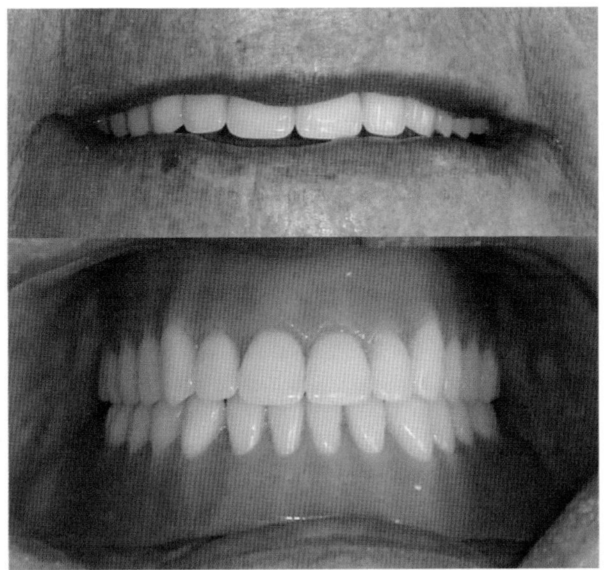

Figure 45.4 Postoperative clinical photograph of the patient's smile and occlusion.

References

Abduo, J., Lyons, K., Bennani, V., Waddell, N. and Swain, M. (2011) Fit of screw-retained fixed implant frameworks fabricated by different methods: a systematic review. *Int J Prosthodont*, **24**, 207–220.

Andreiotelli, M., Att, W. and Strub, J.R. (2010) Prosthodontic complications with implant overdentures: a systematic literature review. *Int J Prosthodont*, **23**, 195–203.

Aparicio, C., Manresa, C., Francisco, K. *et al.* (2014) Zygomatic implants: indications, techniques and outcomes, and the zygomatic success code. *Periodontology 2000*, **66**, 41–58.

Cawood, J.I. and Howell, R.A. (1988) A classification of the edentulous jaws. *Int J Oral Maxillofac Surg*, **17**, 232–236.

Feine, J.S., Carlsson, G.E., Awad, M.A. *et al.* (2002) The Mcgill Consensus Statement on Overdentures. Montreal, Quebec, Canada. May 24–25, 2002. *Int J Prosthodont*, **15**, 413–414.

Gahan, M.J. and Walmsley, A.D. (2005) The neutral zone impression revisited. *Br Dent J*, **198**, 269–272.

Gillings, B.R. (1984) Magnetic denture retention systems: inexpensive and efficient. *Int Dent J*, **34**, 184–197.

Gonda, T., Yang, T.C. and Maeda, Y. (2013) Five-year multicenter study of magnetic attachments used for natural overdenture abutments. *J Oral Rehabil*, **40**, 258–262.

Goodacre, C.J., Bernal, G., Rungcharassaeng, K. and Kan, J.Y. (2003) Clinical complications with implants and implant prostheses. *J Prosthet Dent*, **90**, 121–132.

Heydecke, G., Zwahlen, M., Nicol, A. *et al.* (2012) What is the optimal number of implants for fixed reconstructions: a systematic review. *Clin Oral Implants Res*, **23** Suppl 6, 217–228.

Kim, H.Y., Lee, J.Y., Shin, S.W. and Bryant, S.R. (2012) Attachment systems for mandibular implant overdentures: a systematic review. *J Adv Prosthodont*, **4**, 197–203.

Kim, Y., Oh, T.J., Misch, C.E. and Wang, H.L. (2005) Occlusal considerations in implant therapy: clinical guidelines with biomechanical rationale. *Clin Oral Implants Res*, **16**, 26–35.

Kutkut, A., Bertoli, E., Frazer, R., Pinto-Sinai, G., Fuentealba Hidalgo, R. and Studts, J. (2018) A systematic review of studies comparing conventional complete denture and implant retained overdenture. *J Prosthodont Res*, **62**, 1–9.

Lekholm, U. and Zarb, G.A. (1985) Patient selection and preparation, in *Tissue Integrated Prostheses: Osseointegration in Clinical Dentistry* (eds P.I. Branemark, G.A. Zarb and T. Albrektsson), Quintessence, Chicago, pp. 199–209.

Lynch, C.D. and Allen, P.F. (2006) Overcoming the unstable mandibular complete denture: the neutral zone impression technique. *Dent Update*, **33**, 21–22, 24–26.

Malo, P., Rangert, B. and Nobre, M. (2005) All-on-4 immediate-function concept with branemark system implants for completely edentulous maxillae: a 1-year retrospective clinical study. *Clin Implant Dent Relat Res*, 7 Suppl 1, S88–94.

Morjaria, K.R., Wilson, R. and Palmer, R.M. (2014) Bone healing after tooth extraction with or without an intervention: a systematic review of randomized controlled trials. *Clin Implant Dent Relat Res*, **16**, 1–20.

Patzelt, S.B., Bahat, O., Reynolds, M.A. and Strub, J.R. (2014) The all-on-four treatment concept: a systematic review. *Clin Implant Dent Relat Res*, **16**, 836–855.

Raghoebar, G.M., Meijer, H.J., Slot, W., Slater, J.J. and Vissink, A. (2014) A systematic review of implant-supported overdentures in the edentulous maxilla, compared to the mandible: how many implants? *Eur J Oral Implantol*, 7 Suppl 2, S191–201.

Roccuzzo, M., Bonino, F., Gaudioso, L., Zwahlen, M. and Meijer, H.J. (2012) What is the optimal number of implants for removable reconstructions? A systematic review on implant-supported overdentures. *Clin Oral Implants Res*, **23** Suppl 6, 229–237.

Sadowsky, S.J. and Zitzmann, N.U. (2016) Protocols for the maxillary implant overdenture: a systematic review. *Int J Oral Maxillofac Implants*, **31** Suppl, S182–191.

Sheridan, R.A., Decker, A.M., Plonka, A.B. and Wang, H.L. (2016) The role of occlusion in implant therapy: a comprehensive updated review. *Implant Dent*, **25**, 829–838.

Soto-Penaloza, D., Zaragozi-Alonso, R., Penarrocha-Diago, M. and Penarrocha-Diago, M. (2017) The all-on-four treatment concept: systematic review. *J Clin Exp Dent*, **9**, E474–E488.

Tallgren, A. (2003) The continuing reduction of the residual alveolar ridges in complete denture wearers: a mixed-longitudinal study covering 25 years. *J Prosthet Dent*, **89**, 427–435.

Thoma, D.S., Zeltner, M., Husler, J., Hammerle, C.H. and Jung, R.E. (2015) EAO Supplement Working Group 4 - EAO CC 2015 short implants versus sinus lifting with longer implants to restore the posterior maxilla: a systematic review. *Clin Oral Implants Res*, **26** Suppl 11, 154–169.

Thomason, J.M., Feine, J., Exley, C. *et al.* (2009) Mandibular two implant-supported overdentures as the first choice standard of care for edentulous patients – the York Consensus Statement. *Br Dent J*, **207**, 185–186.

Thomason, J.M., Kelly, S.A., Bendkowski, A. and Ellis, J.S. (2012) Two implant retained overdentures – a review of the literature supporting the McGill and York consensus statements. *J Dent*, **40**, 22–34.

Walmsley, A.D. (2002) Magnetic retention in prosthetic dentistry. *Dent Update*, **29**, 428–433.

Willenbacher, M., Al-Nawas, B., Berres, M., Kammerer, P.W. and Schiegnitz, E. (2016) The effects of alveolar ridge preservation: a meta-analysis. *Clin Implant Dent Relat Res*, **18**, 1248–1268.

Zarb, G.A. and Schmitt, A. (1990) The longitudinal clinical effectiveness of osseointegrated dental implants: the Toronto Study. Part III: Problems and complications encountered. *J Prosthet Dent*, **64**, 185–194.

46

Ridge Defects (Localised)

Ian Brook and Abdurahman El-Awa - Case study

46.1 Introduction

An extraction socket heals in several stages, including blood clot formation (2–3 days), granulation tissue (4–5 days), young connective tissue/osteoid formation (1 week), start of osteoid mineralisation/epithelial coverage (3 weeks), and bone formation (6 weeks). Bone resorption of the walls of the socket occurs after extraction and the alveolar bone width continues to shrink by 30% in 3 months and 50% in 12 months (Schropp *et al.*, 2003). Buccal bone reduction is often more severe than lingual/palatal wall resorption. Horizontal bone loss of 29–63% and vertical bone loss of 11–22% after 6 months following tooth extraction have been reported in a systematic review (Tan *et al.*, 2012).

Various techniques have been suggested to reduce ridge resorption following extraction of teeth (Masaki *et al.*, 2015).

- Flap elevation for complete soft tissue closure
- Placement of connective tissue grafts over the extraction sites
- Placement of bone grafts
- Use of barrier membranes

However, some of the limitations of socket preservation techniques using bone grafts and membranes include the following.

- Long healing period before implant therapy.
- Being invasive and technique sensitive.
- Difficulty achieving soft tissue coverage which may lead to compromised aesthetic results.
- High cost.
- Unable to stop ridge resorption completely (Horvath *et al.*, 2013).

Soft tissue collapse following extraction may be prevented by immediate postextraction placement of an ovate pontic to support the soft tissues. This approach can be particularly helpful in multiple extraction situations.

Localised ridge defects can be classified as follows (Seibert, 1983).

- Class I: reduced buccolingual width of the ridge but normal apicocoronal height
- Class II: reduced apicocoronal height of the ridge but normal buccolingual width
- Class III: a combined loss of the width and height of the alveolar ridge

The following sections describe different surgical techniques for ridge augmentation, including soft and hard tissue grafts.

46.2 Ridge Augmentation by Soft Tissue Grafts

Soft tissue grafting is indicated where bone volume is adequate but soft tissues are deficient. The aim is to increase the bulk of missing gingival tissues around prostheses to improve aesthetics, optimise soft tissue coverage and in some cases to increase the amount of keratinised tissue around restorations. Alternatively, some patients may choose the option of using pink-coloured restorative material to replace the missing soft tissues to avoid surgical ridge augmentation and soft tissue grafting.

Different options for soft tissue grafting procedures include the following.

- *The pedicle graft procedure* such as the roll flap (Abrams, 1980) is used for short-span (single tooth/implant) ridge defects with minor loss of height and width. It involves preparation of a connective tissue pedicle graft from the palatal aspect of the ridge which is then rotated and placed into a subepithelial pouch on the buccal side (Veisman, 1998).
- *Free graft procedures* are mainly indicated for larger soft tissue defects (Lang and Lindhe, 2015). Options include the following.

Diseases and Conditions in Dentistry: An Evidence-Based Reference, First Edition. Keyvan Moharamzadeh.

Companion website: www.wiley.com/go/moharamzadeh/diseases

- Pouch grafts are suitable for class I defects and involve preparation of a subepithelial pouch in the area of the ridge defect, and placement of a free connective tissue graft harvested from the palate or tuberosity into the pouch.
- Interpositional grafts are used for class I and small-to-moderate class II ridge defects. The harvested graft contains both epithelium and connective tissue. The connective tissue part of the graft is inserted into an envelope in the recipient site and the epithelial side of the graft is left exposed.
- Onlay grafts are indicated for class II and III defects to gain additional ridge height and involve placement of an epithelialised free graft (harvested from the palate) on de-epithelialised connective tissue of the recipient site. Onlay grafts are contraindicated when there are additional mucogingival problems such as insufficient gingival width, high frenum and gingival scarring.
- Combined onlay-interpositional grafts have been used for class III defects.

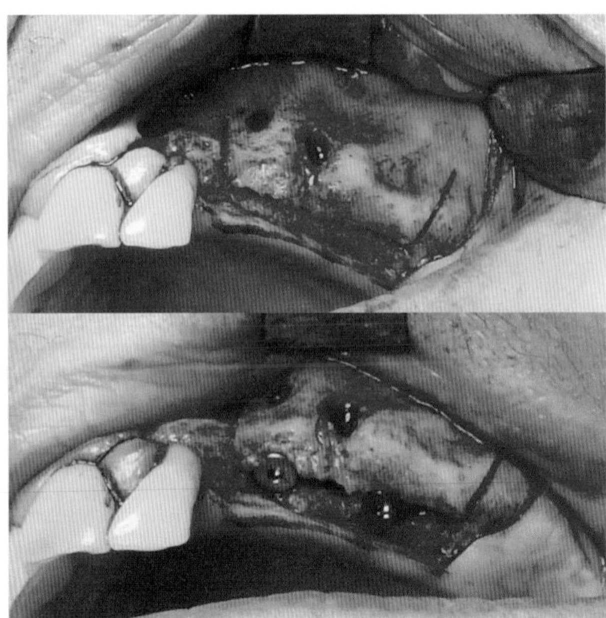

Figure 46.1 Segmental osteotomy in split crest technique to horizontally augment the atrophic maxillary ridge and insert implants within the split ridge.

46.3 Ridge Augmentation with Hard Tissue Surgery

Strategies for augmentation of the alveolar ridge can be divided into two categories: anatomical repositioning techniques and bone grafting procedures (Paknejad *et al.*, 2017).

46.3.1 Anatomical Repositioning Techniques

- *Inferior alveolar nerve repositioning*: in this procedure, the inferior alveolar nerve is freed from its canal, repositioned laterally, implants are placed in the posterior mandible, and then the nerve is placed adjacent to the implants (Abayev and Juodzbalys, 2015a). A major risk of this approach is potential nerve damage and subsequent neurosensory dysfunction (Abayev and Juodzbalys, 2015b).
- *Distraction osteogenesis (DO)*: DO is based on the formation of new bone following gradual segmental bone separation in an osteotomy site without the need for harvesting of bone graft. DO has been used to augment atrophic alveolar ridges in vertical or horizontal directions and it enables simultaneous bone and soft tissue augmentation with predictable outcomes (Yun *et al.*, 2016).
- *Split crest technique (inlay grafting)*: this procedure involves segmental osteotomy of the ridge and placement of bone graft materials within the split ridge (Figure 46.1). Although this can be a difficult surgical technique, it is associated with a high success rate of the augmented bone and survival of the inserted dental implants (Mestas *et al.*, 2016).

46.3.2 Bone Grafting

Other surgical hard tissue grafting techniques for ridge augmentation are listed below.

- *Onlay block grafting* using autologous bone grafts harvested from either intraoral sites (such as the mandibular symphysis, ascending ramus, maxillary tuberosity and anterior palate for the repair of small defects) or extraoral sites (such as iliac crest, calvaria, tibia, femur and fibula for reconstruction of large defects). The onlay block graft is usually placed and fixed onto the prepared recipient site. It has been shown that the survival and success rates of implants placed in resorbed ridges augmented with intraoral onlay block bone grafts are high, ranging from 96.9% to 100% for horizontal ridge augmentation, and 89.5% to 100% for vertical augmentation (Aloy-Prosper *et al.*, 2015).
- *Guided bone regeneration (GBR)* involves using different types of bone substitutes such as allografts, xenografts and synthetic materials, and placement of barrier membranes (resorbable or non-resorbable) over a defect for space maintenance and to provide an ideal environment for new bone formation (Troeltzsch *et al.*, 2016). The most frequently used GBR method is the combination of xenografts and resorbable

membranes (Sanz-Sanchez *et al.*, 2015). Bioactive factors such as platelet-derived growth factor (PDGF), insulin-like growth factor (IGF) and bone morphogenic proteins (BMPs) have been studied to further promote osteogenesis (Almela *et al.*, 2017). It is important to have adequate soft tissue and periosteal release of the buccal/labial flap to ensure full soft tissue coverage of the grafted materials and the membrane.

- *Combination of block grafting and GBR* is a predictable surgical technique as the use of membrane over autologous block grafts reduces its resorption rate (Antoun *et al.*, 2001). Details of this procedure are given in the clinical case at the end of this chapter.

It has been shown that the survival of implants in augmented ridges using GBR is high (above 90% in most studies) and similar to that of normal ridge (Hammerle *et al.*, 2002). It appears that GBR is a predictable technique that allows the placement of implants in atrophic areas (Clementini *et al.*, 2012; Esposito *et al.*, 2009).

Vertical ridge augmentation in the atrophic mandible can be challenging and the use of short implants can be an alternative approach to vertical bone grafting (Esposito *et al.*, 2009). Evidence shows that if around 4 mm vertical ridge augmentation is required in an atrophic mandible, DO, inlay bone grafting, onlay block grafting and GBR are all equally reliable. However, when greater vertical ridge augmentation is required, DO and inlay bone grafting appear to be superior to the other techniques in the atrophic mandible. GBR shows the lowest complications and vertical bone resorption. Implant survival and success are high and similar for all techniques (Elnayef *et al.*, 2017).

Case Study

This clinical case demonstrates horizontal and vertical bone augmentation of a severe localised maxillary alveolar ridge defect in a 21-year-old male patient following resection of a central giant cell granuloma lesion in the UR1–UR4 region.

Radiographic assessment showed significant vertical bone loss (Figure 46.2) and cone beam computed tomography (CBCT) also revealed severe horizontal and vertical alveolar ridge defect (Figure 46.3) in the right maxilla.

Ridge augmentation with onlay block grafting, using autologous bone harvested from the anterior mandible, and simultaneous GBR, using xenograft bone substitute and resorbable membrane, was carried out under general anaesthesia as described below.

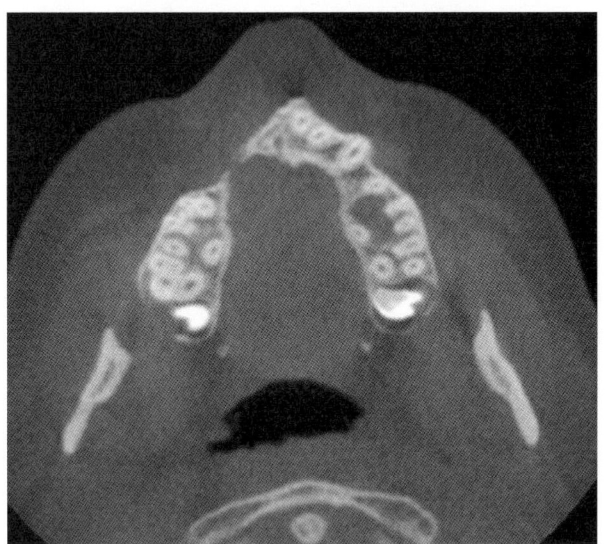

Figure 46.3 Preoperative CBCT showing severe alveolar ridge defect in the right maxilla.

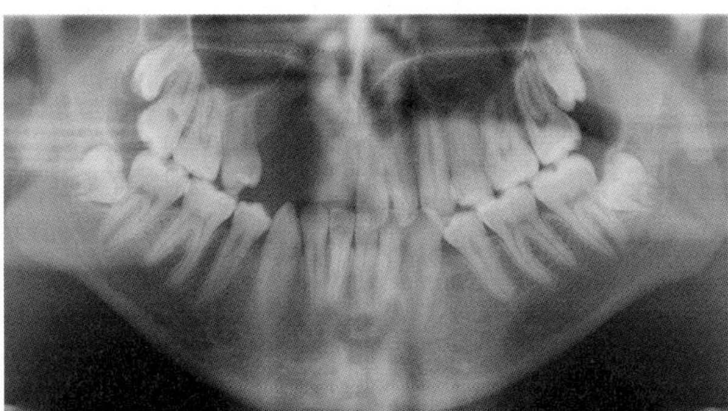

Figure 46.2 Preoperative oral panoramic radiograph showing significant vertical bone defect in the maxillary right canine region and adequate bone height in the anterior mandible suitable for harvesting a block graft.

1) Full-thickness flap elevation of UR1–UR4 and preparation of the recipient site as demonstrated in Figure 46.4.
2) Harvest of autologous bone block grafts from the anterior mandible (Figure 46.5).
3) Fixing the block grafts onto the recipient site using bone screws (Figure 46.6) and simultaneous GBR using bovine-derived bone graft substitute (Bio-Oss®, Geistlich, Wolhusen, Switzerland) and porcine-derived sterile resorbable bilayer collagen membrane (Bio-Gide®, Geistlich).
4) Flap advancement and wound closure.

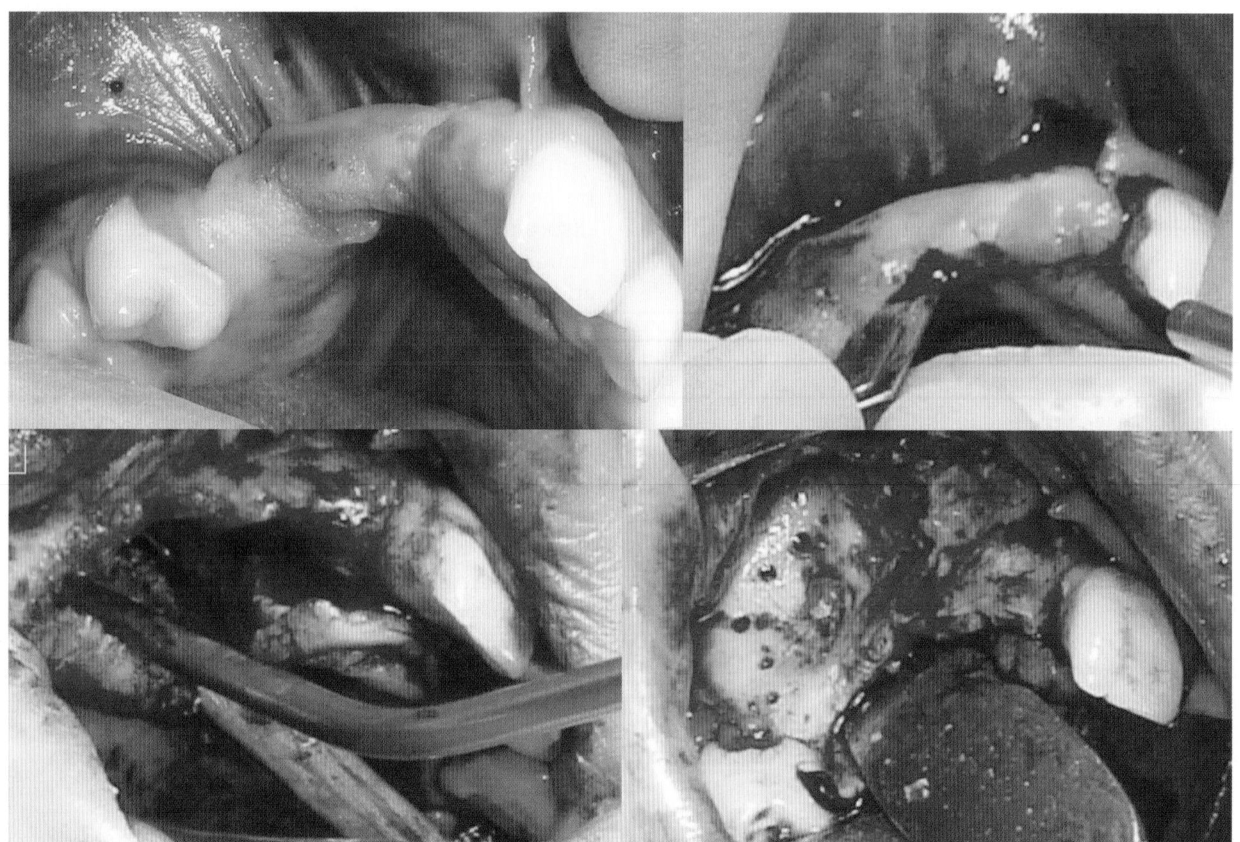

Figure 46.4 Preparation of the recipient site UR1–UR4 involving a crestal incision with two mesial and distal releasing incisions, elevation of full-thickness mucoperiosteal flaps buccally and palatally, periosteal release to mobilise the buccal flap, and piercing the cortical bone on the buccal side.

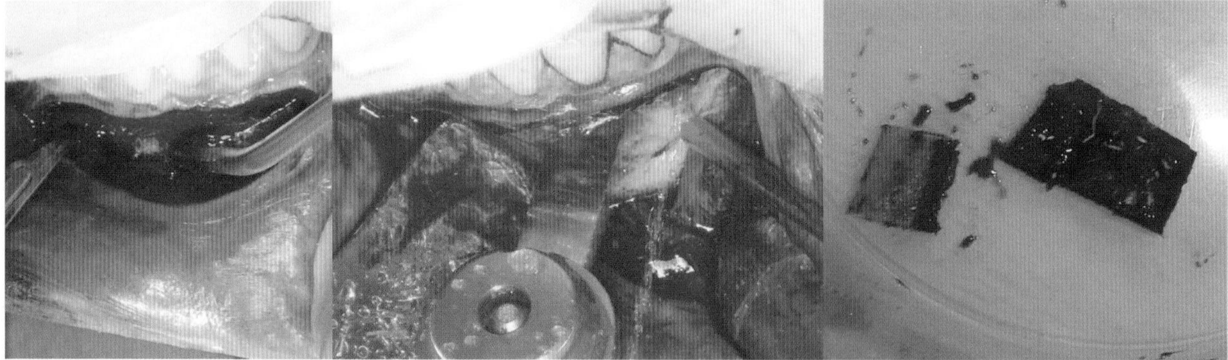

Figure 46.5 Harvesting an autologous intraoral block bone graft from the anterior mandible. Images showing a horizontal incision through the alveolar mucosa in the mandibular incisor region to access the donor site bone below the roots of the teeth, monocortical bone cuts using an osteotomy saw under saline irrigation, and separated block grafts (using chisels).

The augmented ridge healed well and dental implants were placed at the healed site after 6 months to enable prosthetic rehabilitation of the missing teeth in the right maxilla (Figure 46.7).

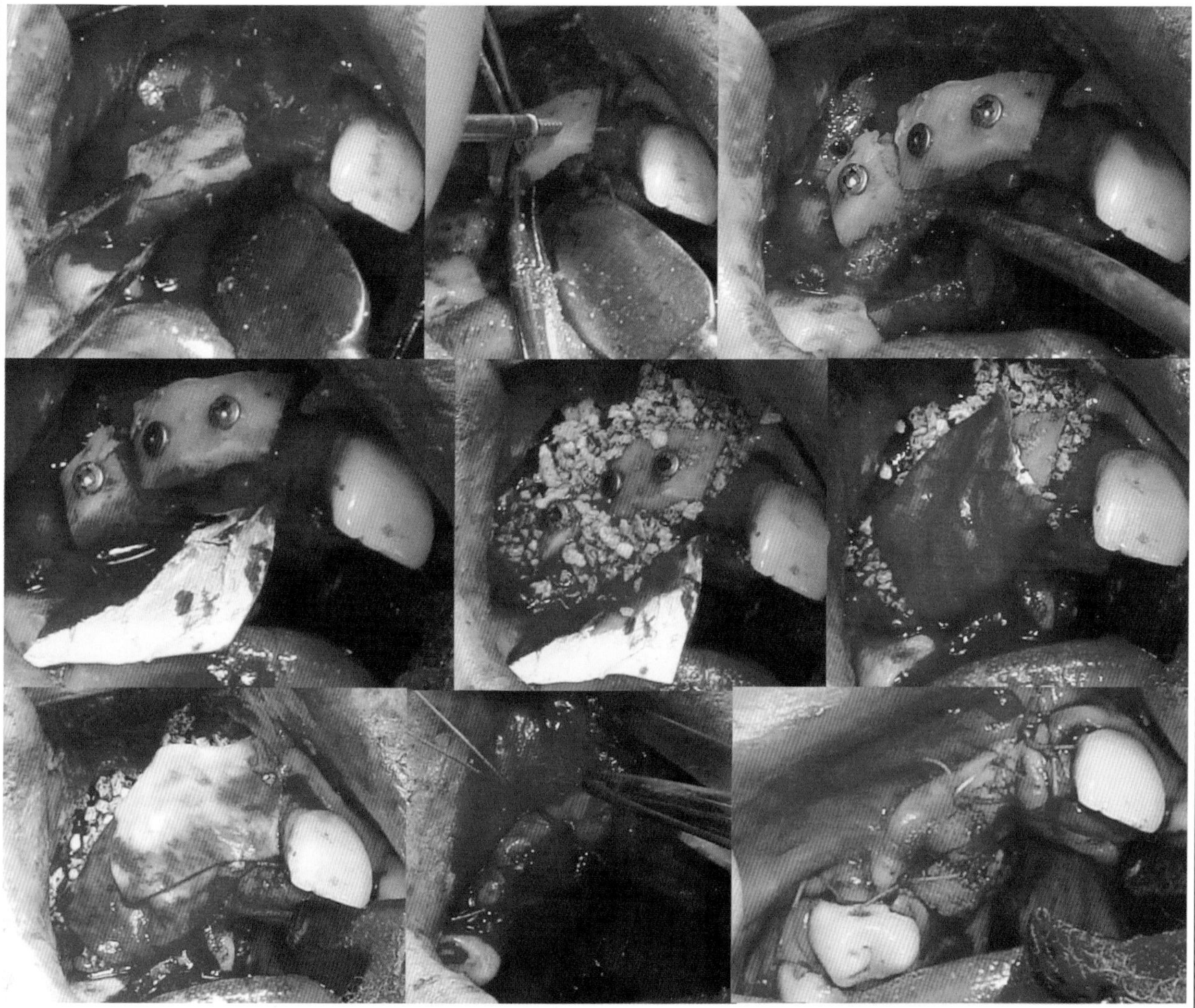

Figure 46.6 Onlay grafting and GBR procedure involving passive adaptation of the block bone graft on the recipient area, fixation of the bone graft using screws, adaptation of one end of the membrane under the palatal flap, packing of particulate bone substitute around the block graft, coverage of the graft materials with double membranes, soft tissue advancement and closure with suturing.

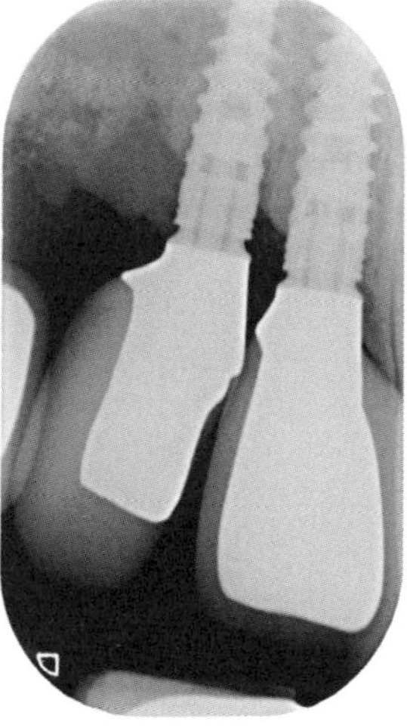

Figure 46.7 Postoperative periapical radiograph of the restored implants placed in the grafted bone.

References

Abayev, B. and Juodzbalys, G. (2015a) Inferior alveolar nerve lateralization and transposition for dental implant placement. Part I: A systematic review of surgical techniques. *J Oral Maxillofac Res*, **6**, E2.

Abayev, B. and Juodzbalys, G. (2015b) Inferior alveolar nerve lateralization and transposition for dental implant placement. Part II: A systematic review of neurosensory complications. *J Oral Maxillofac Res*, **6**, E3.

Abrams, L. (1980) Augmentation of the deformed residual edentulous ridge for fixed prosthesis. *Compend Contin Educ Gen Dent*, **1**, 205–213.

Almela, T., Brook, I. and Moharamzadeh, K. (2017) Bone tissue engineering in maxillofacial region, in *Biomaterials for Oral and Dental Tissue Engineering* (eds L. Tayebi and K. Moharamzadeh), Woodhead Publishing, Duxford, pp. 387–404.

Aloy-Prosper, A., Penarrocha-Oltra, D., Penarrocha-Diago, M. and Penarrocha-Diago, M. (2015) The outcome of intraoral onlay block bone grafts on alveolar ridge augmentations: a systematic review. *Med Oral Patol Oral Cir Bucal*, **20**, E251–258.

Antoun, H., Sitbon, J.M., Martinez, H. and Missika, P. (2001) A prospective randomized study comparing two techniques of bone augmentation: onlay graft alone or associated with a membrane. *Clin Oral Implants Res*, **12**, 632–639.

Clementini, M., Morlupi, A., Canullo, L., Agrestini, C. and Barlattani, A. (2012) Success rate of dental implants inserted in horizontal and vertical guided bone regenerated areas: a systematic review. *Int J Oral Maxillofac Surg*, **41**, 847–852.

Elnayef, B., Monje, A., Gargallo-Albiol, J., Galindo-Moreno, P., Wang, H.L. and Hernández-Alfaro, F. (2017) Vertical ridge augmentation in the atrophic mandible: a systematic review and meta-analysis. *Int J Oral Maxillofac Implants*, **32**(2), 291–312.

Esposito, M., Grusovin, M.G., Felice, P., Karatzopoulos, G., Worthington, H.V. and Coulthard, P. (2009) Interventions for replacing missing teeth: horizontal and vertical bone augmentation techniques for dental implant treatment. *Cochrane Database Syst Rev*, **3**, CD003607.

Hammerle, C.H., Jung, R.E. and Feloutzis, A. (2002) A systematic review of the survival of implants in bone sites augmented with barrier membranes (guided bone regeneration) in partially edentulous patients. *J Clin Periodontol*, **29** Suppl 3, 226–231; discussion 232–233.

Horvath, A., Mardas, N., Mezzomo, L.A., Needleman, I.G. and Donos, N. (2013) Alveolar ridge preservation. *A systematic review. Clin Oral Invest*, **17**, 341–363.

Lang, N.P. and Lindhe, J. (2015) *Clinical Periodontology and Implant Dentistry*, Wiley-Blackwell, Oxford.

Masaki, C., Nakamoto, T., Mukaibo, T., Kondo, Y. and Hosokawa, R. (2015) Strategies for alveolar ridge reconstruction and preservation for implant therapy. *J Prosthodont Res*, **59**, 220–228.

Mestas, G., Alarcon, M. and Chambrone, L. (2016) Long-term survival rates of titanium implants placed in expanded alveolar ridges using split crest procedures: a systematic review. *Int J Oral Maxillofac Implants*, **31**, 591–599.

Paknejad, Z., Jafart, M., Nazeman, P., Rezai Rad, M. and Khojasteh, A. (2017) Periodontal and peri-implant hard tissue regeneration, in *Biomaterials for Oral and Dental Tissue Engineering* (eds L. Tayebi and K. Moharamzadeh), Woodhead Publishing, Duxford, pp. 405–428.

Sanz-Sanchez, I., Ortiz-Vigon, A., Sanz-Martin, I., Figuero, E. and Sanz, M. (2015) Effectiveness of lateral bone augmentation on the alveolar crest dimension: a systematic review and meta-analysis. *J Dent Res*, **94**, 128s–42s.

Schropp, L., Wenzel, A., Kostopoulos, L. and Karring, T. (2003) Bone healing and soft tissue contour changes following single-tooth extraction: a clinical and radiographic 12-month prospective study. *Int J Periodont Restorat Dent*, **23**, 313–323.

Seibert, J.S. (1983) Reconstruction of deformed, partially edentulous ridges, using full thickness onlay grafts. Part I. Technique and wound healing. *Compend Contin Educ Dent*, **4**, 437–453.

Tan, W.L., Wong, T.L., Wong, M.C. and Lang, N.P. (2012) A systematic review of post-extractional alveolar hard and soft tissue dimensional changes in humans. *Clin Oral Implants Res*, **23** Suppl 5, 1–21.

Troeltzsch, M., Troeltzsch, M., Kauffmann, P. *et al.* (2016) Clinical efficacy of grafting materials in alveolar ridge augmentation: a systematic review. *J Craniomaxillofac Surg*, **44**, 1618–1629.

Veisman, H. (1998) 'The palatal roll'. Soft tissue ridge augmentation using a subepithelial connective tissue pedicle graft. *Oral Health*, **88**, 47, 49–51; quiz 53.

Yun, K.I., Choi, H., Wright, R.F., Ahn, H.S., Chang, B.M. and Kim, H.J. (2016) Efficacy of alveolar vertical distraction osteogenesis and autogenous bone grafting for dental implants: systematic review and meta-analysis. *Int J Oral Maxillofac Implants*, **31**, 26–36.

47

Shortened Dental Arch (SDA)

47.1 Definition

The shortened dental arch (SDA) is defined as compromised dentition with reduced number of posterior molar and premolar teeth and is frequently referred to as the absence of molar teeth (Witter *et al.*, 1999).

47.2 History

The concept of the SDA was introduced by Kayser (1981), who showed that four pairs of occluding premolars are sufficient for satisfactory masticatory function and patients maintained adequate (50–80%) chewing capacity with premolar occlusion.

The World Health Organization (WHO) has highlighted that a minimum number of 20 teeth throughout life is required to maintain a natural dentition with an acceptable level of oral function (Armellini and von Fraunhofer, 2004).

The SDA concept has been subject to debate over many years and there have been various opinions in terms of its suitability as a treatment option. However, it still remains a viable management approach in many patients and the majority of the studies support this concept, although there has been a recent attitude shift and increase in studies opposing the concept (Manola *et al.*, 2017).

47.3 Effect of SDA on Oral Health-Related Quality of Life

It has been shown that the patterns of missing occlusal units appear to be related to oral health-related quality of life (OHRQoL) impairment in patients with SDA and the presence of the first molar contact has a particularly high impact (Baba *et al.*, 2008).

A systematic review and meta-analysis by Fueki and Baba (2017) showed that there was no statistically significant difference in oral health impact profile (OHIP) summary scores between SDA and removable partial denture treatment at different postoperative time intervals up to 1 year. Only one non-randomised clinical trial with small sample size showed higher OHRQoL with implant-retained fixed prosthesis in comparison with SDA but the differences in OHIP summary scores were not statistically significant.

47.4 Effect of Tooth Loss on Masticatory Function

The loss of teeth has been associated with reduced masticatory function (Ikebe *et al.*, 2012) and masticatory performance is significantly affected by the position and number of occluding pairs of residual teeth (Gotfredsen and Walls, 2007; Ikebe *et al.*, 2011; Kayser, 1981). It has been shown that subjects with extreme SDA had 30–40% reduced masticatory function and distal-extension removable partial dentures can partially compensate for this reduction by approximately 50% (Liang *et al.*, 2015; Moore and McKenna, 2016).

Studies show that elderly people can maintain acceptable occlusal function with a reduced dentition consisting of 10 or even fewer occluding pairs. The minimum number of teeth required for a functional dental arch varies between individuals and depends on several local and systemic factors, including age, periodontal status of the remaining teeth, occlusal activity, spatial relationship between the maxillary and mandibular teeth, and the adaptive capacity of the patient (Kayser, 1990).

47.5 Effect of SDA on Occlusal Stability

Extreme shortened dental arches with fewer than two pairs of occluding premolars may be at increased risk of tooth movement which can result in changes such as

Diseases and Conditions in Dentistry: An Evidence-Based Reference, First Edition. Keyvan Moharamzadeh.

Companion website: www.wiley.com/go/moharamzadeh/diseases

interdental spacing, vertical overlap and increased contacts on incisor teeth and mobility (Sarita *et al.*, 2003). These changes are often minor, adaptive and self-limiting and remain stable over time (Witter *et al.*, 2001).

Studies show that for most patients, 3–4 functional posterior units with a symmetrical tooth loss pattern or 5–6 units with an asymmetrical pattern are sufficient to provide occlusal support and stability (Gotfredsen and Walls, 2007). However, an SDA with periodontally compromised teeth may show further periodontal breakdown (Witter *et al.*, 1994a).

47.6 Effect of SDA on Temporomandibular Joint

Some studies have reported that patients who lose their posterior teeth may have a higher prevalence of temporomandibular disorders (TMD), especially young women (Tallents *et al.*, 2002; Wang *et al.*, 2009). Other studies show that the SDA is not a risk factor for TMD and can provide sufficient oral comfort in the long term (Witter *et al.*, 1994b), and there is no relationship between SDA and symptoms of TMD (Gotfredsen and Walls, 2007). Therefore, there are continued arguments for and against the effects of the SDA on the temporomandibular joint (Manola *et al.*, 2017).

47.7 Alternative Treatment Options

Although SDA is still a viable, simple and low-cost management approach for many patients, other prosthetic treatment options should also be considered and discussed with patients, including the risks and benefits of each.

- Removable partial dentures (see Chapter 38)
- Resin-bonded or conventional bridges (see Chapter 25)
- Implant-retained fixed prostheses (see Chapter 37)

Case Study

A 78-year-old female patient was referred from the oral medicine clinic for prosthetic rehabilitation of the edentulous maxilla (Figure 47.1) and partially dentate mandible (Figure 47.2). The patient complained of an uncomfortable, unstable and non-retentive upper complete denture and missing many of the lower teeth.

The patient was under treatment for lichen planus in the oral medicine department.

Clinical and radiographic examination confirmed the following diagnoses.

- Edentulous and atrophic maxillary arch with an unstable and non-retentive complete denture.
- Mild chronic periodontitis and gingival recession of the remaining mandibular teeth (canines and premolars).
- Lichen planus and hyperkeratosis.

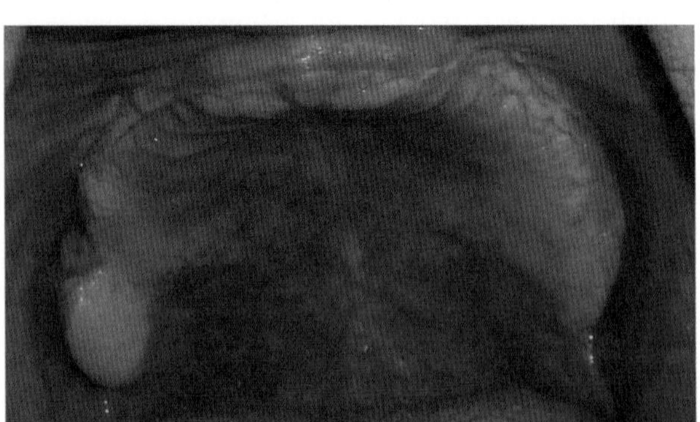

Figure 47.1 Preoperative clinical photograph of the edentulous maxillary arch showing atrophic ridge, reduced sulcus depth and white mucosal lesions.

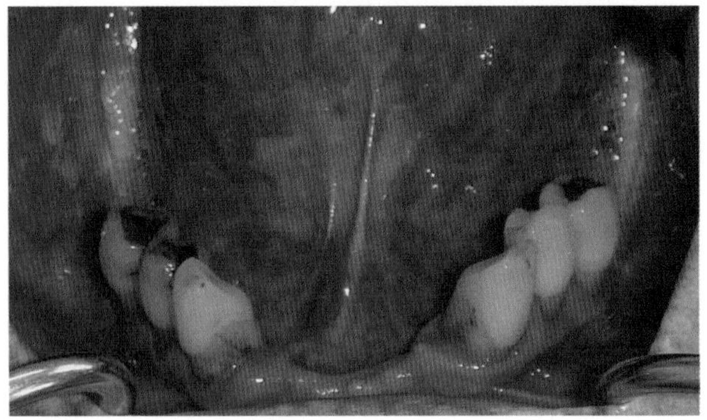

Figure 47.2 Preoperative clinical photograph of the partially dentate mandible showing missing mandibular incisor and molar teeth, gingival recession and white mucosal lesions on the posterior ridge and buccal mucosa.

Restorative treatment strategy included the following points.

- Non-surgical periodontal treatment and preventive care.
- Fabrication of a new maxillary complete denture.
- Resin-bonded bridge from LR3 to LL3 to replace the missing mandibular incisor teeth and maintain a shortened dental arch in the mandible.
- Supportive periodontal therapy (SPT) and maintenance.

The postoperative intraoral photograph is shown in Figure 47.3 and the postoperative smile photograph is shown in Figure 47.4.

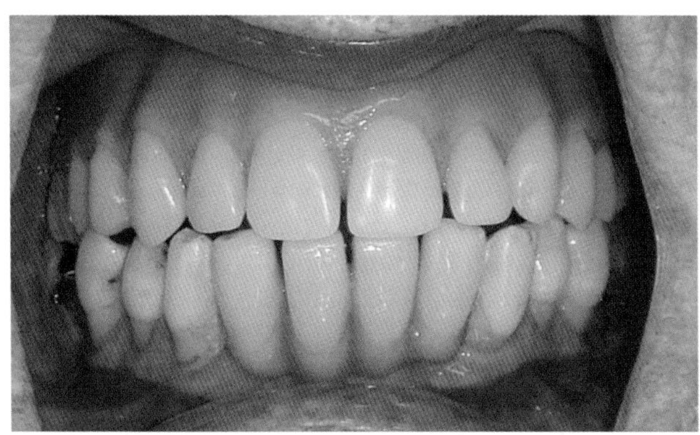

Figure 47.3 Postoperative photograph of the maxillary complete denture against a mandibular shortened dental arch restored with a resin-bonded bridge.

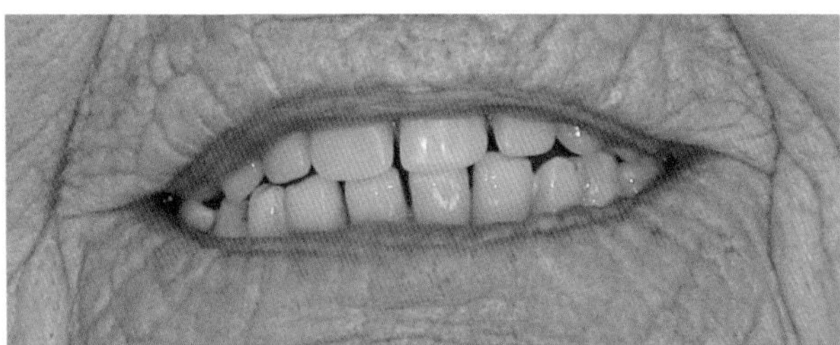

Figure 47.4 Postoperative photograph of the patient's smile.

There were several interesting points in this case.

- Border moulding of the special tray and adequate posterior extension of the denture base resulted in significant improvement of the retention and stability of the maxillary denture.
- The space between the mandibular canines was too wide for four incisor teeth. However, the patient wanted to have spaces between her anterior teeth. This was very helpful in designing the lower anterior bridge as it allowed the placement of spaces between the pontics to address her aesthetic concern.
- There was 3–4 mm gingival recession associated with the remaining mandibular teeth and a marked reduction in the width and height of the alveolar ridge in the lower anterior region. Pink porcelain was used on the gingival margin of the pontics to produce a favourable aesthetic result and also a hygienic pontic design provided access for cleaning under the bridge.

The patient was very satisfied with the outcome of treatment. She reported that significant improvement in the appearance of the teeth had a very positive psychological impact on her, which improved her quality of life and she felt much happier and more sociable. The patient was discharged to her general dental practitioner for long-term dental care and maintenance.

References

Armellini, D. and von Fraunhofer, J. A. (2004) The shortened dental arch: a review of the literature. *J Prosthet Dent*, **92**, 531–535.

Baba, K., Igarashi, Y., Nishiyama, A. *et al.* (2008) Patterns of missing occlusal units and oral health-related quality of life in SDA patients. *J Oral Rehabil*, **35**, 621–628.

Fueki, K. and Baba, K. (2017) Shortened dental arch and prosthetic effect on oral health-related quality of life: a systematic review and meta-analysis. *J Oral Rehabil*, **44**, 563–572.

Gotfredsen, K. and Walls, A.W. (2007) What dentition assures oral function? *Clin Oral Implants Res*, **18** Suppl 3, 34–45.

Ikebe, K., Matsuda, K., Kagawa, R. *et al.* (2011) Association of masticatory performance with age, gender, number of teeth, occlusal force and salivary flow in Japanese older adults: is ageing a risk factor for masticatory dysfunction? *Arch Oral Biol*, **56**, 991–996.

Ikebe, K., Matsuda, K., Kagawa, R. *et al.* (2012) Masticatory performance in older subjects with varying degrees of tooth loss. *J Dent*, **40**, 71–76.

Kayser, A.F. (1981) Shortened dental arches and oral function. *J Oral Rehabil*, **8**, 457–462.

Kayser, A.F. (1990) How much reduction of the dental arch is functionally acceptable for the ageing patient? *Int Dent J*, **40**, 183–188.

Liang, S., Zhang, Q., Witter, D.J., Wang, Y. and Creugers, N.H. (2015) Effects of removable dental prostheses on masticatory performance of subjects with shortened dental arches: a systematic review. *J Dent*, **43**, 1185–1194.

Manola, M., Hussain, F. and Millar, B.J. (2017) Is the shortened dental arch still a satisfactory option? *Br Dent J*, **223**, 108–112.

Moore, C. and McKenna, G. (2016) In patients with shortened dental arches do removable dental prostheses improve masticatory performance? *Evid Based Dent*, **17**, 114.

Sarita, P.T., Kreulen, C.M., Witter, D.J., van't Hof, M. and Creugers, N.H. (2003) A study on occlusal stability in shortened dental arches. *Int J Prosthodont*, **16**, 375–380.

Tallents, R.H., Macher, D.J., Kyrkanides, S., Katzberg, R.W. and Moss, M.E. (2002) Prevalence of missing posterior teeth and intraarticular temporomandibular disorders. *J Prosthet Dent*, **87**, 45–50.

Wang, M.Q., Xue, F., He, J.J., Chen, J.H., Chen, C.S. and Raustia, A. (2009) Missing posterior teeth and risk of temporomandibular disorders. *J Dent Res*, **88**, 942–945.

Witter, D.J., de Haan, A.F., Kayser, A.F. and van Rossum, G.M. (1994a) A 6-year follow-up study of oral function in shortened dental arches. Part I: Occlusal stability. *J Oral Rehabil*, **21**, 113–125.

Witter, D.J., de Haan, A.F., Kayser, A.F. and van Rossum, G.M. (1994b) A 6-year follow-up study of oral function in shortened dental arches. Part II: Craniomandibular dysfunction and oral comfort. *J Oral Rehabil*, **21**, 353–366.

Witter, D.J., van Palenstein Helderman, W.H., Creugers, N.H. and Kayser, A.F. (1999) The shortened dental arch concept and its implications for oral health care. *Commun Dent Oral Epidemiol*, **27**, 249–258.

Witter, D.J., Creugers, N.H., Kreulen, C.M. and de Haan, A.F. (2001) Occlusal stability in shortened dental arches. *J Dent Res*, **80**, 432–436.

48

Supernumerary, Fusion and Gemination

48.1 Supernumerary (Hyperdontia)

A supernumerary tooth is a tooth additional to the normal dentition and can be found in any area in the dental arch.

48.1 1 Prevalence

The prevalence of supernumerary teeth ranges from 0.1% to 3.8% (Rajab and Hamdan, 2002). Most cases present as single tooth supernumerary, mainly in the permanent dentition. The most common area is the maxillary incisor site followed by retromolar, premolar and canine areas. Multiple supernumeraries are mostly found in the mandibular premolar region (Ata-Ali *et al.*, 2014).

48.1.2 Classification

Supernumerary teeth can be categorised based on their position into anterior mesiodens, para-premolars, paramolars and disto-molars (Garvey *et al.*, 1999).

Supernumeraries can also be classified based on their morphology into the following types (Garvey *et al.*, 1999).

- *Conical*, which are peg shaped and sometimes inverted into the palate.
- *Tuberculate*, which possess more than one cusp or tubercle and are barrel shaped, invaginated and often paired on the palatal aspect of central incisors.
- *Supplemental*, which appear like a normal tooth, most commonly the lateral incisor.
- *Odontome*, which can be complex or compound.

48.1.3 Aetiology

Genetic and environmental factors may play a role in the aetiology of supernumerary teeth (Anthonappa *et al.*, 2013). The following conditions and syndromes have been associated with supernumerary teeth (Lubinsky and Kantaputra, 2016).

- Cleidocranial dysostosis
- Gardner's syndrome (familial adenomatous polyposis)
- Cleft lip and cleft palate
- Down's syndrome
- Nance–Horan syndrome
- Rubinstein–Taybi syndrome
- Tricho-rhino-phalangeal syndrome
- Opitz BBB/G syndrome
- Craniometaphyseal dysplasia
- Robinow's syndrome
- Oculofaciocardiodental syndrome
- Orofaciodigital syndrome

48.1.4 Oral and Dental Complications

Supernumerary teeth may cause several complications, such as failure of eruption or delayed eruption of permanent teeth, rotation or displacement of other teeth, crowding, dentigerous cyst formation and root resorption of adjacent teeth (Ata-Ali *et al.*, 2014).

48.1.5 Examination and Diagnosis

Supernumerary teeth can be completely asymptomatic and may be accidentally found during routine radiographic examination. However, several clinical signs may prompt the clinician to suspect the presence of an impacted supernumerary tooth: a wide midline diastema, failure in eruption or delayed/ectopic eruption of permanent teeth, unilateral retained primary incisor and rotated permanent incisor teeth (Shah *et al.*, 2008).

Radiographic examination is indicated if there are suspicious clinical findings. Oral panoramic radiograph in combination with occlusal or periapical radiographs are useful to confirm the presence of a supernumerary tooth and determine its buccolingual location using the parallax technique (Shah *et al.*, 2008).

Diseases and Conditions in Dentistry: An Evidence-Based Reference, First Edition. Keyvan Moharamzadeh.

Companion website: www.wiley.com/go/moharamzadeh/diseases

Cone beam computed tomography (CBCT) provides detailed three-dimensional information regarding the morphology, location and relationship of the supernumerary tooth with adjacent structures and any associated pathology (Noar and Pabari, 2013). However, use of CBCT in the management of supernumerary teeth must be justified based on its relative merits compared to the risks of imaging (Kapila and Nervina, 2015).

48.1.6 Management

Once the supernumerary tooth is localised, it can be monitored annually in the following conditions (Garvey *et al.*, 1999).

- Absence of any related symptoms, pathology or complications.
- Satisfactory eruption of adjacent permanent teeth.
- No active orthodontic treatment plan.
- Removal would jeopardise the vitality of related teeth or hamper development of the roots of erupting teeth.

Indications for the removal of supernumerary teeth include (Parolia *et al.*, 2011):

- delayed or inhibited eruption of the central incisor teeth
- displacement or ectopic eruption of central incisors
- presence of pathology associated with the supernumerary tooth
- prior to orthodontic tooth movement in close proximity to the supernumerary tooth
- prior to secondary alveolar bone grafting in cleft lip and palate patients if its presence would compromise the grafting procedure
- prior to placement of a dental implant in the site of the supernumerary
- spontaneous eruption of the supernumerary.

48.2 Fusion

Fusion is a developmental dental anomaly defined as union of two separate tooth buds during odontogenesis before mineralisation of the crown. Fusion can be complete or partial, depending on the stage of development of the teeth, and the fused teeth can have different crown and pulpal morphology.

48.2.1 Classification

Aguilo *et al.* (1999) classified double teeth into four categories based on their morphology.

- Type I: bifid crown with single root
- Type II: large crown with a large root
- Type III: two fused crowns with a single root
- Type IV: two fused crowns with two fused roots

48.2.2 Aetiology

The aetiology of dental fusion is not fully understood and different theories have been suggested (Hulsmann *et al.*, 1997).

- Physical forces and trauma causing necrosis of epithelial cells of the joining tooth buds, leading to close contact and fusion.
- Prolonged existence of interdental lamina between the two tooth buds during organogenesis.
- Genetic and environmental factors.

48.2.3 Incidence

The incidence of fusion varies depending on race, gender and region (Whittington and Durward, 1996). It ranges from 0.2% to 2.5% and is more common in primary dentition.

48.2.4 Relevant Investigations

The following investigations can be useful in the diagnosis and management of fused teeth.

- Sensibility testing to determine the pulp vitality.
- Percussion test to assess ankyloses and tenderness to percussion.
- Periodontal examination to identify and treat any related periodontal defects.
- Periapical radiograph to investigate pulp morphology, periodontal and periapical hard tissues.
- Three-dimensional imaging such as CBCT can provide detailed information about the fused teeth, their shape and morphology of the root canal system (Zhu *et al.*, 2015).
- Occlusal analysis to assess occlusion and any occlusal interferences caused by the fused teeth.
- Orthodontic assessment to consider space management and correction of any malocclusion (Finkelstein *et al.*, 2015).
- Aesthetic evaluation, as fused teeth may have poor appearance.
- Articulated study models and diagnostic wax-up if restorative treatment is envisaged.

48.2.5 Treatment Options

Treatment of fused teeth can be challenging and often requires multidisciplinary management. Different treatment options for fused teeth include the following.

- Monitoring and maintenance.
- Selective grinding and composite restoration.

- Separation of the fused teeth and extraction of the anomalous part, reshaping/restoration of the remaining tooth and orthodontic closure of the space (Sfasciotti *et al.*, 2011; Steinbock *et al.*, 2014).
- Surgical separation of the fused teeth with restoration of both teeth (Ramamurthy *et al.*, 2014; Sammartino *et al.*, 2014).
- Endodontic treatment may be indicated if the teeth are non-vital or root resection/separation with pulpal involvement is planned (Oelgiesser *et al.*, 2013).
- Extraction and orthodontic space closure.
- Extraction and prosthetic treatment with fixed bridges or dental implants with or without prior orthodontic treatment.

48.3 Gemination

Gemination is characterised by a large single tooth with a partially divided crown and often a common root due to an attempt by a tooth bud to split into two. In gemination, the number of teeth in the dental arch is normal if the geminated tooth is counted as one. However, in fusion, the tooth count is less than normal unless there is fusion of a supernumerary tooth with an adjacent tooth (Grammatopoulos, 2007).

Gemination often involves the primary teeth (Chipashvili *et al.*, 2011), although it may affect the permanent dentition, mainly the incisor teeth (Hamasha and Al-Khateeb, 2004).

Diagnosis and treatment of gemination can be challenging due to aesthetic considerations, space problems and occlusal issues (Neena *et al.*, 2015). Clinical assessment and relevant special investigations for geminated teeth are similar to those of fused teeth as described above.

Treatment options can also vary, from simple crown reshaping and monitoring to complex multidisciplinary treatment involving endodontic treatment, surgical periodontal treatment, orthodontics and restorative management as discussed above (Benetti *et al.*, 2004; Braun *et al.*, 2003).

Case Study

A 54-year-old female patient was referred by her GDP for endodontic retreatment of previously root-treated LL5. The patient presented with history of pain and swelling of the left mandible.

Clinical examination showed that LL5 had a porcelain fused to metal crown and was tender to percussion with grade I mobility. Periodontal examination showed an isolated 7 mm deep periodontal pocket on the distal aspect of heavily restored LL6 which was vital as tested by an electric pulp tester.

Radiographic examination (Figure 48.1) showed a large periapical radiolucency and apical root resorption of root-treated LL5. An impacted supernumerary tooth was found below LL6 with evidence of root resorption of the distal root of LL6, as well as mild periodontal bone loss on the distal aspect of LL6 with deep restoration margin.

The diagnoses were:

- chronic apical periodontitis of LL5
- impacted supernumerary tooth
- root resorption of LL6
- localised chronic periodontitis associated with plaque retention and deep restoration margin on LL6.

Treatment options for LL5 were discussed with the patient, including endodontic retreatment or extraction of the tooth. The patient preferred endodontic retreatment and therefore this treatment was successfully carried out.

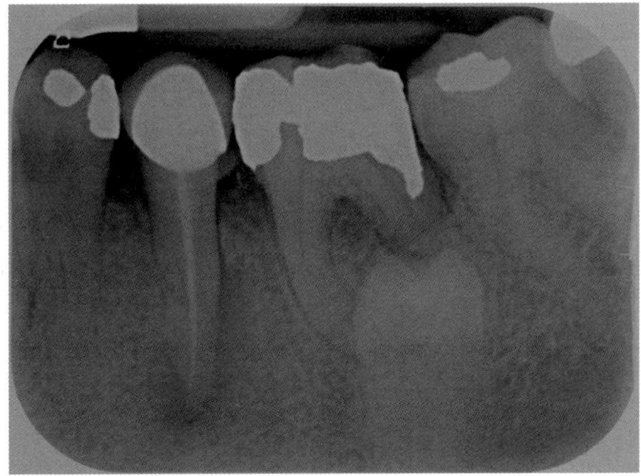

Figure 48.1 Preoperative periapical radiograph of LL5 and LL6 showing large periapical radiolucency and apical root resorption of root-treated LL5, impacted supernumerary tooth below LL6, root resorption of the distal root of LL6, and mild periodontal bone loss on the distal aspect of LL6 with deep restoration margin.

Treatment options regarding LL6 were also discussed with the patient, including:

- non-surgical periodontal treatment (oral hygiene instructions and root surface debridement under local anaesthesia) and monitoring LL6, which was a conservative treatment option. However, it would be challenging to correct the restoration margins on the distal aspect of

LL6 non-surgically due to its deep subgingival position which may require surgical intervention

- endodontic treatment and surgical resection of the distal root of LL6. However, this treatment had doubtful prognosis as tooth restorability was questionable due to a large subgingival restoration
- extraction of LL6 and prosthetic replacement.

Options regarding the impacted supernumerary tooth were either to leave the tooth *in situ* and monitor it or surgical removal of the tooth which carried the risk of inferior alveolar nerve damage.

The patient preferred to keep the tooth and have non-surgical periodontal treatment of LL6 and monitor the impacted supernumerary tooth.

After endodontic retreatment of LL5, the patient was discharged back to her GDP with advice to carry out non-surgical periodontal treatment of LL6, monitor the impacted supernumerary tooth and continue with long-term periodontal maintenance.

References

Aguilo, L., Gandia, J.L., Cibrian, R. and Catala, M. (1999) Primary double teeth. A retrospective clinical study of their morphological characteristics and associated anomalies. *Int J Paediatr Dent*, **9**, 175–183.

Anthonappa, R.P., King, N.M. and Rabie, A.B. (2013) Aetiology of supernumerary teeth: a literature review. *Eur Arch Paediatr Dent*, **14**, 279–288.

Ata-Ali, F., Ata-Ali, J., Penarrocha-Oltra, D. and Penarrocha-Diago, M. (2014) Prevalence, etiology, diagnosis, treatment and complications of supernumerary teeth. *J Clin Exp Dent*, **6**, E414–418.

Benetti, R., Toffanin, A. and Zupi, A. (2004) Gemination of maxillary incisors. *Minerva Stomatol*, **53**, 375–378.

Braun, A., Appel, T. and Frentzen, M. (2003) Endodontic and surgical treatment of a geminated maxillary incisor. *Int Endod J*, **36**, 380–386.

Chipashvili, N., Vadachkoria, D. and Beshkenadze, E. (2011) Gemination or fusion? Challenge for dental practitioners (case study). *Georgian Med News*, 28–33.

Finkelstein, T., Shapira, Y., Bechor, N. and Shpack, N. (2015) Fused and geminated permanent maxillary central incisors: prevalence, treatment options, and outcome in orthodontic patients. *J Dent Child (Chic)*, **82**, 147–152.

Garvey, M.T., Barry, H.J. and Blake, M. (1999) Supernumerary teeth – an overview of classification, diagnosis and management. *J Can Dent Assoc*, **65**, 612–616.

Grammatopoulos, E. (2007) Gemination or fusion? *Br Dent J*, **203**, 119–120.

Hamasha, A.A. and Al-Khateeb, T. (2004) Prevalence of fused and geminated teeth in Jordanian adults. *Quintessence Int*, **35**, 556–559.

Hulsmann, M., Bahr, R. and Grohmann, U. (1997) Hemisection and vital treatment of a fused tooth – literature review and case report. *Endod Dent Traumatol*, **13**, 253–258.

Kapila, S.D. and Nervina, J.M. (2015) CBCT in orthodontics: assessment of treatment outcomes and indications for its use. *Dentomaxillofac Radiol*, **44**, 20140282.

Lubinsky, M. and Kantaputra, P.N. (2016) Syndromes with supernumerary teeth. *Am J Med Genet A*, **170**, 2611–2616.

Neena, I.E., Sharma, R., Poornima, P. and Roopa, K.B. (2015) Gemination in primary central incisor. *J Oral Res Rev*, **7**, 55–57.

Noar, J.H. and Pabari, S. (2013) Cone beam computed tomography – current understanding and evidence for its orthodontic applications? *J Orthod*, **40**, 5–13.

Oelgiesser, D., Zyc, R., Evron, D., Kaplansky, G. and Levin, L. (2013) Treatment of a fused/geminated tooth: a multidisciplinary conservative approach. *Quintessence Int*, **44**, 531–533.

Parolia, A., Kundabala, M., Dahal, M., Mohan, M. and Thomas, M.S. (2011) Management of supernumerary teeth. *J Conserv Dent*, **14**, 221–224.

Rajab, L.D. and Hamdan, M.A. (2002) Supernumerary teeth: review of the literature and a survey of 152 cases. *Int J Paediatr Dent*, **12**, 244–254.

Ramamurthy, S., Satish, R. and Priya, K. (2014) Surgical and orthodontic management of fused maxillary central and lateral incisors in early mixed dentition stage. *Case Rep Dent*, **2014**, 109301.

Sammartino, G., Cerone, V., Gasparro, R., Riccitiello, F. and Trosino, O. (2014) Multidisciplinary approach to fused maxillary central incisors: a case report. *J Med Case Rep*, **8**, 398.

Sfasciotti, G.L., Marini, R., Bossu, M., Ierardo, G. and Annibali, S. (2011) Fused upper central incisors: management of two clinical cases. *Ann Stomatol (Roma)*, **2**, 40–44.

Shah, A., Gill, D.S., Tredwin, C. and Naini, F.B. (2008) Diagnosis And Management Of Supernumerary Teeth. *Dent Update*, **35**, 510–2, 514–6, 519–20.

Steinbock, N., Wigler, R., Kaufman, A.Y., Lin, S., Abu-El Naaj, I. and Aizenbud, D. (2014) Fusion of central incisors with supernumerary teeth: a 10-year follow-up of multidisciplinary treatment. *J Endod*, **40**, 1020–1024.

Whittington, B.R. and Durward, C.S. (1996) Survey of anomalies in primary teeth and their correlation with the permanent dentition. *N Z Dent J*, **92**, 4–8.

Zhu, M., Liu, C., Ren, S., Lin, Z., Miao, L. and Sun, W. (2015) Fusion of a supernumerary tooth to right mandibular second molar: a case report and literature review. *Int J Clin Exp Med*, **8**, 11890–11895.

49

Temporomandibular Disorders

49.1 Definition

Temporomandibular disorders (TMD) are a group of musculoskeletal and neuromuscular conditions that affect the temporomandibular joint (TMJ) complex and the surrounding muscles and bone parts (Gauer and Semidey, 2015). Other names have also been used to identify these disorders such as TMJ pain dysfunction syndrome, myofascial pain dysfunction syndrome and facial arthromyalgia (Lyons, 2008).

49.2 Prevalence

Around 40% of the population show signs of TMD at some stage in life and 20–25% of patients have symptoms of TMD but do not necessarily require treatment; 4% of patients require treatment at some stage (de Kanter *et al.*, 1993; Liu and Steinkeler, 2013).

49.3 Classification

Temporomandibular disorders can be classified into two main categories (Schiffman *et al.*, 2014).

- *Myogenous or extra-articular TMD*, involving the surrounding muscles and including disorders such as myofascial pain, myositis, local myalgia, myofibrotic contracture and myospasm.
- *Arthrogenous or intra-articular TMD* that are temporomandibular joint (TMJ) disorders within the joint such as:
  - disc displacement (with or without reduction) and disc perforation
  - degenerative joint disorders including inflammatory capsulitis, synovitis, polyarthritides and non-inflammatory osteoarthritis
  - joint hypermobility such as dislocation and subluxation
  - joint hypomobility such as ankylosis and trismus
  - developmental condylar hyperplasia and resorption
  - traumatic fracture and intracapsular haemorrhage
  - joint infection and neoplasm.

49.4 Aetiology

Temporomandibular disorders have multifactorial aetiology including biological, environmental, emotional, social and cognitive factors (Gauer and Semidey, 2015) which can be categorised into the following groups (Lyons, 2008).

Predisposing factors include:

- systemic parameters such as biochemical susceptibility, anxiety, stress and depression
- structural factors such as joint laxity and occlusal features including anterior open bite, loss of posterior teeth and increased overbite.

Perpetuating factors can be behavioural, social and emotional problems (Kindler *et al.*, 2012).

Initiating factors include:

- parafunction and habits such as bruxism, clenching, nail biting and gum chewing
- adverse loading
- trauma.

Systematic reviews on the relationship between bruxism and TMD have reached the following conclusions (Jimenez-Silva *et al.*, 2017; Manfredini and Lobbezoo, 2010).

- The studies were characterised by potential bias and confounders at the diagnostic level.
- Self-reported or clinical bruxism diagnosis showed a positive association with TMD.
- Sleep bruxism could be associated with myofascial pain, arthralgia and joint pathology such as disc displacement and joint noises.
- Anterior tooth wear is not a major risk factor for TMD.

Diseases and Conditions in Dentistry: An Evidence-Based Reference, First Edition. Keyvan Moharamzadeh.

Companion website: www.wiley.com/go/moharamzadeh/diseases

49.5 Diagnosis

Diagnosis of TMD is mainly based on the history and clinical examination. A thorough and accurate history is essential to identify any aetiological factors as described above and establish the exact nature of the patient's symptoms. Using an appropriate TMD questionnaire and a visual analogue pain scale can be very helpful.

Clinical examination should include evaluation of the entire masticatory system, assessment of jaw clenching, palpation and auscultation for TMJ sounds, assessment of tenderness of TMJs and muscles of mastication, mandibular range of movement and full dental assessment.

Myogenous TMD is usually characterised by painful muscles and trismus. Pain is usually dull and poorly localised. Jaw movements usually exacerbate the pain which may radiate widely. Trismus may be present due to spasm of the muscles of mastication (Yule *et al.*, 2016).

In some patients, myogenous and arthrogenous problems may co-exist. TMJ disc displacement with reduction is characterised by stable, pain-free and reproducible TMJ clicking in which the disc returns to its normal position after the click and the clicking disappears in protruded mouth opening (Naeije *et al.*, 2013). TMJ disc displacement without reduction can cause TMJ pain and limited mouth opening (painful locking or closed lock) which can be acute or chronic (Al-Baghdadi *et al.*, 2014).

49.6 Special Investigations

The American Academy of Oral and Maxillofacial Radiology states: '*Radiology is not recommended for TMJ clicking in the absence of other signs and symptoms. However, radiographic examination is indicated where there is recent evidence of progressive pathology, recent trauma, a change in occlusion, a mandibular shift, a change in range of movements, sensory and motor alterations*' (Brooks *et al.*, 1997; Martinez Beneyto *et al.*, 2007).

Relevant imaging techniques for TMJ include the following (Al-Ani and Gray, 2007).

- Oral panoramic radiograph which is the most common first-line radiographic examination method.
- Transpharyngeal radiograph provides a lateral view of TMJ.
- Transcranial radiograph provides a modified lateral view of TMJ.
- Transorbital radiograph provides an anteroposterior view of TMJ.
- Arthrography with injection of radiopaque contrast medium to the lower compartment of TMJ allows assessment of the position and morphology of the articular disc, and presence of perforation or adhesions of the disc.
- Computed tomography (CT) scan provides three-dimensional images of the joint with the most accurate assessment of bony components.
- Magnetic resonance imaging (MRI) provides excellent images of intra-articular soft tissues, making it a valuable technique for assessment of disc morphology and its position. MRI is a non-invasive technique without exposure to radiation, but it has high cost, requires special site planning and cannot be used on patients with metal implants or pregnant patients in the first trimester.

Other diagnostic techniques that have been used to aid TMD diagnosis include pressure allometric devices, surface electromyographic (EMG) tools to detect muscle pain, joint sound vibration devices and electronic jaw tracking instruments (Baba *et al.*, 2001).

49.7 Management

Based on literature evidence (List and Axelsson, 2010) and guidelines (Greene, 2010), initial treatment of TMDs should be based on reversible and conservative approaches including patient advice, cognitive behavioural therapy (CBT), physiotherapy, pharmacological therapy and application of intraoral splints (Yule *et al.*, 2016).

49.7.1 Patient Education

Patients should be initially reassured and informed about the aetiology and management of TMD. Advice should be given to maintain a soft diet, avoid wide mouth opening, avoid chewing gums, rest the jaw and apply moist heat to the painful area.

49.7.2 Jaw Exercise and Manual Therapy

Active and passive jaw exercises, postural exercises, neck exercises and manual therapy are simple and safe interventions that can benefit patients with TMD, although the overall level of evidence is low according to a systematic review and meta-analysis (Armijo-Olivo *et al.*, 2016).

49.7.3 Acupuncture

Conventional acupuncture therapy has been shown to be effective in reducing pain, especially in patients with myogenous TMD (Fernandes *et al.*, 2017; Wu *et al.*, 2017).

49.7.4 Pharmacotherapy

Pharmacological agents that have been used to manage TMD-associated pain include the following (Gauer and Semidey, 2015; Mujakperuo *et al.*, 2010).

- Non-steroidal anti-inflammatory drugs (NSAIDs) which are the first-line treatment for acute TMD pain.
- Muscle relaxants can also be prescribed if the patient experiences acute muscle spasm.
- Benzodiazepines can be used initially in the short term.
- Tricyclic antidepressants have been used for the management of chronic TMD pain.
- Anticonvulsants may be prescribed for longer periods in some patients.
- Intra-articular injection of corticosteroids and hyaluronate has been suggested for patients with degenerative joint disease and pain who do not respond to conservative treatment.

49.7.5 Occlusal Stabilising Splint Therapy

Occlusal stabilising splints are widely used for TMD and have proven to be helpful in many patients with myofascial pain (Ebrahim *et al.*, 2012), with some evidence to support the efficacy of splints for reducing TMD symptoms in the short term (Kuzmanovic Pficer *et al.*, 2017).

The Michigan-type occlusal splint is recommended, which provides a hard and flat surface for all the opposing teeth to contact occlusally and anterior guidance to provide posterior disclusion in mandibular protrusion and lateral excursions (Milosevic, 2003).

Studies have shown reduction in EMG activity of the muscles of mastication during splint use, mainly the temporalis muscle (Naeije and Hansson, 1991). Suggested mechanisms of action for stabilising splints are reduction of muscle activity, increase in occlusal vertical dimension, occlusal disengagement and possibly a placebo effect (Lyons, 2008).

It is important to note that soft splints may stimulate additional muscle activity, encourage chewing/clenching and exacerbate the problem.

It is recommended that patients with myofacial pain wear the occlusal stabilising splint mainly at night (Davies and Gray, 1997b).

49.7.6 Anterior Repositioning Splint

The anterior repositioning splint is indicated for treatment of disc displacement with reduction, especially when clicking becomes socially embarrassing or when there is associated pain or locking (Orenstein, 1993).

This splint is usually made of hard acrylic material covering the occlusal surfaces of the mandibular teeth and guides the mandible forwards and downwards into a protrusive position (Simmons, 2006). It provides a favourable condyle–disc relationship and enhances retrodiscal tissue adaptation.

It is recommended that patients wear the anterior repositioning splint 24 hours per day for a 3-month period (Davies and Gray, 1997a).

Factors that can have a negative impact on the outcome of treatment include disc displacement without reduction, presence of inflammatory diseases, change in disc anatomy and severe disc displacement (Kurita *et al.*, 2001).

49.7.7 Occlusal Adjustment

There is no evidence to support occlusal adjustment or complex occlusal therapy in dentate patients as a preventive measure or as a primary treatment modality for TMD (List and Axelsson, 2010). Therefore, occlusal changes in patients with TMD should be minimised and any prosthetic treatment for other reasons should only be provided after reversible treatment has resolved pain and dysfunction (de Boever *et al.*, 2000a, b).

49.7.8 TMJ Lavage

Temporomandibular joint lavage approaches, including arthrocentesis and arthroscopy, are more aggressive and some clinical studies have supported the use of these techniques (Bouchard *et al.*, 2017). However, there is a lack of strong evidence due to the relatively small number of patients included in the studies, the high risk of bias and the heterogeneity of the data. Therefore, the use of this technique for the treatment of temporomandibular disorders should be recommended with caution.

49.7.9 Surgery

Invasive surgery is only rarely considered to treat TMJ pathological conditions and to correct anatomical or articular abnormalities. Options include condylar shave, condylectomy, discectomy and total joint replacement. Patients who undergo TMJ surgery often have significant pain and functional deficit which have been unresponsive to more conservative treatment modalities. A systematic review showed no significant differences between non-invasive conservative treatment and minimally invasive or invasive surgical approaches for the management of TMJ disc displacement without reduction (Manfredini, 2014). Therefore, initial management should be based on the most minimal and least invasive intervention in this group of patients.

Case Study

A 49-year-old female patient presented with tenderness of TMJs and muscular facial pain extending to the neck, back and shoulders. The problem had been going on for 2 years with several acute episodes of pain in the past. The patient had a stressful job and used to grind and clench her teeth. There was no history of trauma or recent dental treatment.

The patient was fit and well and had a clear medical history.

Clinical examination showed both TMJs, masseter and pterygoid muscles were tender to palpation and mouth opening was slightly limited. There was no TMJ clicking or deviation of the mandible.

Intraoral examination showed normal soft tissues and dentate arches with class I occlusion (Figure 49.1). The patient had good oral hygiene and healthy periodontium. There was no evidence of any dental hard tissue diseases.

Based on the history and clinical examination, the diagnosis of myogenous TMD (myofascial pain) in a patient with history of bruxism and clenching was made.

The management strategy was as follows.

- Patient advice to avoid chewing on hard food, avoid wide mouth opening, avoid chewing gums, advice to reduce stress, relax the jaw and face and to apply warm packs to the painful areas of the face.
- Jaw exercises for 5 minutes twice a day when the patient is relaxed (in the morning and at night).
- Prescription of anti-inflammatory medication (ibuprofen) to reduce pain.
- Fabrication and fitting of an upper hard Michigan-type stabilising splint (Figure 49.2) to be worn at night. The clinical procedure involved taking upper and lower alginate impressions, a face-bow record and bite registration at the retruded contact position (RCP). Following laboratory fabrication, the splint was fitted on the teeth in the mouth, occlusal contacts were marked using an articulating paper and the splint was carefully adjusted to achieve even contacts of the splint's flat surface with all the opposing teeth, shared incisor guidance in protrusion and canine guidance with posterior disclusion in lateral excursions.
- Review and further adjustment of the splint.

Significant improvement in symptoms was reported by the patient following the above conservative treatment. The patient was well motivated and managed to wear the splint as instructed. She was very satisfied with the outcome of treatment.

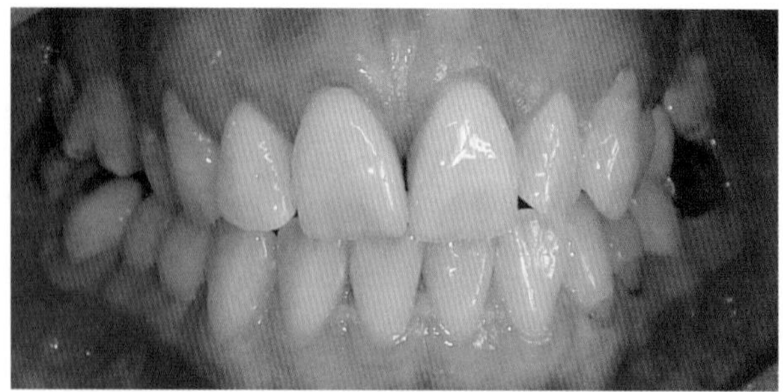

Figure 49.1 Preoperative intraoral clinical photograph.

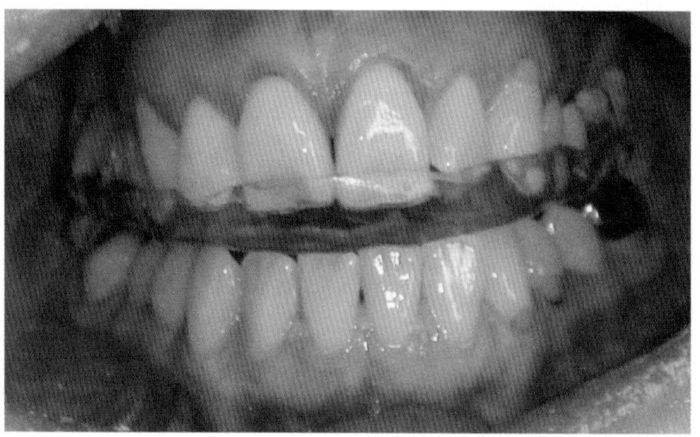

Figure 49.2 Intraoral photograph of the patient wearing the stabilising splint.

References

Al-Ani, Z. and Gray, R. (2007) TMD Current Concepts: 2. Imaging and treatment options. an update. *Dent Update*, **34**, 356–358, 361–364, 367–370.

Al-Baghdadi, M., Durham, J., Araujo-Soares, V., Robalino, S., Errington, L. and Steele, J. (2014) TMJ disc displacement without reduction management: a systematic review. *J Dent Res*, **93**, 37s–51s.

Armijo-Olivo, S., Pitance, L., Singh, V., Neto, F., Thie, N. and Michelotti, A. (2016) Effectiveness of manual therapy and therapeutic exercise for temporomandibular disorders: systematic review and meta-analysis. *Phys Ther*, **96**, 9–25.

Baba, K., Tsukiyama, Y., Yamazaki, M. and Clark, G.T. (2001) A review of temporomandibular

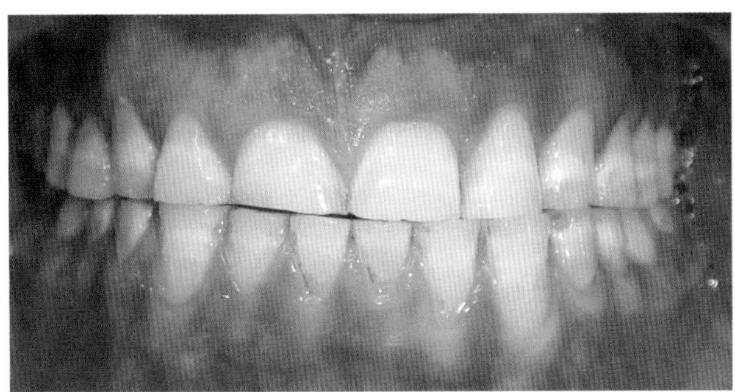

Figure 50.5 Preoperative clinical photograph of the patient's occlusion showing flat edge-to-edge occlusion and lack of space for incisal and occlusal build-up of the teeth.

analysis and diagnostic wax-up (Figure 50.6) of the worn anterior and posterior teeth at a VD increased by 3 mm to ideal crown shape and morphology with canine occlusal guidance.

3) Direct composite build-ups of the worn teeth employing every other tooth technique using a laboratory-made clear stent (Figure 50.7) made over the diagnostic wax-up replicate model. Anterior teeth were built up first to establish canine guidance and then the posterior teeth were built up shortly after to provide posterior support (Figures 50.8 and 50.9).
4) Fabrication and fitting of a maxillary occlusal splint to protect the restorations from occlusal trauma due to bruxism.
5) Review and maintenance.

Case 2

A 32-year-old male patient, referred by the GDP for treatment of tooth wear, complained of shrinking upper teeth, sensitivity and recurrent abscesses.

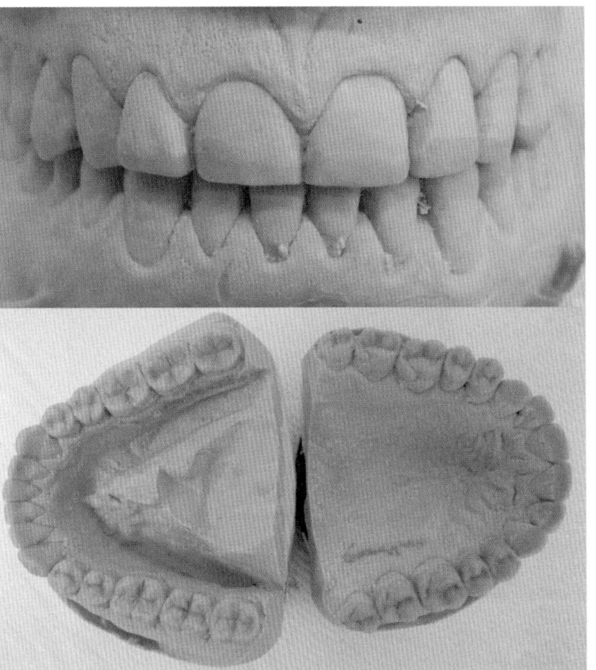

Figure 50.6 Diagnostic wax-up of the worn teeth at an increased VD.

The patient's medical history included acid reflux disease, schizophrenia and paranoia which were all controlled by medications (lansoprazole and clozapine). He was a regular dental attender and had good oral hygiene. He was a former smoker, and drank 5 units of alcohol per week. He was not aware of any grinding habits and had a normal diet.

The patient's preoperative clinical photographs and radiographs are shown in Figures 50.10 and 50.11 respectively.

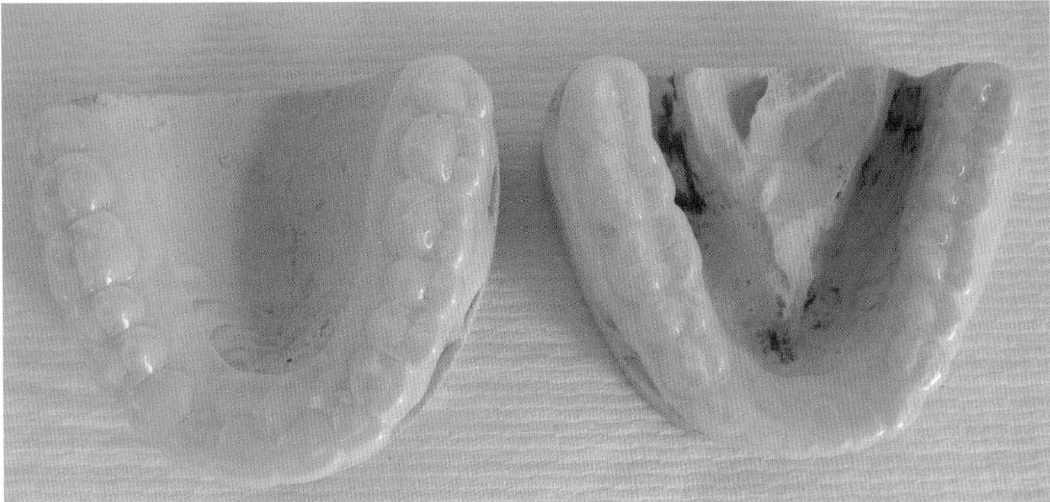

Figure 50.7 Photograph of the laboratory-made clear stent made over the diagnostic wax-up replicate models.

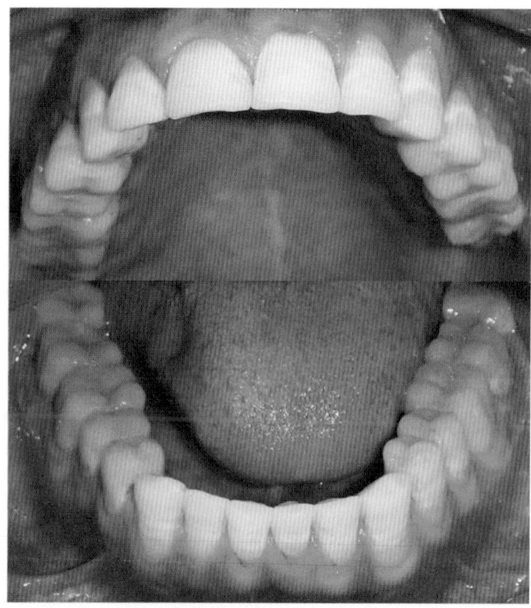

Figure 50.8 Postoperative clinical photograph of the teeth restored with direct adhesive composites.

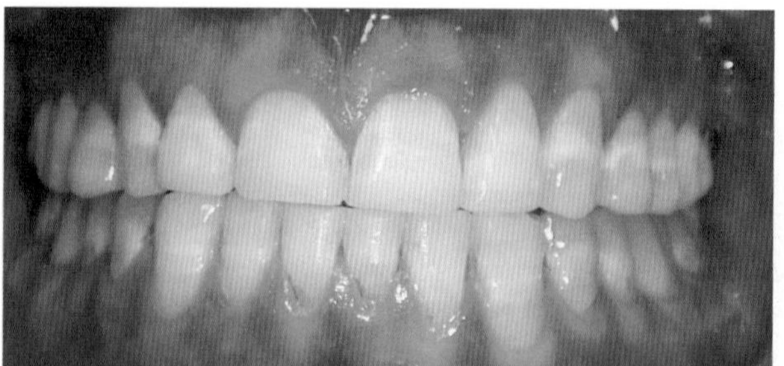

Figure 50.9 Postoperative clinical photograph of the patient's occlusion.

Sensibility testing with an electric pulp tester showed UR3, UR4, UR5, UL3, UL4, UL5 and UL7 were vital.

The diagnoses were:

- severe generalised tooth surface loss in the maxillae mainly due to erosion with some attrition
- chronic apical periodontitis UR2
- lost UL6, LR6, LL4, LL6 and LL7
- failed restoration UR6
- reduced occlusal vertical dimension.

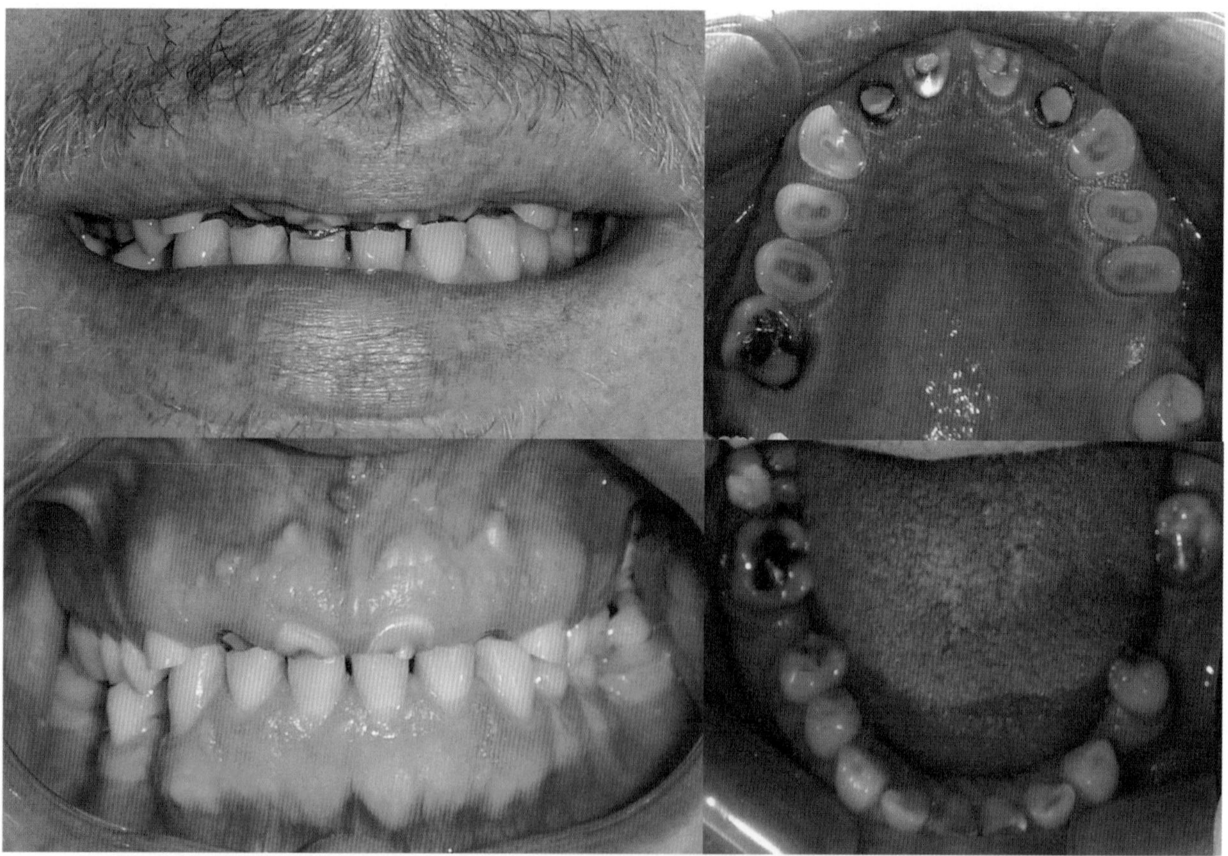

Figure 50.10 Preoperative clinical photographs showing severe tooth surface loss affecting the maxillary teeth with over 90% loss of the clinical crown height of the maxillary incisor teeth, significant tooth wear on the palatal aspect of the maxillary canine and premolar teeth and evidence of dentoalveolar compensation limiting the restorative space in the anterior maxilla.

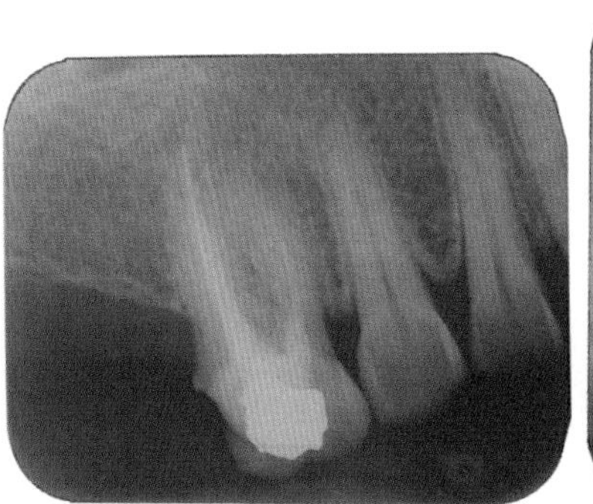
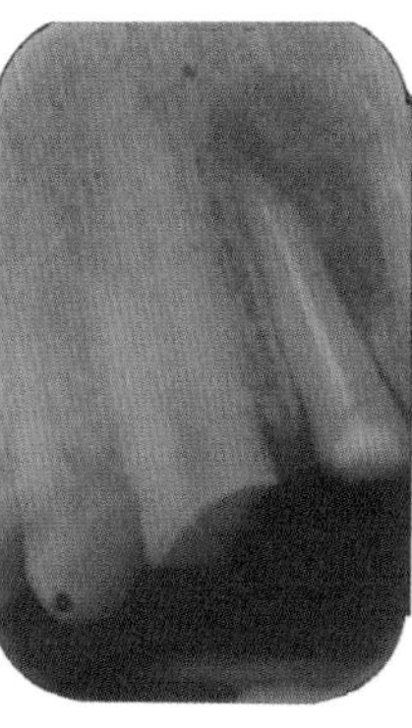
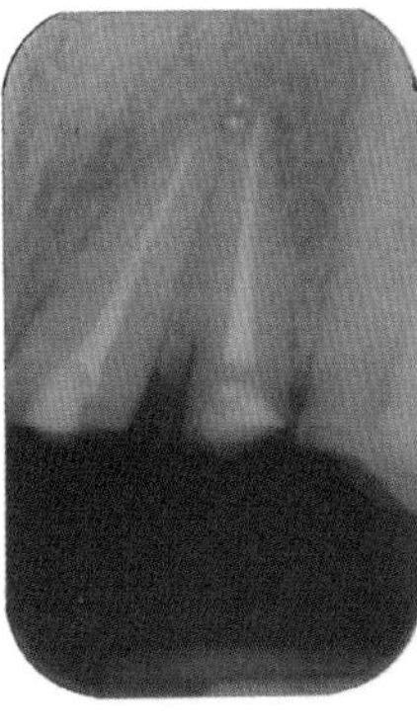
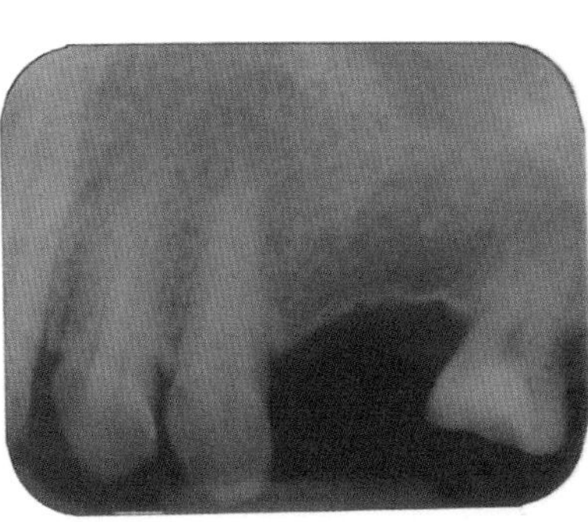

Figure 50.11 Preoperative periapical radiographs of the maxillary teeth showing root-filled UR6 and incisor teeth with a large periapical lesion associated with UR2.

Treatment options included:

- prevention only with no further restorative treatment
- overdenture, which would be too bulky and may not be desirable for the patient
- extraction of the worn teeth and replacement by a removable denture or implant-retained prosthesis
- extraction of UR2 or endodontic retreatment
- composite build-ups of the maxillary canines and premolars and replacement of the anterior teeth with a RPD
- crown lengthening of the maxillary canines and premolars, restoration of these teeth with indirect crowns, and replacement of the anterior teeth with either a RPD (overdenture) or dental implants.

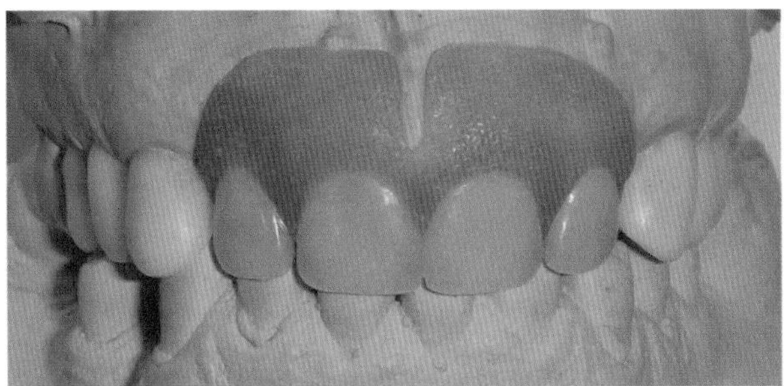

Figure 50.12 Simultaneous diagnostic wax-up of the worn maxillary canine and premolar teeth and a removable wax try-in of maxillary incisor teeth at an increased VD.

The patient preferred to have the UR2 extracted and have crown lengthening of UR3, UR4, UR5, UL3, UL4 and UL5, followed by restorations with full-coverage crowns and a small RPD overdenture to replace the maxillary anterior teeth.

The following treatment procedures were carried out.

1) Impressions, bite registration at the RCP, face-bow transfer, preparation of articulated study models and occlusal analysis.
2) Duplication of the maxillary cast and fabrication of a surgical stent for crown-lengthening surgery.
3) Crown-lengthening surgery on UR3, UR4, UR5, UL3, UL4 and UL5.
4) New impressions 6 weeks after surgery and bite registration with wax blocks.
5) Simultaneous diagnostic wax-up of UR3, UR4, UR5, UR6, UL3, UL4, UL5 and UL7 and removable wax try-in of UR1, UR2, UL1 and UL2 at an increased VD of 3 mm (Figure 50.12).
6) Restoration of UR6 with composite resin.
7) Core build-ups of maxillary canine and premolars with composite resin and preparation of these teeth (Figure 50.13) for full-coverage PFM crowns.

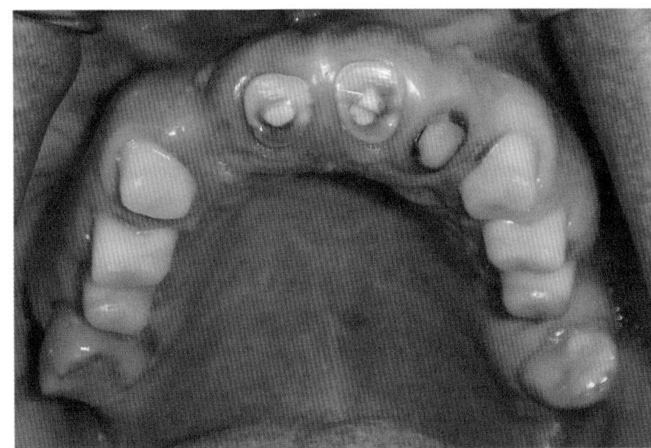

Figure 50.13 Intraoral photograph of the maxillary teeth after crown lengthening of the canines and premolars, composite core build-ups and crown preparations.

8) Temporisation of the prepared maxillary canine and premolar teeth with provisional crowns, fabricated using a stent made over the diagnostic wax-up.
9) Fabrication and fitting of milled PFM crowns on UR3, UR4, UR5, UL3, UL4 and UL5 incorporating the features of a Co-Cr RPD design (Figure 50.14).

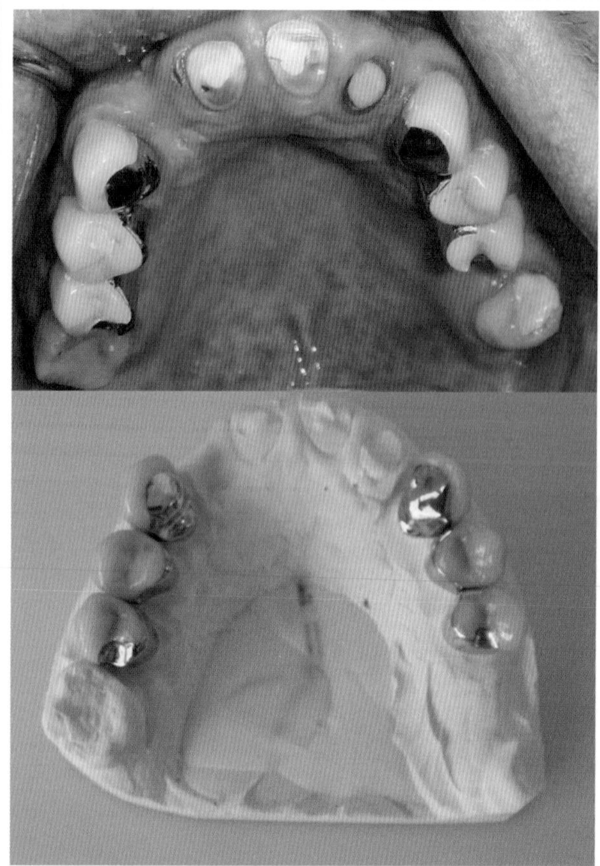

Figure 50.14 Milled PFM crowns on UR3, UR4, UR5, UL3, UL4 and UL5 incorporating the features of RPD design, including cingulum rests on canines, distal occlusal rests on second premolars, parallel palatal guiding planes and appropriate buccal undercuts on premolars.

10) Fitting of a temporary acrylic RPD to replace the anterior teeth.
11) Fabrication and fitting of the final Co-Cr RPD (Figure 50.15) with a short labial flange due to the presence of a prominent alveolar ridge in the anterior maxilla.
12) Review and maintenance.

The patient was very satisfied with both the functional and aesthetic outcome of the treatment. Therefore he was discharged back to the GDP for long-term dental care and maintenance.

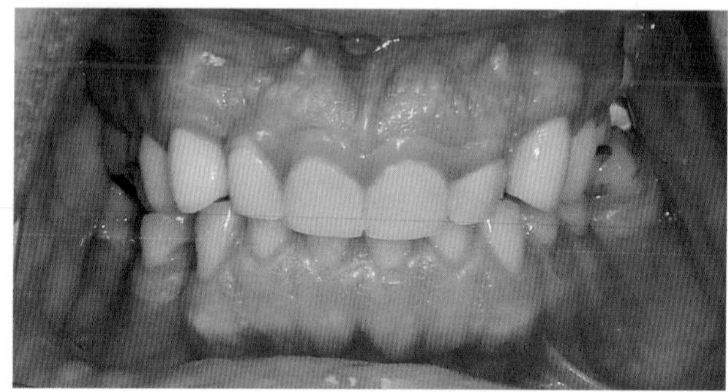

Figure 50.15 Postoperative photograph of the final Co-Cr RPD with a minimal labial flange.

References

Abduo, J. and Lyons, K. (2012) Clinical considerations for increasing occlusal vertical dimension: a review. *Aust Dent J*, **57**, 2–10.

Ahmed, K.E. and Murbay, S. (2016) Survival rates of anterior composites in managing tooth wear: systematic review. *J Oral Rehabil*, **43**, 145–153.

Al-Khayatt, A.S., Ray-Chaudhuri, A., Poyser, N.J. *et al.* (2013) Direct composite restorations for the worn mandibular anterior dentition: a 7-year follow-up of a prospective randomised controlled split-mouth clinical trial. *J Oral Rehabil*, **40**, 389–401.

Ashcroft, A. and Milosevic, A. (2007a) The eating disorders: 1. Current scientific understanding and dental implications. *Dent Update*, **34**, 544–546, 549–550, 553–554.

Ashcroft, A. and Milosevic, A. (2007b) The eating disorders: 2. Behavioural and dental management. *Dent Update*, **34**, 612–616, 619–620.

Bardsley, P.F. (2008) The evolution of tooth wear indices. *Clin Oral Invest*, **12** Suppl 1, S15–19.

Bartlett, D.W. (2003) Retrospective long term monitoring of tooth wear using study models. *Br Dent J*, **194**, 211–213; discussion 204.

Bartlett, D. (2016) A personal perspective and update on erosive tooth wear – 10 years on: Part 1 – Diagnosis and prevention. *Br Dent J*, **221**, 115–119.

Bartlett, D.W. and Shah, P. (2006) A critical review of non-carious cervical (wear) lesions and the role of abfraction, erosion, and abrasion. *J Dent Res*, **85**, 306–312.

Bartlett, D. and Sundaram, G. (2006) An up to 3-year randomized clinical study comparing indirect and direct resin composites used to restore worn posterior teeth. *Int J Prosthodont*, **19**, 613–617.

Bartlett, D. and Varma, S. (2017) A retrospective audit of the outcome of composites used to restore worn teeth. *Br Dent J*, **223**, 33–36.

Bartlett, D., Ganss, C. and Lussi, A. (2008) Basic Erosive Wear Examination (BEWE): a new scoring system for scientific and clinical needs. *Clin Oral Invest*, **12** Suppl 1, S65–68.

Bartlett, D.W., Lussi, A., West, N.X., Bouchard, P., Sanz, M. and Bourgeois, D. (2013) Prevalence of tooth wear on buccal and lingual surfaces and possible risk factors in young European adults. *J Dent*, **41**, 1007–1013.

Bateman, G.J., Karir, N. and Saha, S. (2009) Principles of crown lengthening surgery. *Dent Update*, **36**, 181–182, 184–185.

Burke, F.J. (2007) Four year performance of dentine-bonded all-ceramic crowns. *Br Dent J*, **202**, 269–273.

Burke, F.J. (2014) Information for patients undergoing treatment for tooth wear with resin composite restorations placed at an increased occlusal vertical dimension. *Dent Update*, **41**, 28–30, 33–34, 37–38.

Carvalho, T.S., Colon, P., Ganss, C. *et al.* (2015) Consensus report of the European Federation of Conservative Dentistry: erosive tooth wear – diagnosis and management. *Clin Oral Invest*, **19**, 1557–1561.

Chu, F.C., Siu, A.S., Newsome, P.R., Chow, T.W. and Smales, R.J. (2002a) Restorative management of the worn dentition: 2. Localized anterior tooth wear. *Dent Update*, **29**, 214–222.

Chu, F.C., Siu, A.S., Newsome, P.R., Chow, T.W. and Smales, R.J. (2002b) Restorative management of the worn dentition: 4. Generalized tooth wear. *Dent Update*, **29**, 318–324.

Chu, F.C., Yip, H.K., Newsome, P.R., Chow, T.W. and Smales, R.J. (2002c) Restorative management of the worn dentition: I. Aetiology and diagnosis. *Dent Update*, **29**, 162–168.

Cunliffe, J. and Grey, N. (2008) Crown lengthening surgery – indications and techniques. *Dent Update*, **35**, 29–30, 32, 34–35.

Dahl, B.L., Krogstad, O. and Karlsen, K. (1975) An alternative treatment in cases with advanced localized attrition. *J Oral Rehabil*, **2**, 209–214.

Davies, S.J., Gray, R.M. and Whitehead, S.A. (2001) Good occlusal practice in advanced restorative dentistry. *Br Dent J*, **191**, 421–424, 427–430, 433–434.

Dukic, W., Dobrijevic, T.T., Katunaric, M., Milardovic, S. and Segovic, S. (2010) Erosive lesions in patients with alcoholism. *J Am Dent Assoc*, **141**, 1452–1458.

Eccles, J.D. (1979) Dental erosion of nonindustrial origin. A clinical survey and classification. *J Prosthet Dent*, **42**, 649–653.

Eliyas, S., Shah, K. and Briggs, P.F. (2014) Interactive treatment planning in tooth wear: are we doing it right? *Dent Update*, **41**, 206–208, 210–212, 215–216.

Evans, R.D. and Briggs, P.F. (1994) Tooth-surface loss related to pregnancy-induced vomiting. *Prim Dent Care*, **1**, 24–26.

Fradeani, M., Barducci, G. and Bacherini, L. (2016) Esthetic rehabilitation of a worn dentition with a minimally invasive prosthetic procedure (MIPP). *Int J Esthet Dent*, **11**, 16–35.

Geurtsen, W. (2000) Rapid general dental erosion by gas-chlorinated swimming pool water. Review of the literature and case report. *Am J Dent*, **13**, 291–293.

Green, J.I. (2016) Prevention and management of tooth wear: the role of dental technology. *Prim Dent J*, **5**, 30–33.

Gulamali, A.B., Hemmings, K.W., Tredwin, C.J. and Petrie, A. (2011) Survival analysis of composite Dahl restorations provided to manage localised anterior tooth wear (ten year follow-up). *Br Dent J*, **211**, E9.

Hermont, A.P., Oliveira, P.A., Martins, C.C., Paiva, S.M., Pordeus, I.A. and Auad, S.M. (2014) Tooth erosion and eating disorders: a systematic review and meta-analysis. *PLoS One*, **9**, E111123.

Kanzow, P., Wegehaupt, F.J., Attin, T. and Wiegand, A. (2016) Etiology and pathogenesis of dental erosion. *Quintessence Int*, **47**, 275–278.

Macedo, C.R., Silva, A.B., Machado, M.A., Saconato, H. and Prado, G.F. (2007) Occlusal splints for treating sleep bruxism (tooth grinding). *Cochrane Database Syst Rev*, **4**, CD005514.

Marsicano, J.A., de Moura-Grec, P.G., Bonato, R.C., Sales-Peres, C., Sales-Peres, A. and Sales-Peres, S.H. (2013) Gastroesophageal reflux, dental erosion, and halitosis in epidemiological surveys: a systematic review. *Eur J Gastroenterol Hepatol*, **25**, 135–141.

Mehta, S.B., Banerji, S., Millar, B.J. and Suarez-Feito, J.M. (2012a) Current concepts on the management of tooth wear: Part 1. Assessment, treatment planning and strategies for the prevention and the passive management of tooth wear. *Br Dent J*, **212**, 17–27.

Mehta, S.B., Banerji, S., Millar, B.J. and Suarez-Feito, J.M. (2012b) Current concepts on the management of tooth wear: Part 2. Active restorative care 1: the management of localised tooth wear. *Br Dent J*, **212**, 73–82.

Mehta, S.B., Banerji, S., Millar, B.J. and Suarez-Feito, J.M. (2012c) Current concepts on the management of tooth wear: Part 3. Active restorative care 2: the management of generalised tooth wear. *Br Dent J*, **212**, 121–127.

Mehta, S.B., Banerji, S., Millar, B.J. and Suarez-Feito, J.M. (2012d) Current concepts on the management of tooth wear: Part 4. An overview of the restorative techniques and dental materials commonly applied for the management of tooth wear. *Br Dent J*, **212**, 169–177.

Mesko, M.E., Sarkis-Onofre, R., Cenci, M.S., Opdam, N.J., Loomans, B. and Pereira-Cenci, T. (2016) Rehabilitation of severely worn teeth: a systematic review. *J Dent*, **48**, 9–15.

Milosevic, A. and Burnside, G. (2016) The survival of direct composite restorations in the management of severe tooth wear including attrition and erosion: a prospective 8-year study. *J Dent*, **44**, 13–19.

Mizrahi, B. (2006) The Dahl principle: creating space and improving the biomechanical prognosis of anterior crowns. *Quintessence Int*, **37**, 245–251.

Mizrahi, B. (2008) Combining traditional and adhesive dentistry to reconstruct the excessively worn dentition. *Eur J Esthet Dent*, **3**, 270–289.

Moazzez, R. and Bartlett, D. (2014) Intrinsic causes of erosion. *Monogr Oral Sci*, **25**, 180–196.

Moazzez, R., Bartlett, D. and Anggiansah, A. (2003) Complications of medical management of dental erosion. *Dent Update*, **30**, 83–86.

Monagas, J., Ritwik, P., Kolomensky, A. *et al.* (2017) Rumination syndrome and dental erosions in children. *J Pediatr Gastroenterol Nutr*, **64**, 930–932.

Pace, F., Pallotta, S., Tonini, M., Vakil, N. and Bianchi Porro, G. (2008) Systematic review: gastro-oesophageal reflux disease and dental lesions. *Aliment Pharmacol Ther*, **27**, 1179–1186.

Packer, M.E. and Davis, D.M. (2000) The long-term management of patients with tooth surface loss treated using removable appliances. *Dent Update*, **27**, 454–458.

Patel, M., Seymour, D. and Chan, M.F. (2013) Contemporary management of generalized erosive tooth surface loss. *Dent Update*, **40**, 222–224, 226–229.

Patel, R.M. and Baker, P. (2015) Functional crown lengthening surgery in the aesthetic zone; periodontic and prosthodontic considerations. *Dent Update*, **42**, 36–38, 41–42.

Peumans, M., de Munck, J., Mine, A. and van Meerbeek, B. (2014) Clinical effectiveness of contemporary adhesives for the restoration of non–carious cervical lesions. A systematic review. *Dent Mater*, **30**, 1089–1103.

Poyser, N.J., Porter, R.W., Briggs, P.F., Chana, H.S. and Kelleher, M.G. (2005) The Dahl concept: past, present and future. *Br Dent J*, **198**, 669–676; quiz 720.

Poyser, N.J., Briggs, P.F., Chana, H.S., Kelleher, M.G., Porter, R.W. and Patel, M.M. (2007) The evaluation of direct composite restorations for the worn mandibular anterior dentition – clinical performance and patient satisfaction. *J Oral Rehabil*, **34**, 361–376.

Redman, C.D., Hemmings, K.W. and Good, J.A. (2003) The survival and clinical performance of resin-based composite restorations used to treat localised anterior tooth wear. *Br Dent J*, **194**, 566–572; discussion 559.

Robinson, S., Nixon, P.J., Gahan, M.J. and Chan, M.F. (2008) Techniques for restoring worn anterior teeth with direct composite resin. *Dent Update*, **35**, 551–552, 555–558.

Sailer, I., Makarov, N.A., Thoma, D.S., Zwahlen, M. and Pjetursson, B.E. (2015) All-ceramic or metal-ceramic tooth-supported fixed dental prostheses (FDPs)? A systematic review of the survival and complication rates. Part I: Single crowns (SCs). *Dent Mater*, **31**, 603–623.

Satterthwaite, J.D. (2006) Indirect restorations on teeth with reduced crown height. *Dent Update*, **33**, 210–212, 215–216.

Satterthwaite, J.D. (2012) Tooth surface loss: tools and tips for management. *Dent Update*, **39**, 86–90, 93–96.

Senna, P., del Bel Cury, A. and Rosing, C. (2012) Non-carious cervical lesions and occlusion: a systematic review of clinical studies. *J Oral Rehabil*, **39**, 450–462.

Shellis, R.P. and Addy, M. (2014) The interactions between attrition, abrasion and erosion in tooth wear. *Monogr Oral Sci*, **25**, 32–45.

Smales, R.J. and Berekally, T.L. (2007) Long-term survival of direct and indirect restorations placed for the treatment of advanced tooth wear. *Eur J Prosthodont Restor Dent*, **15**, 2–6.

Smith, B.G. and Knight, J.K. (1984) An index for measuring the wear of teeth. *Br Dent J*, **156**, 435–438.

Talbot, T.R., Briggs, P.F. and Gibson, M.T. (1993) Crown lengthening: a clinical review. *Dent Update*, **20**, 301, 303–306.

Tong, H.J., Rudolf, M.C., Muyombwe, T., Duggal, M.S. and Balmer, R. (2014) An investigation into the dental health of children with obesity: an analysis of dental erosion and caries status. *Eur Arch Paediatr Dent*, **15**, 203–210.

Treasure, J., Claudino, A.M. and Zucker, N. (2010) Eating disorders. *Lancet*, **375**, 583–593.

van'T Spijker, A., Kreulen, C.M. and Creugers, N.H. (2007) Attrition, occlusion, (dys)function, and intervention: a systematic review. *Clin Oral Implants Res*, **18** Suppl 3, 117–126.

van't Spijker, A., Rodriguez, J.M., Kreulen, C.M., Bronkhorst, E.M., Bartlett, D.W. and Creugers, N.H. (2009) Prevalence of tooth wear in adults. *Int J Prosthodont*, **22**, 35–42.

White, D.A., Tsakos, G., Pitts, N.B. *et al.* (2012) Adult Dental Health Survey 2009: common oral health conditions and their impact on the population. *Br Dent J*, **213**, 567–572.

Wiegand, A. and Attin, T. (2007) Occupational dental erosion from exposure to acids: a review. *Occup Med (Lond)*, **57**, 169–176.

Wilson, C. (2015) Multidisciplinary treatment of anterior worn dentition: a staged approach. *Compend Contin Educ Dent*, **36**, 202, 204–207.

Wood, I., Jawad, Z., Paisley, C. and Brunton, P. (2008) Non-carious cervical tooth surface loss: a literature review. *J Dent*, **36**, 759–766.

Woodley, N.J., Griffiths, B.M. and Hemmings, K.W. (1996) Retrospective audit of patients with advanced tooth wear restored with removable partial dentures. *Eur J Prosthodont Restor Dent*, **4**, 185–191.

Yule, P.L. and Barclay, S.C. (2015) Worn down by tooth wear? Aetiology, diagnosis and management revisited. *Dent Update*, **42**, 525–526, 529–530, 532.

Zanardi, P.R., Santos, M.S., Stegun, R.C., Sesma, N., Costa, B. and Lagana, D.C. (2016) Restoration of the occlusal vertical dimension with an overlay removable partial denture: a clinical report. *J Prosthodont*, **25**, 585–588.

Index

Diseases and Conditions in Dentistry: An Evidence-Based Reference, First Edition. Keyvan Moharamzadeh.

Companion website: www.wiley.com/go/moharamzadeh/diseases